FAMILY HEALTH

from

A TO Z

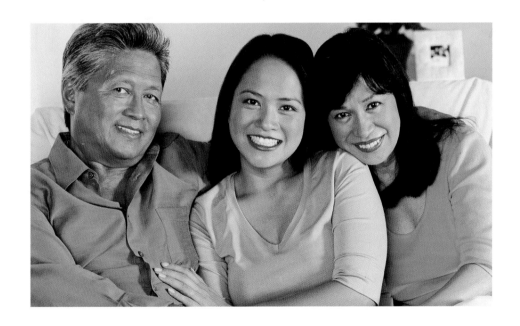

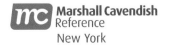 **Marshall Cavendish**
Reference
New York

Published by Marshall Cavendish Reference
An imprint of Marshall Cavendish Corporation

All rights reserved.

No part of this publication may be reproduced, stored in a retrieval system or transmitted, in any form or by any means, electronic, mechanical, photocopying, recording, or otherwise, without the prior permission of the copyright owner. Request for permission should be addressed to Permissions, Marshall Cavendish Corporation, 99 White Plains Road, Tarrytown, NY 10591. Tel: (914) 332-8888, fax: (914) 332-1888.

Website: www.marshallcavendish.us

Other Marshall Cavendish Offices:
Marshall Cavendish International (Asia) Private Limited, 1 New Industrial Road, Singapore 536196 • Marshall Cavendish International (Thailand) Co Ltd. 253 Asoke, 12th Flr, Sukhumvit 21 Road, Klongtoey Nua, Wattana, Bangkok 10110, Thailand • Marshall Cavendish (Malaysia) Sdn Bhd, Times Subang, Lot 46, Subang Hi-Tech Industrial Park, Batu Tiga, 40000 Shah Alam, Selangor Darul Ehsan, Malaysia.

Marshall Cavendish is a trademark of Times Publishing Limited.

All websites were available and accurate when this book was sent to press.

Library of Congress Cataloging-in-Publication Data

Family health from A to Z.
    p. cm.
Includes bibliographical references and index.
 ISBN 978-0-7614-7945-1 (alk. paper)
1. Medicine, Popular.   I. Marshall Cavendish Reference.
RC81.F236 2012
616.003--dc22   2011006782

Printed in Malaysia

15 14 13 12 11 1 2 3 4 5

Marshall Cavendish

Publisher: Paul Bernabeo
Project Editor: Brian Kinsey
Production Manager: Michael Esposito
Indexer: Cynthia Crippen, AEIOU, Inc.

Medical Consultant

Gerald Medoff, MD
Washington University School of Medicine

CONTENTS

INTRODUCTION

Family Health from A to Z provides authoritative information on a wide variety of health care topics that affect individuals on a daily basis. Although the focus in planning this collection of articles was on common subjects that are of interest to young readers, the information provided here is valuable to users of any age.

The 136 color-coded articles are categorized into five major areas of interest: human body; diseases and other disorders; treatments and cures; prevention and diagnosis of disease; and human behavior. Simply comparing the color of the questions-and-answers feature in a given article to the colors shown in the Key will identify the category to which the article belongs.

KEY TO COLOR CODING OF ARTICLES
■ HUMAN BODY
■ DISEASES AND OTHER DISORDERS
■ TREATMENTS AND CURES
■ PREVENTION AND DIAGNOSIS OF DISEASE
■ HUMAN BEHAVIOR

This volume is intended to provide students and the general public with valuable information that is clear, concise, and useful. It also offers an overview of numerous medical topics in such a manner as to allow immediate comprehension of medical conditions and health issues. The volume's easy and attractive style will help readers understand medical terms and issues and thereby assist in preventing problems and encouraging well-being. The substantial level of medical knowledge contained here will allow users to dispel misunderstanding and apprehension associated with health care.

The content in these articles can be accessed in a variety of ways because of their structured organization, cross-referencing, and the simple A-Z format. Therefore, it is easy for the reader to find reliable information about

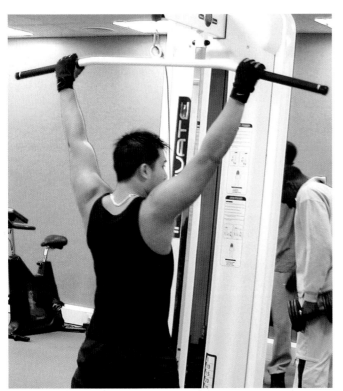

a variety of daily health issues from a trusted source. Valuable information is also conveyed through numerous photographs, charts, graphs, and artworks with clear descriptive captions. The immediately accessible questions-and-answers feature in every article addresses issues that are most likely to be of concern to readers.

At the end of the volume is a comprehensive first aid handbook, along with a medical glossary, resources for further research, and an index. While *Family Health from A to Z* is not a substitute for obtaining advice and treatment from a licensed medical practitioner, the knowledge offered in this reference work will help promote good health.

Additional health care information is available in the single-volume *Human Body from A to Z*, the 18-volume set *Encyclopedia of Family Health*, and the online *Family Health* database at www.marshallcavendishdigital.com.

Abrasions and cuts

Is it better to cover wounds with bandages or not?

As a rule, all wet, weepy wounds need to be covered. Fresh wounds are best protected if you are working in dirty conditions, but fresh, dry wounds should be left uncovered in clean conditions.

Do older people heal as quickly as young people?

Older bodies can heal as quickly as young ones, but there are exceptions. Arterial disease can make the blood flow more slowly, and hinder healing. Infection is more likely, and if circulation is bad, ulcers may develop on the shins and ankles. Cuts on an elderly person's leg need daily attention to prevent ulcers.

If a limb is bleeding severely, should I make a tourniquet?

Tourniquets (strips of cloth wrapped tightly around a limb) stop bleeding by cutting off the blood supply. Once widely used, they are now considered dangerous because low blood and oxygen levels in a limb can cause permanent damage and make infection more likely. They should be used only by a qualified person.

Do I need to get a tetanus shot every time I get cut?

Most children are immunized against tetanus, with three injections (shots) within a year, and a booster every 10 years.
   If you have not had one in the last 10 years (five years if the wound is serious), you will need a small booster if you are cut. This is vital if you puncture the skin in a garden or in the countryside, because tetanus bacteria live in soil and animal manure. Tetanus germs can cause lockjaw, a very serious and often fatal condition.

The skin protects vulnerable internal organs from injury, but as the body's front line of defense, skin often gets damaged. Fast, effective first aid can help to speed the healing process and prevent infection.

Scratches, abrasions, cuts, lacerations, and punctures are all types of abnormal breaks through the skin and are generally referred to as wounds. The body has very efficient mechanisms for stopping bleeding, healing wounds, and fighting infection, but it often needs help. Whenever the skin is broken, blood vessels may be torn and germs can enter the body, so all wounds need to be cleaned, and many need to be dressed.

How the body copes

When tissue is damaged and a wound bleeds, it forms a blood clot. Connective tissue cells called fibroblasts migrate to the area and form a plug of fibrous tissue in the clot, which seals off the broken blood vessels and stops bleeding. At the same time, the muscles in the walls of the damaged blood vessels contract to slow down the flow of blood. If bleeding is severe and constant, blood pressure is lowered throughout the entire body. As soon as skin is broken, special white blood cells, called phagocytes, gather at the site of the injury. They remove

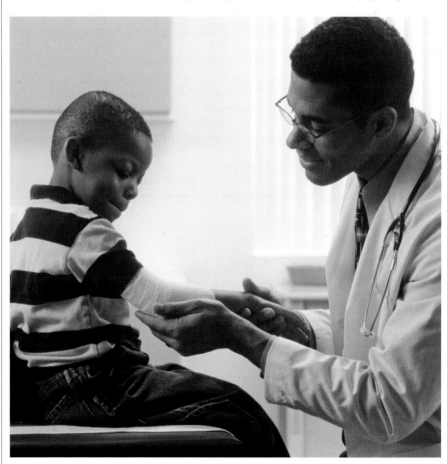

▲ *If a cut or abrasion is likely to be exposed to dirt, it should be cleaned with soap and water, and any grit should be removed before covering it with a sterile dressing.*

First aid for minor injuries

HOW TO STOP BLEEDING

Sometimes it is better to let a wound bleed for a while, because the flow of blood can help to wash dirt and bacteria away. This is particularly important with puncture wounds, which are difficult to clean thoroughly. However, if bleeding is heavy, it should be stopped.

Unless you suspect a broken limb, in which case it should not be moved, raise an arm or leg so that the blood pressure is reduced slightly. Then, using a clean bandage, apply firm pressure to the wound. The pressure needs to be constant for at least five minutes to be effective. If blood seeps through the bandage, do not change it, just add more on top;

dabbing a wound, or changing a bandage, removes the protective blood clot.

If blood is flowing with a pumping, squirting motion, an artery has been damaged. In this case, get medical help immediately. In the meantime, continue to apply firm pressure. Locate the local artery and press on it, for no longer than 15 minutes at a time.

There is one exception: scalp wounds bleed heavily, but if you suspect a skull fracture, do not apply direct pressure. Instead, make a dressing in the shape of a ring, so that the pressure is applied around the wound, but not directly on it.

CLEANING WOUNDS

While you prepare to clean the wound, cover it with a clean piece of cloth or a towel so that no more germs can enter it. Then wash your hands thoroughly, taking special care to scrub under your nails.

Wounds can be cleaned with a variety of liquids, from mild antiseptics to soap and water or mild detergents and water, depending on what you have available.

If you use an antiseptic other than hydrogen peroxide, which is completely safe to use straight from the bottle, be sure to dilute it following the instructions on the bottle. Using a solution that is too strong may damage tissues and make the wound worse rather than better.

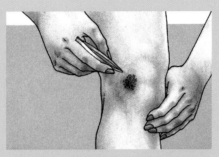

▲ *If there is any grit in the wound, scrub gently with a clean brush under running water: this is an effective, though painful, way of removing grit. Extract large pieces of grit and splinters with a pair of tweezers. If a large splinter will not come out easily, leave it until you can get the patient to a doctor or emergency room.*

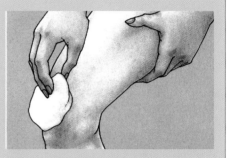

▲ *Brush any remaining bits of dirt from the surface of the wound with small swabs of gauze or cotton soaked in antiseptic. Then, working away from the wound, clean around it using fresh antiseptic swabs. Finally, clean the wound itself using separate swabs for every stroke. Work from the center outward.*

APPLYING A DRESSING

A small, clean cut can be covered with adhesive bandages. These thin strips of gauze set in fabric or plastic are used to hold a wound closed. The strips should be placed diagonally across each other, pulling the edges of the wound together. The sticky part should not touch the wound.

A nonstick dressing is the best protection for a small wound, because it can be removed without harming the scab.

Never use a dressing of fluffy cotton, because this material will stick to wounds and be difficult to remove later.

Large wounds should be covered with sterile gauze dressings that also cover the surrounding skin.

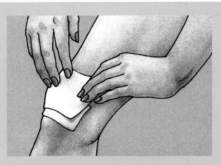

▲ *Next, pad the dressing with either cotton or additional layers of gauze; these will absorb any discharge and will also act as a protective buffer. When the dressing is changed, the layers should be peeled off individually to avoid disturbing any scab that has formed.*

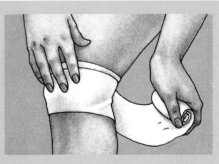

▲ *Wrap the area firmly with a cotton or crepe bandage. Crepe stretches, so it fits around awkward shapes easily. Change dressings regularly. If a dressing is stuck to the wound, soak it in a mild antiseptic solution until it comes off easily. Never pull it off quickly; this can damage the scab.*

DIFFERENT TYPES OF WOUNDS

▶ *Abrasions are usually not as serious as they look, though they may be very painful and leave scars. They should be cleaned thoroughly.*

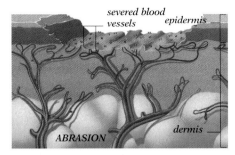

▶ *Cuts may bleed heavily. They must be kept closed to heal properly, and may need to be stitched, especially when they occur on the face.*

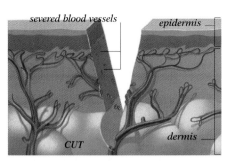

▶ *Lacerations are often serious wounds and take the longest time to heal. They should usually be treated by a doctor and kept covered in the meantime.*

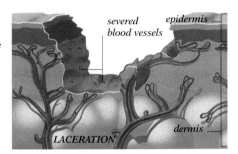

▶ *Puncture wounds are more serious than they look, especially those to the abdomen or chest. Unless they are tiny, get medical help quickly.*

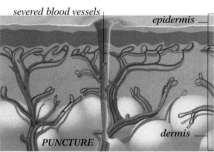

microscopic particles, like bacteria, and so make up the body's first line of defense against infection. The larger the damaged area, the more likely it is to be contaminated with bacteria, and the greater the risk of infection.

When bleeding has stopped and the wound is clear of infection, a fibrous scab begins to form, under which new skin tissue forms. The scab shrinks over the next few days and forms an extremely strong bond between the cut surfaces.

Scratches

There are five different types of wounds: scratches, abrasions, cuts, lacerations, and punctures. A scratch is a minor tear through the outer layer of the skin, called the epidermis. The edges of the skin are not separated, and the small amount of bleeding comes from the tiny blood vessels within the skin itself. A scratch stops bleeding quickly, but it can still become infected, especially if the skin is scratched by something dirty.

Abrasions

An abrasion is an area of skin that has been torn away by force. Light scuffing of the skin is called a graze, but sometimes a large, deep area of skin is affected, and the abrasion is more like a severe burn. Occasionally, an abrasion is so severe that a skin graft is needed. Because millions of tiny nerve endings are exposed, abrasions can be more painful than cuts. They are often full of dirt or grit, so the main problem is infection. After the abrasion is cleaned thoroughly to remove dirt particles, it should be covered with dry gauze.

Cuts

Any clean division through layers of the skin is called a cut. Cuts are usually caused by sharp edges such as glass, razor blades, knives, or even paper. They often bleed freely, especially if any of the large blood vessels under the skin have been damaged. Many cuts gape open slightly; to help them heal, the edges should be kept together

with an adhesive plaster or surgical tape. This is particularly important for cuts on the elbows, knees, and fingers, which are constantly being bent.

If the cut gapes so badly that it cannot be held together with tape, or if it is deep enough to expose a layer of fat or muscle, it needs to be stitched. All cuts on the face, however small, should be

Wounds that need medical attention

Wounds that will not stop bleeding.
Any very large, deep, gaping, or jagged wounds.
Any wounds with dirt or grit embedded under the skin.
Puncture wounds caused by dirty or rusty objects.
Any cut on the face.
Any wound that is infected.
Even when the greatest care is taken, there is always a danger of infection. Localized infection is common and produces a discharge of yellowish pus. If the wound is relatively small, the body's natural defense mechanisms will probably cope with any infection. However, if the area around the wound becomes very red, irritated, and inflamed, or if the patient develops a fever, a doctor should be consulted; antibiotics may then be prescribed. Any pus that has formed should be allowed to drain. If the infected wound has been stitched, it may be necessary for your doctor to take out some of the stitches to release the pus. Infected abrasions should be washed and dressed each day.

Recognizing and treating serious wounds

Apart from specific wounds that require a doctor's attention, there are some obvious signs that indicate when medical attention is needed urgently. Ideally, one person should apply first aid, while a second calls for help. If you are alone, you will have to decide what immediate first aid is necessary and call for help. All the examples below require medical attention, but this may become obvious only after first aid has been applied. Do not lose time in getting help—never feel you should try to cope with an emergency alone.

SYMPTOMS	POSSIBLE CAUSES	ACTION
Bleeding persists.	An artery may have been severed, in which case the blood will spurt out with every heartbeat; alternatively, there may be a deep puncture wound.	Apply pressure in the normal way for at least 10 minutes. If an artery is severed, try to locate a pressure point, a place where a main artery can be pressed against a bone. Pressure can be applied at these points to stop arterial blood loss, but it should be applied for no longer than 15 minutes without a break.
Patient shows signs of shock. Usually all of the following symptoms will be present: pale face and lips, cold and clammy skin, faint or dizzy feeling, and weak and rapid pulse.	Caused by a combination of low blood pressure, constriction of blood vessels, and blood loss. The body diverts the remaining blood to the essential organs, such as the kidneys, heart, and brain. If shock is present but there is no visible blood loss, there may be internal bleeding.	Place the patient comfortably on his or her side. If possible, raise the feet so that blood is concentrated in the area of the vital organs. Loosen tight clothing. It is important to reassure someone in shock, so stay by the person if possible. Never give the patient any liquids.
Patient experiences tingling in the wounded area, or loss of movement.	A tendon or nerve may be severed (tendons attach muscles to the bone at the joints).	Apart from general first aid, there is no immediate treatment for this.

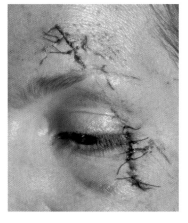

◄ *Cuts on the face should always be stitched to prevent scars. A doctor should carry out this procedure.*

stitched by a medical practitioner to minimize scar formation.

Lacerations

A laceration is a tear in the skin, usually caused by a hard blow or a serious accident. The skin edges are jagged, there is often extensive bruising, and infection is a risk unless the wound is cleaned thoroughly as soon as possible. This type of wound should be seen by a doctor.

Lacerations often bleed heavily and may be made worse if there are foreign objects embedded in them, such as pieces of metal or large splinters. Attempts to pull these out should be left to a doctor; trying to remove them may cause massive bleeding. A thick, ring-shaped dressing can be built up around them to stop them from working deeper into the wound, but a doctor or nurse should treat the wound.

Puncture wounds

A puncture or stab wound is a small, deep wound of unknown depth, caused, for example, when the prong of a metal rake is run through the foot. It is most important that the wound is allowed to bleed—

this is the only way it can clean itself. Once the bleeding has stopped, the wound can be washed and covered with a clean, dry dressing.

Except for wounds made by a small clean object, such as a thumbtack, all puncture wounds need swift medical attention, because there can be a danger of internal bleeding and damage to tendons and nerves. There is also an increased chance of infection and tetanus, because tetanus germs thrive in deep, closed wounds where there is no oxygen. A puncture wound is always worse than it looks, so for anything more than a very small wound, medical help should be sought without delay.

What the doctor will do

Although minor wounds do not usually need medical attention if first aid is applied, major wounds, or very dirty ones, need to be treated by a doctor.

The doctor will clean the wound thoroughly and examine it to ensure that there are no remaining foreign bodies or dirt. If there is any risk that splinters of glass or pieces of metal are still embedded in the wound, an X ray may be taken. The doctor will check that the nerves and tendons are all functioning normally and decide whether a tetanus injection is necessary or whether the wound requires stitching (suturing). Stitches are used to pull the edges of a gaping wound together. This closes the wound to prevent further contamination and decreases the chances of an ugly scar.

However, stitches will not be used if the wound can be held closed without them, because stitches themselves can sometimes injure the surrounding tissue and may leave extra scars. If stitching is needed, it should be done as soon as possible. A local anesthetic will be given to numb the area.

See also: **Bacteria; Tetanus**

Acne and pimples

Almost all teenagers and young adults suffer from some form of acne or pimples, but the majority grow out of both. In the meantime, there are preventive measures and treatments that can help these common problems.

Many people suffer from occasional pimples, but it is only when these become widespread and persistent that they really cause a problem. Pimples most commonly occur after blockages form in the pores of the skin. Blackheads are blockages that form when oily sebum from the oil-producing glands within the pores clogs at the pore openings, hardening to form dark plugs. Whiteheads are hard lumps of sebum that form under the skin when the pores are blocked by an excess of keratin (the tough protein produced by skin cells). Both types of blockage (called comedones) encourage bacteria that are normally found on the skin to multiply in the sebum; ultimately, this can lead to the development of inflamed and pus-filled

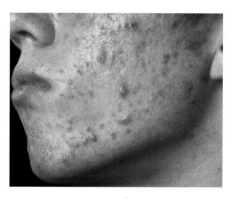

▲ *Teenagers are particularly prone to acne—which is triggered by the upsurge in hormone output that occurs at this time.*

pimples. Inflammation and the buildup of oil can also cause oil glands to rupture. Widespread blackheads and whiteheads, accompanied by the pink or reddish inflammation that follows bacterial infection, are the hallmark of the condition called acne. Acne vulgaris is the most common form, and it tends to affect areas of the skin where the sebaceous glands are larger and more numerous, such as the face, the back of the neck, the upper back, and the chest. The condition can vary from very mild to severe.

It was once thought that the bacteria that naturally thrive on sebum, such as *Propionibacterium acnes*, were the underlying cause of acne, but they are now known to cause the inflammation rather than the acne itself. When a pore becomes clogged, oxygen is excluded, creating an environment that is ideal for the growth of these bacteria. In response to chemicals produced by these microorganisms, the body mobilizes its defense forces: white blood cells. The white cells multiply in number, the blood vessels expand to bring more infection-fighting cells to the infected area, and the tissues become red and inflamed. As the white cells work at neutralizing and then engulfing the bacteria, they themselves die, accumulate, and form pus. At the same time, dead bacterial matter also builds up. Inflammation may also be aggravated by substances produced by the cells lining the oil duct, and by fatty acids and sebum penetrating the lower layer of the skin (the dermis) after an oil duct has ruptured.

People with acne may also develop large tender cysts (saclike growths) beneath the skin that have no obvious head, and inflamed red lumps, which are painful to touch. These deep-seated lesions can persist for months and may leave scars even after they have healed. Secondary infections can also lead to scarring. Scars may be flat and thin, or they may be crater-like pits that form when pores fail to regain their original size and shape after the swelling has disappeared. Other lesions include excoriations (picked spots), red marks from recently healed pimples, and areas of brown or white pigmentation from old spots.

Common causes of acne

Acne vulgaris is most common in young people between the teen years and the early twenties, and it tends to occur more frequently and be more severe in boys. It is often triggered by puberty, the time of life when hormone production by the sex organs and the adrenal glands increases, transforming a child into a sexually mature adult. This type of acne may appear as early as age 10 and usually begins to improve by the end of adolescence.

Normally the oil-releasing sebaceous glands in the skin produce just enough sebum to lubricate the surface of the skin, reducing water loss from the skin surface and protecting it from bacteria and fungi. In some adolescents, however, the influence of the sex hormones—particularly that of the androgens, or "masculinizing" hormones—causes the sebaceous glands to become overactive. They then enlarge and release too much sebum—a condition called seborrhea. Excessive sebum output can cause pores on the surface of the skin to become blocked. The female hormones, the estrogens, stimulate production of a more fluid sebum, which explains—at least partly—why girls are generally less prone to acne than boys.

Sometimes acne vulgaris can continue for many years, and it can also appear in older people who did not previously have a problem. Research has shown that genetics plays a big part in the development and persistence of the disease.

In some women, the hormonal fluctuation that occurs during a normal menstrual cycle can trigger outbreaks: pimples often occur just before the period. Acne can also occur or worsen in early pregnancy. Researchers have also found that women with polycystic ovary syndrome (a sex hormone imbalance which causes the ovaries to become enlarged with numerous cysts, and which may cause an excessive growth of body hair) may be more prone to the condition. Stress may be another important triggering factor in both teenagers and older sufferers, because of its influence on hormone levels; in particular, there appears to be an increasing incidence of acne in older women with high-pressure jobs. Fetal hormones are thought to be responsible for infantile acne that sometimes occurs on the faces of babies; this usually settles down within a few months but may require treatment.

Other types of acne

Acne conglobata and acne fulminans are two severe types of acne that more usually develop in men. Acne conglobata is characterized by large recurrent cysts, interconnecting abscesses, and pronounced scarring. It can affect the neck, arms, chest, and buttocks. Acne fulminans is even more severe; the symptoms are ulcerated nodules,

fever, and painful joints. Hypersensitivity to *P. acnes* is thought to be a possible cause. Both types can be caused by taking testosterone or anabolic steroids. Expert treatment should be sought urgently.

Other, more unusual forms of acne include occupational acne and drug-induced acne. Occupational acne may develop in people who are constantly exposed to certain industrial oils and greases, such as those cooking at fast-food restaurants or working in car repair shops. In these cases, the pores are constantly being clogged by oil in the air or on oily clothes that come into close contact with the skin. Acne can also be aggravated by high humidity, because continual sweating makes the skin swell and blocks the pores. Drug-induced acne may occur when people take certain prescription drugs, such as corticosteroids, anabolic steroids, testosterone, and certain contraceptives, antiepileptics, and antidepressants.

Chloracne is a rare form of acne caused by exposure to certain toxic chemicals found in some fungicides, insecticides, and wood preservatives. In these cases, the skin is not usually oily.

Managing the condition

On a day-to-day basis, washing the affected areas with a gentle soap or foaming cleanser is all that is needed to keep the skin clean. Contrary to popular belief, acne is not a symptom of poor hygiene, and overzealous washing can aggravate the condition. Neither are antiseptic washes likely to help much. Using a soft brush—kept scrupulously clean to avoid reinfection—may help to loosen the top layer of skin, taking with it some, if not all, of the plugs of sebum. Drying with a rough towel will have the same effect. Most pimples will eventually rupture of their own accord, and it is most important not to pick the blemishes, or to scrub aggressively at the skin, since this can cause more inflammation and make any scarring worse.

Creams and lotions

Various topical preparations (those that are applied to the skin) can help to reduce acne. The most commonly used are those that loosen the blockages of sebum in the pores; they contain agents such as benzoyl peroxide, azelaic acid, salicylic acid, glycolic acid, sulfur, and

HOW A PIMPLE FORMS

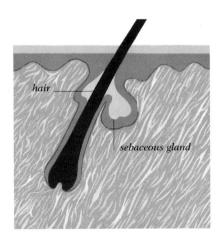

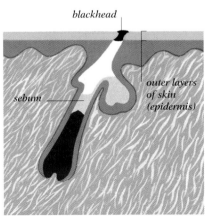

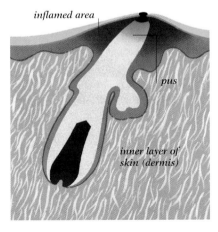

▲ In acne, extra sebum (oil) first clogs up the pores through which sebum is released to the skin surface.

▲ The sebum is trapped and forms a plug with a raised top. When exposed to air, this becomes a blackhead.

▲ The surrounding skin then becomes inflamed and infected, resulting in a pimple filled with pus.

Helping to alleviate acne

DO

Do wash the affected area gently twice a day (and after vigorous exercise) with warm water and a gentle cleanser, and dry with a clean towel

Do consult your doctor if the acne is persistent or widespread

Do apply topical acne products thinly to the entire area affected

Do get out in the fresh air and sunshine

Do use a concealer to disguise individual pimples

AVOID

Avoid washing the affected area too often with harsh soaps and cleansers; this can overdry and irritate the skin and damage the skin's natural protective barrier; it may even increase the number of *P. acnes* bacteria

Avoid heavy moisturizing creams and oily cosmetics such as foundation or sunscreen, which can block the pores; avoid leaving makeup on overnight

Avoid abrasive skin treatments; these can rupture the blocked pores and lead to inflamed pimples

Avoid squeezing pimples; this can cause infection and scarring

Avoid worrying about your condition; stress may actually cause pimples

Avoid excessively humid conditions

Avoid giving up on treatments too soon; acne may take months to respond

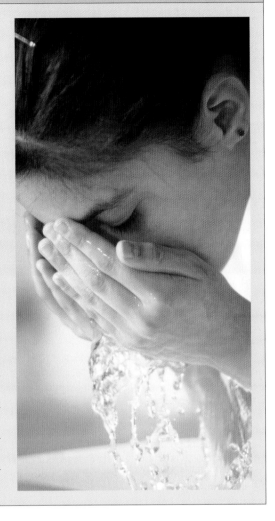

resorcinol. These preparations tend to dry the skin and may cause some peeling of the top layer, which helps rid the skin of dead or damaged tissue. They are often successful in controlling milder forms of acne, although the whole area should be treated regularly to keep the blemishes under control. However, they can cause mild side effects, such as redness or itching.

The most commonly used preparation is benzoyl peroxide, which can be bought from a druggist or may be prescribed by a doctor. Not only does this loosen the keratin that blocks the pores, but it also reduces the number of bacteria on the skin surface, and has an anti-inflammatory action. It can be used for many months without causing any kind of bacterial resistance.

Topical antibiotics such as clindamycin or erythromycin may be prescribed to treat mild forms of acne, but they may cause allergies or cause bacteria to become resistant to the drug.

Stronger lotions derived from vitamin A, called retinoids, also require a prescription. These can be used locally to unblock pores and encourage skin shedding, but they can cause redness, inflammation, and sensitivity to the sun.

Other treatments

A doctor may also be able to prescribe oral treatments (taken by mouth) that are not available over the counter. Antibiotics such as tetracycline or erythromycin may be prescribed for a few months to cut down the growth of bacteria and calm the inflammation in the blemishes; these are most effective if combined with a topical treatment that unblocks the pores. Women may be prescribed oral hormones to counteract the effects of male hormones on the skin.

Severe acne may require treatment under the supervision of a dermatologist. An oral retinoid called isotretinoin can halt acne by shrinking the sebaceous glands, but it has to be used with care because it can cause fetal abnormalities and affect liver function.

If deep-seated skin infections develop, a doctor may have to lance them to release the pus. Other surgical treatments to remove persistent blockages include electrosurgery (cautery or diathermy), cryotherapy (freezing), and microdermabrasion. Large cysts may be treated with corticosteroid injections or removed surgically. Dermabrasion, chemical skin peeling, laser resurfacing, and skin grafting may help to reduce scarring.

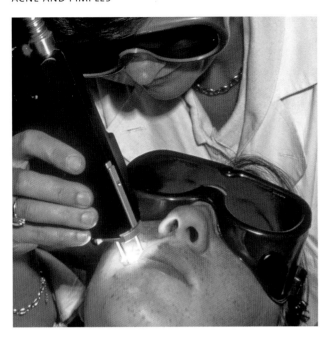

▲ *Laser treatment is showing promising results in the treatment of mild to moderate acne.*

The benefits of light

Many acne sufferers find that their pimples and scars clear up more quickly when exposed to sunlight. This is because the ultraviolet (UV) light in sunshine helps dry up grease on the skin, and aids the peeling of the top layer; other blue wavelengths have been shown to kill the bacteria within the skin, and certain red wavelengths actively promote skin healing.

At one time, ultraviolet lamps were sometimes advised for acne sufferers, but these can cause burning and can result in an increased risk of skin cancer. However, new types of light treatment that omit the damaging UV rays have shown promising results in people suffering from mild or moderate acne. Some systems expose the skin to a high-intensity blue-violet light which starts a chemical reaction that destroys *P. acnes* in the skin, and reduces inflammation. Another system combines the bacteria-killing blue light with a red light that promotes healing. Laser treatment is also being used; it appears to work by heating up blood vessels in the skin and temporarily damaging the sebaceous glands, reducing the oil supply. It is also thought to stimulate the formation of large amounts of new collagen, which aids the healing process. Compared with conventional treatments, all these methods appear to cause minimal side effects—but they are expensive.

Emotional and psychological problems

Acne can have severe mental effects on sufferers. People who are badly affected can be so embarrassed by their appearance that they find it difficult to form relationships and may limit their social behavior to avoid exposing the affected areas. This lack of confidence can also affect academic performance, career choices, and success in employment. Extreme cases can lead to social phobia and depression. For this reason, one of the most essential and important treatments for acne is understanding and sympathy from friends and parents, so that physical scars do not become psychological ones. In extreme cases, counseling, psychological treatments to overcome negative thinking, and antidepressant medication may be necessary.

Other causes of pimples

Certain other conditions can cause symptoms similar to acne. For this reason, is it is worth consulting a doctor if persistent pimples occur. One of these is folliculitis, a name given to a group of conditions in which the hair follicles become inflamed.

Folliculitis

Bacterial folliculitis is an infection of the hair follicles, often by *Staphylococcus aureus*. Boils can sometimes result. Using an antiseptic cleanser can help, but it may be necessary for antibiotic lotions or tablets to be prescribed in severe cases.

Spa pool folliculitis is caused by a bacterium that thrives in warm water that is not adequately disinfected. Itchy red spots and pustules occur a few hours or days after exposure but usually clear up within a few days.

Another type of folliculitis, more common in people with curly hair, occurs when hairs regrow into the skin after shaving, waxing, or plucking. Moisturizing the skin, shaving in the direction of the hair follicle using a single blade, and using lotions containing glycolic acid to exfoliate the surface skin cells can help alleviate the problem.

Folliculitis can also be caused by an overgrowth of a yeast that is normally found on the skin and is associated with a tendency to dandruff. The itchy pink spots and pustules may be made worse by humid environments, by synthetic clothing, and by using oily creams. The condition is linked to oily skin, stress, fatigue, diabetes, and the use of oral contraceptives. Treatment may include antifungal lotions or tablets.

Contact with mineral oils or tar can cause oil folliculitis, resulting in the formation of comedones and small pustules, particularly on the forearms and thighs. Diesel mechanics, sheep shearers, road workers, and people working in engineering and in oil refineries are most at risk. Washing with mild soap and water and using acne treatments usually prove effective.

Rosacea

Rosacea is a facial rash of dome-shaped red spots and pustules that occurs in middle age. There are no blackheads or whiteheads, and the affected skin may be hot and swollen. Other symptoms may include frequent flushing, sensitive skin, "gritty" eyelids, and an enlarged and thickened nose. Oil-based creams, sunlight, and hot and spicy food and drink may aggravate the condition. Oral and topical antibiotics and lasers may be used to treat the condition.

Keratosis pilaris

Keratosis pilaris occurs when the old skin cells stick in the hair follicles, forming scaly plugs; the blockages may then turn red. The condition is most common in younger people and tends to affect the upper arms, the thighs, the buttocks, and occasionally the face. The condition tends to be worse when the skin dries out. Moisturizing, exfoliating with a pumice stone or loofah, or using a prescribed tretinoin cream can help.

See also: **Adolescence; Antibiotics; Infection and infectious diseases**

Adolescence

In adolescence, young people undergo the physical and mental changes that take them into adulthood, and this can be a difficult time. It is vital that parents show understanding—and can judge when help is needed.

Questions and Answers

We used to have a very close relationship with our son. Now he has turned completely against us. Where did we go wrong?

It is often the case that the closer the relationship, the more sudden the rebellion in adolescence. Just remember that this does not mean rejection. A child who rages against his or her parents obviously still cares what they think—probably more so than a child who just ignores them.

My 16-year-old daughter wants to go on the Pill, although she swears she is not having a sexual relationship. She says it is "just in case." Should I let her?

Although you may be worried, the fact that she has consulted you is a compliment to your relationship with her. If you prevent her from taking the Pill, you won't stop her from having sexual relationships in the future, and she could easily become pregnant. Talk to her calmly and sympathetically. Point out that the Pill is a drug that should not be taken unnecessarily. Tell her how you feel about early sexual relationships and the need for commitment, but remember that she needs to make her own decision once she has as many opinions and as much factual information as possible. After all, she will soon be an adult.

My 15-year-old son is often rude to my husband, but I'm afraid that if I put my foot down, he will turn against us. Will he grow out of this phase or should I be firm with him now?

Do put your foot down—firmly. In the long run, he'll respect you for it, and that means you will be doing him a favor; children who have no regard for their parents often never develop any self-respect themselves.

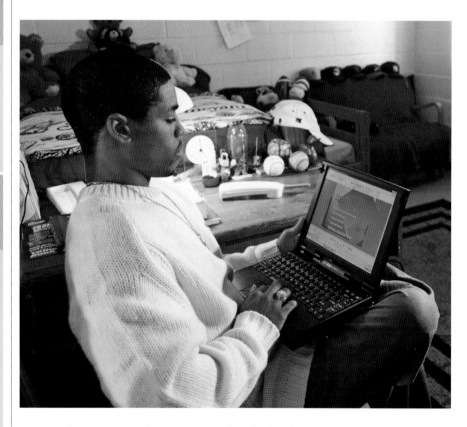

▲ *An adolescent may prefer to remain undisturbed in the sanctuary of his or her room.*

Adolescence is the period between childhood and adulthood when the body begins to develop rapidly and the physical changes of puberty occur. Boys grow taller and more muscular at a rapid speed. Girls, too, increase quickly in height; body fat begins to be redistributed to breasts, buttocks, hips, and thighs; and the menstrual periods start. In boys, the penis and testicles grow larger. Both sexes develop body hair in the armpits and on the pubis and limbs; boys begin to grow facial hair.

These changes are brought about by a complex interaction of hormones, or chemical messengers, which are released into the bloodstream by the sex glands. Their effect is not only physical but also mental and emotional.

On average, adolescence starts at around age 11 for girls and 13 for boys, but it can begin at any time from 10 to 16 in both sexes. Girls mature physically, emotionally, and mentally about two years ahead of boys. By the mid-teens, boys overtake girls in physical prowess and appear to catch up with them in academic skills, although many boys do not go on to reach their full academic potential. Studies are continuing in an effort to discover why this should be the case and what can or should be done to remedy the matter. Both sexes share a surging physical, emotional, and mental strength, coupled with an extremely powerful sexual drive and a growing sense of independence and self-awareness. In most developed societies, teens are considered to be adults at the age of 18, although psychological maturing can continue for several more years.

A time of conflict

In the past, Western society expected boys to work toward developing careers in order to support spouses and families, and girls to learn homemaking skills and prepare to be mothers. However, in the latter half of the 20th century and the beginning of the 21st century, male and female roles and life goals were constantly changing. The rapid pace of these changes in expectation for both sexes can result in feelings of confusion. Girls who want to compete in the workplace and also start a family may not be sure which way to proceed at school, or whether to get married and have children.

Boys, who are expected to be successful providers and have all the traditional masculine traits, such as physical strength, are also under pressure to behave with an understanding of the more traditionally feminine traits, such as sensitivity and empathy. Indecision about the future and fear of failure may also lead to rebellious behavior.

How can parents help?

Contradictory and confused behavior can worry and annoy parents, who have perhaps forgotten that they went through a similar kind of turmoil. Great patience is required to cope with an individual who demands to be treated like an adult one minute and then has a temper tantrum or demands help and reassurance the next.

The most important thing that parents can do to help adolescent children is to become less obviously their protectors and disciplinarians, while still remaining a safety net should problems arise. This change has to take place over a period of time, ending when children have reached a recognized state of adulthood and feel they are ready to leave home and become independent. Although

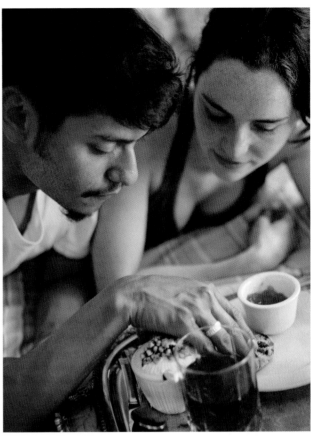

▲ *Interest in the opposite sex usually starts at adolescence or even earlier. Sexual attraction is controlled by factors such as physical appearance and social influences.*

adolescents are reluctant to admit it, they really do rely very much on their parents. This is the time of life when they are trying to work things out for themselves, but they still need someone to turn to for support when a situation becomes difficult for them to cope with.

What is normal behavior?

Because young people have to adjust to physical changes, confusion, and unfamiliar feelings, sometimes various kinds of adolescent experimentation or rebellion can get out of control, yet teens often find it difficult to admit anything to their parents. Although sexually mature, a teen is still emotionally immature, and this can cause conflict. It is sometimes difficult to tell when things have gotten out of hand. The mental state of adolescents is often confusing to an outsider. Moodiness, an entirely normal but usually temporary stage, can result in a teen's expressing unconventional or outlandish opinions. It may be obstinacy that makes a teen expound controversial ideas to parents who hold opposing views.

Teens often change their ideas about eating: some prefer to become vegetarians or vegans; others may become anorexic because they aspire to a body shape they regard as the norm. Some teens overeat and become obese; obesity has its own health problems. Parents have to be aware of these possibilities and take steps to deal with them.

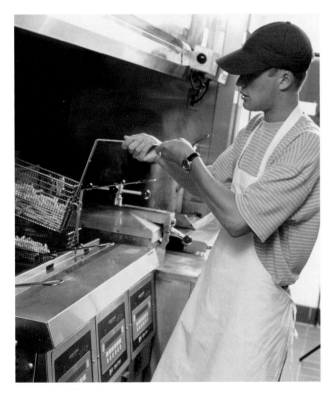

▲ *Experience in a restaurant can help introduce a young person to the world of work.*

Our eldest daughter was difficult to deal with all through her teens, but our second daughter is very quiet and doesn't cause us any problems. Is this significant?

Not really. The amount of trouble adolescents cause is not always an indication of how they will behave in the future. Parents often worry about their first child. This is mainly because they are adjusting to the new responsibilities of parenthood, so the child may be under constant pressures that make him or her react strongly. A younger child is not under as much pressure and is likely to behave differently. If you think your daughter is too quiet, seek advice from a counselor.

I found a collection of dirty magazines under my son's bed. What should I do?

Adolescents tend to be very preoccupied with sex. All you need to do is point out that they offend you and that you would rather he did not leave them where you can find them. If you make too much of a fuss, they could take on the attraction of forbidden fruit. However, you may ask yourself why you were looking under his bed. After all, they were out of sight. It sounds as though he's more considerate of you than you are of him—and that he is probably more able to handle adult thoughts than you give him credit for.

My cousin has begun to ask the most bizarre questions about God, the meaning of life, and so forth. Is this normal?

Yes, in fact it is probably the sign of a lively, inquisitive mind, struggling with some of the fundamental questions of life.

Adolescence is a period when growing children begin to be fascinated by obscure questions. Questions concerning religion, death, and the state of the world and the environment can be of profound interest to adolescents aware of them as relevant topics for the first time.

Danger signals

The most common problem in adolescence is depression. This can be either a reaction to an upsetting life event—such as failing an important exam, being unable to find a job, or breaking up with a boyfriend or girlfriend—or it can simply happen for no apparent reason. The most evident symptom is deep apathy. The young person shows no interest in anything, is listless, is uncommunicative, and mopes around the house. Sleeping habits are disturbed; he or she may wake early in the morning, continue to lie awake, and then stay in bed for hours.

Because of depression, many young people commit suicide or attempt suicide. Danger signals are deep introspection, furtive behavior, drinking, and outbursts of aggression and violence. Suicide attempts may be impulsive and a cry for help, but some attempts are successful. Suicide attempts or the suggestion of suicide should always be taken seriously. If there appears to be any real cause for concern, outside help should be requested from a doctor or counselor.

Drug abuse can be a worry for parents of adolescents. Although marijuana use among teenagers is very common, it has not been associated with a significant increase in truancy or lowered grades. Marijuana use does not necessarily lead to the use of other, hard drugs. Nevertheless, the use of ecstasy, cocaine, and crack among adolescents continues to be a serious problem. Some so-called designer drugs may also have serious medical consequences in addition to the usual problems of addiction.

Alcohol abuse is also a concern. Although experimentation seems to be a normal part of adolescence, heavy and daily use of substances should be dealt with. Parents should also be aware of the effect of their own drug and alcohol consumption on their children.

Social problems

Rowdiness and vandalism can cause problems for parents and for the general public. Such antisocial activities can be part of growing up and proving independence. The adolescent, having rejected the security of the family home, but not yet ready to take on the adult world, finds security in a group of friends who have devised their own rules about dress and conduct.

Gangs are bound by strong ties to each other; hostility to other groups can, in extreme cases, erupt in gang warfare. However, those who become involved in serious violence often come from

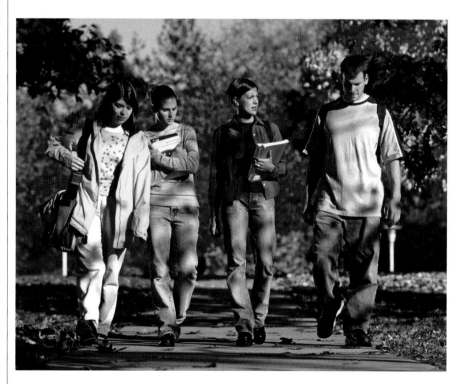

▲ *While adolescents are attempting to come to terms with society, they identify with their peers and often form close relationships at school or college.*

Problems that may affect adolescents

PROBLEM	REASONS	SIGNS	HOW PARENTS SHOULD REACT
Depressed behavior	Inability to make friends; academic problems; loss of boyfriend or girlfriend; bad self-image; anxiety about the state of the world; no apparent reason	Apathy; introspection; secrecy; tiredness; bad grades; disturbed sleep; surliness; difficulty in communicating or refusal to communicate at all; suicide threats	Consult the school about the situation; ask advice from family doctor or psychologist; bolster child's self-esteem in terms of appearance and ego; never shout "Snap out of it!"; ask yourself if you are expecting too much or not caring enough
Promiscuity (sleeping around)	Insecurity; anxiety; curiosity; confusion about the part sex plays in forming relationships	Staying out very late or all night; contraceptive devices hidden or obvious taking of the Pill; secrecy concerning a close relationship; rebelliousness	Try to talk about it calmly; never react with horror; be supportive and discuss responsibility and contraception; if you know you cannot discuss the subject without embarrassment, find someone who can—a friend, your doctor, or a counselor
Excessive dieting (affects girls more often than boys)	Possible psychological rejection of female sexuality or fear of male sexuality	Bad self-image; consistent weight loss; starvation due to dislike and refusal of food; self-induced vomiting after being persuaded to eat	Consult a doctor or a psychologist; be reassuring; do not panic
Alcohol and drug abuse	Depression; the example of parents; easy access to substances; defiance of parents; bravado; insecurity; boredom; like the taste; like its effect; identification with drug cultural lifestyle; denial of or escape from real life	Alcohol: drunken behavior Marijuana: cough, sore eyes, lethargy Stimulants: overactivity; fast, incoherent speech Hard drugs: needle marks in arms, scratching due to itching skin, yawning, sweating Glue: sores around mouth and nose, drunken behavior	Check with the school; consult a doctor, a psychologist, or a counselor
Member of a gang	Proving independence; rejection of home rules in favor of gang's rules; rejection of society's values; indifference to environment	Aggression; acts of violence against property and individuals	Consult a psychologist or a counselor

violent or deprived homes, and adolescence is not always the root cause or the only cause of such antisocial behavior.

Sexual problems

To adolescents themselves, sex poses perhaps the biggest problem of all. Many are confused by their awakening sexual instincts, and some may react either by becoming introspective and shy or by behaving outrageously. Young adults need time to adjust their self-image to accommodate this new factor in their lives.

An important part of the adolescent's development is a growing interest in the opposite sex. Dating, going out, and getting to know a number of different boyfriends or girlfriends are ways of helping to relate to people in adult life.

Part of any relationship with the opposite sex will invariably involve some sexual experimentation as both sexes explore their own, and each other's, physical and emotional responses to sex.

In a context of media sexual exploitation, many teens are bound to become involved in premature sexual relationships. But good sex education, both at home and at school, may be a way of ensuring that adolescents fully understand about sex, responsibility, and birth control. This means that parents and teachers need to be sympathetic, sensitive, and able to discuss sexuality in a straightforward and caring manner. Abstinence programs are gaining in popularity among adolescents; increased government funding has been made available to promote them.

Many parents worry that their teenage son or daughter may be exposed to a variety of sexually transmitted diseases, including HIV and AIDS. The increase of the disease among young people makes it essential that adolescents are taught about safe sex. Because HIV is transmitted through body fluids, safe sex means always using a condom, preferably with a spermicide. The way HIV is transmitted accounts for its incidence among users of hard drugs, who run a high risk of contracting the virus through shared hypodermic needles. This is another compelling reason for ensuring that adolescents are educated about the health risks and consequences of drug abuse.

> *See also:* AIDS; Anorexia and bulimia; Depression; Suicide

AIDS

Since AIDS was recognized as a medical problem in the United States in 1981, scientists the world over have tried to find a cure. Many strides have been made in understanding the disease, but the toll in human lives has been enormous.

Questions and Answers

Where can I get more information and advice regarding AIDS?

The U.S. Public Health Service operates an AIDS hotline. The toll-free number is 1-800-342-AIDS. Information is also available from your local Red Cross chapter.

Can someone contract AIDS from being bitten by a mosquito?

A good deal of research has been conducted on this possible route of infection, mostly in Africa, where the mosquito is well-known for its ability to carry and transmit the organism that causes malaria. All the evidence indicates that people cannot be infected with the AIDS virus from the bite of any insect.

How are hospitals going to be able to handle all the AIDS cases predicted in the years ahead?

There is no easy answer to this question. In some major cities entire hospitals have been converted into facilities devoted only to the care and treatment of AIDS patients. However, many new hospitals and clinics are likely to be needed in the near future.

Is it possible to get AIDS from donating blood?

No. At no time does a person giving blood come into contact with the blood of another person.

How can I tell if someone has been infected with the virus that causes AIDS?

A nonmedical person has no way of knowing if another person has been infected with HIV until AIDS actually develops, up to 10 years later. Three months after an infection, however, or often earlier, an antibody test can show whether the virus is present.

In 1981 doctors in both San Francisco and New York found themselves dealing with an unusual outbreak of a type of cancer rarely encountered outside of Africa. The malignancy, called Kaposi's sarcoma, primarily affects the blood-vessel tissues of the skin. Up until that time, its infrequent occurrence in the United States usually involved older males of Italian or Jewish background. The patients in New York and San Francisco, however, were mostly young white men, and the majority were homosexual.

Preliminary findings

It was also noticed that many of these men were particularly susceptible to a variety of infections. One of these, pneumocystis carinii, was caused by a one-celled organism that is normally harmless in humans. The search for explanations for the cancers and infections led to a surprising discovery: all the patients had a severely depressed immune system. In late 1981, the new disease was described and given a name: acquired immunodeficiency syndrome, shortened to the acronym AIDS.

Members of two other groups, intravenous drug users and individuals who had received frequent blood transfusions, were also found to be susceptible to the disease. This suggested that some sort of infectious agent in the blood might be responsible. The search for the possible cause of AIDS began in earnest.

The cause

It is now known that AIDS is caused by a retrovirus, designated HIV (human immunodeficiency virus), one of a small family of viruses that reproduce in a particular way in host cells. HIV is able to invade several different kinds of cells in the body, but its affinity for certain white blood cells of

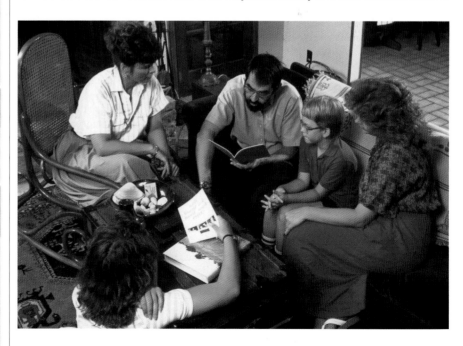

▲ *Family members educate themselves at home about the dangers of AIDS.*

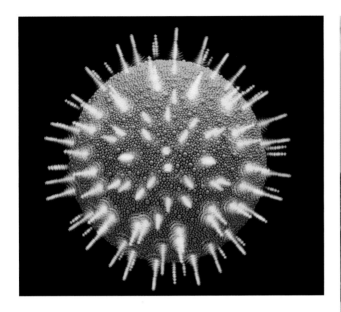

▲ *A computer-generated image of the virus that causes AIDS.*

the human immune system, T4 lymphocytes, is what lies behind the virus's ability to cause the syndrome. T4 cells, sometimes called helper T cells, help regulate the activity of other components of the immune system.

Once inside a T4 cell, the AIDS virus uses an enzyme called reverse transcriptase to translate its genetic message, which is in the form of RNA (ribonucleic acid), into DNA (deoxyribonucleic acid). The viral DNA then inserts itself into the host cell's chromosomes, where it may remain inactive until it is "triggered," perhaps by a new infection, to instruct the host cell to begin rapidly making numerous copies of the virus. The T4 cell dies, probably from perforations of the cell wall by the escaping viruses. The decline in the number of helper T cells cripples the immune system and makes the body vulnerable to the many infections that characterize AIDS.

Who is at risk?

Anyone who comes into intimate contact with the body fluids of an individual carrying HIV is at risk of becoming infected and then possibly developing full-blown AIDS in the future.

Initially, sexually active homosexual and bisexual men accounted for half of the recorded cases of AIDS in the United States. A 2005 UNAIDS assessment of the United States showed the proportion of AIDS cases attributed to heterosexual transmission had increased and accounted for 32 percent of newly diagnosed cases (15 percent of cases among men, and 80 percent of cases among women).

In Africa, more than 80 percent of cases are acquired heterosexually. More than one-third of AIDS patients are intravenous drug users, who acquired HIV by sharing contaminated hypodermic needles.

In 2001, 39,400 new cases of AIDS were reported to the Centers for Disease Control (CDC) in Atlanta. By 2006, a new method of measuring incidence had been implemented by the CDC, and that year it was estimated that 56,300 new HIV infections occurred.

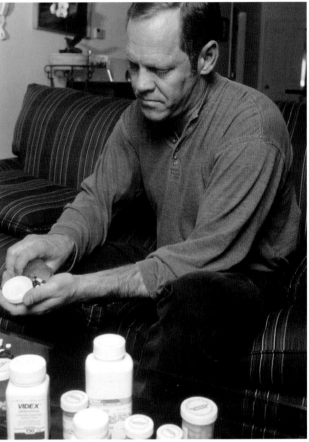

▲ *This HIV-positive man takes a range of pills to help protect him from developing AIDS.*

Before a test for screening donated blood was developed in 1985, a small number of recipients of blood transfusions became infected. A relatively high percentage of hemophiliacs acquired HIV through injections of clotting factors, which are derived from thousands of donors. New techniques for removing viruses from such material have greatly reduced the risk for this group.

A pregnant woman infected with HIV can give the virus to her child during the pregnancy or at the time of birth. Researchers believe that there is a 50 percent chance that a baby born to an AIDS patient will become infected. Medical therapies reduce the risk of passing HIV to the baby.

All present evidence strongly suggests that casual nonsexual contact with an infected individual in the home, workplace, or school does not pose a threat.

Symptoms

A person can be infected with HIV for years before suffering symptoms or developing a full-blown case of AIDS. The earliest signs of infection might be the swelling of lymph nodes in the neck and armpit, sometimes called persistent generalized lymphadenopathy (PGL). A later development may be a condition called AIDS-related complex (ARC). Symptoms include fever, fatigue, loss of weight, diarrhea, and attacks of shingles or herpes.

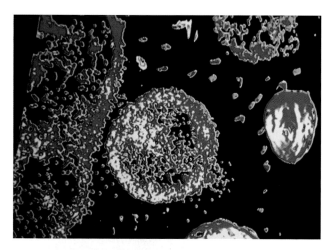

▲ *An electron microscope image of the AIDS virus.*

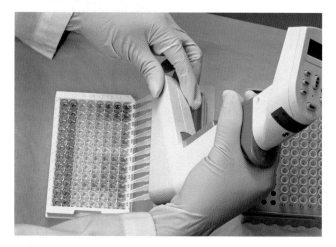

▲ *HIV testing involves checking the blood for antibodies, which will indicate whether a person is HIV-positive.*

Full-blown AIDS is characterized by the collapse of the immune system, which leads to severe opportunistic infections and cancers, such as Kaposi's sarcoma, that eventually may prove fatal. HIV can also invade the cells in the brain. Dementia (similar to Alzheimer's disease) and even schizophrenia, which is a psychotic personality disorder, may occur as a result either early or late in the disease.

It is believed that not all infected individuals will develop AIDS. Several explanations have been proposed. For example, some strains of the virus may be more virulent than others, or certain cofactors—another infection or even a genetic susceptibility—might enhance or trigger the virus's ability to cause disease.

Testing

People infected with HIV develop antibodies, and the infection is usually confirmed by testing a blood sample for these HIV-specific antibodies. The test most commonly used is an enzyme-linked immunosorbent assay (ELISA) test, which, if positive, is then confirmed by a blood test called a Western blot. It may take up to 2 weeks to get the results for these tests. Diagnosis can also be made

by checking for the HIV viral p24 antigen or, less commonly, by culturing HIV.

Rapid HIV testing is also available. One such test uses a drop of blood from a finger prick and another uses secretions collected from a pad rubbed against the gums. This oral test has a sensitivity of detecting the presence of HIV that is very close to that for blood testing. Results are available within 20 to 60 minutes. In addition, there is a Food and Drug Administration (FDA) home test available to check for HIV. In this test, a drop of blood placed on the specified testing media is mailed, and the results are available by calling a toll-free number. However, the CDC recommends confirmation of positive test results with standard laboratory tests for HIV infection.

Treatment

Early treatment is important because it helps preserve immune function, reduces the frequency and severity of opportunistic infections, improves well-being, and prolongs survival. Antibiotics, antifungal drugs, and antiviral drugs for opportunistic infections play a major role in therapy, but more important, there are antiretroviral drugs available to fight HIV. Highly active antiretroviral therapy (HAART), which was introduced in the 1990s, involves treatment with three or more drugs active against HIV. HAART can be used in all stages of HIV infection or AIDS. Although there is a risk of toxicity with HAART, the benefits are remarkable. During the first three years of HAART, a 60 to 80 percent reduction was noted in AIDS-defining diagnoses, deaths, and AIDS-related hospitalizations. However, HAART treatment is prohibitively expensive for most people with HIV infection or AIDS. Although treatment provides great benefit—people living with HIV are able to lead longer, healthier lives—it is not a cure and may be needed lifelong.

Prevention

Until a vaccine that protects against the AIDS virus becomes available, the only way to prevent infection is to avoid practices that spread the disease. The use of condoms among homosexuals and heterosexuals has become commonplace, and promiscuous contact with numerous sex partners is discouraged. Steps to reduce the use of contaminated needles among drug users, who represent a major method of transmission, have been widely undertaken.

Because the AIDS virus mutates easily, coming up with a vaccine that is effective against all potential strains is very difficult. There are two main varieties, HIV-1 (United States) and HIV-2 (West Africa), and more than 10 subtypes of the virus. It is unlikely that an HIV-1 vaccine, if one were available, would give any protection against other varieties. An enormous research effort is in progress to produce anti-HIV vaccines, and there have been many disappointments. As knowledge grows, however, the prospect for an effective vaccine is steadily improving.

The World Health Organization estimated in 2009 that about 33 million people worldwide—31 million adults and 2 million children—had HIV infection or AIDS; almost 2.7 million people acquired HIV infection; and 2 million people died from AIDS. It was estimated that about 1.2 million people in the United States had HIV infection or AIDS, and about 22,000 people in the United States died from AIDS.

> *See also:* **Antibiotics; Cancer; Contraception; Drug abuse; Hemophilia; Infection and infectious diseases; Viruses**

Alcoholism

Questions and Answers

I have heard that women are more at risk when they drink than men. Is there any truth in this?

Although drinking among women is on the increase, women still drink less than men. However, if a woman becomes an alcoholic, she is more vulnerable to the ill effects than a man—her liver may be affected earlier than a man's, and treatment is often less successful. There are also problems for an alcoholic woman who becomes pregnant—she risks causing mental retardation in her baby; the child may also be born with congenital deformities, such as dislocated hips or a cleft palate.

My uncle drinks very heavily, and in the past year I have noticed a change in his personality. He used to be pleasant and outgoing; now he is surly and introverted. Could his drinking be the cause?

Almost certainly. Heavy drinkers can become moody, violent, jealous, and paranoid. They often forget things, and they may hear imaginary voices, see visions, and become unable to cope with life.
   Withdrawal from alcohol can result in delirium tremens (the "DTs"), the symptoms of which include trembling, visual hallucinations, and a general feeling of panic. If you recognize any of these danger signs in your uncle, encourage him to seek help.

Where can I go to get help for alcoholism?

Go to your family doctor for advice on the physical aspects of alcohol addiction—he or she will refer you to a rehabilitation clinic, if necessary. For family problems see a social worker or your rabbi, minister, or parish priest. There are also self-help groups, such as Alcoholics Anonymous; these can provide long-term support to people who want to stop drinking.

Most people drink moderately, enjoy drinking, and experience no ill effects. However, some individuals become so dependent on alcohol that they can no longer lead a normal life. It is important to be able to recognize the danger signals and to know when to seek help.

When people talk about alcohol, they are usually referring to drinks that contain varying amounts of pure alcohol, such as wine, beer, and hard liquor (whiskey, vodka, and rum, for example). Alcoholic drinks have a restricted food value in the form of sugar—as in sweet wines, for example—and carbohydrates found in liquor and beers made from grain. Alcohol is basically a drug—a substance that affects the working of the mind and body in a variety of different ways.
   Taken in moderation, alcohol can encourage the appetite and produce a feeling of well-being, because the alcohol stimulates the blood flow to the skin; this has the effect of making the

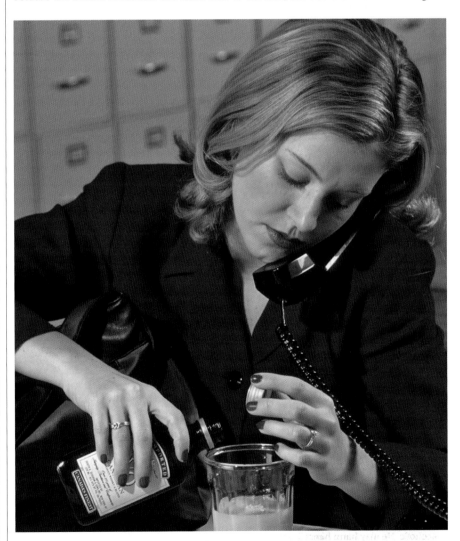

▲ *The stresses and anxieties of modern life can lead men and women from all social and economic backgrounds to turn to alcohol as a source of relaxation and escape.*

Questions and Answers

What is the best cure for a hangover? I get a really awful headache after drinking alcohol, and everyone has different ideas on what I should do about it.

The only real cure for a hangover is rest. Acetaminophen may be used to treat a bad headache, but aspirin should not be taken; it will only cause further disturbance to an already irritated stomach. The "hair of the dog" remedy (having another drink) is not a good idea, as it will lead to you spending the rest of the day drunk. Drink as much water as possible before going to sleep after a drinking session. Dehydration is one of the causes of a hangover, and water will help to reduce this effect. However, it is better still to try not to drink too much in the first place; this way you avoid having a hangover altogether.

As you say, most people have a favorite cure—orange juice, vitamin pills, milkshakes. However, a good rule to follow is that prevention is better than cure.

Are some people more vulnerable to alcohol than others? I seem to get drunk on one glass of wine.

It used to be thought that people who found themselves suffering the effects of drink very quickly were different in their physical and psychological makeup, but this idea is now discounted. Anyone can become an alcoholic, although some studies have suggested a genetic basis for alcoholism. If you have a bad reaction to alcohol, it is better to avoid it, or at least be very careful to stay within your known limits.

My sister says her husband has a drinking problem but denies that he is an alcoholic. Is this possible?

No. A person with a drinking problem and an alcoholic are one and the same thing. A person whose drinking has gotten out of control and who has become dependent on alcohol is an alcoholic. He may harm himself and others, so it is best to be truthful about the situation and get help.

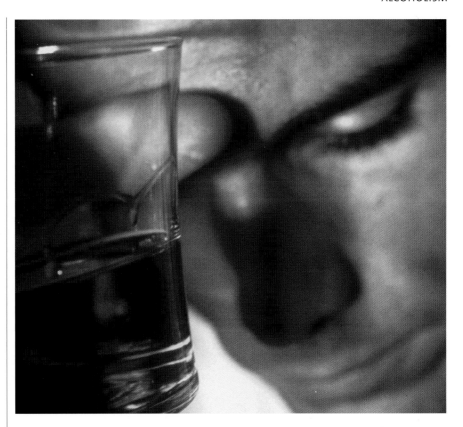

▲ *Because of the feeling of well-being it produces when taken in moderation, some people think alcohol is a stimulant; in fact, when taken in excess, it is a depressant.*

drinker feel pleasantly warm. When the alcohol reaches the brain, anxiety is reduced and self-confidence increases. Shyness disappears, and the world seems to become a friendlier place.

Dependency

Heavy drinking is entirely different from taking alcohol in moderation. When heavy drinking is repeated over any period of time, subtle changes can occur in the personality. It is thought that these changes have a chemical basis and can lead to the need to continue the drinking pattern. When the feeling becomes so persistent that every time an alcoholic drink is delayed the drinker suffers a desperate and urgent desire to have one, he or she has reached a state that is known as alcohol dependency.

In the early stages of heavy drinking, this dependency tends to be psychological rather than physical. This is because anxiety and stress usually lead people to drink in the first place. Later, heavy drinkers come to rely on alcohol physically as a prop to relax them.

If the drinking becomes much heavier, so too does the drinker's psychological need. In the transitional period, this may not be noticeable; however, as physical dependence grows, withdrawal will become more and more difficult and uncomfortable. Eventually, alcohol deprivation for any length of time will result in trembling, sweating, and acute stress. The first drink will relieve these feelings—until the next time.

Alcohol and personality changes

Alcohol tends to affect different people in different ways. The same amount can turn one person into the life of a party, bring out violent aggression in another, and send a third quietly to sleep.

Although it reduces tension, alcohol is not a stimulant; it is, rather, a depressant. As soon as it enters the bloodstream, it begins to impair judgment, self-control, and skill. Research has shown that workers with blood-alcohol levels of between 0.03 percent (30 mg, or the equivalent of two cans of 6.4 percent alcohol beer) and 0.1 percent (100 mg) have more accidents than those with less than 30 mg. With driving, the likelihood of an accident increases when the blood-alcohol level reaches 30 mg; at 80 mg, the likelihood of an accident is four times greater; and at 150 mg, it is 25 times greater. This is because the coordination between hand and eye and the ability to judge distances accurately deteriorate progressively the more alcohol a person drinks.

The problems of alcoholism

Once an excessive or heavy drinker is unable to stop drinking without outside help, he or she can be classified as an alcoholic. It is in this situation that social, economic, and medical problems—often already evident in a heavy drinker—can become worse. Eventually these problems will bring despair and confusion to the alcoholic and everyone else with whom he or she has contact. Alcohol breaks up marriages, sets children against parents and vice versa, and costs individuals their jobs and their reputation in the community. Ultimately, alcoholism can also kill.

When most people think of alcoholics, they visualize the stereotypical street-corner inebriates. However, it is not just the deprived and inadequate members of society who resort to drinking as a means of escape. There are children too inebriated to attend school after lunch, businessmen and women incapable of working in the afternoons, and mothers and fathers barely able to prepare a meal for their children at the end of the day.

Alcoholism can strike irrespective of age, class, creed, race, or gender. Once afflicted, alcoholics may mix only with like-minded friends; they may neglect their families altogether, break promises, lie and steal, and live only to drink.

Reasons for heavy drinking

Drinking is an accepted and approved cultural activity. Thus it appears that some people are more exposed to the risk of becoming alcoholics than others simply because of social pressures and conditioning. For example, studies of national groups reveal that the Irish have a high rate of alcoholism; this is in contrast to the rate in Jewish communities, which is very low. Certain professions seem to encourage alcoholism—traveling salespeople, bar attendants, waiting and catering staffs, and company directors, among others, are particularly at risk because of frequent socializing and the availability of alcohol.

Housewives are increasingly victims of this form of addiction. These women are often isolated, either with small children or with too little to do once their families have grown up and left home, and drinking can provide them with a welcome escape from a seemingly tedious existence. The fact that most grocery stores stock alcohol makes it only too easy for people to buy.

In most cases drinking starts at an early age; as with smoking, children frequently copy the habits of their parents. It is statistically proved that the children of alcoholic parents have a higher than average risk of developing alcoholism themselves. Teenagers also tend to be strongly influenced by their friends' behavior. The largest population of problem drinkers in the United States is single urban males under the age of 25.

Today so much socializing is built around the consumption of alcohol that it is hard for people to avoid drinking. It is easy to find other people who drink and to go to the same bar or restaurant regularly. In addition, advertising suggests that men are not men unless they drink, and being able to "hold one's liquor" is considered

The effects of alcoholism

PHYSICAL

Cirrhosis of the liver: there is no cure for this; it is the most common disease associated with alcoholism.

Other diseases: alcoholics commonly develop kidney trouble, heart disease, and ulcers; these conditions fail to respond to normal treatment if a person continues to drink.

Frequent appearance of bruises and cuts, resulting from falls and bumping into things.

Persistent, vague physical complaints with no apparent cause, such as headaches and stomach upsets.

Inexplicable trembling of the hands; sweating.

Loss of appetite and loss of sleep (insomnia).

Pins and needles in hands and feet.

Delirium tremens: this is a psychotic disorder typical of withdrawal in chronic alcoholics; symptoms include tremors, anxiety, and disorientation. It is also sometimes accompanied by visual hallucinations.

EMOTIONAL AND SOCIAL

Increasing anxiety, depression, remorse, and phobic or paranoid fears.

Obsession with drinking begins to override everything else in life; the need for alcohol increases as tolerance grows.

Disruption or breakdown of family life; persistent marital arguments and other problems.

Loss of friends and interests—alcoholics increasingly seek the company of others like themselves.

Frequent absenteeism from work and repeated job changes; a loss of efficiency and reliability that can lead to job loss.

Lack of concentration; loss of memory.

Impaired behavior and social adjustment.

Shabby appearance; poor hygiene.

Sneaking drinks; gulping drinks.

Arrests for drunken driving.

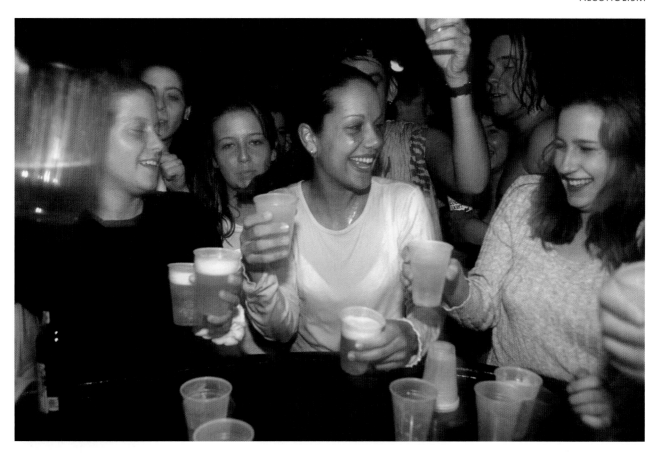

a sign of masculinity. Finally, a refusal to drink is often thought to be abnormal and sometimes seen as an antisocial action. All these factors can combine to make it difficult for a person to maintain a responsible attitude toward alcohol and to keep drinking habits moderate.

Danger signals

The human body develops a tolerance to alcohol, and the danger lies in the fact that a heavy drinker soon needs more drinks to reproduce the original feeling of relaxation and well-being. The higher the daily intake becomes, the more difficult it is for him or her to give it up. If an individual drinks to relieve worries, this too can lead to more drinking—more worries mean more alcohol, and fewer worries become the reason for a round of celebratory drinks.

It can take several years for someone to develop an addiction to the point where he or she would be classified as an alcoholic. Symptoms to watch for are an obvious obsession with alcohol and the inability to give it up, or even restrict drinking to a reasonable level; moral and physical deterioration; and increasingly obvious problems with work, money, and family. A typical alcoholic will probably need a drink early in the morning and may need continual boosters to keep going during the day.

Safe drinking

In a situation where an individual wants to drink but not to excess, alcohol should be consumed as slowly as possible. He or she should always consume some food before the first drink so that the alcohol will be absorbed more slowly into the bloodstream.

▲ *Drinking with friends can be an enjoyable way to unwind. However, drinking for its own sake, and showing a marked reluctance to stop—no matter how much has been drunk— are danger signals. Young people are particularly vulnerable to pressure from their peers to take alcohol and to keep drinking even after they have had enough.*

Consumption can also be kept down by alternating alcoholic drinks with non- alcoholic ones. It is better not to drink alone, because it is all too easy to consume more than usual to combat feelings of loneliness.

If a person does not want to drink an excessive amount, he or she can also set a personal limit as to the number of drinks that can be drunk before inebriation occurs, and then stick to this resolution.

Finally, the combination of drinking and driving—or handling any type of heavy machinery—is extremely dangerous. Research has found that elevated blood-alcohol levels are present in 16 percent of individuals involved in accidents at work, 22 percent of those in home accidents, and 30 percent of those in highway accidents.

People who know they will be drinking should leave the car at home and take a taxi or get a ride from a friend. Not only is driving while inebriated illegal; a large percentage of accidents and deaths on the road are caused by drunken drivers. There can be no compromise; it is clear that drinking and driving do not mix.

See also: **Drug abuse; Stress**

Allergies

Allergies can cause considerable discomfort and inconvenience. Although there are at present no cures, medical research is making progress in discovering the main causes and alleviating the symptoms of allergies.

An allergy is a sensitivity to a substance that does not normally cause people any discomfort or harm. Hay fever, which is caused by a sensitivity to pollen, is an example. Asthma, eczema, rashes, and a variety of other complaints can also be caused partly or entirely by an allergy. Allergies can affect almost any part of a person's body and can be triggered by a vast range of both natural and artificial substances.

Allergies are seldom life-threatening, although they can be dangerous and are often very uncomfortable for the sufferer. Much has been discovered in recent years about the underlying cause of allergies and about the genetic basis of hypersensitivity. However, these discoveries have not yet led to a cure.

Allergies are reactions to allergens; this is the name given to those substances, such as pollen, that spark off symptoms in someone who is sensitive to them. Among the most common allergens are foods (notably eggs, milk, and fish), pollens, spores, insect bites (especially bee and wasp stings), animal hair and dander, and chemicals. One type of allergy is caused by contact with metal; therefore, some people get a rash when wearing certain pieces of jewelry next to their skin. A common allergen found in even the cleanest homes is the dust mite; this is a tiny creature, invisible to the naked eye, that lives in bedding, carpets, and draperies.

Questions and Answers

I love the taste of shrimp, but when I eat it, I break out in a nasty rash. Is there any cure?

There are several ways of relieving the symptoms of allergies, but these are not cures. Whatever treatment you receive, it is not going to change your basic sensitivity to the food in question. It is best to avoid foods that you know you are allergic to.

My best friend has just developed an allergy to penicillin, and she is now really worried in case she catches a disease. Surely there are alternative drugs to penicillin?

There is really no need for her to worry. Although a penicillin allergy does reduce the number of antibiotics that a doctor might consider prescribing, there is still a range of antibiotics available for people with this type of allergy.

My younger brother is allergic to cats, and touching one makes him break out in a rash. Will he grow out of this problem?

Possibly. Children who suffer from either allergic rashes or eczema often do grow out of the problem. However, they may suffer from other forms of allergy—asthma, for example—when they are older, because they have a basic tendency to be allergic.

I suffer terribly from hay fever and am now pregnant. Could my child inherit the condition?

This could happen. It has been discovered that hay fever, like eczema and asthma, is a genetic disorder caused by mutations in one or more of several genes. The resulting state is called atopy. Although atopic parents are more likely to have an atopic child, this state—and hence an allergy—is not necessarily inherited.

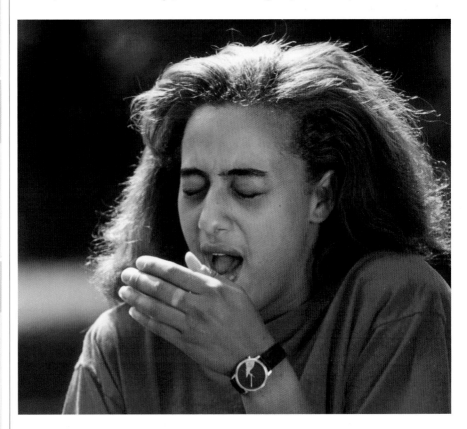

▲ *Allergies are a common complaint. Distressing as the symptoms are, a lot can be done to improve the situation. Runny eyes and sneezing are typical of hay fever.*

HOW ALLERGY-PRODUCING HISTAMINE IS RELEASED

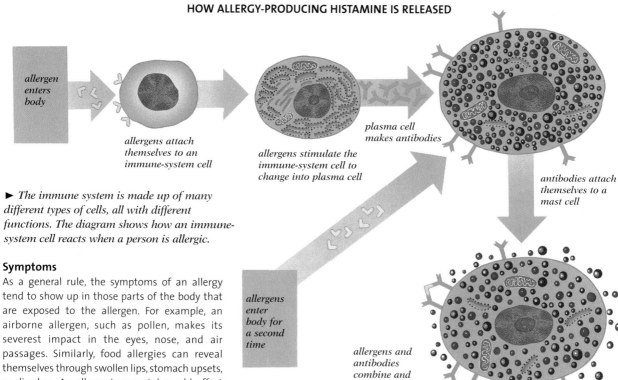

allergen enters body

allergens attach themselves to an immune-system cell

allergens stimulate the immune-system cell to change into plasma cell

plasma cell makes antibodies

antibodies attach themselves to a mast cell

allergens enter body for a second time

allergens and antibodies combine and histamine is released

▶ *The immune system is made up of many different types of cells, all with different functions. The diagram shows how an immune-system cell reacts when a person is allergic.*

Symptoms

As a general rule, the symptoms of an allergy tend to show up in those parts of the body that are exposed to the allergen. For example, an airborne allergen, such as pollen, makes its severest impact in the eyes, nose, and air passages. Similarly, food allergies can reveal themselves through swollen lips, stomach upsets, or diarrhea. An allergy to a metal would affect the part of the skin the metal touches, and an allergy to rubber would result in a rash on the part of the body where, for example, elastic in underwear or swimwear came into contact with the skin.

However, this is only a very general rule, because if an allergen gets into the bloodstream, it can cause reactions almost anywhere on the body. This is particularly true of food allergens, which are absorbed through the digestive tract into the blood. As a result, food allergens can cause a wide range of reactions in sufferers, including itchy skin, eczema, hives (red bumps on the skin), asthma, and even, in some cases, mental disorders.

Types of allergies

Skin allergies: There are three basic forms of allergic reaction that affect the skin. The most common, particularly in children, is eczema. This appears as a rash or as scaly skin, found mostly on the hands, face, and neck, and in the creases of the forearms and behind the knees, although it can affect any body part.

Contact dermatitis, often caused by metal jewelry or by chemicals in detergents, is a blistery, itchy inflammation of skin that has come into direct contact with the allergen.

The third reaction is urticaria, best described by its popular name, hives. This is a red, irritating swelling that often has a small white point in the middle that makes it look like a nettle sting.

Eye, ear, and nose allergies: Eye allergies generally show up as an irritation in the white part of the eye, accompanied by redness. Severe swellings can occur, but generally the symptoms are watering of the eyes and soreness.

The ears may also be the target of allergens. When this happens, fluid builds up inside the ear, and may affect hearing temporarily.

Hay fever can affect the eyes and ears, although its principal target is the nose, which becomes stuffy, runny, or sneezy. Unlike a common cold—which is caused by a virus and should clear up after four or five days in an otherwise healthy person—hay fever will last for as long as a sufferer is exposed to the particular pollen to which he or she is allergic. If a person is unsure whether he or she has a cold or an allergy, it is worth waiting for several days to see if the condition clears up. If it does not, the sufferer should consult a doctor for advice and possible treatment.

Food allergies: These have a wide variety of symptoms. The most obvious symptom of an acute food allergy is stomach upset, followed quickly by nausea, vomiting, or diarrhea. People who are acutely sensitive to a food may also get a swollen tongue and lips.

Sometimes the sufferer gets two kinds of symptoms; for instance, a child who is allergic to cow's milk may get both diarrhea and a skin rash. Apart from rashes, which may appear hours or even days after a particular food is eaten, food allergy symptoms become apparent almost immediately afterward, usually within one hour. This makes it quite easy for the sufferer to identify the allergen concerned.

Asthma attacks can also be brought on as a result of an allergic reaction to foods; such attacks are characterized by wheezing and difficulty in breathing.

Doctors now believe that a wide variety of other physical and mental symptoms can also be caused by food allergies, although the exact cause of a reaction is often difficult to identify. Depression, anxiety, headaches, schizophrenia, hyperactivity in children, and even convulsions have all been (not always correctly) attributed to food allergies. There have also been cases of bed-wetting and cystitis (a urinary tract infection) that have been blamed on food allergies.

Another complaint, which is caused by food intolerance—and so is not strictly an allergy—is celiac disease. This is a disorder of the

Questions and Answers

I am worried that I may become addicted to the drugs I am taking to treat an allergy. Is this possible?

No. Nor do these drugs lose their effect if you have to keep taking them for a long time. However, they may have side effects—antihistamines, for example, can make you drowsy. Like all drugs, those that treat allergies should be used with caution.

Whenever my father is near my mother, her eyes run and she can't stop sneezing. Can you be allergic to people, places, or animals?

You cannot be allergic to a person, but allergy to body fluids or material on the skin is possible. Allergy to seminal fluid has been described. Some people who are acutely allergic to fish can get swollen lips from kissing someone who has just been eating fish. Allergy to animals is common, though it is the fine pieces of hair or feathers from the animal that are to blame. You can be allergic to a place only if you are allergic to something found in that place, such as pollen.

I sit next to a girl in school who has eczema, and sometimes the rash is severe. Could I catch the condition from her, and are there any precautions I should take?

Allergies are not infectious. You cannot catch an allergy from another person, nor can you pick up an effect—in this case eczema—of that allergy.

My parents both suffer from food allergies, but I have shown no signs of any allergies yet. Is there any way to prevent an allergy?

Some specialists say there is little that can be done; others believe that some can be prevented. The risk of a child's developing a milk allergy, for instance, may be reduced by breast-feeding him or her as a baby. Some experts believe that it is possible to reduce the risk of other food allergies by eating as varied a diet as possible.

digestive system, and its symptoms are gas and pain in the stomach after eating. Soft, smelly feces, which are full of undigested fat, and weight loss result from the sufferer's inability to absorb food properly. Celiac disease is an intolerance to gluten, one of the proteins found in wheat, so sufferers must avoid foods containing gluten.

The most severe—though quite rare—symptom caused by allergy is known as anaphylaxis. The patient's air passages swell and close, and the blood pressure falls abruptly. A severe allergy to nuts or strawberries is associated with this symptom. Anaphylaxis is an acute and life-threatening condition; however, it can be reversed quickly by an injection of adrenaline.

Causes

The immune system is a collection of several different classes of cells with different functions. These cells are constantly on the lookout for foreign substances, such as bacteria, viruses, and other proteins that are different from the body's own proteins and may pose a threat. When immune-system cells come across a potentially dangerous foreign protein, they form a substance called an antibody; this combines with the foreign substance and neutralizes it.

A slightly different antibody is created to deal with each foreign substance. Once an antibody has been formed for the first time, the body is able to produce the same antibody again to deal with any future "attack" by that substance. This explains why infectious diseases such as measles and chicken pox occur only once in a person's lifetime—after the first attack, the body has supplies of antibodies that can deal with the virus whenever it appears again.

By checking identifying surface markers, the immune system of a normal, healthy person is able to tell the difference between dangerous foreign matter—such as a virus—and a harmless one, such as a food protein. However, in an allergic person, the immune system reacts to a harmless foreign protein as if it were a dangerous one and starts forming an antibody. This antibody attaches itself to cells called mast cells. Mast cells contain a number of chemicals, the most important of which is called histamine.

People who are allergic produce much larger quantities than normal of a particular class of antibodies known as immunoglobulin,

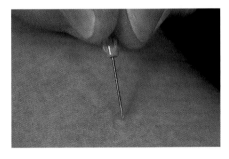

▲ *In the scratch test, a doctor scratches the skin of the patient's arm several times with a needle. Drops of solution containing possible allergens are dropped on the scratches to test for a reaction.*

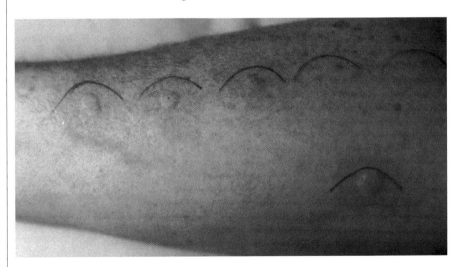

▲ *This allergy sufferer has undergone the scratch test and found that the cause of her allergy is the dust mite. The positive reaction to this allergen is shown in the large welt at the bottom. The marks above it show no reaction and represent negative results.*

		Common allergies		
ALLERGY	**ALLERGENS**	**SYMPTOMS**	**TREATMENT**	**PREVENTION**
Asthma	Dust mites. Animal hair. Pollen. Some foods and food additives.	Difficulty in breathing; wheezing.	Drugs by inhalation, including steroids, bronchodilators, and mast cell stabilizers.	Keep house dust-free as much as possible. Avoid pollen. Keep clear of allergenic foods.
Contact dermatitis	Contact with allergen, e.g. jewelry, chemicals in detergents.	Itchy, blistery skin inflammation.	Steroid creams given on doctor's prescription.	Avoid contact with allergen.
Eczema	Some foods, especially cow's milk, flour, eggs; possibly some seafoods.	Rash on hands, face, neck, arms, and legs; looks like scaly skin.	Moisturizers and steroid creams; sometimes anti-histamines or antibiotics.	Take dietary precautions to avoid allergen.
Food allergy	Could be caused by almost any food—more commonly milk, flour, eggs; also nuts, strawberries, shellfish; and some food additives.	Upset stomach and general nausea; acute reaction produces swollen tongue and lips, as well as diarrhea. If food is absorbed into bloodstream, it can produce skin rashes similar to eczema.	Sometimes scratch test, elimination test and/or provocation test for diagnosis of the allergen.	Keep to diet; avoid allergenic foods.
Hay fever	Pollen; may react to just one pollen or to several different types.	Sore, itchy eyes, runny or stuffy nose, prolonged sneezing.	Scratch test to confirm allergy. Injections and antihistamine pills to relieve symptoms; mast cell membrane stabilizers.	Injections before season begins; listen to pollen count on weather report. Avoid open air when the pollen count is high.
Hives	Certain foods. Handling certain plants. Hot and cold water.	Red, irritating swelling on skin with small white point in center.	Skin condition treated with antihistamine cream, if necessary.	Avoid the allergens.

class E (IgE). These antibodies attach themselves firmly to receptors on the surface of the mast cells. A gene on chromosome number 13, which regulates the B cells producing IgE, was identified in 2003. Several other mutations of the genes that code for the IgE receptors on the membranes of mast cells have also been discovered. The gene mutations are believed to be the cause of a state known as atopy; this state is associated with the allergic disorders hay fever, asthma, and eczema.

When allergens, such as pollen grains, lock on the IgE molecules on the mast cells, they impose strain between adjacent molecules, and this leads to a tearing of the cell membrane and the release of the powerfully irritating mast cell contents; the most irritating of these is the chemical histamine.

The surge of histamine produces an effect very much like the inflammation that follows a wound—it makes tiny blood vessels dilate. As they dilate, the blood vessel walls become leaky, so that fluid from the blood escapes into the surrounding tissues.

The dilation of the tiny blood vessels causes redness and itching on the skin's surface; at the same time, the escaping fluid makes the surrounding tissues swell. In hay fever, the mucous glands in a sufferer's nose and sinuses are also stimulated to produce fluid; it is this that causes the characteristic stuffiness and runny nose.

Diagnosis

The diagnosis of pollen allergies—and sometimes of food allergies, too—is still sometimes performed with the help of a technique called the scratch test. A doctor or nurse gently scratches the skin of the patient's arm with a needle, then drops a watery solution onto the scratched spot where the skin is broken. This solution contains a very small amount of a particular allergen.

Up to 40 of these little scratch tests may be performed at one session, usually without much discomfort for an adult. If a person is allergic to one of the allergens, a round, red welt will show up on the skin in that spot within about 15 minutes.

A special diet, called the elimination diet, is sometimes used to identify which food or foods are the cause of a food allergy. Sufferers are asked to exclude some of the most common allergy-producing foods from their diet. If they get better after being on this diet for several days, it is likely that one or more of the foods that have been eliminated are the cause of the problem. The individuals may then be asked to reintroduce these foods into their diet, one at a time, to see if the symptoms return.

This process of elimination eventually reveals the identity of the allergenic food. As elimination diets can take a long time, some doctors now use provocation tests; this involves injecting a weak

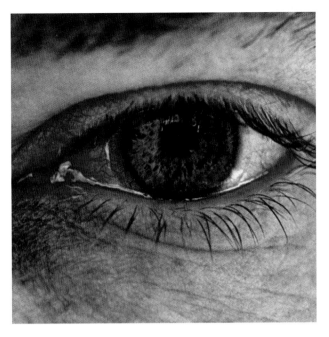

▲ *Red, swollen, itchy eyes are one of the common symptoms of an allergy; an eyewash or drops may help relieve discomfort.*

solution of various foods under the skin or dropping the solution under the tongue to see if it provokes symptoms. In addition to testing for food allergies, a doctor may also test an allergy sufferer's reaction to some of the chemicals that are commonly found in the home, or that are used as flavoring, coloring, or preservatives in food.

Treatment

People who have an acute allergy to a food that makes them sick whenever they eat it—for example, strawberries or shellfish—hardly need a doctor to diagnose the problem. The cause and the effect are obvious, and the simplest way to deal with the allergy is also the most obvious—avoiding the allergen completely.

In the case of pollen allergies, a doctor will first try to establish which pollen is causing the allergy, sometimes by means of a scratch test. Having identified the culprit, the doctor may then prescribe a set of injections. These injections also contain small amounts of the allergen, and their aim is to desensitize the sufferer by encouraging the immune system to produce a harmless "blocking antibody." This kind of antibody intercepts the allergen before it sets off symptoms by alighting on the mast cell antibodies. Injections can be given during the pollen season, although giving injections before the pollen season begins is usually more successful. These injections do not work for everybody, but they can give about 70 percent of sufferers protection that lasts throughout the pollen season.

However, sufferers should be aware that both provocative testing and desensitizing injections can be dangerous. Doctors who perform them must be skilled in resuscitation and must have the necessary equipment and drugs on hand. In the past, deaths have been caused by injection of substances to which the patients were highly allergic.

Several different kinds of drugs may be prescribed to deal with the symptoms of allergy. Antihistamines combat the inflammatory effects of histamine when it is released. They are available as pills, liquid medicine, and nose drops or eyedrops; there are also injectable antihistamines that can be used to treat serious allergic reactions. However, these drugs do tend to make people feel drowsy.

Another drug, disodium cromoglycate, works at the beginning of the process by preventing the mast cell membranes from tearing. Because it acts as a preventive, it must be taken before symptoms occur; it can do nothing about histamine that has been released. This drug is given in various forms: as an inhalant for asthma; as eyedrops for allergic symptoms in the eye; as pills for stomach allergies; or via a device called an insufflator, in which it is sniffed.

Corticosteroid drugs, such as cortisone, are very powerful anti-inflammatories. They are sometimes prescribed for skin allergies or via an inhaler to combat asthma. Asthma can also be controlled by a group of drugs known as bronchodilators, so called because they dilate (open up) the bronchi (the air passages in the lungs). These drugs are not cures; they simply relieve the symptoms of an allergy. Nor are they problem-free. Corticosteroids, for example, have to be used sparingly and for short periods only. It is even possible to develop an allergy to antihistamines. It is important that patients tell a doctor about any unpleasant side effects from a medication.

There are many antiallergenic drugs, and a doctor should be able to prescribe a brand that suits a particular individual better while having the same beneficial effects.

Food allergies can sometimes be relieved by drugs. However, some doctors prefer to recommend diets to ensure that a sufferer eliminates all foods that set off an allergic reaction. This type of diet should always be planned in conjunction with a doctor so that the new diet is not deficient in any essential nutrients.

Self-help

There is quite a lot that sufferers can do to help themselves. If they suffer from a food or chemical allergy, they should make every effort to avoid known allergens. This means reading the labels on food packages carefully to see if the product contains even small amounts of the substance causing a particular allergy. Sufferers should also be very careful about food eaten in restaurants and other people's homes, where it is difficult to identify the ingredients.

People with hay fever should be careful about going out in the open air during the pollen season, especially in midafternoon, when the pollen count is highest. Weather reports often forecast the pollen count for the following day. Goggles can protect the eyes against pollen or spores. It might also be worth thinking about buying a small air conditioner for the home or an automobile that can extract pollen from the air. Some vehicles now have filters in the ventilation system that are designed to catch pollen.

Anyone who is taking a vacation in the late spring or early summer should keep in mind that there is usually much less pollen in seashore or desert air than there is in the middle of the country. Alternatively, traveling in late autumn or winter is ideal.

Dust mites are difficult to eliminate from the home altogether, but regular vacuuming of carpets, draperies, and mattresses, along with washing of bedding, including blankets, will help to keep their numbers down. Pillows and comforters stuffed with artificial fibers are less likely to harbor dust mites than those with feathers, and make bedding easier to wash.

See also: **Genetics; Hay fever; Rashes**

Alternative medicine

As more people use alternative medicine, interest in it grows. Is it a healthy alternative, or, as some critics claim, are there too many unregulated therapies that have only anecdotal evidence to support them?

Questions and Answers

I suffer badly from stress. My friend told me that meditation might help. Would it?

Research shows that meditation affects the body's ability to relax and resist disease. More doctors are recommending it as a safe and simple method to help conditions such as high blood pressure, asthma, and insomnia, and the general stresses of life.

Meditation techniques can be performed anywhere; meditation involves listening to the breath, attempting to detach from thoughts, repeating a mantra, and focusing the attention in an attempt to induce calm and self-awareness. Physiological effects include a slowed heart rate and a state of relaxation.

Is acne influenced by diet, and are there alternative treatments for it?

Diet is not thought to be an important factor in causing acne, however, some people do find that sweet and fatty foods tend to exacerbate the condition. If conventional medicines do not help clear acne, there are some alternative treatments to try. Aromatherapy practitioners recommend applying one drop of tea tree oil to the blemish after cleansing the face. Tea tree is a natural antiseptic and can speed healing. Herbal medicine, vitamin therapy, homeopathy, and ayurvedic medicine all claim to have remedies for acne.

How can I choose a reliable alternative practitioner?

You could ask your local hospital for a list of practitioners in the area. Or contact a professional organization that will tell you if the practitioners of the therapy are licensed in your state. State health departments can give you information so that you can be sure a practitioner is competent.

Alternative medicine uses medical systems, therapies, and techniques that are not considered to be part of mainstream or conventional medicine. Although there is proven scientific evidence in favor of some such therapies, many of them still require substantial studies to determine whether they are safe and whether they are effective in treating the conditions and diseases for which they are used.

Therapies that have been proved to be safe and effective are gradually becoming adopted into conventional health care. Conventional, or orthodox, medicine is that practiced by holders of M.D. (medical doctor) or D.O. (doctor of osteopathy) degrees. Other conventional medical health professionals include registered nurses, psychologists, and physical therapists.

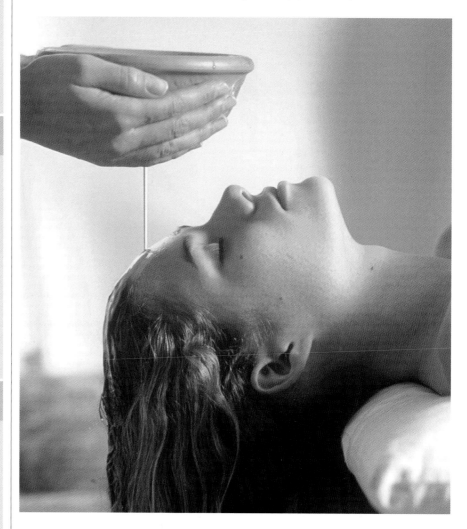

▲ *Warm sesame oil is dripped onto the forehead of a person undergoing* shirodhara, *an ayurvedic treatment that is said to profoundly relax the nervous system.*

Questions and Answers

Will my health insurance cover alternative medicine?

As alternative medicine becomes more popular, health insurers are becoming more willing to cover these therapies and are experimenting with coverage for alternative treatments. It will vary from company to company, but some pilot schemes cover homeopathy and naturopathy. There are wellness plans, for which the premiums are lower than for more traditional plans. The rationale for these schemes is that if people take care of themselves and take preventive measures against ill health, everyone will save money.

Are alternative therapies reasonably safe?

Obviously the skill, training, and experience of the practitioner have a bearing on safety, but all therapies, even conventional ones, may have risks attached. Factors such as the patients' state of health, their belief in the therapy, and how the treatment is used can all affect the safety of a treatment. The quality and type of ingredients in an alternative product also affect the safety of the treatment.

Any claims made for the supplement or therapy, such as claims that the product is able to diagnose, treat, cure, or prevent disease, must be substantiated by scientific proof. If this is not provided, the product is on sale illegally and can be removed by the authority of the FDA.

Where can I get information about an alternative therapy?

First, talk to your health practitioner and ask for advice, or for a referral to someone who knows about the therapy. Second, use the Internet to search for information. Check the database "CAM on PubMed" developed by the National Center for Complementary and Alternative Medicine and the National Library of Medicine. Third, visit your library for relevant books or publications.

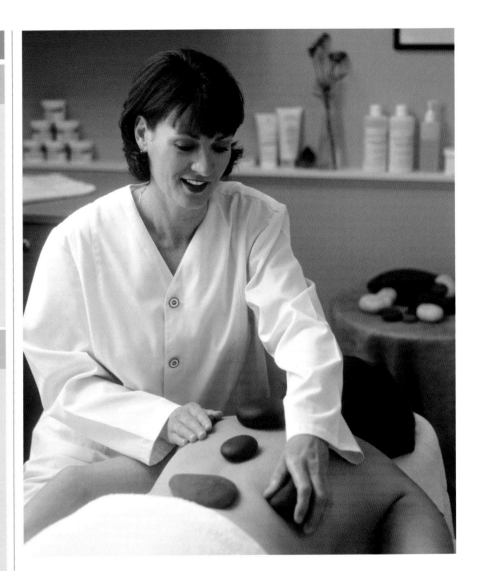

▲ *This patient is undergoing heat therapy at a spa. Heated stones are placed at intervals on the back; this helps stressed muscles to relax.*

Alternative and complementary medicine

Many people think that the terms "alternative medicine" and "complementary medicine" are synonymous, but in fact there is a significant difference between them. While alternative medicine is used in place of conventional medicine, complementary medicine is used in conjunction with conventional medicine. An example of a complementary therapy is the use of massage or aromatherapy to attempt to alleviate a patient's discomfort after surgery. An example of an alternative therapy to treat cancer is a holistic ayurvedic diet in place of conventional treatment such as surgery, chemotherapy, and radiation. Both alternative and complementary medicine are now more commonly referred to as nonconventional medicine. Although alternative medicine and complementary medicine are different, they are usually both mentioned in descriptions of medical practice and products that are not part of conventional medicine.

Integrative therapies

A third style of therapy is available, called integrative therapy; this combines conventional medical therapies with alternative and complementary therapies for which there is scientific evidence of safety and effectiveness. Thus, the patient takes advantage of a wide range of tried and tested treatments for his or her condition.

Why are alternative therapies gaining in popularity?

There are various reasons why patients resort to consulting alternative practitioners.

Some patients turn to alternative treatment because they have already had traditional medical treatment that they feel has not been effective, while others feel that their own doctors have too little time to discuss their complaints. Another prevailing feeling experienced by some people is that modern medicine uses too much technology. Some patients would prefer to revert to what they think are less invasive and more natural methods. One perception appears to be that alternative practitioners promote health but conventional medicine concentrates on illness. Other people believe that healing comes from God.

With the swing toward nontraditional systems, many doctors have been forced to examine these therapies, with the result that some conventional doctors now work with practitioners of complementary medicine. Some doctors will refer their patients to complementary practitioners if they think they can be helped by these practitioners' treatment.

Although there has been huge success in orthodox medicine in the field of vaccination, infectious diseases, and certain types of surgery, recovery rates for other illnesses have not improved so dramatically, especially in the area of psychiatric illnesses and degenerative diseases. Some diseases are actually caused by medical treatment.

All these factors could explain the growing interest in alternative medicine.

Critical consumers

Before using alternative therapies, a patient should consult his or her doctor to find out if there are possible risks involved in the therapy, and to ask the doctor if he or she can recommend a registered practitioner who has a known successful record of treatment.

Potential patients should ask the practitioner for his or her credentials in the form of qualifications and experience, and ask whether he or she is confident that the treatment will improve the condition. It is vital that a treatment such as chiropractic is carried out by a skilled practitioner, because some conditions can be made worse by an inexperienced operator.

Treatment programs

A treatment plan should be discussed with the practitioner, who should provide a clear idea of the length of the treatment and when an improvement in the condition can be expected. The practitioner should inform the patient of possible side effects and risks and what to do if there is no improvement, and discuss with the patient any supplementary treatment that could be useful.

When patients decide to use alternative medicine, they should first be sure that orthodox medicine cannot cure the problem. There is a danger that patients will undergo alternative treatment, which may not be effective, and then find that the condition has advanced beyond the help of orthodox treatment.

Three groups of therapies

Alternative therapies can be loosely divided into three broad categories, depending upon how acceptable they are to orthodox medicine.

Therapies in the first group

The first group consists of treatments that are governed by professional bodies, have training systems for their practitioners, and have scientifically proved effectiveness. The disciplines of the first group are as follows.

Acupuncture: This is based on the traditional Chinese practice of inserting fine needles into the skin to regulate or correct the flow of energy (chi) in the body. Western acupuncture aims to affect nerve impulses, using the same technique: the insertion of needles. Sometimes heat, pressure, friction, suction, or impulses of electromagnetic energy are also used to stimulate the acupoints. Practitioners of acupuncture are familiar with the basics of Chinese philosophy; the philosophies of the Dao or Tao, yin and yang, the eight principles, the three treasures, and the five elements are the basics of Chinese acupuncture and the role it has in helping to maintain health and well-being.

Chiropractic: A chiropractor uses special techniques to treat muscular and skeletal problems. This may involve soft tissue work and manipulative therapy, probably with a rapid thrust to the

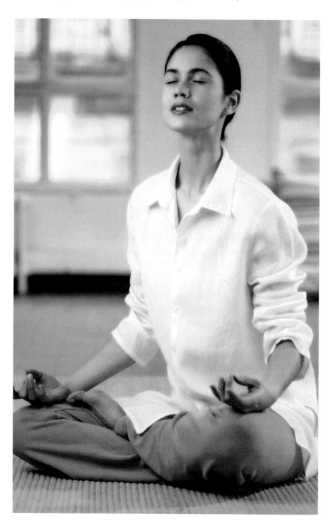

▲ *The benefits of meditation are claimed to be relaxation, reduction of stress, and relief from insomnia.*

vertebrae. Chiropractic focuses on the relationship between the structure of the spine and its function, and how that function affects the health of the individual. The type of technique depends on age, build, and general health. Massage and trigger points are often used to loosen knots and to warm up tense, painful muscles.

Herbal medicine: The use of herbs for medicines has been known since 3000 B.C.E., and 75 percent of people in the world still use herbs as the main treatment of sickness. In the West, the use of herbs declined with the rise of the pharmaceutical industry. However, many people still believe that herbs, correctly used, are more effective than synthetic chemicals; the varied ingredients in herbs can work together more effectively than a single ingredient chemical.

Homeopathy: In homeopathic medicine, "like cures like." Highly diluted quantities of homeopathic remedies are prescribed to cure symptoms. Homeopathic remedies are selected for their ability to replicate the symptoms of an illness; the same substance in a concentrated dose would cause the same symptoms. Homeopathic practitioners take a holistic approach; the whole person is seen to be important in choosing a remedy. Homeopathy is considered to be very safe, and no harm can come to someone if the wrong remedy is selected.

Osteopathy: This is now a fairly well-accepted treatment of the musculoskeletal system. Osteopaths believe that all the body's systems work together and that problems in one system will affect the others. They use manipulation and other techniques to restore function, alleviate pain, and promote health and well-being.

Therapies in the second group

The second group comprises therapies which lack regulation and have not been subjected to rigorous scientific investigation, but which are known to give help and comfort to many people.

Alexander technique: The Alexander technique is a process of reeducation of the body. Its aims are to treat, and also to prevent, a wide range of disorders by teaching people to become aware of how they use their bodies and to make the changes that they find necessary in order to feel some physical or psychological benefit. The conditions that respond best to the Alexander technique include back pain, stress-related disorders such as headaches and fatigue, breathing difficulties, and neck and joint pain. It has also been found to be helpful in such diverse conditions as high blood pressure, spastic colon, asthma, osteoarthritis, and neuralgia. Improved posture often results from the use of the Alexander technique, because students are taught to use their body in a relaxed, balanced, and efficient way. Teaching is often on a one-to-one basis; 30 lessons are usually needed at weekly intervals.

Anthroposophical medicine: This type of medicine aims to treat the soul as well as the body. It was founded by the Austrian scientist and philosopher Rudolf Steiner and a Dutch doctor, Ita Wegman. Anthroposophical medicine is practiced by medically qualified doctors who believe that the body has a spiritual as well as a mental dimension. Steiner said that the body is made up of earth, fire, water, and air, which are connected through three structures; the nerve–sense system (brain, nerves, and senses); the metabolic system (liver, digestive organs, and muscles); and the rhythmic system (heart, lungs, respiration, and circulation).

Anthroposophical medicine aims to achieve a balance between these three structures, through a mixture of medicines and therapies. As well as using metals and essential oils, anthroposophical medicine also uses mistletoe therapy (Iscador), which in some patients has been found to specifically attack cancer cells. Mistletoe also stimulates the immune system, increasing the amount of white cells that attack malignant cells. The therapy can be taken alone, or in conjunction with orthodox radiation therapy.

Spiritual and physical healing are also effected by counseling, art therapy, music, hydrotherapy, and movement therapy, or eurythmy, which consists of a series of movements to energize the immune system. Proponents of anthroposophical medicine believe the patients are empowered because they are given control over their own recovery and are not just passive participants in their treatment. Many patients have gained great benefit from mistletoe treatment, but there is little published evidence to back up claims, because the treatment has not yet been tested with full trial methodology.

Aromatherapy: For this therapy, essential oils, extracted from flowers, herbs, and trees, are used as extracts or essences during a massage, on a compress, in a bath, or as a steam inhalation, to induce health and relaxation. Essential oils appear to have an effect on the central nervous system, and there is also an emotional response to the scent of the oil that can induce positive feelings.

Bach flower remedies: Made from the flowers of wild plants, bushes, and trees, flower essences are intended to be used for mental symptoms rather than physical symptoms. Flower remedies were first prepared by Edward Bach, a medical doctor and homeopath who believed that negative emotions were the cause of physical disease. By treating negative aspects through the remedies, positive characteristics are allowed to develop. Bach discovered 38 remedies that could treat negative emotions, such as anxiety or apathy. Because they do not produce side effects, the remedies can be used for babies, the elderly, the sick, and animals.

Hypnotherapy: A trancelike state or hypnosis is produced in the patient and suggestions are then made to change behavior patterns to help overcome anxiety and stress-related illnesses.

Massage: Massage is an ancient therapy based on the instinct to use the hands to soothe, heal, and comfort. It is known to reduce the effects of stress on the nervous system, by calming and soothing an anxious person, while it can also stimulate and energize someone who is depressed. As well as increasing the circulation of blood and lymph, massage can restore strength and

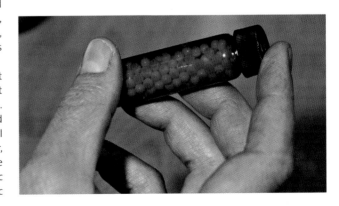

▲ *Homeopathic remedies are extremely diluted. They replicate the symptoms of illness to stimulate healing.*

mobility after injury and surgery and can help to break down scar tissue and adhesions. After vigorous exercise, when lactic acid buildup in the muscles causes pain, massage can increase the recovery rate of sore, aching muscles. It also stimulates the production of endorphins, the body's natural painkillers, and reduces muscle tension and spasm.

Meditation: This is the act of achieving a state of consciousness in which the mind, although still alert, becomes completely still. Many medical benefits have been noted, such as a reduction or stabilization of blood pressure, a lowering of heart rate, a reduction of muscle tension, and changes in brain-wave activity that show an alert but relaxed state. Other reported benefits of meditation are an improvement in memory, an increase in energy levels, and increased feelings of well-being and self-esteem. Anyone can meditate anywhere, indoors or outdoors. No equipment is needed, just a quiet place to sit undisturbed. The methods of achieving a meditative state are various. During focused breathing, the person gives full attention to the air flowing in and out of the nose. In breath counting, each inhalation is counted from one to 10 and if the mind wanders, beginning from one again. Mantra or sound meditation involves mentally repeating a word or phrase in time with natural breathing. Another method is concentrative meditation, in which the person focuses on a lighted candle, then closes the eyes and holds the image in the mind. In time it becomes easier to calm the mind and gain benefit from meditation.

Reflexology: This is a system of treating the whole body through a comprehensive foot massage, working on the principle that there are reflexes in the feet that correspond to all the systems and organs in the body. When pressure is applied to the reflexes in the feet, the body can be restored to a state of balance.

Shiatsu: The term "shiatsu" means finger pressure, and the practice is based on the same principles as acupuncture and acupressure, although practitioners also use thumbs, palms, forearms, and even feet and knees to apply pressure. Shiatsu has its origins in the massage techniques of Japan and traditional Chinese medicine and has evolved into the form now generally used. Shiatsu also uses manipulative techniques, stretches, joint rotations, and massage. Treatment is carried out with the recipient, clothed in loose pants and shirt, lying on a futon.

Yoga: Yoga exercises are balanced stretching movements that increase the flexibility of the spine and improve flexibility, posture, and muscle tone. As well as helping relaxation, yoga is a good stress reducer. It is suitable for any age group.

Therapies in the third group

The third group of alternative therapies have insufficient research studies and evidence to support their claims for safety and effectiveness. This is only a selection of the many therapies available.

Ayurvedic medicine: This ancient alternative medical system has been practiced on the Indian subcontinent for 5,000 years. It is based on holistic diets and herbal remedies, and it concentrates on employing the body, mind, and spirit in the treatment and prevention of disease.

Chinese herbal medicine: This is an ancient form of medicine, which involves using combinations of herbs to treat ill health and applies the concepts of Chinese philosophy. These include yin and yang, chi or energy, and the five elements and their role in maintaining good health.

Crystal therapy: The use of crystals is not new. Indigenous people in Australia and America used them for religious ceremonies as well as for healing. The theory behind crystal therapy is that the human body is made up of energy fields and energy centers or chakras. Crystals emit vibrations that affect the energy flow in the body and are said to redress energy imbalances in the body's energy field.

Cupping: Cupping is used to treat blood stagnation in the channels. The cups are warmed and placed on the skin, a vacuum is created, the resulting pressure encourages the flow of chi and blood in the area beneath the cup, and local stagnation clears. The technique should be applied only by licensed practitioners.

Iridology: Practitioners claim to be able to diagnose illness by studying the iris of the eye. They believe that each area of the body is represented by an area in the iris, and that someone's state of health can be diagnosed by looking at pigment flecks in the eye. Some practitioners claim that a patient's past medical history can be shown by interpreting eye markings. Iridology has not been proved to be effective by any scientific tests, and many medical doctors are skeptical of it.

Kinesiology: The term "kinesiology" refers to the study of human movement and physical activity. Applied kinesiology uses a system of muscle testing to help to diagnose what is functioning abnormally. Among other problems, this could be the nervous system that controls the muscle, a nutritional deficiency or excess, malfunctioning of the lymphatic drainage system, or a problem with the vascular supply to a muscle or organ. Treatment for the problems that have been diagnosed include chiropractic manipulation, acupuncture, and cranial osteopathic techniques.

Naturopathy: This alternative medical system uses natural forces in the body to help the body heal and become more healthy. Naturopathy recognizes that the patient's mental, emotional, and physical condition must be taken into account and treated appropriately. A naturopath will look for the cause of the disease and treat it, rather than simply treat the symptoms of the disease. Various practices are used; they include diet, herbal medicine, hydrotherapy, homeopathy, massage, acupuncture, physical therapy, and exercise therapy. Some naturopaths can practice natural childbirth. Naturopaths are able to work in an integrative manner with conventional and alternative medicine.

Chi kung or qigong: This is an ancient Chinese system of physical training, philosophy, and self-healing intended to direct one's internal energy through the body. The technique combines aerobic conditioning, meditation, breathing, and movement to enhance the flow of chi or qi (vital energy) in the body, help the immune system work more efficiently, and improve circulation. Chinese doctors have used qigong to treat a variety of ailments, including allergies, arthritis, asthma, headaches, hypertension, and many more. The technique improves delivery of oxygen to the cells in the body, reduces stress, and improves bowel functioning.

Reiki: This is an ancient Tibetan healing system, adapted in the 19th century in Japan. It involves the laying-on of hands. The aim of reiki is to channel energy where it is most needed in the body, leading to an increase in physical, emotional, and mental strength. Reiki is said to benefit anyone. It is thought to boost the immune system, to help insomnia, to reverse the loss of self-confidence, and to release stress and anxiety.

See also: **Stress**

Alzheimer's disease

First described by the neurologist Alois Alzheimer in 1906, Alzheimer's disease affects the brain's transmission process. The disease causes mental confusion and memory loss, and almost always affects older people.

Alzheimer's disease is a progressive deterioration of the brain that usually affects people over 60 years of age. Its onset is gradual, usually beginning with problems remembering events, particularly recent events. People who are affected may be able to recall vividly events from their childhood or early adult life but may be unable to remember what they had for breakfast or where they left their eyeglasses only a few minutes before.

As the disease progresses, confusion may become so crippling that patients wander about in a daze and cannot safely be left alone. Constant supervision is then required. Ultimately, total mental and physical incapacitation will follow, and institutionalization becomes necessary.

The German neurologist Alois Alzheimer first described the disease in 1906. Initially, the term was used only when the condition occurred in people under 60, when it was also called pre-senile dementia. As autopsy studies progressed, however, it was found that the changes in elderly people affected by the disease were essentially the same as those in younger patients.

Diagnosis

Diagnosing Alzheimer's disease is often a matter of eliminating other possible causes, since other diseases, such as high blood pressure, diabetes, and alcoholism, also cause dementia. Some drugs also cause mental confusion. Various blood tests may be done to rule out these other causes.

Contrary to what is widely believed, dementia is not a part of normal aging; it occurs because a person is suffering from a disease of the brain. Alzheimer's disease is the most common cause of dementia in the elderly. For people under age 75 the rate is about 3 percent. Thereafter, the rate

EFFECTS OF ALZHEIMER'S DISEASE ON NERVE IMPULSES

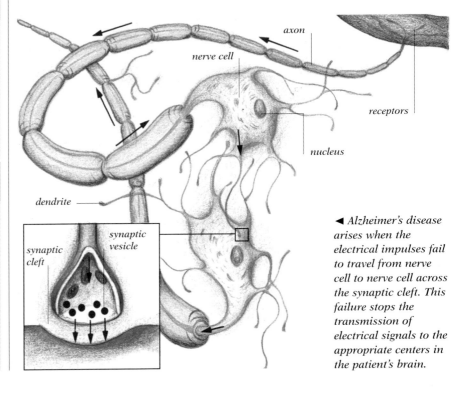

◀ *Alzheimer's disease arises when the electrical impulses fail to travel from nerve cell to nerve cell across the synaptic cleft. This failure stops the transmission of electrical signals to the appropriate centers in the patient's brain.*

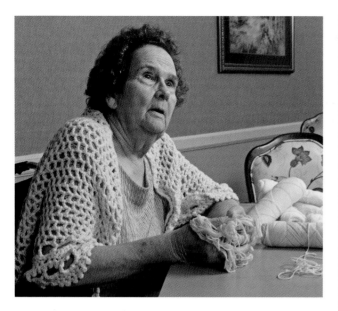

▲ *Alzheimer's disease is the most common cause of dementia.*

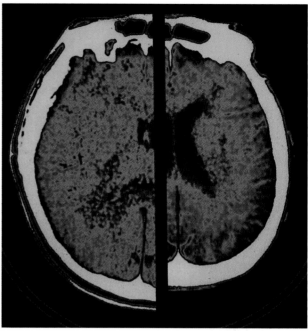

▲ *Scans of a healthy brain (left) and one with Alzheimer's (right); the dark areas of low activity are typical of the disease.*

rises steeply. For people age 75 to 84 the rate is 19 percent, and for those over 85 the rate is 47 percent. Almost all people with Down syndrome who live beyond 45 years develop Alzheimer's disease.

The first indication of the disease is an insidious impairment of the higher intellectual functions; it becomes more difficult for a sufferer to understand new concepts, and he or she loses mathematical and other mental skills. Following this stage are subtle, then progressive, indications of deterioration in behavior and sometimes in standards of personal care. Over the next five to 10 years the progress of the dementia is steady and inexorable. Suspicion of the diagnosis may be aroused when a patient's loss of memory gives rise to disorientation regarding place and time. An affected person may get lost in an area that has been familiar for years.

The essential feature of Alzheimer's disease is extensive loss of nerve tissue in the brain, called cerebral atrophy. In advanced cases this is readily apparent in computed tomography (CT) or magnetic resonance imaging (MRI) scans; these show extensive widening of the deep grooves on the surface of the patient's brain (the sulci) and enlargement of the spaces within the brain (the ventricles). However, by the time these changes have developed, the diagnosis is usually obvious on purely clinical grounds.

Cause

Some cases of Alzheimer's disease that appear very much earlier in life have a strong genetic basis. There is a gene on chromosome 21 for an essential brain protein called amyloid precursor protein (APP); in familial cases, this gene has a mutation. It is probably relevant that Down syndrome is caused by an additional chromosome 21 in every cell (trisomy 21).

At postmortem, two distinctive brain lesions provide a definite diagnosis. One is plaque, a group of dead brain cells; the other is called neurofibrillary tangle. The tiny plaques that form in the brain are of amyloid-rich material; these are derived from APP. The amyloid plaques lie outside brain nerve cells and mainly affect the parts of the brain concerned with memory—that is, the amygdala and hippocampus. They have been found to be consistently present in patients suffering from Alzheimer's disease. Neurofibrillary tangles are bundles of fine protein filaments within the nerve cell bodies. These are seen in all senile brains, but they are invariably present in enormously increased numbers in victims of the disease. The basic cause of nonfamilial Alzheimer's disease is unknown.

Treatment

No cure for Alzheimer's disease is currently available. However, a feature of the condition is a reduction in the levels of the chemical messenger acetylcholine that conveys nerve impulses across synapses. This neurotransmitter is normally broken down rapidly by an enzyme called acetylcholinesterase. Several drugs are known to inhibit the action of this enzyme, and so prevent acetylcholine breakdown in Alzheimer's patients. These drugs include donepezil, galatamine, and rivastigmine.

Another neurotransmitter, glutamate, malfunctions in Alzheimer's disease. The drug memantine allows activation of glutamate receptors during the formation of memories but blocks the toxic effects of abnormally high glutamate levels. It, too, is proving of some value in slowing the progress of the disease.

Free radicals are involved in the causation of nerve cell destruction in Alzheimer's; antioxidant treatment with vitamins C and E may help.

In the United States, the annual cost of taking care of patients with Alzheimer's disease is estimated at more than $50 billion. It is projected that as many as 14.3 million Americans will have the disease by 2050; a 350 percent increase from 2000. This could rapidly cause a crisis in medical care.

See also: **Genetics**

Anemia

People who look pale and feel run-down often assume they are anemic, but this is not necessarily so. If anemia is diagnosed, treatment is usually simple, quick, and effective, resulting in a rapid return to health.

Questions and Answers

I am pregnant and getting paler and paler. Could I be anemic?

During pregnancy, the body's demand for essential nutrients, such as iron and folic acid, is increased. The developing fetus depletes the mother's store of nutrients via the placenta, and the mother may then become deficient in one or more of them, causing anemia, unless extra iron and folate are given. Check with your doctor, who will give you a prescription for supplements.

Can stress and strain cause anemia? I'm in high school and have an after-school job, and seem to be tired all the time.

Anemia cannot be caused by emotional problems alone; there is always an organic basis. Chronic depression, for instance, may be accompanied by a poor diet. This may lead to anemia through vitamin and iron deficiency. It is best to discuss this with your doctor. You may just need a break from your normal routine.

Can anemia be prevented by taking various vitamins?

If the cause is vitamin deficiency, anemia is often treated with vitamin supplements in the form of pills and injections. If not, a balanced diet will provide all the chemicals needed to make blood cells.

My mother has anemia. I am worried that I might have inherited it. Is this possible?

You cannot inherit common anemias like iron deficiency, but some rare anemias, for example thalassemia, can be passed on from generation to generation. In cases of pernicious anemia, the disease is not transmitted, but family members are more likely to have it.

Anemia is the name given to a disorder of the blood, in which there is a deficiency or an abnormality of hemoglobin, which is the oxygen-carrying pigment of red blood cells. Hemoglobin picks up oxygen in the lungs and then distributes it to body tissues, where, together with glucose, it is needed to provide energy. Red blood cells are produced in the bone marrow and circulate in the bloodstream before being broken down in the spleen. The marrow produces two million red cells a second—these survive in the bloodstream for 120 days. If the level of blood cells in circulation is reduced from normal levels for any reason, a lack of oxygen will result in the tissues, producing the symptoms of anemia: lack of energy, fainting, shortness of breath after mild physical exertion, and skin pallor.

Iron deficiency

In general, anemia is a superficial symptom of some other disorder in the body. There are a number of causes of anemia; one of the most common is a lack of iron. Iron is a mineral and an essential component of hemoglobin because it attracts oxygen to the blood. When the supply of iron is reduced, the production of hemoglobin and its inclusion in the red blood cells in the bone marrow is also reduced, and there is less hemoglobin to pick up oxygen in the lungs and to distribute oxygen to the tissues in the body.

ROLE OF RED BLOOD CELLS IN ANEMIA

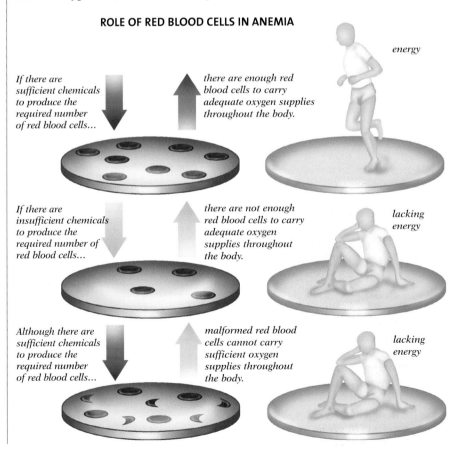

If there are sufficient chemicals to produce the required number of red blood cells...

there are enough red blood cells to carry adequate oxygen supplies throughout the body.

energy

If there are insufficient chemicals to produce the required number of red blood cells...

there are not enough red blood cells to carry adequate oxygen supplies throughout the body.

lacking energy

Although there are sufficient chemicals to produce the required number of red blood cells...

malformed red blood cells cannot carry sufficient oxygen supplies throughout the body.

lacking energy

Types of anemia

TYPE	CAUSES	TREATMENT
Iron deficiency	Heavy menstrual loss; acute blood loss; bleeding duodenal ulcer; poor diet	Iron tablets or injections over several months
Pernicious anemia	Failure of stomach lining to secrete a substance called intrinsic factor	Vitamin B12 injections once a month for life
Anemia of chronic diseases	Certain kidney diseases and some other chronic complaints	Anemia usually disappears upon treatment of underlying disease
Aplastic anemia	Bone marrow fails to make required number of red blood cells; can be brought about by cancer	Long-term; isolation; antibiotics and transfusions; drug treatment of marrow; marrow transplant
Sickle-cell anemia	Abnormally shaped red blood cells due to defective hemoglobin; genetic	If severe, transfusion; occasionally drugs
Thalassemia	Defective hemoglobin; genetic	If severe, regular transfusions; occasionally removal of spleen
Hemolytic (many types)	Red cells are killed off too early or in too great numbers in spleen	Drugs or removal of spleen, depending on type of anemia

This deficiency is often the result of eating the wrong foods, when insufficient quantities of iron are eaten as part of the diet. It can also be caused by severe blood loss. Women are particularly prone to this problem because of the amount of blood they lose each month during menstruation, a loss that, if heavy, depletes the body of its store of iron. The problem also occurs during pregnancy when the mother loses iron during the development of the baby.

Iron deficiencies can also be caused by peptic ulcers, in which there is slow, steady bleeding, and by parasites such as tapeworms, which compete with the host for vitamin B12. Cancers of the digestive tract lead to blood loss and anemia.

Other causes

Another condition, known as pernicious anemia, occurs when the stomach lining fails to create a substance called intrinsic factor. This results in a deficiency of vitamin B12, a vitamin which is essential for the production of red blood cells. Vitamin B12 can be absorbed into the body only with the help of intrinsic factor. If its secretion comes to a halt, the number of red cells is reduced, resulting in an anemic condition. Untreated pernicious anemia leads to a serious spinal cord disorder called subacute combined degeneration.

Chronic diseases, such as rheumatoid arthritis and certain kidney diseases, may also cause anemia. The reason is not clear, but it appears that the body's ability to utilize iron breaks down. Instead of passing to the bone marrow, iron is retained in the tissues. The lack of iron in the marrow then reduces the output of red blood cells.

The most serious form of anemia is aplastic anemia. This occurs when the bone marrow's ability to make red blood cells (as well as white cells and platelets, two further constituents of blood, both of which are made in the marrow) is halted. Again, the cause is not fully known, but it does appear to be brought on by chemicals contained in

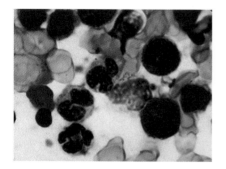

▲ *The large, solid-looking red blood cells (stained purple) in this bone marrow are typical of pernicious anemia.*

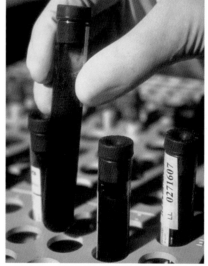

▲ *Glass test tubes holding labeled samples of blood, ready for testing in a hematology laboratory.*

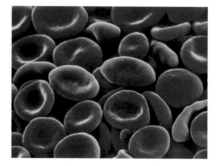

▲ *This scanning electron micrograph shows red blood cells distorted into a sickle shape.*

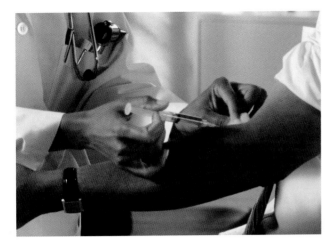

▲ *Blood is taken from a patient's vein for testing.*

some medicines, or by cancer. This is a very serious form of anemia, as not only do the body tissues lose their vital source of oxygen, but the body also loses its ability to ward off infection, owing to a lack of white cells.

Hereditary and hemolytic anemias

There are many types of hemolytic anemias in which the red cells carry too little oxygen and break down prematurely, often because of abnormal fragility. These anemias also occur either as a result of a bad blood transfusion or from a complication with a Rh-positive fetus and a Rh-negative mother. There is a tendency for some types of hemolytic anemia to run in families.

Other types of anemia include those of a genetic nature. Sickle-cell anemia, common among African American communities, arises because of an abnormality of hemoglobin, in which the red cells become distorted into a sickle shape. In severe cases, a blood transfusion may be necessary. Thalassemia, which is common in Greek and other Mediterranean communities, also involves abnormal hemoglobin and is similar to sickle-cell anemia.

Symptoms

The symptoms depend on the severity and type of anemia, and this depends on the initial cause. Common symptoms are lethargy, paleness, and breathlessness, and sometimes heart palpitations. Severe cases of anemia resulting from rapid loss of blood will cause fainting, dizziness, and sweating. Symptoms of pernicious anemia may include pins and needles in the hands and feet, nosebleeds, and in severe cases heart failure. When children suffer from iron deficiency, they may show irritability and hold their breath. In severe cases of iron deficiency, as well as the usual symptoms there may be thirst, and some loss of control, owing to reduced oxygen to the brain.

Aplastic anemia can develop slowly, becoming obvious only weeks or months after exposure to a poison. It has all the normal symptoms of anemia but is also accompanied by infections due to the deficiency of white blood cells.

Most types of anemia are impossible to guard against, as they result from a malfunction of the blood-making system, but steps can be taken to prevent the onset of iron deficiency anemia. Eating a good balanced diet of milk, meat (especially liver), fresh fruit, and vegetables, all of which contain a good supply of the necessary vitamins and are rich in iron, will contribute to good health and keep anemia at bay. Taking vitamins is of little or no value unless they are recommended by a doctor for those who have difficulty following a balanced diet. However, because of the demands made on their systems, pregnant mothers may be advised to boost their iron and vitamin intake.

Dangers

It is important that the origin of the anemia is diagnosed as soon as possible to ensure that the patient can make a fast recovery. With most forms of anemia, the dangers are not immediate, but the condition can deteriorate progressively if left untreated. However, in the case of acute blood loss, if the condition is not quickly controlled it may lead to a fall in blood pressure. In extreme cases, the reduction in the oxygen supply to the blood may be life-threatening.

Chronic anemia may become worse if there is an already existing disease, and this is particularly true for elderly patients. Anemia can be dangerous during pregnancy, as it will be passed on to the baby and deprive the baby of oxygen, which is needed for healthy development.

Treatment

Treatments vary according to the type of anemia, but usually the patient will be treated to counteract the initial symptoms while undergoing tests to discover the underlying causes of the condition.

Simple iron deficiency anemia is normally treated with a course of iron pills or injections, often lasting several months. At the same time the patient is also checked for gastrointestinal bleeding. In the case of pernicious anemia, B12 has to be given on a regular basis—usually once a month. Since the cause of the missing vitamin is the stomach's failure to secrete the intrinsic factor—a disorder that will never improve—the treatment lasts for life.

Anemia associated with a chronic disease can be treated only by resolving the underlying disease. Once this is done, the anemia usually disappears. The treatment for aplastic anemia is normally long-term. The patient is treated in a special isolation unit designed to prevent infection. The treatment consists of an intravenous infusion of antibiotics to fight infection and regular blood transfusions to keep fresh blood in circulation. The patient's bone marrow may be encouraged to recover with the use of certain drugs. In some cases, bone marrow transplants have been successful as a treatment for this type of complaint.

Outlook

The future for sufferers of anemia depends on the type of anemia and on any underlying disorder that may affect it. In some cases, such as pernicious anemia, improvement from medication may be dramatic. Iron deficiency anemia is usually cured relatively quickly; the patient gradually gains strength and energy, but the underlying cause will still be treated by drugs, diet, or surgery. The outlook for the sufferers of aplastic anemia is not as good; bone marrow transplants are not always a guaranteed cure. Nor are drugs always successful. However, future research offers some hope.

In some cases of hemolytic anemia, hospitalization may be needed, but patients usually respond well to supervised medical treatment.

See also: **Iron; Minerals; Oxygen; Vitamin B**

Anorexia and bulimia

Questions and Answers

Sometimes I eat a bag of cookies. Then I'm sorry, so I make myself vomit afterward. Am I suffering from bulimia?

Not unless these binges have become uncontrollable and frequent. Many dieters go on an eating binge after they have been on a strict diet for some time, because they have been starving themselves. This is not good for the body, but it does no lasting harm. Only when it becomes a way of life should you seek treatment. You seem to feel guilty about overeating, but try to be less emotional about it and attempt to lose weight in a more sensible way.

Are parents to blame for anorexia in a girl?

Not in a deliberate sense. A girl with this problem may have very loving and protective parents, but sometimes they can be so repressive that they stunt the normal process of growing up. A girl may use control over her weight as the only form of rebellion possible.

Can a person really die from dieting?

Yes, if it turns into anorexia nervosa—a disease from which about a quarter of victims die. Understanding and early treatment of this condition have helped to cure many sufferers.

My friend has been told she is anorexic but doesn't believe it. Why can't she realize how emaciated she looks?

She is suffering from an abnormal mental state. When she looks in a mirror she sees a distorted body image that initiates, and prolongs, the disease. Your friend should get help from a counselor or doctor.

When young people have an obsessional interest in food and body weight and body size, they may be suffering from anorexia nervosa. Bulimia, binge eating followed by vomiting, is another type of eating disorder.

Anorexia nervosa is commonly known as the dieter's disease, but its cause is much more complex than a simple desire to lose weight. The need to refrain from eating is more compelling than it is in ordinary dieting. Anorexia nervosa almost always strikes young people between the ages of 11 and 30, and it affects more girls than boys. Statistics show that those from middle-class homes are more prone to the disorder than those from less affluent homes. This suggests that anorexia nervosa is largely a problem of the developed Western world.

Dramatic loss of weight is the most obvious sign that something is very wrong, and sufferers may need hospital treatment if it has reached a really serious stage. A doctor will try to find the reasons for attempting to lose weight, may arrange for blood tests to discover any hormone imbalance, and will investigate any psychological disorders, such as depression, that may be the underlying cause of the disorder.

Causes of anorexia

Anorexia nervosa has become a common problem. The parents of victims may find it difficult to understand its cause, but sometimes the problem actually lies within the family. A teen who never rebels or gives trouble, who delights his or her parents in every way and seems part of a perfect family, may have a basic lack of confidence and self-esteem. If the family is concerned with achievement, the teen may be under huge pressure to succeed. Refusing to eat may be the only area of life that he or she can control.

Because a slim body is important in Western culture, many young people strive to attain acceptance by fitting in with what they perceive as the norm. Added to this are feelings of inadequacy and fears of the demands that maturity may bring. These feelings can lead to seeing extreme thinness as a desirable goal.

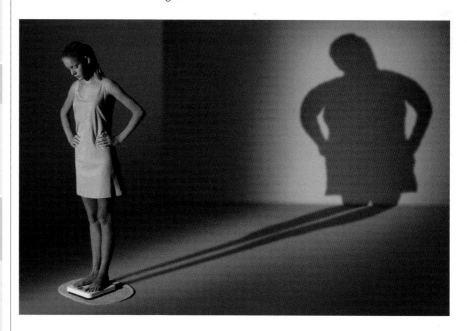

▲ *A distorted body image is common in anorexia nervosa. The sufferer, although extremely thin, thinks of herself as fat and feels the need to diet drastically.*

If young people lose substantial amounts of body fat and retain a childish figure, then they may feel that the problems of adult life will not have to be faced. The popular image of slimness and superficial prettiness that is promoted by films, advertising, and television may justify their rejection of food. In fact, they may not be overweight at all. They may diet drastically to increase their sexual confidence, and cling obstinately to the distorted idea that their extreme emaciation is beautiful, ignoring the evidence to the contrary that is only too obvious to everyone else who knows them.

Dangers of anorexia

Experience has shown that the more distorted an idea victims have of themselves, the more difficult it is to cure anorexia nervosa. The longer the condition goes untreated, the more uncertain the outcome will be. The National Institute of Mental Health (NIMH) has reported that 0.5 to 2 percent of women under the age of 20 suffer from anorexia nervosa and, of these, 5 to 10 percent will die from it. Because of this statistic, anorexia nervosa must never be dismissed as a passing phase that time and maturity will cure. Anorexics are not mature, nor are they suddenly likely to become so. Spontaneous cures rarely happen, because the victims take a positive pride in sustaining their hunger strike. The longer the illness lasts and the more weight is lost, the greater the sense of achievement. This reinforces the illusion that being thin is a significant and outstanding achievement. It also succeeds in focusing attention on the anorexic, and providing a form of personal rebellion against parental authority that should have been made much earlier—and in a less dangerous form—as part of growing up.

Compulsive dieting and anorexia

When normal people embark on drastic dieting, they can stop when they choose. Most find it so unpleasant to be hungry or deprived of favorite foods in the midst of plenty that the real problem is keeping to the diet. But anorexics, once set on a course of self-starvation, cannot reverse it. It is as though they are suffering from feelings similar to those caused by alcohol or drug addiction—with some of the same light-headedness. It has been suggested that anorexics may have a different body chemistry from normal people, but this has never been proved. It seems far more likely that they just have a different mental outlook, with confused motives that involve not only self-punishment but also punishment of their parents.

Symptoms of anorexia

It is vital that the illness is recognized and that treatment is started as early as possible. The illness is often neglected until the weight loss becomes so obvious that it is clear that something is severely wrong and a visit to the doctor is necessary. An unmistakable symptom in a girl, once her weight has fallen below 100 pounds (45 kg) or thereabouts, is that her periods stop.

It may be discovered that she is making herself vomit, either to get rid of food she has been coaxed to eat or as part of a binge-and-vomit pattern, enabling her to indulge in food without putting on weight. Constant vomiting of stomach acid causes damage to the teeth, and the backs of the hands may show scarring from the teeth caused by the attempts to induce vomiting. The body eventually becomes so accustomed to existing on a greatly reduced amount of food that it has difficulty in coping with a large meal. In a few cases, anorexics use emetics, laxatives, diuretics, and enemas. Over a period

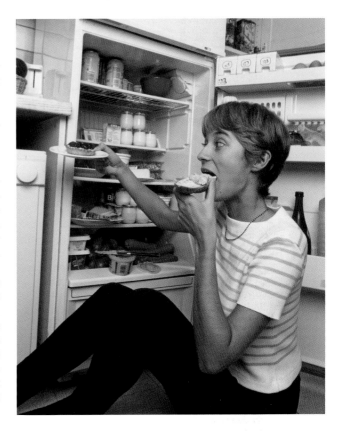

▲ *If a person is suffering from bulimia, there will be episodes of binging followed by self-induced vomiting.*

of time, these can badly disturb body chemistry and greatly increase the risk of a fatal outcome. Prolonged starvation causes weakening of health and a greater susceptibility to infection.

Treatment of anorexia

Alert families should call for medical help long before symptoms are acute. The first job is to restore weight to at least above danger level, before psychiatric treatment can begin. Research suggests that there is a critical weight that must be achieved, between 90 and 95 pounds (41 and 43 kg), before psychotherapy can penetrate the mental isolation that starvation brings.

Weight gain for anorexics often requires a prolonged stay in the hospital or a clinic, with intravenous feeding in the early stages. To coax patients to eat normal food and gain a set amount of weight, a system of rewards and withdrawal of privileges is often used. The basis for rewards is often a list made up by patients; it can include such things as being allowed to get up to go to the toilet, having extra visitors, wearing day clothes, going home for a weekend, and finally leaving the hospital or clinic for good.

Future action and anorexia

Once enough weight has been gained and patients are out of immediate danger, the more difficult part of the treatment can begin. Some family counseling is required so that parents can understand the nature of the illness and its causes. Initially victims have to be convinced that anorexia nervosa is not just a matter of

Questions and Answers

How is it that my daughter seems to eat normally but loses weight?

She may be pretending to eat but actually smuggling food out of the room or house in her pocket or purse. Suggest that she visit the doctor to rule out any other cause of weight loss. He or she will understand the potential dangers and take the necessary preventive steps.

My new boyfriend says that I'm too fat. In fact, I've always tended to be overweight and would like to do something about it, but I'm worried that I might overdo things and even develop anorexia nervosa and get really sick.

Anorexia nervosa is not something that you catch or that sneaks up on you in the night. Although it is the result of excessive or compulsive dieting that pays no attention to the body's basic needs, it is fundamentally due to a disordered state of mind with regard to weight, in particular, and the rest of life in general. If you use a scientifically formulated diet, you will not be in danger of becoming anorexic. The diet should allow you to lose weight but still ensure that you get enough of all the important food groups your body needs. You will be able to reach your target weight in perfect safety.

My grandmother, who is 72, was in the hospital for tests, and I overheard the doctor say that she had anorexia. I thought this happened only to people my age—am I totally wrong?

There is a confusion of terms here. The anorexia you have in mind is called anorexia nervosa, which is common in adolescent girls and is sometimes called anorexia for short. But as a medical term, anorexia means a poor appetite or a complete loss of appetite. Many older people suffer from this for different reasons, and this is what the doctor meant when discussing your grandmother.

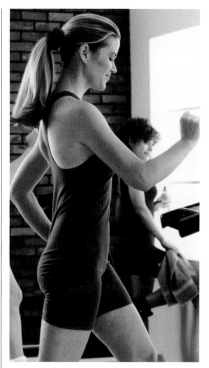

▲ *Anorexics may exercise frequently, for long periods of time, even if they are an average size.*

weight loss. The victims, helped by a therapist, can then begin their own search and fight for identity. This includes dealing with the inner doubts and fears that haunt them, accepting the challenges, and appreciating the real promise of their own sexuality and maturity. They must be helped to realize that their old ideas about themselves were distorted, and gradually replace those ideas with a truer picture. This improved image will give them the confidence to grow.

Bulimia

Bulimia is a different eating disorder that involves the compulsive eating of large quantities of food in a short time. These binges are usually followed by periods of strict dieting. Sufferers from bulimia may also indulge in strenuous exercise in an attempt to counteract the effects of overeating. In addition to making themselves vomit, many will take large quantities of laxatives or diuretics (which help rid the body of water). Bulimia is more common in women between the ages of 18 and 30, and sufferers often have low self-esteem.

Bulimia, which means insatiable hunger, has much in common with anorexia. Both involve an obsession with food and weight. However, although many people with anorexia do binge from time to time, most of those whose bulimia is their main problem do not suffer from anorexia. Indeed, bulimics tend to be of normal weight or a little overweight. Therefore, if they are secretive about their compulsive eating, as is usually the case, it may take a long time for the problem to be detected.

The female connection and bulimia

Bulimia affects mainly women, often following a period of strict dieting. Researchers are not clear as to the causes. It does not seem to be associated with any particular personality type, but it may be initiated by a very stressful event.

It is estimated that over half those affected by bulimia induce vomiting either during or after the binge to prevent the food from being absorbed into the body. Many bulimics do this secretly, using bags or other containers, which are later disposed of so that other people will not discover the secret. Even more bulimics, it seems, use large quantities of laxatives in the mistaken belief that they will clear the food out from the body before it has a chance to be converted into fat. A large number use diuretics, which have no real effect on permanent weight loss.

Treatment of bulimia

Successful treatment of bulimia depends on awareness by the people concerned that they have an eating problem that may endanger both their physical health and their emotional well-being. They need to be motivated to change their eating habits and to be aware that there may be a period of adjustment while new routines and attitudes are developed.

Treatment by a doctor or therapist should aim to help sufferers adopt new and more sensible attitudes to food, weight, and their own body image. Bulimics need to cooperate by eating regular meals to maintain an agreed-on weight; they must avoid extreme forms of dieting, as well as any other inappropriate methods of weight loss.

Finally, bulimics need to recognize the triggers that start them on an eating binge and then find other, less harmful ways of releasing tension and dealing with stress and emotional problems.

See also: **Diet; Dieting; Stress**

Antibiotics

Antibiotics fight a wide variety of infections, have conquered or controlled many deadly diseases, and have made possible some of the most dramatic advances in modern medicine. How do these "miracle drugs" work?

My doctor never prescribes antibiotics when I go to her with a sore throat or a cold. Why?

Antibiotics work only against diseases caused by bacteria. Colds, the flu, and most sore throats are carried by viruses, which are different types of germs.

I have some antibiotics left from last year. Can I take them now for the same condition I had then?

No. You should never take old antibiotics. Nor should you take any drugs prescribed for someone else. They could be dangerous. Always see a doctor with every new illness, even if it seems to be the same as a previous condition.

I am taking the contraceptive pill. Will antibiotics affect it at all?

Most antibiotics do not affect the action of the Pill. However, one, rifampin, destroys the Pill in the body, making it ineffective. Another, ampicillin, makes the Pill less effective. Always remind your doctor if you are on the Pill.

Can I drink alcohol while I am on antibiotics?

Most antibiotics have no side effects when combined with alcohol. Any warnings about their use with alcohol will be printed on the label of the bottle.

Can I take antibiotics during pregnancy?

No drug should be taken during pregnancy unless it is essential for the mother's health. There is no certain way of testing whether drugs are safe for the unborn child. For example, tetracyclines taken during pregnancy can cause discoloration in the teeth of a child. Your doctor will advise you.

The search for and discovery of new types of antibiotics has been constant since the first antibiotic, penicillin, was introduced during the 1940s. The antibiotics that have been discovered since then have dramatically reduced the mortality rates of several of the world's most deadly diseases.

Because of antibiotics, pneumonia is no longer a killer. The sexually transmitted diseases syphilis and gonorrhea can be cured if detected early enough. People who catch typhoid fever can usually expect a complete cure. Patients with bronchitis can be helped a great deal. Deaths from meningitis—an inflammation of the membranes of the brain and spinal cord—are fewer than ever before. Antibiotics are also used to combat infection in patients who have undergone surgery and patients with serious body wounds. The number of lives that have been saved since the advent of antibiotics, then, is countless. The drugs can also cure many relatively minor problems such as throat infections, tonsillitis, cystitis, abscesses, carbuncles, and blood poisoning.

What antibiotics can do

Humans are continually exposed to what doctors and scientists call microorganisms—in other words, germs. These are present in the food people eat, the air they breathe, plants, the soil, and the body. Most are harmless to human beings, and many are even beneficial; however, a few are not, and it is these that cause diseases.

The microorganisms that cause disease are divided into a number of different types. The four most commonly encountered are bacteria, viruses, fungi, and protozoa. These attack the body in different ways to cause different illnesses. Among the many conditions caused by bacteria are pneumonia and tuberculosis. Viruses cause such ailments as the common cold, flu, chicken pox, and smallpox. Fungi cause tinea, thrush, and other infections. Finally, protozoa bring about, among other things, amebic dysentery and various vaginal irritations.

Antibiotics are drugs that kill bacteria. They have no effect on viruses and are not prescribed for them. Strictly speaking, they are not used against fungal or protozoal infection either.

How antibiotics work

Antibiotics actually attack microorganisms; they break bacteria down and prevent bacterial growth and multiplication within the body. One of the most important aspects of antibiotic action is that it is selective: any given antibiotic drug works only against certain types of

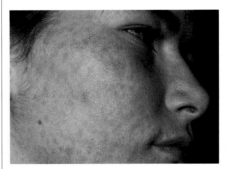

▲ *A penicillin allergy rash.*

▶ *Penicillin (center, each section) acting against different bacteria. The dark areas show where it has the strongest effects.*

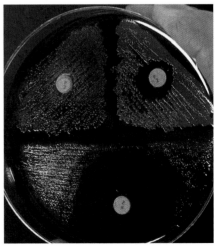

Antibiotics and their uses

ANTIBIOTIC	USES
Penicillins: penicillin G, flucloxacillan, ampicillin, amoxycillin, and ticaricillin.	Some forms of tonsillitis, pneumonia, meningitis, syphilis, gonorrhea (although many gonococci are resistant to the older penicillins), cystitis, urinary infections, septic fingers, bronchitis, and carbuncles.
Tetracyclines: demeclocycline, doxycycline, minocycline, and limecycline.	Chronic bronchitis, acne, and chlamydial infections, especially pelvic inflammatory disease.
Cephalosporins: cefaclor, cefotaxime, cefuroxime, cephodoxime, cephalexin, cephamandole, and cephradine.	Upper respiratory tract infections and a wide variety of other infections that are resistant to penicillins.
Macrolides: axithromycin, clarithromycin, and erythromycin.	For patients with penicillin allergy; also for respiratory, skin, and soft tissue infections, campylobacter infections, and Legionnaires' disease.
Sulfonamides: co-trimoxazole and trimethoprim.	Urinary infections, *Pneumocystis carinii* pneumonia, and toxoplasmosis.
Aminoglycosides: gentamicin, amikacin, neomycin, tobramycin, and netilmycin.	Used internally and externally.
Quinolones: ciprofloxacin, levofloxacin, moxufloxacin, and nalidixic acid.	Infections caused by a wide range of bacteria, including some that resist other antibiotics.
Nitroimidazoles: metronidazole and tinidazole.	Anaerobic bacterial infections, *Gardnerella vaginalis* infections, *Trichomonas vaginalis* infections, and Vincent's angina.
Glycopeptide: vancomycin.	Used to treat colitis (inflammation of the intestine caused by bacteria).

microorganism; it homes in on the foreign bacteria it is intended to kill but leaves the other bacteria in the body unharmed.

Different classes of antibiotics function in a variety of ways to kill germs. The penicillins and cephalosporins, for example, attack the bacterial cell wall by binding to proteins involved in the cell wall construction. The effect is to break down the cell walls so that the bacteria are killed. However, some (gram-negative) bacteria have impermeable waxy outer protective envelopes that prevent penicillins from acting in this way.

Tetracyclines, aminoglycosides, macrolides, and some other classes of antibiotics attack ribosomes (minute particles of RNA and protein) within bacteria where bacterial protein is formed. Sulfonamides act by interfering with bacterial folate metabolism. Quinolones act by directly inhibiting DNA synthesis in bacteria.

Drawbacks

Bacteria can reproduce in 20 minutes, so evolutionary changes in their characteristics can occur much more quickly than with most living things. In any population of bacteria there are likely to be some individuals that are inherently (genetically) more capable of resisting antibiotics than others. Thus the susceptible bacteria will be killed first. If the antibiotic is stopped too early or is incapable of killing these more resistant organisms, they will survive to reproduce differentially. In this way, the original population of mainly susceptible bacteria will be replaced by a population that is wholly resistant to the antibiotic.

In theory, antibiotics should be used as little as possible. If a bacterium becomes resistant to a certain antibiotic, as happened, for example, with the first penicillins, an alternative antibiotic has to be used. The development of alternative and synthetic antibiotic types makes this possible.

Side effects

Some people are allergic to penicillin, usually breaking out in a rash when they take the drug. In such cases, the doctor who prescribed the penicillin should be told so that he or she can treat the allergy.

Antibiotics can have side effects, ranging from indigestion and diarrhea to deafness and loss of balance. In most such cases patients must tolerate some temporary discomfort for the sake of a cure. However, if an antibiotic has a persistent, worrying side effect on an individual, he or she should see a doctor without delay.

Antibiotics really are "miracle drugs." However, like all precision instruments, they need to be used properly. Medically, the prescribing doctor tailors the drug to the patient's infection. Bronchitis or urinary problems may, for example, be caused by one bacterium in one attack and a slightly different one in the next. Each new attack needs a specific antibiotic to treat it.

The side effects of taking the wrong antibiotic can, in some cases, be unpleasant and even dangerous. If treatment is being prescribed by a new doctor, the patient should tell him or her of any antibiotic or any other drug that has an allergic effect.

An individual should never take another person's antibiotics; nor should he or she take antibiotics that were prescribed for a previous illness. People should always take a full course of antibiotics; if they do not, the bacteria may become immune, and an infection could get worse.

See also: **Bacteria**

Antioxidants

Questions and Answers

Which foods contain antioxidants?

Vitamin A and beta-carotene (a precursor of vitamin A that can be enzymatically converted into vitamin A) are found in liver, egg yolk, spinach, carrots, broccoli, yams, tomatoes, peaches, butter, and margarine. Vitamin C can be found in citrus fruits, strawberries, kiwi fruit, green peppers, and spinach. Vitamin E can be obtained from whole grains, fish-liver oils, dried apricots, nuts, and seeds.

When did medical science become aware of free radicals and the role of antioxidants in combating them?

Research began to emerge in the 1970s about chemical groups called free radicals that damage the body's cells and tissues. This research was spearheaded by the American chemist and Nobel Prize winner Linus Pauling (1901–1994). In his book *Vitamin C and the Common Cold* (1970), he proposed, on the basis of his own experience, that people who took large, regular daily doses of vitamin C had a striking decrease in the number and severity of colds they caught. Many scientists dismissed his claims, but interest in the topic grew. In the late 1990s a number of studies found that antioxidants like vitamin C and vitamin E can limit the damaging effects of free radicals.

I heard that smoking cigarettes produces free radicals. How?

Cigarette smoke contains a mixture of free radicals which, if inhaled, can produce more free radicals in the body and cause much of the damage associated with smoking, especially the free radical oxidation that deposits cholesterol in the walls of the arteries and damages DNA. Some doctors advise smokers to take large doses of beta-carotene or vitamin C to reduce this risk of damage by free radicals.

Antioxidants are known to mop up harmful free radicals generated in the body during metabolism, and when the body is exposed to infections and environmental factors such as radiation, UV light, and pollution.

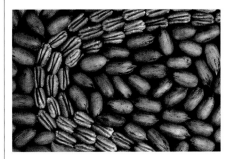 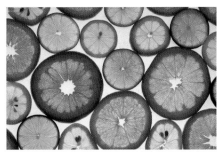

▲ *The antioxidant vitamin E can be found in nuts (left); the antioxidant vitamin C exists in citrus fruits such as oranges, lemons, and limes (right).*

During normal metabolism, when oxygen is metabolized or burned, by-products are produced by the cells, which are known as free radicals. They attack the cells, setting up chain reactions in cell membranes and in other tissues that have the effect of disrupting cell structures. This damage is thought to accelerate aging and to contribute to many major health problems such as cancer, heart disease, and the degenerative diseases associated with aging.

The body's primary and secondary antioxidant defense mechanisms neutralize free radicals, but they are not 100 percent effective. When the production of free radicals exceeds the ability of the body to deal with them, free radicals can cause widespread molecular damage to proteins, lipids, DNA, and carbohydrates. The primary defense system is believed to combat free radicals and includes vitamins such as vitamin A, vitamin E, and vitamin C; carotenoids such as beta-carotene; flavonoids from teas and grape skins; and some enzymes. The body's secondary defense system includes enzymes that are involved in the repair of damaged proteins and lipids.

Antioxidants work by boosting the immune system, stopping nitrosamine (a carcinogen) formation, assisting in maintaining cell membranes, and repairing DNA. It seems that each antioxidant works by acting in synthesis with others, but this process is still being researched.

Antioxidants and disease

Studies have shown that there is a link between higher intakes of certain antioxidants and a lower risk of contracting certain degenerative diseases.

Antioxidant vitamin supplements such as vitamin E, beta-carotene, and vitamin C have been shown in clinical studies to reduce the risk of certain cancers and heart disease. Fruits and vegetables, which are the main source of antioxidants, are thought to reduce the risk of cancer, and people who consume the most dietary antioxidants have the greatest reduction in disease. What seems likely is that eating a balanced diet rich in antioxidant nutrients is the best way of improving health and staving off disease.

The medical view

Some health organizations such as the American Medical Association and the American Cancer Society support the recommendation for increased consumption of fruits and vegetables but have not gone so far as to say that they recommend supplementation. According to one school of thought, more research is required into other factors in fruits and vegetables that may contribute to preventing disease.

See also: Diet; Genetics; Protein; Vitamin A; Vitamin C; Vitamin E

Appendicitis

The appendix is a small organ that was useful to our ancestors but is now obsolete. It can still cause problems and sometimes has to be removed, but the operation, called an appendectomy, is both speedy and safe.

Questions and Answers

I am a model for a swimwear company and have to have my appendix removed. Will I have an ugly scar after the operation?

This rarely happens. Various ways of sealing wounds improve the appearance of an operation scar. The scar from your surgery will be below the bikini line, so your job should not be affected.

Do people always pass gas after an appendix operation? I would be embarrassed if this happened.

Gas is a sign that the bowels are returning to life, so you should not be embarrassed about it. After any abdominal operation, the bowels stop working for a while and food and drink cannot be taken until "bowel sounds" return. The bowels are full of gas, and as they gain strength, it is expelled.

My brother, who is a sailor, has a grumbling appendix. What would happen if it got worse at sea?

If he is away from medical help, some treatment has to be tried. Painkillers are essential and antibiotics may help. A large ship will probably have a doctor on board to deal with such an emergency; otherwise, air-sea rescue services can be called to cope with any crisis that may occur. If the problem continues, his appendix could be removed.

I am going on a long trip and have had appendicitis in the past. Can I have my appendix removed as a preventive measure?

This is sometimes done, but rarely. The dangers of an unnecessary operation may outweigh the risks of sudden appendicitis, but in your case, it may be a sensible precaution. A doctor will be able to advise you.

AN INFLAMED APPENDIX AND ITS POSITION IN THE BODY

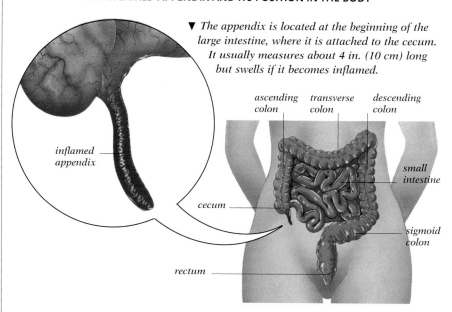

▼ *The appendix is located at the beginning of the large intestine, where it is attached to the cecum. It usually measures about 4 in. (10 cm) long but swells if it becomes inflamed.*

inflamed appendix

ascending colon   transverse colon   descending colon

small intestine

cecum

sigmoid colon

rectum

The appendix is a narrow, tubelike piece of gut resembling a tail. It is located at the start of the large intestine. The tip of the tube is closed, and the other end joins onto the large intestine. It can measure up to 4 inches (10 cm) long and about ⅝ inch (1.5 cm) in diameter. The appendix is found only in humans, certain species of apes, and the wombat, an Australian mammal. Other animals have an organ in the same position as the appendix that acts as an additional stomach, where cellulose, the fibrous part of plants, is digested by bacteria. It seems that as humans evolved and began to eat less cellulose in favor of more meat, a special organ was no longer needed for its digestion. The appendix can be thus described as a relic of evolution.

Occurrence

Facts about the appendix appear to contradict one another. On one hand, nature appears to have adapted it to act as a watchdog for infection at the lower end of the gut. Like the tonsils and adenoids, it contains a large collection of lymph glands for this purpose; but if the appendix does become inflamed, a condition called appendicitis results, and the organ may have to be removed. On the other hand, the appendix seems by no means essential to health. It can be dispensed with at an early age, making no apparent difference, and has nearly shriveled up completely by the age of about 40. Appendicitis can occur at any time, from infancy to old age. However, it is rare under the age of two, is more common among teenagers, and then becomes increasingly rare again over the age of 30. Why it should reach its peak in youth remains a mystery.

Causes

The history and incidence of appendicitis remain puzzling. Up to the end of the 19th century, appendicitis was relatively unknown. This is still the case in places like Asia, Africa, and Polynesia. However, in the 21st century in North America, Europe, and Australia, for example, appendicitis is a common complaint.

A great-aunt of mine died of appendicitis some years ago. Could this happen nowadays?

It is most unlikely. In the past any operation was fraught with dangers. As a result, an appendix operation was often delayed until perforation occurred, and the patient might then become rapidly ill and even die.

Several members of my family have had their appendixes removed. Is this a coincidence, or can a tendency to appendicitis be inherited?

It is possible that you have an inherited tendency. It may be that you have all inherited a similarly shaped appendix. One that is long and thin will block more easily than one that is short and stubby, and so cause appendicitis.

I am 45 and have heard that it is highly unlikely that I will ever have appendicitis at my age. Is this true?

Yes, it is. If you have reached middle life without having had appendicitis, the chances are that you are unlikely to get it now. The appendix shrivels as you get older, so it should be completely shriveled by the age of 45—and unlikely to become irritated and inflamed. This is why appendicitis tends to be a complaint only of young people.

I have heard that swallowing cherry pits leads to appendicitis. Cherries are my favorite fruit, so I am worried that this might happen. Is it possible?

When appendectomies were first performed years ago, surgeons thought that the small hard lumps they found in the appendix were cherry pits. In fact they were fecaliths—that is, small lumps of feces trapped in the appendix because it leads nowhere. Swallowed fruit pits are usually excreted from the body in the normal way; only rarely do they cause irritation to the appendix.

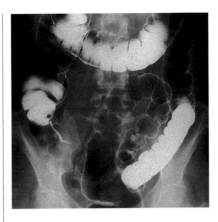

◀ *This is how a healthy appendix appears when X-rayed.*

The reason for this is thought to be directly related to changes in eating habits. The modern Western diet has become so refined that it now lacks sufficient fiber. This deficiency causes the food to slow down in its passage through the intestines, and the sluggishness can lead to blockages, which may be a contributory cause of appendicitis. Food residues can occasionally collect in the appendix and form an obstruction. Fruit pits and other foreign bodies that may have been swallowed accidentally can also aggravate the appendix, but these are among the rarer causes of appendicitis. Worms, which can result from eating contaminated food, are another danger to the appendix. These intestinal parasites may lodge there and eventually cause an obstruction. Whatever their origin, obstructions of any kind can lead to the onset of appendicitis.

The "grumbling" appendix

Recurrent attacks of appendicitis, each lasting a day or two, can sometimes occur. As the appendix gets inflamed, the intestines nearby close around it to contain the infection. If the inflammation clears up, the intestines may still be left stuck around the appendix. These adhesions can restrain the normal movement of food around the system, resulting in colicky pains (griping, or spasms in the bowels), which may then be felt in the appendix region during normal digestion. This leads to a "grumbling" appendix, which will settle if it does not become inflamed again.

Serious symptoms

For various reasons, a bout of appendicitis may not clear up on its own: if the appendix is blocked, further action may be necessary. The early symptoms of appendicitis are not easy to distinguish from any other form of stomachache. The pain, which is of sudden onset and intermittent, is felt around the umbilicus (navel) as the appendix muscles contract while they attempt to drive any obstruction out. If there is no obstruction, then there will just be a constant ache. Sometimes the person will have diarrhea, mild fever, and nausea, with or without vomiting. After six to 12 hours, the symptoms will change, as inflammation builds up around the appendix. The overlying peritoneum (lining) of the abdomen becomes irritated, and as this is well supplied with nerves, more pain is felt around the appendix. Usually, this is in the lower right abdomen. If treatment is not given, or it is delayed, the appendix can rupture, leading to serious inflammation of the peritoneum, which can be fatal if untreated.

Diagnosis

A rectal examination by the doctor may be necessary to establish whether pain is, in fact, caused by an inflamed and tender appendix. The doctor may also do a blood test to establish whether the white cell count is raised, indicating infection. If the doctor diagnoses appendicitis, the patient will be admitted to a hospital. There, an ultrasound scan or CT scan may be done to confirm the diagnosis.

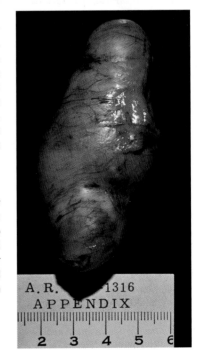

▶ *An enlarged and inflamed appendix that was removed during minimally invasive surgery.*

Recognizing appendicitis

EARLY SYMPTOMS	ACTION
Colicky (griping, or spasmodic) stomach pain that comes and goes.	Give mild painkiller such as acetaminophen.
Loss of appetite.	Try a soothing drink: warm milk or weak tea.
Constipation.	Give a hot water bottle. DO NOT GIVE A LAXATIVE—this causes painful contractions of the appendix, increasing the chance of perforation.
In children, a respiratory infection may show symptoms imitating appendicitis, but these could also be genuine.	Tell the doctor about stomach symptoms in a child—just in case.

LATER SYMPTOMS	ACTION
More pain in appendix area (right lower abdomen), which may move up or down from navel.	
Slight rise in temperature, for example to 99.5°F (37.5°C).	
Slight increase in pulse rate.	
Patient lies with right leg bent up. Stretching it down produces pain.	GET MEDICAL HELP AT ONCE
Diarrhea is possible, but constipation is more common.	
Nausea and vomiting.	
Foul-smelling breath.	

The inflamed appendix often lies on the right leg muscle where it joins the back. Because this makes the leg stiff, the patient naturally bends the leg up to gain relief. Stretching down causes pain. The muscles in the front wall of the abdomen go into spasm to protect the appendix from any painful movements the patient may make.

It may be difficult for a doctor to diagnose appendicitis in a child. The child may have a chest infection, with symptoms that imitate appendicitis; these may disappear as the respiratory infection improves, but the appendicitis may be brought on by the other infection swelling the glands. Even if a child has clear signs of chest trouble, the doctor must be told if he or she also has a stomachache. If the pain has continued for a whole day or night and has become increasingly severe, and if the patient is vomiting and unable to get up, then medical help must be sought. It may be quicker to take the patient to the doctor's office rather than wait for a house call. Home treatments, such as painkillers or soothing drinks, should not be tried at this stage. Surgery may be urgently needed, and the stomach must be empty of food and liquids before an anesthetic can be given.

Dangers of appendicitis

If the problem is neglected, the condition can become worse. The tip of the appendix can become gangrenous, causing perforation. If pus spreads into the abdominal cavity, the result can be a serious inflammation called peritonitis, which can happen within hours. This can be localized in adults, but in children under 10 it can turn into general peritonitis. When the appendix is removed, a plastic drain has to be inserted to allow any infected matter to drain away. Intravenous fluids (a drip) and antibiotics will also be given to combat the infection and speed recovery.

Appendectomy

Because the risks of neglecting appendicitis are greater than the risks of an unnecessary operation, the surgeon will operate even if in doubt. However, if the symptoms are inconclusive, the patient may be put to bed and kept under observation. If the condition does not improve, an operation will be performed. The operation is usually done by minimally invasive surgery and takes only about half an hour, under general anesthetic. Modern drugs and antibiotics have greatly reduced the risk of complications. When the appendix has been removed, the patient feels much better and is ready to leave the hospital a few days later. The stitches at the site of the operation are removed after a week. Once the stitches have been taken out, the scar still has to heal, but the patient can soon lead a reasonably normal life again, though active sports like football or boxing are out of the question for several weeks.

Aftereffects

Some twinges of pain will be felt during healing, but these will disappear within a month or so. However, the patient may develop severe flatulence after the operation because the abdomen has been opened during surgery, and air can enter the intestine. After any abdominal operation, the bowels cease working, so temporary flatulence is a good sign, because it indicates that the digestive system is returning to normal, so that the patient will soon be able to eat and drink normally again. The patient should be assured that this is the best possible sign that he or she is on the way to complete recovery.

See also: Pain; Parasites

Arthritis

Questions and Answers

A relative told me that he avoided arthritis by keeping a piece of potato in his pocket. Is there any truth in this, and should I try it?

It is unlikely to have any basis in fact. Although many plants have proven medicinal properties, the potato is not one of them. Your relative was just lucky enough not to develop arthritis.

Is it safe to take a lot of aspirin to ease pain caused by arthritis?

Yes and no. Because aspirin reduces inflammation and temperature and eases pain, it is often used as a first-line treatment for arthritis. However, when aspirin is taken for a long time, there are two possible side effects: tiny gastric ulcers can bleed or an existing ulcer can flare up. If you vomit blood or anything that resembles coffee grounds, or excrete black, tarlike bowel movements, stop taking aspirin and seek medical help. If you get ringing in the ears, you are taking far too much aspirin and are endangering your hearing.

Are some occupations more likely to cause arthritis than others?

Yes. There are occupational effects, such as "baker's cyst" (fluid at the back of the knee, produced by constant bending when getting bread in and out of the oven), "porter's neck" (osteoarthritis of the neck joints, caused by constantly tilting the neck), and even "ballet dancer's toe," which looks like a bunion.

Will liniment help to relieve the pain of an inflamed joint?

Not much, but it may be soothing. Vegetable oil is as effective as products costing more. Massaging a bruised joint with emollients may help relieve the pain.

"Arthritis" is the umbrella name for several conditions, in which the symptoms vary from temporary discomfort to a more serious disability. Medical treatment and physiotherapy can help relieve most types of arthritis.

Arthritis is an inflammation of the joints, and its causes are as varied as the condition itself. It affects people of all ages and is a common complaint in temperate climates. It can be mild or severe, affecting one joint or several; the different types include rheumatoid arthritis, osteoarthritis, rigid spine disease (ankylosing spondylitis), and arthritis that is due to an injury or an infection. The study of arthritis is a well-established specialty called rheumatology, but medical research does not yet have all the answers.

Rheumatoid arthritis in adults

Although it is a common condition, why rheumatoid arthritis occurs is unknown. What is known is that it is an immune disorder in which the body produces antibodies that act against the lining membrane of the joints—the synovial membranes—and these membranes become heavily infiltrated by immune system lymphocytes. Sometimes other tissues are also affected. High levels of an antibody known as rheumatoid factor appear in the bloodstream. This is used as a test for rheumatoid arthritis.

The disease affects three times more women than men and affects mainly people of a particular tissue type. Because the condition is common in some families, a genetic factor may be involved. Rheumatoid arthritis is most common in adults between the ages of 40 and 60. Inflammation of the knuckles of both hands is the usual symptom, and the joints of the toes are affected in a similar way. At the same time, the sufferer may lose weight, feel sick, and become

▼ *An X ray of an arthritic hip. A suitable treatment would be to replace the hip joint.*

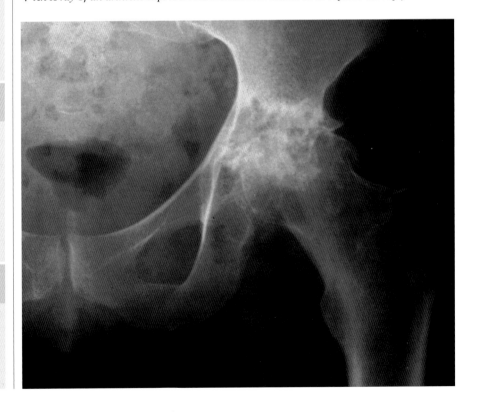

COMPARISON OF A NORMAL AND AN OSTEOARTHRITIC KNEE JOINT

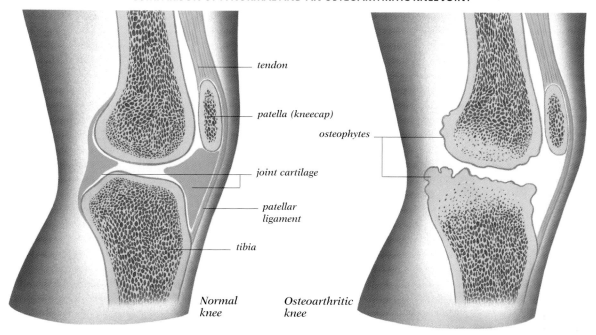

tendon

patella (kneecap)

osteophytes

joint cartilage

patellar
ligament

tibia

Normal
knee

Osteoarthritic
knee

▲ *In osteoarthritis some cartilage, which lines the bones of the knee joint, forms into lumps (osteophytes) and some wears away. As it wears, bones lose their protection; this is what causes the pain.*

lethargic. The symptoms may be acute, starting suddenly with a fever or rash, or may happen gradually over several weeks.

The areas most often affected are the knees, hips, shoulders, wrists, elbows, ankles, and bones of the neck. The stiffness is usually at its worst in the mornings, and in acute cases the sufferer may be confined to bed or have great difficulty with movement.

In about one-quarter of cases, attacks will last about six months, but they may happen only every few years. Some cases are persistent and vary in severity but tend to burn out after many years.

Rheumatoid arthritis in children

Rheumatoid arthritis can occur in children; the condition is called Still's disease, but it is rare. Two main age groups are affected—between one and three and 10 and 15. The inflammation starts gradually, and in about one-third of cases it occurs in one joint only, most commonly the knee joint. It can also affect the hands, wrists, feet, and ankles. The disease is slow to progress but burns itself out in late adolescence. The chance of a cure depends on the severity of the case, how early it is diagnosed, and how quickly treatment is begun. Treatment should be started early to prevent permanent stiffening and joint deformity.

Osteoarthritis

Osteoarthritis occurs as part of the aging process. It happens mainly in weight-bearing joints: hips, knees, and spinal joints. In women, the hands are also often affected, particularly the top joints of the fingers and the base of the thumb. This condition is caused by a degeneration of the cartilage, which is a tough, elastic tissue that protects the surface of the joint. The cartilage is normally glistening and smooth, but osteoarthritis causes it to roughen and become dry. This change has two effects: it compresses the underlying bone surface that the cartilage should protect, and it inflames the synovium lying over it. The first symptoms are pain and loss of use. Stiffness and swelling follow, and the joint eventually changes shape. There may be only one joint involved, such as the right hip in a right-handed person (because in such a person the right side of the body is more active and bears more weight than the left); but in many cases, the knees, spine, shoulders, hands, and neck are affected. This condition is also slow to progress, but disability rarely happens unless the arthritis in a weight-bearing joint is severe. Any injury is likely to cause the condition to flare up.

Rigid spine disease

Ankylosing spondylitis is a form of arthritis that affects the pelvic joints and spine. This, too, involves immune system activity similar to that in rheumatoid arthritis, and there is a tendency for it to run in families. It is about four times more common in men, and it usually begins between the ages of 15 and 30. In this condition, inflammation causes calcium to be deposited in the ligaments, which are the fibrous bands that connect joints. The calcification causes stiffness, which can lead to a fusion of the spinal bones (vertebrae) if the inflammation is not alleviated by both medical treatment and exercise—hence its common name "poker back." The illness progresses slowly for a few years; it often spreads to the whole spine and involves the hip joints before the active inflammation ceases.

Other causes of arthritis

An injury can trigger a type of arthritis called traumatic arthritis. The injury can result from a blow to a joint or can result when a joint such as the knee is hurt by a person falling heavily on it. Traumatic

Questions and Answers

My doctor says I have a "frozen shoulder." Is that a form of arthritis, and should I be worried about it?

Frozen shoulder is not a form of arthritis but simply a condition that mimics it. Other conditions in this category include tennis elbow and nerve pain in the wrist, which is called carpal tunnel syndrome. What these conditions have in common is inflammation of the tissues around a joint—but in each case, evidence confirming arthritis is absent. If you follow your doctor's instructions for treatment, you should make a recovery.

My sister is severely affected by arthritis, but she is planning to get married. What are her chances of enjoying a fulfilling sex life—or starting a family?

When either partner has arthritis, the couple will want answers to many questions before starting a family. An important point is whether their children will be prone to this condition. Only one type of arthritis, caused by hemophilia, is clearly inherited. With many other forms, the chance that an affected parent will hand down the disease is low. In an acute phase of the disease, it would be painful to attempt sex, but otherwise it is quite safe to have intercourse.

My grandmother always wears a bandage made of fabric wound tightly around her arthritic knee. Is this really helpful?

It can be of some help. Bandaging or supporting an acutely inflamed joint can stop jarring movement and, therefore, ease some of the pain. When a joint is swollen, the tissues feel stretched—a support under these circumstances gives a sensation of stability. Wearing a bandage also serves to warn other people that being bumped or knocked would not be appreciated. However, she should always be careful not to make the bandage too tight, as this risks reducing the circulation of blood to the lower part of the leg.

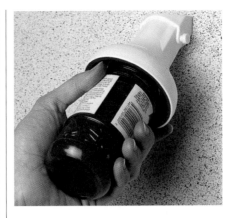
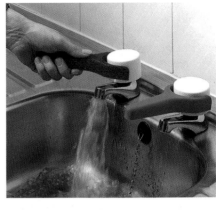
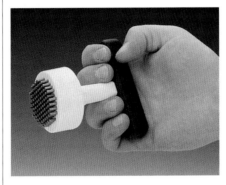
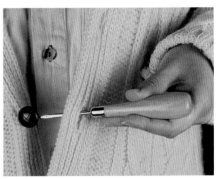

▲ *A range of devices to help arthritic people. Clockwise from top left: a wall-mounted bottle opener; handles to make faucets easier to turn; a long-handled hook to button clothing; a device to grip small knobs.*

arthritis usually develops in men, although women are not immune. The knee, ankle, and wrist are the joints most commonly affected. A few hours after the injury, the joint becomes inflamed, painful, and swollen. An X ray is needed to determine whether a fracture has occurred, but rest, bandaging, and painkillers may be all that is necessary.

Physiotherapy can also help restore mobility and muscle power to the affected limb. Occasionally, the injury causes bleeding into the joint, which becomes very tense and painful; the blood may have to be drawn out with a needle (aspirated) under a local anesthetic.

Bacteria can also cause conditions such as septic arthritis, which is caused by bacteria in the joint fluid. This happens either because of an injury to the joint or because it is transmitted from the blood. Half of such cases involve the knee, but the condition can occur in any large joint. Both children and the elderly can be affected; however, it is a rare condition.

Another rare form of arthritis can result from an attack of rubella. This can happen to adults, who may experience a swelling of their finger joints, knees, and ankles. The swelling usually subsides after a few weeks. Arthritis from tuberculosis (TB) is now also rare, except in people in developing countries. Other infections, such as rheumatic fever, gonorrhea, dysentery, and the skin disease psoriasis, are also associated with arthritis.

Diagnosis and treatment

If some form of arthritis is suspected, the worst thing a person can do is to suffer without consulting a doctor. Self-diagnosis should not be attempted; the family doctor should be visited. Any delay might increase the risk of permanent deformity, especially in the case of a child with Still's disease, which is a condition that needs hospital care.

The doctor will ask for a history of the illness and undertake an examination. He or she may prescribe drugs such as aspirin, indomethacin, and ibuprofen, which combat inflammation and ease pain; and painkillers like synthetic narcotics, which are stronger. Gold compounds may be injected in the affected joints, but these can have unpleasant side effects and are used only when considered absolutely necessary. The patient may have to rest the affected joints or wear an individually made splint to keep the affected area in the best position and to prevent deformities from occurring. Swelling in joints can be treated by drawing off excess fluid under a local anesthetic or by injecting an anti-inflammatory drug into the joint. The patient may be feeling generally ill and be advised to cut down on some everyday activities and to rest.

Steroid drugs (such as cortisone) may be prescribed to suppress the inflammation in the joints, but because they have side effects they are used only when all other forms of treatment have been tried and found unsuccessful. Doses must always be kept at the lowest possible level at which they will control symptoms, and progress must be carefully monitored by a doctor.

If the symptoms persist, the doctor may recommend a visit to the rheumatic clinic of a local hospital for further investigation. An acute attack of arthritis with fever, swollen joints, and a general feeling of being unwell may require immediate hospital treatment, including splinting and rest on a special vibrator bed—an electric current vibrates through a plastic mattress, producing a cushioning effect. Blood tests are done to establish the type of arthritis involved, to see if the patient is anemic, to check the amount of inflammation in the body at regular intervals, and to assess the progress of the disease. Other tests will show whether the condition is caused by septic arthritis, gonococcal (STD) arthritis, or bleeding into the joint.

Another technique, called arthroscopy, involves a narrow viewing instrument that is inserted into the knee and allows the doctor to look inside the knee joint under local anesthetic. Both the cartilage and the lining tissue can be examined by this means, and small pieces of tissue can be removed for further microscopic examination to help establish the exact cause of the condition.

Exercise and physiotherapy

Physiotherapy plays an important part in the treatment of all forms of arthritis. For affected joints that are in a quiescent phase—that is, free of inflammation—exercise is essential to prevent stiffness and loss of mobility and to restore those muscles around the joint that may have deteriorated. There is no evidence that exercising an arthritic joint in the quiescent phase causes it to flare up.

The physiotherapist at the local hospital will teach the patient exercises that can be continued at home. Heat can be used to ease painful joints. These treatments can include short-wave diathermy, in which a heat pad is placed near the affected joint; or hydrotherapy (exercising in a small, very warm swimming pool). The effect of the heat is to relax tense muscles, and because the water supports the weight of the body, movement is increased and free.

If the doctor or physiotherapist advises it, an infrared lamp can be used at home. A paraffin wax bath for hands and feet is another treatment that can be used very easily at home once the technique is learned. On the other hand, some therapists favor ice packs as a form of pain-relieving therapy.

The benefits of surgery

Great advances have been made in the replacement of badly damaged joints with artificial ones. In the first instance, the decision that an arthritic joint needs surgery will be made by a specialist in the field, an orthopedic surgeon who has been consulted by either a patient's own doctor or a rheumatologist. The results of such an operation can be a dramatic relief of pain, correction of deformity, and increased movement. The benefits to the patient may include regained enjoyment of sexual intercourse, which previously may have been very difficult.

Coping with arthritis at home
Build a ramp to replace outdoor steps
Make door openings wide enough for a wheelchair, if necessary
Attach a handrail on both sides of the stairs
Replace worn carpets; keep floor space clear for walking aids
Raise electric sockets about 3 ft. (1 m) above floor
Replace light switches with cords that can be easily reached
Fix the mailbox at a convenient height to avoid bending when retrieving the mail
Raise heights of chairs with blocks attached to ends of chair legs; raise height of seat with firm cushions
To increase leverage on refrigerator handle, slip a loop of leather or strong string over handle
Pad handles of utensils (e.g., potato peeler) with foam rubber; also pad brush and broom handles
Use a basket on wheels to carry things from one room to another
Install handrails in the bath and around the toilet; invest in an elevated toilet seat
Attach an iron and ironing board to the wall to avoid carrying
Install wall-mounted jar and bottle openers and can openers
Use long-handled garden tools
Use an adjustable seat in the bathtub
Use a lightweight carpet sweeper
Extend the toilet seat for wheelchair users
Position the washing machine and kitchen surfaces at convenient heights
Use an adjustable bed that can flex into any position; these beds also have an optional vibrating effect

Types of arthritis and their treatment

TYPE	CAUSE	SYMPTOMS	TREATMENT
Rheumatoid arthritis	Unexplained immune system disorder more common in women. Affects adults usually between 40 and 60, also children (Still's disease).	Lethargy, high temperature, rash (occasionally). Pain, swelling, redness, stiffness, and loss of function in joints of fingers or toes.	Anti-inflammatory drugs, painkilling drugs, gold injections, or steroid drugs. Immediate hospital treatment for children. Reducing swelling by drawing off (aspirating) fluid, physiotherapy, exercise, splinting, joint replacement. Potent immunosuppressive agents and antibodies to tumor necrosis factor.
Osteoarthritis	Wear and tear due to aging; degeneration of cartilage over joint.	Pain, followed by stiffness, swelling, change of shape.	Basic principles as above.
Ankylosing spondylitis	Strongly linked to a particular tissue type. More common in males between 15 and 30. Calcium deposited in joint ligaments.	Stiff lower back in mornings, pain on bending spine.	Anti-inflammatory drugs, exercise.
Traumatic	Injury—for example, falling heavily.	Joint becomes inflamed, painful, and swollen a few hours after injury.	Rest, bandaging, painkilling drugs, then physiotherapy. X ray in case of fracture, possible aspiration of fluid.

Surgery can relieve pressure around a joint, free gummed-up ligaments, or remove inflamed lining tissue of a joint (synovectomy) if it is greatly affected. An extremely painful and useless joint, such as one that may occur with osteoarthritis of the cervical spine (neck) or an arthritic knee, is sometimes surgically fused (arthrodesis) to give relief, although this does involve some loss of movement.

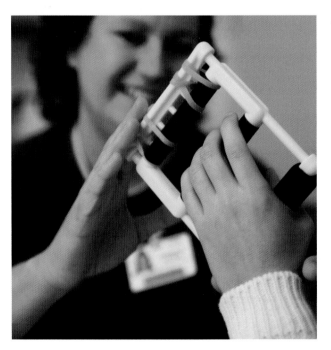

▲ *A physiotherapist can help a person with arthritis to practice special exercises.*

Available help

An active person who has become seriously disabled must first come to terms with feelings of dependence and helplessness. Although there is no cure yet for every disability caused by arthritis, better general care and physical aids can make life more tolerable and movement easier in many ways.

Aids such as splints, surgical collars, walking sticks and frames, elbow crutches, wheelchairs, and some of the more complicated electrical hoisting aids can all be matched to the individual needs of arthritics by physiotherapists.

Replacing one kind of lifestyle with another, although not always easy, is always possible. Adjusting employment to the disability is a priority. An arthritic may need to change shifts, use specially adapted equipment, or generally take on lighter duties. The doctor may write to the disabled person's employer to explain any specific problems that may need to be resolved.

Practical pursuits

Structural changes in an affected person's home may be necessary, and there are many helpful adaptations that can be made. Living on one level in a ranch house or apartment is obviously more practical than living in a conventional two-story house; but when this is not possible, the problems caused by steps or stairs can usually be overcome by using special equipment, such as a chair lift.

Hobbies, activities and pastimes such as card playing, gardening, or needlecraft are all possible for someone who is arthritic. Occupational therapists can give advice about the many devices and techniques that allow arthritics to continue enjoying these pleasures, and how to develop new ones.

See also: Anemia; Bacteria; Infection and infectious diseases; Rubella

Aspirin and analgesics

Questions and Answers

Do painkillers act as sleeping pills?

Strictly speaking, no. Milder painkillers may relieve pain that has been disrupting sleep. Some of the stronger ones obtainable on prescription do also act as sedatives and can induce sleep.

I am taking an analgesic. Is it safe to drink alcoholic beverages?

If you are using a mild analgesic such as aspirin or acetaminophen, it should be safe to have an occasional drink. However, both aspirin and hard liquor can cause bleeding in the gut, so it is wise to avoid the combination.

Alcohol should never be taken at the same time as a strong painkiller, because both substances slow breathing down, and the interaction of the two substances could be dangerous.

My husband gets migraine; if he doesn't take a pill right away, it doesn't work. Why is this?

When a migraine attack occurs, the intestine shuts down. Once this happens, there is little chance of a drug's being absorbed. Get your husband to take his pill as soon an attack starts. If this is impossible, your doctor may prescribe an analgesic in suppository form or an oral drug that will help absorption.

Can aspirin work as a male contraceptive pill?

This is not as unlikely as it sounds. Aspirin inhibits the production of prostaglandins, which are linked to sperm production. In a study of analgesic abuse, few men became fathers while taking large doses of aspirin; in animal tests, large doses inhibited sperm production in males. However, despite these findings, aspirin is an unreliable contraceptive.

There are many easily obtainable analgesics, or painkillers, of which aspirin is the best-known. It is important to know which is the right analgesic to take to relieve a particular pain.

The range of painkilling drugs available can be confusing. Some are fairly mild whereas some are dangerous; many can be bought at drugstores or supermarkets, but others can be obtained only by prescription. The most common analgesic is aspirin. It is used for ailments ranging from flu to fevers, from menstrual pains to rheumatism, and it is also, of course, the standby analgesic for a tension headache.

However, aspirin is not suitable for pain in the heart, gut, or urinary tract, or for those who develop rashes and breathing difficulties when they take it. Acetaminophen, another analgesic, is not suitable for people with liver trouble. If there is any doubt, a pharmacist in a drugstore would be able to suggest a suitable product. If pain persists, a doctor should be consulted.

Painkillers are best taken before the pain gets bad; enough should be taken for the painkiller to work, without exceeding the recommended dose stated on the label of the bottle. For aspirin, the dose is one to two tablets (each tablet is 325 mg) every four hours, or 12 pills in 24 hours. Research shows that it is unsafe to give aspirin to children under 12 years old, because the aspirin can lead to Reye's syndrome, which causes swelling of the brain and inflammation of the liver.

Types

Analgesics fall into two categories—those that act locally on a specific pain and those that act centrally, from within, and affect the whole nervous system. The first group of analgesics, known as peripheral painkillers, includes aspirin, acetaminophen, and the once popular phenacetin—now no longer used because of its effect on the kidneys. The analgesics in this group are used to relieve mild to moderate pain in muscles, joints, or bones; they work by reducing the body's production of substances called prostaglandins, which cause muscles to contract, making the person more susceptible to pain.

The centrally acting group of painkillers are much more powerful and are therefore more strictly controlled by law. This category includes codeine, Demerol, and dilaudid. Also included are all the opiates, both natural and synthetic, such as morphine, heroin, and opium.

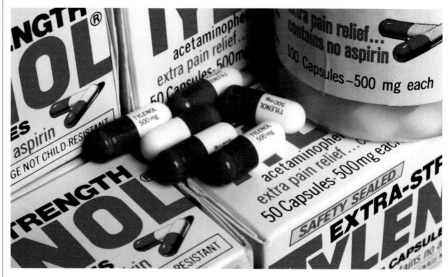

▲ *Acetaminophen is a popular analgesic available in drugstores and other stores. It is included in a group of analgesics that relieve mild to moderate pain.*

Painkillers: Their uses and effects

DRUG	USED FOR	EFFECTS
Aspirin	Acute or chronic aches and pains (tension headache, menstrual pains, neuralgia, toothache); flu; fevers; rheumatism.	Fast-acting; reduces fever and inflammation; does not cause dependence. Can irritate stomach.
Acetaminophen	Aches and pains; flu; fevers.	Reduces fever but does not reduce inflammation. No gastric irritation. Effects less prolonged than those of aspirin. Can possibly affect liver function.
Codeine	Aches and pains; coughs; mild diarrhea.	Slightly constipating; in large doses can slow down breathing and cause nausea.
Phenylbutazone	Rheumatic and joint disorders.	Reduces inflammation and swelling. Can cause fluid retention, nausea, and blood disorders.
Morphine	Diarrhea (with kaolin as liquid mixture); severe pain (in injuries, heart attack, coronary thrombosis, after surgery).	Swift and effective. Can cause constipation, nausea, slow breathing. Derived from opium and therefore addictive.

Dos and don'ts of pain relief

DO

Do take a painkiller soon after the pain begins; otherwise, it will be more difficult to relieve.

Do find out how painkillers interact with any other medicines.

Do take painkillers with food or milk to reduce the risk of stomach irritation.

Do give children smaller doses, as indicated on the label. If in doubt, ask the pharmacist about the correct dosage. Soluble painkillers are best for children; mix with fruit juice or milk.

Do buy medicines in childproof bottles and keep all drugs out of children's reach.

Do call a hospital or poison control center for professional guidance if you suspect that someone has overdosed on painkillers.

DON'T

Don't take painkillers often or in large doses without advice.

Don't take more than the stated dose.

Don't store painkillers such as aspirin in humid places like the bathroom; they will deteriorate. A cool dry place is best.

Don't give aspirin to children under 12.

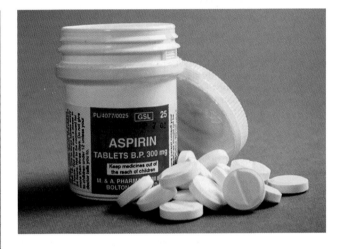

▲ *Aspirin is an analgesic, and also prevents blood clotting.*

Opiates dull pain by interacting with the brain's own naturally produced morphinelike substances called endorphins. Opiates all tend to produce side effects, such as slowed breathing, nausea, vomiting, constipation, and—most serious of all—tolerance and addiction. Codeine is an opiate, and it is obtainable only by prescription.

Alternatives

It is also worth noting that analgesics are not the only way to relieve pain. Nonchemical methods, such as applying cold water (for burns and bruises to the skin), or heat and massage (for painful, aching muscles), can bring significant relief. Alternative techniques on the fringes of orthodox medicine, such as acupuncture, electrical stimulation, meditation, and biofeedback, are well worth trying in both mild and chronic cases.

See also: Pain

Athlete's foot

Athlete's foot is an annoying and unpleasant condition. It is easily transferred but usually responds well to treatment. If attention is paid to basic hygiene, recurrences can be prevented.

Questions and Answers

I have a severe form of athlete's foot that keeps recurring. Will my feet be permanently scarred?

The fungus causing athlete's foot lives only on the superficial layers of the skin, eating dead skin cells, so it will not cause scarring. In chronic cases, the nails may become affected and need treatment with special drugs; but with correct treatment, the foot should return to normal.

I am tired of trying to get rid of athlete's foot. It keeps coming back. What is the reason for this?

The most common reason for reinfection is that the fungus has never been properly gotten rid of in the first place. For this reason, it is important to dust your shoes and socks, as well as your feet, with antifungal powder, as they can also carry the fungus. It is also important to keep up the medical treatment for a few weeks after the symptoms have disappeared.

I have suffered from athlete's foot for some time now and have just found a similar type of irritation on my hands. Can athlete's foot spread to other parts of the body?

The athlete's foot fungus belongs to a group of fungi known as trichophytons, which can live on various parts of the body but are not very contagious and are unlikely to spread. However, there is a condition similar to athlete's foot that can affect the hands, and this should be diagnosed and treated by a doctor.

My sister has athlete's foot. Can she infect the rest of the family?

Not if precautions are taken. Everybody must wash and dry his or her feet carefully, using separate towels, and use antifungal powder on the feet and in the shoes.

Athlete's foot is a fungal infection. It is probably the most common foot complaint that doctors treat. It can affect almost anyone, though small children seem to be immune.

Causes
The only real cause of athlete's foot is a failure to observe the proper personal hygiene, along with carelessness in drying the feet after a shower or bath. People who suffer from sweaty feet are the most prone to the complaint and can aggravate the situation by wearing airless plastic shoes, which prevent sweat from evaporating.

The fungus likes to settle on the soggy skin in the moist, sweaty areas between the toes. It lives by digesting the dead skin that the body sheds each day; in this way it causes inflammation and damage to the living skin. There is a risk of picking up the fungus in bathrooms and in public changing rooms.

Symptoms and treatment
The first sign of athlete's foot is irritation and itching between the toes. This is followed by peeling skin and, possibly, bad foot odor.

In worse cases, painful red cracks called fissures appear between the toes. In severe cases, the toenails become affected, becoming either soft or more brittle as the fungus invades the nail substance. It may be possible to see the nail thickening beneath the outer shell. In extreme cases, the foot swells and blisters, requiring a doctor's prompt attention.

Successful treatments include antifungal creams and powders. Substances such as terbinafine and clotrimazole, in ointment or cream form, should be applied daily while the condition lasts and for two or three weeks after symptoms have disappeared. When the nails have been affected, the doctor may prescribe griseofulvin to be taken orally—if necessary, for months—until the fungus is eliminated. Athlete's foot is treatable at home, but if it spreads or does not respond to treatment a doctor must be consulted.

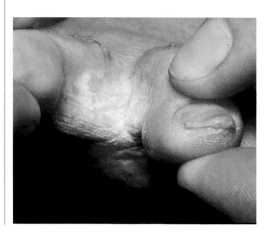

◄ *The white, peeling skin of athlete's foot can be treated with an antifungal cream or powder.*

See also: Hygiene; Infection and infectious diseases

Preventing athlete's foot

The risk of developing athlete's foot can be reduced by following a few guidelines on foot care:

Wash the feet daily with soap; clean all dirt from under the nails and between the toes.

Dry each toe thoroughly with your own towel, paying particular attention to the gaps between the toes.

Treat your feet with antifungal powder or cream. To prevent reinfection, also powder shoes.

Put on clean cotton or wool socks daily. Avoid nylon socks and plastic shoes. Wear open shoes if feet feel sweaty.

Attention deficit hyperactivity disorder

Attention deficit hyperactivity disorder (ADHD) is a mental health disorder commonly diagnosed in children. As its name implies, it is characterized by symptoms of inattention and hyperactivity, as well as impulsivity.

Those affected by ADHD find it difficult to maintain attention, and they will be hyperactive, fidgety, unorganized, or impulsive—symptoms that can lead to poor grades in school and can impair social skills. The disorder occurs not only in children but also in adolescents and adults, persisting in many cases. People who have the condition have described it as similar to living in a fast-moving kaleidoscope of thoughts, sounds, and images that distract them and drive them from one thought or activity to the next, disrupting their daily lives and consuming energy. Although they are usually bright and creative, people with ADHD often feel unable to focus on the tasks they need to complete. This inability can diminish their self-esteem and cause a lifetime of frustration.

Varying symptoms

Although the symptoms of ADHD vary widely, they fall into three broad categories: inattention, hyperactivity, and impulsivity. People who are inattentive tend to be easily distracted, fail to pay attention to detail, often lose or forget things, and may seem only partially aware of what is going on around them. They may concentrate effortlessly on something they enjoy but find it difficult to complete other tasks or to learn something new.

People who are hyperactive cannot sit still. They may dash around, wiggle their feet, talk incessantly, or touch everything. They often feel restless, have difficulty waiting, and may try to

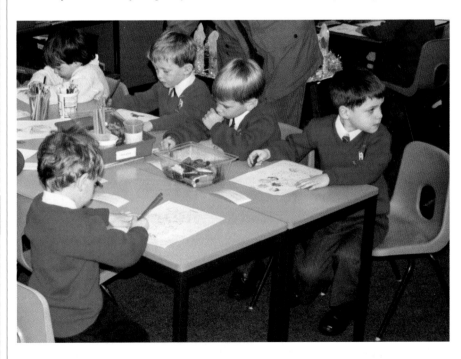

▲ *A child with ADHD may find it difficult to sit still in a chair and focus on a task, being easily distracted by anything that is going on in the background.*

do several things at once. People who are impulsive seem unable to think before they act. They may blurt out inappropriate comments, interrupt when others are speaking, or run into the street without looking.

Most people with ADHD display significant symptoms in all three categories. However, some people are predominantly hyperactive and impulsive; they are capable of paying attention to a task but lose focus because they cannot control their impulsive behavior. Others are predominantly inattentive; they have little trouble sitting still but find it difficult to maintain their attention. Such people are often seen as daydreamers or just lazy. This second type of ADHD, which is sometimes known simply as attention deficit disorder (ADD), is therefore more difficult to spot, but it is estimated that ADD affects about one in seven sufferers.

Similar symptoms

In the past many experts expressed doubts as to whether ADHD was a real medical condition, especially as many other factors can produce similar behaviors. For example, disruptive or unresponsive behavior may be due to anxiety or depression; underachievement may be caused by frustration or boredom; and attention lapses may be caused by allergies, minor epileptic seizures, or infections.

Another problem is that ADHD often occurs with other conditions. Some people also have a learning disability; others have a rare disorder called Tourette's syndrome (which causes uncontrolled movements or utterances); and many boys have also been diagnosed with oppositional defiant disorder or conduct disorder. Those with oppositional defiant disorder tend to be contrary and argumentative, and they may lash out when they feel bad about themselves. Those with conduct disorder tend to be reckless, destructive, and aggressive, and they may steal, set fires, destroy property, and run away from home continually. All these other possibilities must be considered in making a diagnosis.

Diagnosis

Pediatricians, psychiatrists, and psychologists can all help diagnose ADHD. If they are assessing a child they may ask for input from the child's family or teachers; adults may be asked to describe their own experiences. People with ADHD typically exhibit several characteristic behaviors. These almost always appear before age seven, persist over a prolonged period of time, and occur more frequently than would be expected in other people at the same stage of development. To confirm the diagnosis of ADHD, the aberrant behavior should occur in several settings rather than be a response to a specific situation, and it should create a real handicap in at least two areas of a person's life.

What causes ADHD?

The precise causes of ADHD remain unclear. For many years scientists called it "minimal brain dysfunction," believing that minor brain damage caused the condition—a theory now rejected because it could explain only a tiny number of cases. Another popular theory was that refined sugar and food additives caused the symptoms, but this theory is still a topic of heated debate.

More recently scientists using brain-imaging techniques have made several interesting discoveries. They have found that the structure connecting the two sides of the brain and the area that controls memory and emotions often seem to be smaller in people with ADHD. They have also found that there seems to be less activity in the frontal areas of the brain, and lower levels of some neurotransmitters (the chemicals that carry brain messages). On the basis of these findings, some researchers are trying to determine factors that might affect these nerve cells, such as a woman's use of cigarettes, alcohol, or other drugs during pregnancy, or the effect of environmental toxins.

Other research suggests that ADHD may have a strong hereditary component, since children with ADHD often have at least one close relative with the condition, and 75 percent of identical twins share the trait.

Drug treatment

The most common treatment for ADHD is a stimulant drug such as Ritalin, Dexedrine, or Cylert. These only temporarily control the symptoms of ADHD but can dramatically reduce impulsive and overactive behaviors, improving a person's ability to focus, work, and learn. The drug most frequently used is Ritalin, which works in about 70 to 80 percent of cases.

Prescribing stimulants has sparked a great deal of controversy. Some critics argue that too many doctors prescribe the drugs unnecessarily for children who do not have a true attention disorder, while others point to potential side effects such as weight loss, reduced appetite, and disrupted sleep.

Another factor to consider with drug treatments is that while these medications are not addictive in children, they can be in teenagers and adults if misused. Some doctors feel that the potential side effects should be carefully weighed against the benefits, but others believe that these stimulants are relatively safe when used under medical supervision.

Other types of medication may be prescribed to alleviate other symptoms, if stimulants fail to work or if ADHD occurs with another disorder. For example, antidepressants such as Imipramine or Desipramine may be used to control any accompanying depression or anxiety, and Clonidine may be tried when stimulants do not work or when people have both ADHD and Tourette's syndrome.

Psychosocial and behavioral approaches

Many specialists recommend that medications should be combined with other approaches. For example, special education programs can shelter children from distractions, provide encouragement, and divide tasks into more manageable chunks. Parents can also be taught to encourage good behaviors and to be clear about unacceptable actions. One such technique is to remove an unruly child from an agitating situation for a short time to calm down.

Support system

Emotional and practical support may also help adults who suffer from ADHD. Counseling, for example, may help them deal with upsetting feelings, pinpoint self-defeating patterns of behavior, and learn alternative ways of handling their emotions. Behavioral therapy can help them think through tasks or encourage new ways of behaving. People may also find it useful to join support groups, where they can share their frustrations and successes and obtain help with referrals to specialists.

See also: **Autism; Heredity**

Autism

Autism is a broad spectrum of disorders that affect thought, attention, and perception. Specialist teaching and a constructive approach can do much to help autistic children and adults reach their maximum potential.

The word "autism" is used to describe an extremely complex developmental disability. It is taken from the Greek *autos*, "self," and means being turned in upon the self. Autism typically appears during the first three years of life in the form of severe behavioral problems such as tantrums, destructiveness, aggressiveness, and self-injury. It occurs in two to six of 1,000 individuals and is more prevalent in boys than girls. Race, ethnicity, social standing, income, lifestyle, and educational level are all irrelevant. There are a number of misconceptions about autism: for example, it is not caused by bad parenting or psychological developmental factors, nor is it a mental illness.

Autism has been a recognized—that is to say, medically classified—condition for more than 50 years. In 1943 an American psychiatrist, Leo Kanner, first coined the word to describe the symptoms of a group of children whose common abnormalities of behavior distinguished them sharply from other mentally handicapped children in his care. He identified what he considered the most important symptoms common to this group, and from then on the condition became known as Kanner's syndrome or infantile autism. Some years later, a working party of psychiatrists discovered more symptoms, which they added to those identified by Kanner. For many years doctors referred to these symptoms in attempting to diagnose the condition.

What causes autism?

No single cause for autism has been isolated, but the disorder is generally thought to be due to abnormalities in brain structure or function. Research is being conducted to determine whether there is a genetic basis to the disorder, and to investigate the link between genetics and medical

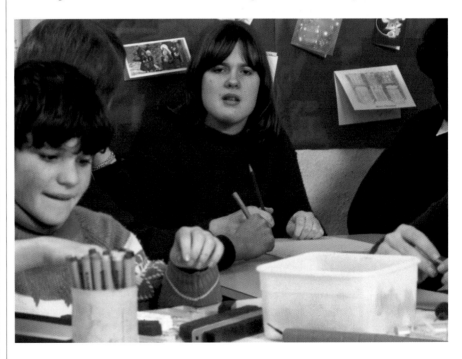

▲ *Autistic children generally need special education with creative, supervised play. Support and understanding are required to prevent them from becoming withdrawn.*

disorders. No gene has yet been identified as causing autism, but researchers are looking for irregularities of the genetic code that may have been inherited by autistic children.

It seems that some children are born with a tendency to autism, but no trigger has been identified that induces autism to develop. Other theories under investigation are that problems during the mother's pregnancy or during delivery can be relevant. Environmental factors such as exposure to chemicals, viral infections, and metabolic balances are also possible causative factors.

Symptoms

What most parents usually notice first in a young autistic child is that the infant cannot show normal responsiveness; he or she does not want to cuddle, make eye contact, or respond to affection.

As the toddler develops, he or she has difficulty mixing with other children and expressing needs. Language skills will be poor or even nonexistent, and the child will repeat words or phrases (echolalia) rather than answering a question using normal language.

The child may also use gestures and point instead of using words. Repetitive activities, such as spinning or rhythmic body movements, are another feature of the disorder.

An autistic child's fits of screaming and tantrums far outdo in length and volume those of even the most violent normal toddler. It is possible that autistic children, even if they see and hear normally, often do not understand what people are saying to them and find it difficult to express themselves through language. These problems can lead to confusion and frustration, which frequently culminate in behavioral problems.

Strange responses

Autistic children also exhibit strange fears—usually of totally harmless objects, such as a bush or a box—but do not register fear when there is real danger. This response is probably connected to their inability to make sense of the impressions they receive. Other aspects of autism are not as easy to explain. Such children tend to be very sensitive to certain sounds—something as everyday as the

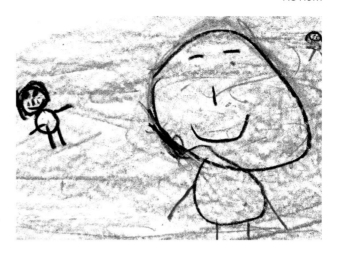

▲ *Autistic children lack motivation and natural interest common to children of their age; this drawing by an autistic six-year-old is typical of a child of four.*

sound of water gushing into a washing machine can frighten them. In addition there is sometimes an inappropriate fascination with bright lights or with objects such as bits of broken plastic or elastic bands. An autistic child may show a dangerous indifference to heat and cold—being capable, for instance, of staying in a very hot bath without showing any adverse reaction. Strangest of all, perhaps, are the odd body movements—grimaces, arm- or hand-flapping, jumping, or hopping from one foot to the other—which no one can satisfactorily explain. If all autistic children displayed all these symptoms, the condition would be much easier to diagnose. They do not, however, and a worried parent or relative can be even more confused by the fact that a child looks perfectly normal and seems to be intelligent.

Autistic savant

Some people with autism have unusual and uncommon skills. Such a person is known as an autistic savant, and about 10 percent of autistic people fall into this category. These people have extraordinary abilities in math, music, and are capable of astonishing feats of memory. They may have perfect pitch or be able to multiply and divide large numbers in their head. They show amazing concentration and can focus their complete attention on a subject. The reason why some autistic people are savants is unknown, but some researchers in psychology think that a full knowledge of the autistic savant will provide an understanding of memory and cognition.

Degrees of autism

Some autistic children may develop a certain amount of useful speech and acquire many practical skills but be unable to tolerate the pace of everyday modern life. While such children will always need to live in a sheltered environment, they are, however, still quite capable of making important positive contributions to that environment, and of living full lives. At the other end of the scale, there are those who are so severely disturbed that their parents will probably always have to make decisions for them. At their worst, these children can quickly damage a normal home—tearing

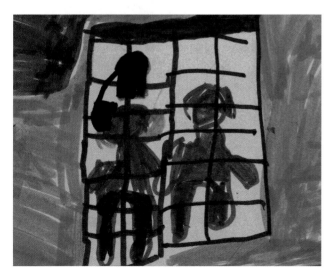

▲ *This drawing by a six-year-old autistic child shows a reasonably well developed sense of color.*

clothing, curtains, bedding, and even their own skin and hair. Many sleep very little and remain hyperactive throughout the night, causing their parents or caregivers to become stressed and to lose sleep and patience. Still others—and these are perhaps the most difficult to help—may be autistic in addition to other handicaps.

The cause of autism must be identified before it is possible to find a cure. Most autistic children remain handicapped for life. Rarely, the severity of the symptoms suddenly eases, usually when the child has been severely affected in the first instance.

Diagnosis

Autism is difficult to diagnose. Once a diagnosis has been reached, a child's development, social skills, and communication skills are assessed and evaluated regularly. Medical tests can aid diagnosis. An audiologist tests for any hearing impairment, and an electroencephalogram (EEG) measures brain waves and will show abnormalities or tumors. Because some autistic disorders can be helped by special diets, a range of blood and urine laboratory tests can be made, to measure how food is being metabolized. To examine the brain in minute detail, magnetic resonance imaging is used; to diagnose structural problems in the brain, a CT (computer assisted axial tomography) scan is carried out. Genetic testing looks for gene abnormalities that could cause a developmental disability.

Teaching methods

No single teaching method (like braille for the blind or sign language for the mute) or technique can be applied to all autistic children. Each child's highly individual needs and problems have to be assessed and treated. Different abilities have to be developed in individual learning programs.

To start with, long-established techniques for behavior management are used to cope with autistic abnormalities. The worst behavioral problems, such as tantrums, screaming fits, hyperactivity, and obsessions, usually have to be dealt with first, since they tend to stand in the way of real progress. There are many calming techniques including vigorous exercise, vestibular stimulation (slow swinging), and deep pressure from a hug machine.

Language problems present the most fundamental obstacles to teaching, since they are linked with the problems of behaving properly and learning to think. They are, therefore, given constant attention. Advice and help are sought from audiologists at hearing clinics and speech therapists, who test comprehension and expression levels and consider articulation problems. After this preliminary testing, a language program is set up for the individual child. Language is concentrated on at all times—not just in the classroom. It is essential that teachers at all levels should speak simply, using short sentences, and about things rather than ideas.

If autistic children remain mute beyond age eight or nine, there is little hope that they can be taught any useful speech. Rarely, a child can be taught sign language, but such a child is exceptional. Because autistic children lack natural interest, motivation, and ordinary concentration, they demand the teacher's careful organization of all daily situations.

Normal children are taught to motivate themselves. Autistic children are unable to motivate themselves; they must be taught to move from one step to the next. The degree of success depends upon the severity of the handicap, but some degree of ability is possible for all autistic children.

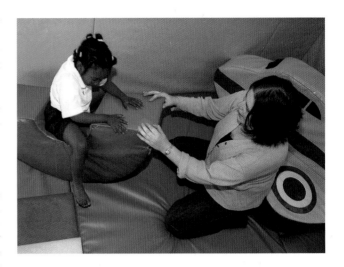

▲ *Observing an autistic child at play can provide information about social, emotional, and cognitive development.*

Autistic children at home

It is very important for parents to be closely involved in the work and techniques of the school. Sometimes either the teacher or a parent may have devised an effective strategy to deal with a behavioral problem, so it is vital that parents and teachers coordinate their treatment of the child to make it constant as well as consistent. If the parents continue the special education at home, the autistic child will obtain the maximum benefit from it.

Therapy and treatment

It has been shown that autistic children do improve with special education, and parents should therefore do everything possible to see that the children receive it. A structured treatment program that includes speech therapy to help improve communication skills is essential. Traditional approaches to speech therapy are not appropriate for someone who is autistic, because training such a person to speak will not affect his or her behavior. Emphasis is therefore placed on teaching the autistic person how to use language to communicate effectively. Behavior therapy can help to modify abnormal behavior and substitute more appropriate behavior.

Physical and sensory skills can be helped by occupational therapy. The aim of this therapy is to improve fine motor skills, such as writing or brushing teeth, and sensory motor skills, including touch, awareness of body position, and balance. Physical therapy is used to improve the function of the body's large muscles, to strengthen, and to help coordination and movement.

Sometimes in addition to autism, a person suffers from food allergies, and these can make behavior worse. If food allergies are suspected and tested for, the foods that test positive are eliminated from the diet. Some parents give autistic children nutritional supplements such as vitamin B6 with magnesium and dimethylglycine. Almost half of the families studied have reported improvement and a noticeable reduction in the children's behavioral problems when supplements are given.

See also: **Child development**

Bacteria

Bacteria are everywhere. They live in the air, the water, and the soil. Some of them can cause diseases, but many more are extremely useful to humans, breaking down organic matter and fixing atmospheric nitrogen.

Bacteria are minute living things, too small to be seen with the naked eye. At their largest, they measure only 10 microns across. They are microscopic single-celled organisms with rigid cell walls, and they are found in every environment.

Mainly harmless

Although they are so small, bacteria are one of the most successful groups of living things. They are found in or on the bodies of animals and people. Bacteria have a bad reputation because they are known to be a cause of disease; but on the whole, they probably do more good than harm, because certain kinds help in the production of foods and the manufacture of important vitamins within the human intestine.

However, it is the disease-causing bacteria that are of most concern to everyone and that need to be effectively controlled to keep contagious diseases at bay.

Different types

Microbiologists—the scientists who make a study of these creatures—usually divide disease-causing bacteria into four main groups based on their shape. The cocci are spherical bacteria, averaging about 1 micron in diameter. They arrange themselves in different ways: staphylococci, responsible for infections such as boils and abscesses, are massed in bunchlike groups, whereas the streptococci that cause, for example, middle ear infections and scarlet fever, are found in chains. Gonococci, the bacteria responsible for gonorrhea, group themselves together in pairs, as do bacteria that cause some types of meningitis and pneumonia. Bacilli are rod-shaped bacteria that average about 30 microns long by 5 microns wide. Typhoid, cystitis, and tuberculosis are all caused by bacilli. The third group, called vibrio, are comma-shaped and cause cholera. The fourth

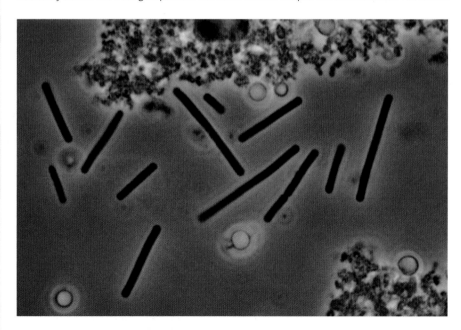

▲ *Not all bacteria are harmful; species of the bacteria* Lactobacillus *shown here are used to ferment milk to make yogurt and sour cream.*

HOW THE BODY FIGHTS BACTERIAL INFECTION

▼ *White blood cells engulf bacteria by phagocytosis: (1) the cell comes into contact with the foreign body; (2) two pseudopods are produced; and (3) join around the invader; (4) the invader is ingested and killed.*

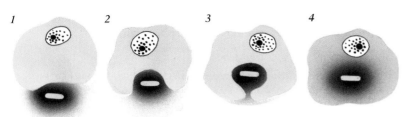

group, the spirochetes, are shaped, as their name suggests, like minute spirals. Syphilis, Lyme disease, and relapsing fever are the three best-known examples of diseases caused by spirochetes.

How they move
Apart from the cocci, which are immobile, most bacteria can move, either by waving their flagella, which are lashing hairlike processes, or, in the case of spirochetes, with twisting movements.

Bacteria are remarkable because they can reproduce without having any form of sex. In the right conditions, they multiply at great speed simply by splitting in two. At blood heat (a temperature of 98°F or 37°C) and in places rich in materials on which they can feed, they will divide in this way once every 20 minutes. In eight hours, one bacterium will multiply to produce over 16 million offspring.

When, on the other hand, conditions for growth are unfavorable, some bacteria—notably the ones that cause tetanus—react by going into a kind of hibernation state. They change into what is known as a spore, with an extra-tough outer wall. These spores are particularly dangerous, because the toughened wall is extremely difficult to destroy.

Bacteria and the human body
The body is able to cope with the presence of thousands of bacteria, because over centuries of human development a mutual tolerance has built up. It is also to the advantage of the bacteria not to kill the host that is providing them with a constant supply of nourishment. However, there are many disease-causing, or pathogenic, bacteria to which the body is susceptible.

Methods of entry
To cause disease, these bacteria must first enter the body. They do this in contaminated food or water, through wounds in the skin, or by being breathed in, especially in the minute droplets of water that are pushed out of the lungs at each breath or shot out at great pressure by coughs and sneezes by other people. Some bacteria, particularly those that cause sexually transmitted diseases, are acquired by direct person-to-person contact. Unless these bacteria gain easy access to the bloodstream through an open cut or scratch, most push their way into the tissues of the digestive, respiratory,

urinary, or genital system in order to do any damage. The bacteria must also survive the body's various defenses against infection.

Bacteria at work
When bacteria enter the blood or tissues, they do not show their effects at once. Before they can do this, they must survive a growth or incubation period—taking from a few hours up to more than a year, depending on the type.

They cause illness because they damage body tissues, as in wound infections, typhoid, meningitis, and whooping cough, by releasing powerful chemical poisons called toxins.

Toxins are the cause of food poisoning and of diseases such as tetanus. In food poisoning the toxins irritate the intestine, causing vomiting and diarrhea; in tetanus and diphtheria, they cause severe damage to the nervous system.

The body's defenses
In response to infection, the body reacts by mobilizing its defense systems. The first of these is inflammation, which means that the blood supply to the affected area is increased and the white cells in the blood try to attack and engulf the invaders within the area of the immediate infection. At the same time, the body starts making what are known as antibodies, which have the ability to attack the invaders. However, antibodies are not produced in sufficient numbers to be effective for several days. Once bacterial infection has set in, of course, medicines can also come to the body's aid. The groups of drugs called antibiotics, prescribed by doctors, are the most effective. Even after a bacterial infection has passed (and it may have been very mild), some bacteria can still be potentially harmful. People who harbor such bacteria are called carriers, and the most dangerous are carriers of typhoid and diphtheria.

Precautions
Bacterial infection can be prevented by getting rid of breeding grounds, by killing the bacteria, or through immunization. The improvement of hygiene standards in the West has done much to wipe out the dwelling places of bacteria, such as contaminated water and open sewers. Improved housing has helped eliminate the bacteria reservoirs that build up when people live together in unhygienic surroundings. These developments reduced disease dramatically in the 19th century. Even today, however, dirty handkerchiefs, sponges, and towels can still represent a paradise for bacteria.

Boiling and the ultraviolet radiation in sunlight kill most bacteria. Disinfectants can be used to get rid of bacteria on inanimate objects, and antiseptics will kill bacteria on the human body without damaging the body itself, but bacterial spores themselves can only be completely destroyed at high temperatures, produced under conditions of high pressure, as in an autoclave or other sterilizing equipment.

BACTERIAL INVASION THROUGH CUT

▲ *Here, at the site of a cut, infection may set in because the bacteria greatly outnumber the white cells.*

Handling food

Hygiene in the home and care in handling food prevent bacterial infections. However, refrigeration and freezing do not kill bacteria but just prevent them from multiplying. This is why it is essential to defrost frozen poultry thoroughly before it is cooked. If the center of the meat is still frozen, cooking will not kill harmful bacteria, since these are the perfect conditions for them to grow and multiply.

Immunization

Immunization or vaccination is available against some, but not all, bacterial infections. It works by stimulating the body to produce antibodies without actually catching the disease. If infectious bacteria do enter the body, antibodies are then mobilized immediately. The exact amount of immunization depends on the disease. For tuberculosis, the injection contains live, but altered, versions of the actual disease-producing bacteria or closely related bacteria that produce tuberculosis in animals but not in people. To prevent diseases such as whooping cough and typhoid, the injection contains bacteria that have been killed but can still stimulate antibodies. With tetanus, the toxin is produced in animals and chemically treated, so that it will then safely promote antibodies in humans.

See also: Antibiotics; Hygiene; Infection and infectious diseases

Bacterial diseases

TYPE	METHOD OF TRANSMISSION	BACTERIUM
Abscess	Through skin contact with contaminated object	Staphylococcus
Acute tonsillitis	Droplets in air	Streptococcus
Anthrax	Contact with infected animal	*Bacillus anthracis*
Bacillary dysentery	Contaminated food or water	*Shigella*
Bartonellosis	Through sand fly bite	*Bartonella*
Boils	Through skin contact with contaminated object	Staphylococcus
Botulism	Contaminated food and water	*Clostridium botulinum*
Brucellosis	Contact with infected cattle or their products	*Brucella*
Cholera	Contaminated food and water	*Vibrio cholerae*
Diphtheria	Droplets in air	*Corynebacterium diphtheriae*
Food poisoning	Contaminated food and water	*Salmonella*, staphylococcus, and others
Gastroenteritis	Contaminated food and water	*Salmonella* and others
Gonorrhea	Sexually transmitted	*Neisseria gonorrhoeae*
Hansen's disease (leprosy)	Droplets in air	*Mycobacterium leprae*
Infectious arthritis	Through wound or injury or from other infected site	Numerous organisms
Leptospirosis	Contact with infected animals or their products	*Leptospira*
Meningitis, bacterial	Droplets in air	*Hemophilus* and *Neisseria*
Middle ear infection	Droplets in air	Staphylococcus and others
Osteomyelitis	Through wound or injury or from other infected site	Staphylococcus and others
Pharyngitis	Droplets in air	Streptococcus
Plague	Contact with infected animals and droplets in air	*Yersinia pestis*
Pneumonia	Droplets in air	Pneumococcus
Relapsing fever	Lice or tick bite	*Borellia* and others
Scarlet fever	Droplets in air	Streptococcus
Syphilis	Sexually transmitted	*Treponema pallidum*
Tetanus	Contaminated soil entering wound	*Clostridium tetani*
Toxic shock syndrome	Mostly infected tampons	Staphylococcus
Tuberculosis	Droplets in air or (rarely) contaminated food	*Mycobacterium tuberculosis*
Tularemia	Contact with infected animal	*Francisella tularemia*
Typhoid	Contaminated food and water	*Salmonella*

Bedbugs

Bedbugs are so named because they bite people in bed during the night. These bugs are often thought to be a thing of the past, but in fact they are on the increase, and they can live as easily in a clean home as in a dirty one.

Bedbugs do not actually live in beds, but they do feed at night—and this is why people are likely to encounter them in bed. They spend the day in cracks in walls, furniture, or behind wallpaper, where they are difficult to find. However, they can be seen with the naked eye, especially when they huddle together in clusters.

Identifying bedbugs

It is highly unlikely that a home will be infested without the occupants knowing it. But people may come across bedbugs without recognizing them for what they are. Bedbugs are wingless, a rusty brown color, and approximately 3/16 inch (5 mm) long. If they have not fed recently, they are flat, but they swell up and become round after a meal of their chosen food—human blood—which they take by biting a small hole in the skin, then sucking out the blood.

▲ *Bedbugs feed at night on human blood. This magnified example is hungry, but when gorged, its flat body will become round and distended.*

If a bedroom is infested, the inhabitants will probably first notice a smear or two of blood on their bedding, then find they are suffering from bites. Although some people seem to be unaffected by the bites, many find them extremely uncomfortable. They can result in swollen, itchy sores, which irritate so much that it is difficult to sleep. Even if someone is one of the lucky people who do not react to bites, he or she will almost certainly be able to smell the bugs, since they produce a strong and unpleasant odor.

Although bedbug bites usually cause no more than local skin discomfort, research has shown that bedbugs can transmit relapsing fever and possibly hepatitis. Under experimental conditions they have been found capable of transmitting hepatitis B virus to nonhuman primates.

Living conditions

In the past, bedbugs were associated with slum conditions, but it is now clear that they can live in the cleanest of homes, as long as there is some nook or cranny into which they can retreat during the day. They are hardy creatures with considerable survival power. In a cold, empty house, they can survive for more than a year without food by going into a kind of hibernation. They can even live for several months at freezing point. The female lays her eggs in the cracks of walls or furniture at the rate of about three a day, and if well-fed will produce up to 100 eggs in all. These hatch after three weeks, and the creatures reach the adult stage about 12 weeks after that.

Getting rid of bedbugs

Moving out of a room infested by bedbugs is unlikely to solve the problem. Nor will moving house, because they will almost certainly be lodging in the furniture. Killing them one by one is hopeless, since too many get away. The answer is to contact a professional exterminator—through either the public health office or a commercial company. The exterminator will apply a powerful insecticide to kill all the bugs. Some bedbugs have developed a resistance to certain chemicals, so it is important to use an expert who has access to appropriate insecticides.

See also: **Bites and stings; Hygiene**

Birth defects

Around 3 percent of babies are born with a birth defect, which can occur in virtually any part of the body. This may not be surprising in view of the fact that the development of a child is a very complicated process, involving millions of cells, and there are many chances for abnormalities to occur.

Birth defects are abnormalities present at birth that are visible or detectable in the first week of life. Some, such as cleft palate, clubfoot, spina bifida, and extra fingers or toes, are obvious; but others, such as heart problems, deafness, hemophilia, phenylketonuria, or cystic fibrosis, are less easy to detect. These conditions may become apparent only through diagnostic tests such as CAT scans, X rays, blood tests, or hearing tests.

What causes birth defects?

Some birth defects are inherited and some are the result of damage sustained during birth. Others can be attributed to the effects of environmental factors or a lack of adequate nutrition during pregnancy, particularly during the first three months. The cause of about 70 percent of birth defects is unknown, however.

Environmental factors

Certain environmental factors increase the risk that a pregnant woman will have a child with a birth defect. These include exposure to radiation, an illness such as rubella during pregnancy, certain drugs, alcohol, smoking, and certain infections. Anything that causes or increases the risk of a birth defect is called a teratogen. Pregnant women should avoid smoking and drinking and should consult a physician before taking any drugs. X rays should also be avoided, but if they are absolutely necessary, the radiologist should be informed so that every care is taken to protect the fetus. If possible, women who have not had rubella (German measles) should be vaccinated against the disease before trying to conceive.

Nutritional factors

Pregnant women should eat a nutritious diet that includes the B vitamin folic acid, known to be essential for the healthy development of the fetus. A lack of folic acid increases the risk that the fetus will develop spina bifida or a similar defect. To avoid this danger women should take at least 400 micrograms of folic acid daily while trying to conceive, and during the first 12 weeks of pregnancy.

Genetic birth defects

The genes that help determine a person's physical makeup are contained within 23 pairs of chromosomes. Some birth defects occur when a fetus inherits certain genes from one or both parents. If a woman carries the gene for hemophilia, for example, she has a 1-in-2 chance of passing it on to her children. A daughter who inherits the gene will simply be a symptomless carrier, but any son who inherits it will develop the disease.

Defects may also occur if a fetus has missing or extra chromosomes, or chromosomal mutations. The older a woman is when she becomes pregnant, the greater the chance that an abnormality will occur. Symptoms caused by chromosomal abnormalities include fragile-X syndrome, which can cause mental retardation; and Down syndrome, which causes delayed physical and mental development and a characteristic physical appearance. (Also, about one-third of children with Down syndrome suffer from heart defects.) Fortunately, many chromosomal abnormalities can be detected early in pregnancy.

Common birth defects

Heart defects account for between one-third and one-fourth of all birth abnormalities. About 1 in every 120 babies will be born with some sort of abnormal formation of the walls, blood vessels, or valves of the heart. These defects may initially be discovered by a doctor hearing

Questions and Answers

How does Down syndrome occur?

Down syndrome is caused by a chromosomal abnormality in the genes of the father or, more often, the mother. People usually have 23 pairs of chromosomes. If the number, size, or arrangement of chromosomes differs from the norm, abnormalities may occur. Down syndrome occurs when the 21st chromosome makes three copies of itself instead of two. This syndrome affects one in 800 babies. Older mothers have a greater chance of giving birth to a baby with Down syndrome—20 percent are born to mothers over 35 years of age.

When I was growing up in the 1960s I saw other children my age who had short, deformed arms, and I was told that it was a birth defect. What caused this?

You are probably referring to a condition caused by a prescription drug called Thalidomide given to pregnant women in the late 1950s and early 1960s as a cure for morning sickness. Thalidomide was found to cause arms or legs, or sometimes both, to be foreshortened and malformed in almost 100 percent of babies whose mothers took the drug in their first three months of pregnancy. It started to be taken off the market in November 1961.

I am pregnant and about to travel to a country that advises visitors to get a tetanus vaccine. However, I have heard that vaccinations in pregnant women can cause birth defects in the baby. Is this true?

It depends. Vaccines such as those for tetanus and hepatitis are made from dead viruses and do not cause infection in the mother and should therefore not harm the baby. Other vaccines, however, such as MMR for measles, mumps, and rubella, could harm the baby.

an abnormal sound through a stethoscope. Ultrasound scanning, electrocardiography, and chest X rays are then used to determine exactly where the problem lies. Many heart defects can be repaired surgically, but some are too severe to be corrected—for example, if part of the heart is underdeveloped or absent.

Defects of the brain and spine are called neural tube defects and occur in about 1 in 1,000 pregnancies. These defects are often severe, causing fetal and infant deaths. Fetuses with conditions such as microcephaly (a smaller than average brain circumference), anencephaly (small or missing brain hemispheres), or hydraencephaly (water on the brain), cannot be put right through surgery; and if the babies survive, they are usually retarded. However, surgery can improve other brain defects, including hydrocephalus and encephalocele, which causes the brain to bulge out of the skull. Spinal defects cause abnormal curvatures of the neck and spine and can be treated with braces or surgery. The most common defect of the spinal cord is spina bifida, which can lead to bladder and kidney abnormalities and other physical deformities.

The body systems most frequently affected by birth defects are the kidneys and the urinary tract. Kidneys may be missing or in the wrong position or place, or they may contain abnormal tissue. The ureters, which connect the kidneys to the bladder, may be too narrow, too wide, or in the wrong place. Likewise, the bladder may be abnormally shaped or the outlet may be too narrow. Any defect that prevents urine from flowing can cause infection, kidney stones, or kidney failure. Some of these conditions can be corrected surgically; others, such as polycystic kidneys, which can cause kidney failure, can be treated only by dialysis or kidney transplant. Defects of the urethra—such as a urethral opening in the wrong place, called hypospadias in boys; or a urethra that is open rather than enclosed, a condition known as epispadias—can be corrected by surgery.

Some children are born with ambiguous genitals that are not obviously male or female. Defects may also occur along the length of the gastrointestinal tract, often causing an obstruction, but these defects can usually be corrected surgically.

Defects of the bone and muscle most commonly affect the skull, face, spine, hips, legs, and feet. The most common defects of the face are cleft lip and cleft palate. These affect about 1 in 1,000 babies but can usually be corrected surgically. Defects of the lower limbs include hip or knee dislocation and clubfoot, which can be improved using splints, orthopedic surgery, and physical therapy.

Eye defects include glaucoma—although this is relatively rare at birth—which raises pressure in the eyeballs and causes them to enlarge, and congenital cataracts. Glaucoma surgery must be performed promptly after birth to prevent blindness. Congenital cataracts are caused by chromosomal abnormalities or exposure to rubella and should be removed as quickly as possible so that the infant can develop sight.

Detection

One way of preventing birth defects is to test people with known hereditary problems to see if they carry the genes for a particular disease. They can then talk to a genetic counselor to determine what the chances are of a child's inheriting the defect before deciding if they want to risk a pregnancy.

If a woman is already pregnant, chorionic villus sampling or amniocentesis can detect a wide range of genetic defects, giving the parents vital information that will help them decide whether or not to continue the pregnancy. The volume of amniotic fluid, which surrounds the fetus in the womb, is another important indicator of birth defects. For instance, a lack of amniotic fluid may indicate a kidney problem that is slowing down the production of urine, causing the limbs and lungs of the fetus to develop abnormally. Too much amniotic fluid, on the other hand, may suggest that the fetus has a severe brain disorder. Amniocentesis and ultrasound examinations can also help detect brain and spinal cord defects.

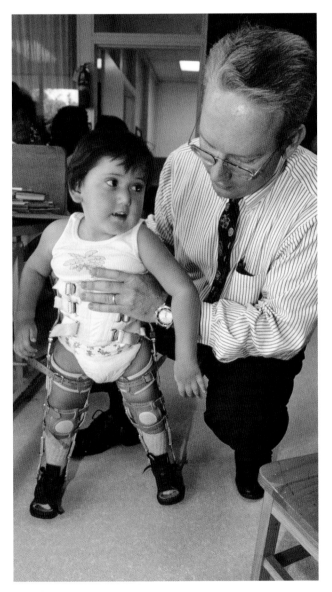

▲ *A doctor examines a child at a clinic near Brownsville, Texas, on the U.S.–Mexican border. The child is suffering from spina bifida, believed to be caused by pollution in the area.*

> **See also:** Environmental hazards; Genetics; Hemophilia; Heredity; Rubella; Vitamin B

Bites and stings

Is it all right to take an aspirin or another form of painkiller for pain relief after being stung by a wasp?

Aspirin and other forms of painkiller won't do any harm, but a soothing ointment would probably relieve the pain better. The pain should soon go away.

How can I tell the difference between a bee sting and a wasp sting?

The best method is to find the insect itself, which has probably died after stinging in self-defense. If this is impossible, remember that a wound with a stinger inside it is more likely to be a bee sting. If you have no idea whether the insect was a bee or a wasp, or indeed anything else, it is a good idea to apply a cold compress to reduce pain and swelling. If you are in real discomfort, or if the discomfort lasts for some time, see your doctor for treatment.

My son was bitten by a neighbor's dog. Should I take him to the doctor to get it checked?

Animal bites should be checked by a doctor if the skin is broken. With a severe cut, stitches may be needed. If the skin is unbroken after a bite, clean the skin and apply soothing ointment. Check that no swelling or symptoms of infection develop later.

When I was on vacation last year, a mosquito bite on my arm swelled into a big lump. Am I allergic to mosquitoes?

The bite may have been infected and then healed, or a mild allergic reaction occurred. Taking an antihistamine can help to counteract such a reaction. When a bite or sting swells a lot, get medical help as soon as possible.

Basic first aid is usually adequate for treating most bites and stings, but sometimes allergic reactions, infection at the site, or disease develop later. Any of these complications require medical help.

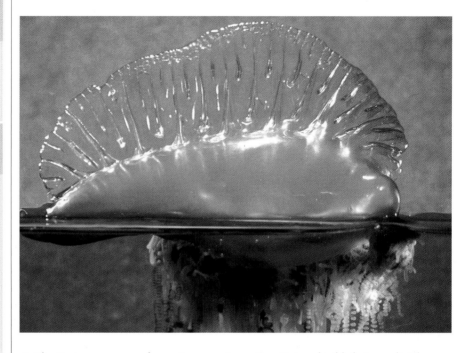

▲ *The Portuguese man-of-war gives a serious sting. Get medical help immediately.*

Many insects, some plants, and some marine creatures can sting. Many animals and insects and some reptiles can bite. In some countries, poisonous insects are dangerous. Deaths from such bites or stings are rare, but prompt action is important. The victim should be taken at once to the nearest hospital or poison control center with the dead insect or animal, if possible, or a good description of it, because this will help identify the appropriate treatment. When traveling abroad, it is best to obtain information about harmful pests beforehand. Recommended inoculations and other precautions should be taken.

Keeping pests away
The greatest risk of being bitten or stung comes from insects, such as bees or hornets; parasites, such as mosquitoes or fleas; and creatures, such as venom-secreting snails and jellyfish. Keep unwanted insect visitors out of the house by using screens and maintaining a general level of cleanliness.

Any bite or sting can lead to infection, so you must always clean the wound thoroughly. Warm water and soap make the best cleanser. If possible, the soap should not contain a detergent, perfume, or other similar irritants.

After cleaning, the wound should be rinsed in clear water. If you have an antiseptic, it can now be applied.

Remember to check the bottle for the correct dilution of a disinfectant or similar substance.

Cover the clean wound with a dry, sterile dressing or a laundered handkerchief. If there is increased pain and inflammation over the next day or two, infection has set in and you must see your doctor.

During hot, damp weather, when insects breed most rapidly, a hanging insecticide will kill winged insects for several months. In the backyard, if mosquitoes are a problem, drain stagnant water. When picnicking on grass, always sit on a ground cloth, and avoid eating sweet, sticky foods, which attract wasps. It is best not to sit too close to flowers where bees gather. A swarm of bees, wasps, or hornets should never be approached—an expert should be called. At the beach, learn to recognize stinging jellyfish and poisonous snails.

Insects living in gardening clothes or shoes normally kept outside are a common source of stings. Shake gardening clothes and boots before putting them on, in case there is anything lurking in them.

Domestic pets

Dogs should be obedience-trained to reduce the risk of their biting people. Other people's pets should not be touched until they have had a chance to get to know you, and you them.

Children should be taught to treat all animals with caution, respect, and kindness—household pets should not be treated like toys. Mauled kittens, puppies, and even hamsters can turn into potentially dangerous biters through abuse. Special care should be

taken when dealing with guard dogs, such as German shepherds, rottweilers, Doberman pinschers, and bull terriers. Children should be taught to stay away from them.

Bee stings

Bee stings can cause severe pain and are among the most dangerous of stings in temperate climates. Young children, old people, and people who are prone to allergies are particularly vulnerable to unpleasant results from bee stings. When a bee stings the flesh, the puncture area will be surrounded by a pale area of skin, and then a reddish area, which is usually swollen into a bump. The black stinger embedded in the center can often be seen. This should be scraped away gently using something firm like the edge of a credit card or a fingernail. Do not use tweezers, because pinching the stinger releases more venom. A bee sting has acid venom, so once the stinger has been removed and the wound cleaned, it should be treated with a paste of baking soda or diluted ammonia. If these are not available, rubbing alcohol or a cold compress can be used. The victim should rest during treatment. Be on the lookout for signs of shock. If there are multiple bee stings, a doctor should be called immediately.

Common bites and stings

SOURCE	PREVENTION	FIRST AID	LATER TREATMENT
Jellyfish and similar creatures	Do not swim in water where jellyfish or similar creatures are known to live.	Get victim to shore and pick off jellyfish tentacles with care. Cleanse sting, and take antihistamine.	Seek medical help, especially for the sting of Portuguese man-of-war.
Dog bites	Avoid strange dogs and train your own dog not to bite.	Wash and dress the wound and see your doctor if the skin is broken.	Stitches or tetanus shot. Treatment for rabies may be required.
Lice	Keep hair and body clean; comb hair with a fine-tooth comb daily.	For head lice, wash hair with insecticide shampoo or cream rinse. For body lice, boil linen and take daily hot baths; then put on clean clothes treated with powder.	Continue treatment until all lice and nits (eggs) have vanished.
Mosquitoes	Cover yourself after dark. Avoid stagnant water. Burn a mosquito stick by the bed. Apply insect repellent.	Take antihistamine, or apply rubbing alcohol; cologne or cold water will do if these are not available. Repeat.	Avoid scratching. Take antihistamine tablets if swelling is severe.
Ants	Do not sit on uncovered grass or disturb ants' nests.	Treat stings with baking-soda paste or dilute ammonia.	None is usually necessary.
Ticks	Check for ticks on scalp and body after walking in wooded areas. Keep dogs and cats free of ticks.	If the tick is embedded in the skin, use petroleum jelly, oil, or alcohol to suffocate it then remove it carefully with tweezers. Kill harvest mite ticks with weak ammonia.	Soothe tick bites with calamine lotion. Treatment for rickettsial infection, ehrlichia infection, and lyme disease may be required.
Fleas	Keep dogs and cats free of fleas.	Treat bites with calamine or take antihistamine. Badly affected children should see a doctor.	Use a suitable powder on animals, clothes, bedding, and cushions.
Poison ivy, oak, or sumac	Teach children to recognize and avoid poison plants.	Wash area of contact immediately with soap and water.	Itchy rash may be coated with calamine or topical steroid cream from the drugstore.

Stings in the mouth are also dangerous because swelling can prevent proper breathing. The patient should be given a mouthwash of one teaspoon of baking soda to a glass of water, followed by ice to suck. Then he or she should be taken to the hospital, along with the dead bee, if it can be found.

Wasp stings

When a person is stung by a wasp, the puncture may or may not contain a black stinger. If the stinger can be seen, it should be carefully taken out with tweezers or a sterilized needle. It should not be squeezed, as this might push the venom further into the skin. The surrounding area will be whitish, then red and probably swollen.

Wasp stings contain alkali venom. After cleansing, the wound should be dressed with vinegar or lemon juice, as the acid content neutralizes the venom. Rubbing should be avoided.

If no vinegar or lemon juice is available, antihistamine can be taken; then the wound can be washed and dressed again. If the swelling is severe, a cold compress should be added.

If there are multiple wasp stings and the person is in shock, a doctor must be called or the patient brought to the hospital. The patient should be put on his or her side and given ice to suck in the meantime. With a single wasp sting, the patient should start to feel better after an hour or so.

Snakebites

There are at least 20 species of venomous coral snakes and pit vipers in North America alone, and Australia is home to several varieties including the world's most poisonous snake, the inland taipan. Bites from many species are extremely dangerous, although few need be fatal if medical attention is obtained promptly.

If a person is bitten by an unidentified snake, it is best to assume that the snake was poisonous. First aid should include applying a broad constricting band to the bitten limb. This is not the same as a tourniquet and should be tight enough only to interfere with the venous return of blood to the heart, not with the arterial flow from the heart.

It is important to act fast in cases of snakebite. Attempting to suck out the poison may not work, and time should not be spent on this. If the snake can be killed easily, it is advisable to do so, and to take it along to the hospital to aid in identification. However, it should be remembered that even a dead snake can reflexively inflict a venomous bite. The bitten limb should be immobilized, and the victim should be transported to the hospital without delay.

First-aid essentials
Antiseptic wipes for use in the absence of soap and water
Antiseptic cream
Calamine lotion
Antihistamine
Aspirin

Spider bites

There are thousands of different kinds of spiders throughout the world, some deadly and others harmless. Two dangerous spiders live in parts of the United States: the female black widow spider and the brown recluse spider.

The black widow spider inhabits dark corners of sheds, cellars, and woodpiles. Its body is about 0.5 inch (1 cm) in diameter, with a red or yellow hourglass mark on the abdomen that serves as a warning to predators. The bite may be felt as a sharp prick or it may be painless, but the poison travels quickly through the body. The victim soon develops severe stomach cramps and the entire abdomen becomes stiff. Other symptoms may include nausea, vomiting, delirium, and convulsions. On rare occasions, the victim dies. Treatment includes an antivenin injection and some painkillers.

The brown recluse spider is slightly smaller than the black widow spider and has a white, violin-shaped marking on its back. It lives mainly in tree bark or under stones but sometimes makes its way into cellars or closets. The area around the bite becomes swollen and tender. After around 12 hours, the victim develops a fever, with chills and vomiting. Later a rash develops, and the bite becomes extremely painful. Treatment includes powerful painkillers, antihistamines, and antibiotics.

Sea urchin stings

Sea urchins are found in many coastal waters and in some countries are considered good to eat. However, their spikes can break off in human skin, causing intense pain and the risk of infection, so it is wise to avoid swimming near them. If a sea urchin is stepped on or touched, a sharp burning pain will be felt and the area where the spine broke the skin will be numb. The spine should be removed from the skin; it is essential to wear gloves for this to prevent a further wound. The wound should be covered with a dry dressing—a clean handkerchief will do—and a doctor seen as soon as possible.

It is necessary to see a doctor because of the high risk of infection from a sea urchin sting. The victim should be kept quiet and still during the journey to the hospital, and measures should be taken immediately if signs of shock occur.

Shock

Shock can result from a bite or sting when the victim also has a severe allergy or experiences extreme pain or deep emotional stress, such as fear. In most cases, shock victims recover well within an hour or so. But because shock can be dangerous, and even fatal in some cases, it is important to be able to recognize it when it occurs, and treat it correctly while waiting for the doctor. The symptoms of shock are pale skin, restlessness, confusion, anxiety, quickened pulse, and rapid breathing. The victim may complain of thirst and may vomit or even lose consciousness. The treatment is to lay the victim flat on his or her back, raise the feet 8–12 inches (20–30 cm), and cover him or her with a coat or blanket. The bitten area should not be elevated, and the victim should not be placed in this position if there are suspected head, neck, back, or leg injuries. Stop any bleeding that would make shock worse and loosen tight clothing, such as a collar, waistband, or belt. Drinks should not be given, and the victim should not be kept too warm. Medical help should be sought quickly.

See also: Rabies; Shock

Blisters

Blisters can be extremely painful, but if left alone, most will heal by themselves. If a blister becomes badly infected, however, or is the symptom of another illness, medical treatment may be required.

The skin has two layers. The outer one, the epidermis, consists of layers of mainly dead skin cells and contains no nerve cells or blood vessels. The deeper one, the dermis, contains both vessels and nerves. When fluid collects between the two layers, a blister forms. A small, well-defined buildup of fluid is called a vesicle; larger ones, often up to 3 inches (7.5 cm) across, are called bullae.

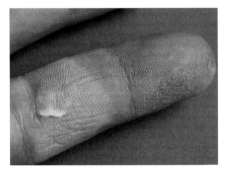

▲ *The blister on this finger was covered with an adhesive bandage for protection.*

Causes

The most common cause of blisters is friction. Rubbing or chafing produces friction and heat, and in response, a blister forms. New shoes can chafe areas of tender skin, and walking long distances will often raise blisters. A person unused to heavy manual labor can get blisters within 30 minutes of beginning work. On the other hand, someone accustomed to manual labor who has thickened skin can work for many hours without any trouble.

All types of burns, including severe sunburn, can raise blisters. The heat and damage to the deep layer of the skin causes an almost immediate outflow of fluid from the blood capillaries, which then lies in the form of blisters under the skin. Sunburn blisters tend to be small and numerous; the skin will start to peel a few days later.

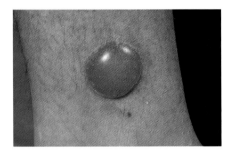

▲ *This blister on a woman's leg is the result of an insect bite.*

Tiny blisters may also form around the site of an acutely inflamed insect bite or jellyfish sting. In more severe cases, large blisters may form, or blisters may become infected and fill with pus.

Another common cause of blisters is the inflammation produced by viruses. Chicken pox in children and shingles in adults are caused by the same virus. Shingles blisters are usually confined to one area of the body and may be painful and uncomfortable. Medical attention should be sought, particularly if the patient's eyes or ears are affected. Chicken pox blisters are far more widespread, covering the trunk and back, and in severe cases the scalp, the inside of the mouth, the ears, and the genitals. They may cause intense itching. When healing, both types of blisters burst. Scabs are then formed, which eventually fall off. The virus that causes smallpox, another blister-producing condition, is no longer active in any part of the world. The herpes simplex virus, which can live within the deep layer of the skin, produces blisters called cold sores. These appear on the lips or side of the mouth after a cold. If the cold is severe or the skin is exposed to too much sunlight, the virus will multiply, and crops of blisters will form. Bacterial infections can also produce blisters. In impetigo, the bacteria breed quickly in the deep layer of the skin. Small blisters form, usually on the hands, legs, or face; these soon burst and form crusty, yellow-brown scabs.

In rare cases medical conditions, such as deep vein thrombosis or severe edema caused by heart failure, will produce blistering. More commonly, blisters that result from skin conditions, such as allergic eczema or chemical irritation, will appear without any history of rubbing or burning. Medical treatment is needed in these instances. Two other conditions produce blisters.

How to avoid blisters on hands

DO	DON'T
Wear soft, thick gloves.	Don't work with abrasive materials, such as bricks, without wearing gloves.
Change grip, and put a bandage on the hand when blisters appear.	Don't let caustic substances, such as mortar, to come into contact with hands.
Harden skin with methylated spirit three times a day for three weeks before doing heavy manual work.	Don't grip tools loosely, since this allows more movement and friction.

How to avoid blisters on feet

DO	DON'T
Wear well-fitting footwear. Too tight a shoe causes pressure. Too loose a shoe produces friction where the foot slides inside.	Don't wear new shoes for the first time on a long walk. Break them in gradually.
Wear comfortable, substantial footwear for long-distance walking.	Don't choose walking shoes with internal ridges or ankle supports that rub.
Wear additional wool socks in rigid walking boots.	Don't walk in sandals with tight, thin straps or flip-flops, where the shoe is held on only by a single strand between the toes.
Choose soft socks without ridges.	Don't wear old, hard socks for walking; clean, soft, wool socks are ideal.
Wash and powder feet regularly.	

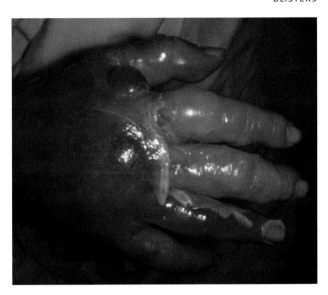

▲ *This severe burn has penetrated to the more sensitive lower dermis layer of the skin, causing what is known as a second-degree burn and painful blistering.*

skin. Chicken pox begins as small, dark red pimples, which within a few hours turn into blisters that look like droplets of water. Where there are multiple blisters with no symptoms, the cause is more likely to be eczema. With large blisters, pemphigoid or pemphigus may be the cause, particularly if the blisters arise painlessly, with little or no attendant itching.

The common friction blister is rarely dangerous, but in other types of blister there is a danger of infection. Bacteria can enter and breed, forming pustules, which delay healing or spread infection. If large areas of the skin are blistered, there is also a risk that the body will become fluid-deficient, causing the patient to become seriously ill.

Treatment

Blisters filled with blood should not be burst, and other blisters should be burst by a doctor only if they are painful or large. Small blisters are usually reabsorbed, but large blisters generally burst on their own. To treat a friction blister, cool and clean the area. If it is small, cover it with an adhesive bandage. If new shoes have caused the problem, pad the area with cotton. If the friction has ceased, friction blisters will heal within three or four days. A new epidermis will develop, and hard pads may form. If there is further friction, release some fluid using a sterile needle, before recovering and repadding the area.

Medical treatment is required for blisters caused by skin inflammations or other illnesses. Antiviral lotions may help in virus infections such as shingles; bacterial infections, such as impetigo, require antibiotic treatment. The blisters should heal once the cause has been treated, but with chicken pox, new crops may develop while the virus is still alive. Pemphigus is a chronic condition and is controlled by the use of steroid drugs, which should be taken only under medical supervision.

Pemphigoid causes blistering on the forearms of elderly people, and though the blisters rarely spread or are harmful, they do require some treatment. Pemphigus is a rare but potentially fatal blistering disease. It is an autoimmune disorder in which there is a defect in a type of protein (desmosome protein) that forms adhesion sites between adjacent cells. It can be of genetic origin or acquired, and onset is usually in middle age. The condition requires urgent treatment with steroids.

Symptoms

The common friction blister causes feelings of heat and pain, and by the time these have been noticed, a blister will have formed. Similarly, a blister arising from a direct burn will appear a few minutes after the accident. Blisters from stings and bites appear more slowly and cause itching and a swelling of the surrounding

See also: **Bacteria; Burns; Sunburn; Viruses**

Body structure

On average, men are 6 in. (15 cm) taller than women and have several internal differences in body structure. Most men have larger hearts and lungs than women, made of 42 percent muscle, compared with 36 percent in women. A woman's body contains about 4 percent less water than a man's, because she has more fat beneath the skin, and fat is a water-free substance.

Is it true that some people have their appendix on the wrong side?

Yes, some people are born with their appendix on the left rather than the right side of the body. Such people have transposition of the whole intestine, a condition known as situs inversus. Their hearts also tend to be reversed so that the apex points to the right rather than to the left. This is called dextrocardia.

My husband and I are both much taller than average. Does this mean that our son will be tall too?

The environment as well as genes has a great effect on height. Your son will probably be taller than average, but his final height will also depend on his diet and the proper functioning of many of his internal organs.

Your son will not grow properly if his diet is deficient in proteins or the mineral calcium, which is needed for building bones. Even with a perfect diet, his growth would be retarded if he had something wrong with his supply of the growth hormone, somatrophin. This is a substance that is necessary if his body is to be able to use the food he eats to enlarge his bones and other internal body structures.

Many people find the human body a fascinating subject, but for a better understanding of the discoveries made about it, a working knowledge of its structure is required.

Structure simply means the way something is put together. In the case of the human body it is possible to talk about an enormously complicated structure by reducing its many parts to a set of simple labels, or medical shorthand. Doctors must do this when they talk to each other. They may say something about a skeletal defect or problems with the digestive system, and unless the patient understands what a doctor means, being treated for an illness can be a mystifying experience. Some of the terms in this basic shorthand are concerned with differences such as race, but most terms make up a picture of what every human body is like under the skin.

For purposes of classification people can be divided into three large groups, or races: the Mongoloids, Negroids, and Caucasians. Each of these groups has certain structural characteristics, and each, in turn, can be divided into many subgroups. People of the Mongoloid group are typified by their yellow skin, straight black hair, and eyes with folded lids that give the eye an almond-shaped appearance. The Mongoloid body has little hair, and the height of the average male ranges from 5 feet 2 inches (1.57 m) to 5 feet 8 inches (1.73 m). The Chinese and the Inuit are typical Mongoloid types.

BODY CAVITIES AND URINARY SYSTEM

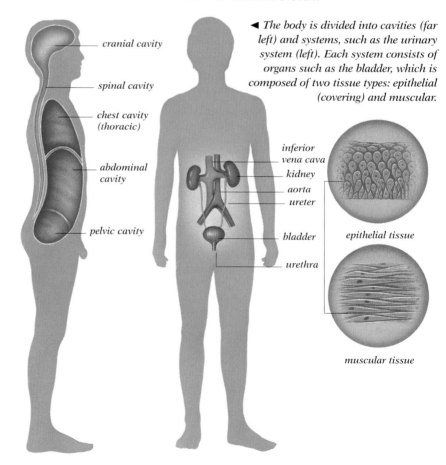

◄ The body is divided into cavities (far left) and systems, such as the urinary system (left). Each system consists of organs such as the bladder, which is composed of two tissue types: epithelial (covering) and muscular.

cranial cavity

spinal cavity

chest cavity (thoracic)

abdominal cavity

pelvic cavity

inferior vena cava

kidney

aorta

ureter

bladder

urethra

epithelial tissue

muscular tissue

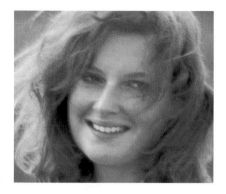

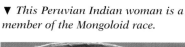

▼ *This Peruvian Indian woman is a member of the Mongoloid race.*

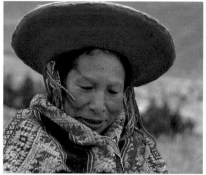

▲ *This Caucasian female has the pale skin of the Nordic group of the race.*

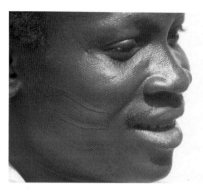

▲ *This man from Nigeria is a Yoruba, one of the groups of the Negroid race.*

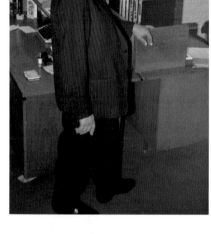

▲ *An endomorph tends to have excess body weight and a rounded build.*

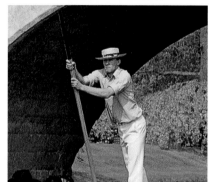

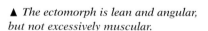

▲ *The ectomorph is lean and angular, but not excessively muscular.*

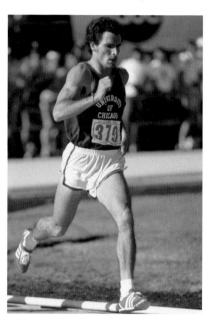

▲ *This athlete is a prime example of the muscular mesomorph.*

Negroids have brown to black skin and woolly hair. Like Mongoloids, they have very little body hair, and they have broad noses, although the Mongoloid nose is narrower at the base. Negroids vary in height—from the Bushmen, averaging 4 feet 8 inches (1.42 m), to the Nilotes, whose adult males average 5 feet 10 inches (1.78 m). Most African Americans are classified as Negroids.

Caucasians, the so-called white races of the world, are actually very mixed, with skin colors ranging from the brown of Indian peoples to the pale coloring of the Nordic (meaning generally found in the north) subdivisions of the race. Their hair may be any shade of brown, black, red, or blond. The body of a Caucasian male is much more hairy than that of members of the other two races, and the face and nose are narrower. One of the least variable Caucasian features is average height, which ranges (for the adult male) from 5 feet 3 inches (1.6 m) in Mediterranean peoples to 5 feet 8 inches (1.73 m) in Nordic types. As well as these three major groupings and their subdivisions, there are many mixed, or composite, races.

Shape

People can also be divided into three groups according to their body shape: endomorph, ectomorph, or mesomorph. A typical endomorph is heavily built and well rounded, with a higher than average proportion of body fat and a tendency toward obesity. The ectomorph is lean and angular with less fat and muscle than average and is capable of a high degree of physical endurance. The mesomorph is muscular and agile—having the typical athlete's body shape—and is the strongest of the three. Not everyone conforms exactly to a standard pattern—most people are a mixture of all three—but each person has an overall leaning toward one of the three body shapes.

Each body type tends be associated with a certain behavior pattern. Extreme endomorphs tend to be very relaxed, with a slow heartbeat and breathing rate. They are tolerant and good company but are inclined to overindulge in food and drink. Extreme ectomorphs are the exact opposite. Hypersensitive and very aware of everything that is happening, they tend to react quickly to new situations. But they are likely to be obsessive and easily thrown off balance by personal setbacks. Between the two are the mesomorphs, who are typically dominating, aggressive, and successful.

Body systems

Whatever a person's race or shape, the body is divided into four sections: the neck and head; the chest or thoracic cavity, which contains the heart and lungs; the abdomen, housing the alimentary canal, kidneys, liver, and various other organs; and the limbs. To understand how these parts link up and work together, the body can be studied as systems—groups of organs that work together. One of these is the digestive system; others include the nervous and reproductive systems. Each organ is made up of tissues formed from cells. These tissues are complex collections of chemicals, including such components as the chromosomes that carry the genes. Many of the body organs have familiar names, such as the adenoids, appendix, or tongue, but the tissues are less well-known. There are four main types, and each organ contains at least one of them. Epithelial tissues cover or line body organs and may secrete substances such as hormones. Connective tissues—which include bones and tendons—link, support, and fill out body structures, including the blood. Muscle tissue enables the body and internal parts to move. Nervous tissue helps the body parts to work in harmony by providing communication and control.

Body fluids

About 60 percent of the body is made up of water, or body fluids, but these are not like tap water. Body water contains a huge variety of dissolved salts that make it more like seawater—where the first living things evolved. A 154-pound (70-kg) man contains an average of 18.5 pints (8.7 l) of body fluids. Of these, 12.5 pints (5.9 l) are inside the cells and are called intracellular fluids. The other 6 pints (2.8 l) are extracellular fluids. Of these, 1.3 pints (0.6 l) are in the blood plasma. The remaining 4.7 pints (2.2 l) are divided between the interstitial fluid, which bathes the cells and body cavities; the lymph fluid; the fluid around the spine and in the joints; and the fluid in places such as the eyes. All this fluid moves constantly in and out of the cells. The body's fluid is even more important to survival than food. It is essential for carrying oxygen, food substances, and hormones around the body and getting rid of wastes. The body maintains a constant check on its fluid level, and if this level becomes too low, endangering body functioning, the water-monitoring center in the brain generates a sensation of thirst, so the person drinks to rebalance body fluids.

See also: **Genetics; Heredity**

A guide to body systems		
SYSTEM	**MAJOR ORGANS**	**MAJOR TISSUES IN TYPICAL ORGAN**
Digestive	Mouth, teeth, tongue, salivary glands, esophagus (tube from back of throat to stomach), stomach, small and large intestines, anus, liver, gallbladder, pancreas	Stomach—epithelial, muscular
Urinary	Kidneys, ureters (tubes joining the kidneys and bladder), bladder, urethra	Bladder—epithelial, muscular
Muscular	All body muscles, some under conscious control (skeletal or striped muscles), others working unconsciously (smooth muscles)	Biceps muscle—muscular, connective
Skeletal	All the body's bones and the connecting joints	Connective
Respiratory	Lungs, bronchi (tubes to lungs), trachea (windpipe), mouth, larynx (voice box), nose, diaphragm	Lungs—epithelial, connective
Circulatory	Heart, arteries, veins, capillaries, blood	Heart—muscular
Nervous	Brain, sense organs (eyes, ears, taste buds, smell and touch receptors), nerves, spinal cord	Nervous
Endocrine	Hormone-producing glands: pituitary, thyroid, parathyroid, adrenals, pancreas, thymus, parts of testes and ovaries, and small areas of tissue in the intestine	Pancreas—epithelial, connective
Reproductive (male)	Testes, penis, prostate gland, seminal vesicles, urethra	Penis—muscular, vascular
Reproductive (female)	Ovaries, fallopian tubes, uterus (womb), cervix (neck of womb), vagina	Uterus—muscular, epithelial
Immune	Structures involved in the body's defense against disease, including lymph nodes, lymph vessels, spleen, tonsils, adenoids, thymus (gland in chest)	Spleen—connective, epithelial

WHAT WE ARE MADE OF

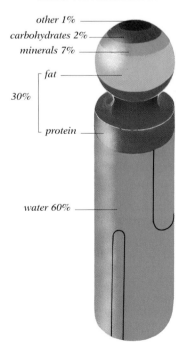

other 1%
carbohydrates 2%
minerals 7%
fat
30%
protein
water 60%

Bruises

If a person is hit by a blunt or solid object, bruising usually occurs around the site of the blow. Severe bruising can lead to complications, but most bruises, although painful at first, will disappear within a few days.

A bruise, the result of damage to surface blood vessels, is a patch of dark or discolored skin. If the skin is unbroken, the bruise is known technically as a contusion. However, if it is more extensive, leading to the formation of a clotted lump of blood beneath the skin, it is called a hematoma.

Bruising can happen as the result of any sudden contact with a solid or blunt object. A single bump will result in a single contusion; the violent impact of a car accident, for example, could cause multiple bruises. If an accident occurs, causing bruising, the force may damage the small blood vessels—the capillaries—within the lining of the skin. If an even greater force is applied, small veins may be broken. This, in turn, could lead to the more massive form of bruising, a hematoma.

Symptoms

When a capillary breaks, blood oozes out—it is this internal bleeding that gives bruised skin its familiar dark-red color. Any bluish tinge is partly caused by a loss of oxygen in the red blood cells, although the thickness of the skin can also distort the color.

The puffiness of bruises is caused by the release of the serous fluid (white blood cells and platelets) in plasma. The platelets initiate a process called coagulation or clotting. This limits the spread of the bruise and produces fibrin, a substance that helps plug the leaking blood vessels. A bruise takes between three and 14 days to clear, changing from reddish blue to greenish blue, and then yellow. These color changes arise from the body's efforts to reclaim the blood that has leaked into the tissues. It is this process that causes the bruise to slowly fade.

Treatment

Small bruises are best left to heal on their own. The only exception is a bruise under a toe- or fingernail, a condition known as subungeal hematoma. In this case medical advice should be sought because the end bone under the nail (the terminal phalanx) could be broken. The doctor may decide to release blood from under the nail, so relieving pain and reducing the risk of infection. When bruises occur with open wounds or lie over bony structures such as the skull and ribs, they may conceal a fracture. In the case of bruises to the face and scalp especially, it is always advisable to consult the doctor to rule out any underlying fracture or other damage.

For a contusion, first aid in the form of gentle compression to the injury, using either an ice pack or a cloth soaked in cold water, will limit the pain and swelling if applied quickly. Painkillers such as acetaminophen will ease discomfort and help reduce bruising. Aspirin, which is an anticlotting agent, should be avoided, since it can delay the healing process.

Larger bruises that result in hematoma should be seen by a doctor, who may decide to release the pressure of the blood by simple surgery. This will deprive bacteria in the damaged tissue of any nourishment. Failure to treat a boxer's hematoma can lead to a deformity called cauliflower ear.

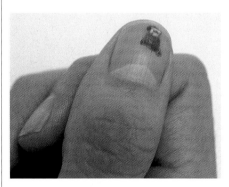

▲ *Sometimes, a bruised fingernail may cover a small broken bone.*

See also: **Aspirin and analgesics; Bacteria; Fractures; Hemophilia; Infection and infectious diseases; Vitamin C**

Burns

Questions and Answers

My mother always believed in putting butter or olive oil on a burn she got while cooking. Is either any good as a burn dressing?

No. Both oil and butter act as food for bacteria, which can develop and increase the risk of infecting the burn. For the same reason, you should never use ointments on burns; use clean, dry dressings on their own instead.

How do I know when a burn is serious enough that I should call a doctor or go to a hospital?

If in any doubt, seek medical help immediately, particularly for burns on the face or genitals, over a joint, or in the mouth or throat; burns larger than 3 sq. in. (20 cm²); burns that are wet and oozing; burns that continue to hurt in spite of first aid; burns caused by electricity; and burns in someone very young or old.

I read that it is not a good idea to drive a burn victim to the hospital yourself. Wouldn't this save time?

Not if you were stopped by the police on the way—remember, you do not have the same priority in traffic as an ambulance. Besides, your patient may need to be lying down and could vomit or lose consciousness as you drive, when you couldn't do anything to help.

Should I see a doctor if I get sunburned on vacation?

Yes, if the sunburn is severe or is combined with sunstroke. You should take care to get used to the sun gradually if you are fair-skinned or unused to strong sunlight. You can even get sunburned on ice and snow on a mountaintop, owing to the reflected ultraviolet radiation from the sun. Also, if you are on a beach, the sun is more intense near the sea and sand than elsewhere.

The best way to deal with burns is to take all the necessary precautions to prevent them. However, if an accident does happen, knowing what to do could mean the difference between life and death.

Every day, countless people die from or are severely injured by burns. Although it is generally assumed that the main cause is fire, burns can also result from touching hot objects or be caused by scalding, harsh friction, electric shock, or accidental contact with corrosive chemicals. The injury can be even greater if the victims are either very young or old. Very old people have the poorest chance of recovery from severe burns, but children are also vulnerable, especially toddlers who do not understand the dangers involved in playing with fire.

Lesser burns

A burn is classified medically according to the depth that it reaches in the skin. There are three types: these are usually referred to as first-, second-, and third-degree burns. In the first group, also called superficial partial-thickness burns, the epidermis (outer layer) of the skin is destroyed and the dermis (thicker, underlying tissues) may also be affected. But the hair follicles, sweat glands, and basic structure remain to form a basis for the growth of healthy new skin. The minor burns that happen in the kitchen or from sunburn fall into this category. The pain will stop within a few days, and the skin will soon recover. Sometimes a blister is formed; this protects the underlying wound from infection and should not be pricked. All the affected part needs is to be covered with a clean, dry dressing and allowed to heal.

More serious burns

In the second group—deep partial-thickness burns—all but the deepest cells, hair follicles, and glands are destroyed. With this type of burn, healing is slow, and the new skin that is produced is likely to be rough and not as elastic as before.

The most serious type of burn is classified as a third-degree burn. Here the whole thickness burns, completely destroying the cellular structure of the skin; there is nothing from which the new skin can reform, unless it is at the very edges of the burn. In this event healing is extremely

SKIN DEPTHS OF FIRST-, SECOND-, AND THIRD-DEGREE BURNS

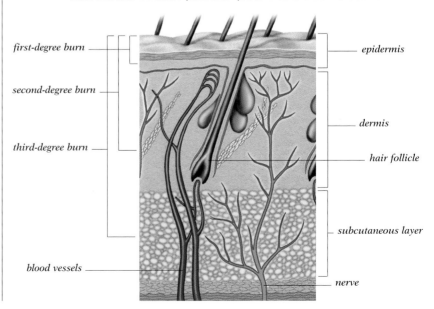

first-degree burn

second-degree burn

third-degree burn

blood vessels

epidermis

dermis

hair follicle

subcutaneous layer

nerve

TREATING BURNS

▼ *The first treatment for every burn is to cool it off. For scalds, remove any clothing that has become hot from boiling fluid, fat, or steam. However, if the clothing has already cooled, do not remove it.*

▼ *A chemical burn can be very nasty, so quickly remove any soaked clothing without touching the chemical yourself. Immediately wash away the chemical by flooding the area with water for at least ten minutes.*

▼ *An electrical burn requires fast action. Do not touch the victim until you have switched off the current. If this is impossible, call the power company or 911 immediately. Do not touch anything in contact with a downed wire.*

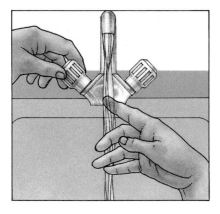

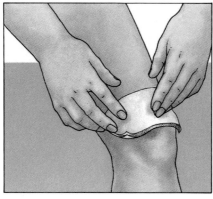

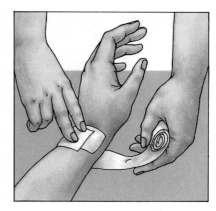

Always begin by cooling the burn. Heat from a burn can cause major damage that penetrates deep into the body. Applying cold water helps reduce this effect. A small part, like a fingertip or wrist, can be held under a running tap; a larger area should be plunged into a bucket or sink full of cold water.

Areas like the face or chest that cannot be kept under water should be covered by a thick cloth soaked in cold water for at least ten minutes. This quickly relieves pain and reduces the formation of blisters. If the cloth gets warm and dry, renew cold water and reapply. If much pain persists, repeat the procedure.

A large burn or a burn on the face should be covered with a nonfluffy dry dressing after cooling. Use the inside of a sterile surgical dressing or a clean handkerchief, handling it as little as possible. Do not apply lotion or ointment, and avoid touching the burn. Cover with more folded padding, and bandage loosely.

slow and uncertain. The whole area is more or less free of pain because the nerve endings have been destroyed. But pain cannot be entirely absent, for at the edges of the burn there are likely to be some areas where nerve endings remain.

The loss of plasma (the colorless, liquid part of the blood) is one of the major problems with severe burns. Burns can form blisters that are filled with plasma which oozes out from the damaged blood vessels in the surrounding area. The blood cells are left behind. From this point of view, the area covered by a burn is more significant than the depth. Plasma, although it is colorless and without its cells, is still blood fluid, and a dramatic drop in its volume contributes to the condition known as shock. To make matters worse, the remaining blood in the body is now thicker, since its cells are concentrated in a smaller amount of plasma—this increases the difficulties of the heart, which may already be under stress.

Another problem is that a surface coating of plasma on the wound makes infection by bacteria much more likely. A great deal of protein is also lost, together with the plasma.

Hospital treatment

Deep and extensive burns require hospital treatment. Relief of pain is, of course, important, but the primary concern is to combat shock.

The percentage of skin area that has been burned is also an important factor in deciding what treatment is to be given—for example, the back or front of the trunk represents 18 percent of the whole surface of the body, while a hand represents 1 percent.

A transfusion is likely to be needed when the burned area represents more than 15 percent of the total skin surface in an adult or more than 10 percent in a child. The fluid is generally plasma, but sometimes whole blood is included to replace red blood cells that have been destroyed. Also, the patient's general condition must be closely watched, as the burned area will have lost much of its natural defense against bacteria. Not only does infection delay healing; it also increases the risk of disfigurement from scarring, and scars may contract and interfere with the movement of any joint they overlie. Antibiotics will be prescribed to combat any infection and thereby help the healing process.

A partial-thickness burn is generally allowed to heal spontaneously, either by being left exposed or by being covered with a dressing. Healing may take between two and three months.

A full-thickness burn will not mend in this way, because the regenerating tissue has been destroyed. The dead material eventually separates off as dark, hard slough, leaving a raw area below. Frequently, it has to be helped off gently by doctors and nurses, and a skin graft will be necessary to close up the wound.

When a skin graft is performed, small pieces of skin are removed from another part of the patient's body (usually from a place that is ordinarily covered by clothing). This healthy skin is implanted into the burned area and gradually grows to reform a new skin surface. Skin grafting demands several months of skillful care; and it is especially important to ensure that the grafted skin does not contract, since contracting can affect the joint below.

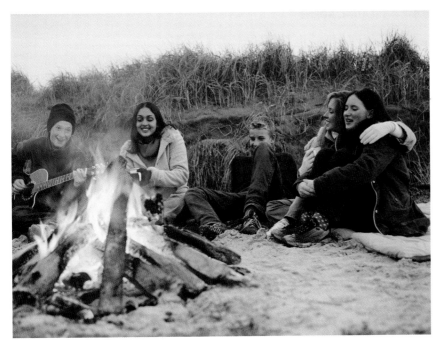

▲ *People often congregate around a campfire to keep warm, but care should be taken. If a person is standing too close to the flames, any loose clothing can catch fire. In such cases, douse the flames with water or smother them with a heavy material.*

Preventing fires and burns

Smoking: Stub out cigarettes thoroughly in ashtray. Do not throw cigarette stubs into a wastepaper basket. Do not smoke in bed or near inflammable material—for instance, in a garage.

Cooking: Light match before turning on gas tap. Never hang cloths over oven. Fill deep fryer no more than halfway and watch constantly; have large metal lid handy to smother flames in case of fire, and keep fire blanket by cooker for same purpose. Never put a hand in front of steam from kettle.

Heating: Have sturdy fireguards. Sweep chimneys regularly. Do not use paraffin or gasoline to light fires. Keep rugs away from fireplace. Ban toys from mantelpiece, and never place mirror on wall above fire. Be sure oil heaters are firmly based, and don't fill or carry them when they are lit.

Clothes: Beware of light cotton fabrics. Buy flameproof nightwear for children and old people.

Wiring: Replace frayed electric wires, loose connections, and trailing leads. Fit correct fuses. Switch off to disconnect apparatus not in use; always pull out plug. Do not connect heaters or irons to lamp sockets.

General planning: Keep a fire extinguisher handy. Clear papers and rags from attic or under stairs.

Victims of severe burns may need a high-calorie diet rich in protein and vitamins, with extra iron to replace what has been lost in the plasma. Other organs, located far away from the burn, such as the liver, stomach, intestines, gallbladder, and kidney, may also have been damaged. This is because shock following the burn reduces blood supply to vital organs, causing damage that will not appear immediately. These organs are kept under surveillance while the patient is in the hospital. Physiotherapy will be given as soon as possible to maintain movement and the health and fitness of undamaged limbs.

What to do in case of fire

If someone is trapped by a fire, a rescuer should cover his or her nose and mouth with a wet cloth. It is better to reach the victim by crawling on the floor, where smoke is less dense, and guide or pull the victim out. If the victim is choked by hot fumes, artificial respiration should be given. Victims may panic and run around beating at their clothes—actions that are likely to fan the flames. The rescuer should try to stop this by getting the victim on the floor, with the burning area uppermost to allow flames to rise away from the body. Flames should be extinguished with water if possible; or, the flames can be smothered with thick material such as a rug, heavy towel, or coat. This should be thrown toward the victim's feet, directing the flames away from the face. Air can be excluded by pressing down gently but any hot, smoldering cloth should not be pressed against the victim's skin. The cloth should be pulled away, but without tearing away any material sticking to the skin. The victim must not be rolled; this would expose different areas to the flames.

Other forms of treatment

With a bad burn, the risk of shock is high. Shock is treated by lying the victim down, loosening any tight clothing, and covering him or her lightly. The victim can be given a cupful of water, to be sipped every 15 minutes. Rescuers should aim to be reassuring and calm, but they should send for an ambulance immediately. Any charred but cold material sticking to the skin should be left in place, but jewelry, such as a ring, bracelet, or necklace, that could constrict the burned area (which may swell) may be removed. A blister must be left alone and nothing but cold water applied to it. If no surgical dressings are handy, a clean handkerchief or towel may be used. For maximum hygiene, the dressing should be handled by one corner and the inside surface used on the burn, followed by a padding of more folded material (another clean handkerchief or small towel) and secured with an improvised bandage, such as a necktie or panty hose. If the face is burned, holes can be cut in the dressing to let the patient see. However, badly swollen eyelids may keep the eyes closed. The victim must be moved only to raise a burned limb; this helps to reduce swelling. The victim should be constantly reassured.

See also: **Blisters; Physical therapy; Protein; Shock**

Calcium

I have heard that too much calcium is harmful. Would it be dangerous if I ate too much in my food?

No. The body regulates how much calcium it requires and absorbs the correct amount from your blood, if you eat an adequate diet. Excess calcium is passed out in the urine. However, taking too many vitamin D pills can upset the balance. If the absorption system goes wrong, kidney stones can result. A low-calcium diet helps to avoid this.

I am pregnant. Do I need calcium tablets to help my baby develop healthy bones and strong teeth?

No, not unless your diet is lacking in protein-rich food and fruit and vegetables. The intestine compensates for you and your baby's requirements and will absorb more calcium from your food as necessary. However, it does no harm to drink extra milk.

My grandmother, who is in her sixties, recently broke her arm in a minor accident. She believes that her bones have weakened since menopause. Is this possible?

Yes. The estrogen present in women before menopause helps build up calcium in the bones. After menopause, osteoporosis (thinning of the bones) may develop. Make sure that your grandmother has an adequate diet. Exercise, extra calcium, and biphosphonate drugs will also improve her condition.

How much milk should my three-year-old drink?

Three glasses of milk contain about 0.018 oz. (0.5 g) of calcium—an adequate daily intake for a one- to nine-year-old. There is calcium in other foods, so a balanced diet should provide enough calcium.

Calcium is essential to the human body—and it is present in amounts that are finely balanced so that we have neither too much nor too little. This balance can sometimes be upset, but treatment will correct the imbalance.

Bones and teeth contain a large proportion of calcium. Calcium crystals form solid building blocks that are held together by a fibrous network. The result is a strong, resilient material for supporting the body—bones. However, calcium is not permanently located in the bones, for it is constantly being mobilized to help maintain the correct levels in the body tissues elsewhere.

Small amounts of calcium regulate the impulses from the nerves in the brain and influence muscle contraction. Blood clotting also relies on a set amount of calcium in the blood.

Calcium balance

We absorb calcium from our food, and it passes, via the intestine, into the bloodstream. Some is lost in the urine. But some is stored in the bones or reabsorbed into the bloodstream.

A balanced level of calcium in the blood is maintained by an elaborate control system. This is located in the parathyroid glands in the neck. Their product, parathyroid hormone (PTH), acts on the bones and kidneys to release more calcium and also to decrease loss in the urine.

When calcium levels are low, more PTH is passed into the bloodstream, whereas high calcium levels will result in less PTH being sent out. In this way, a constant balance is maintained. Vitamin D is also essential for maintaining the balance of calcium. Without it, calcium cannot be absorbed from food. It also acts with PTH to release calcium from the bones.

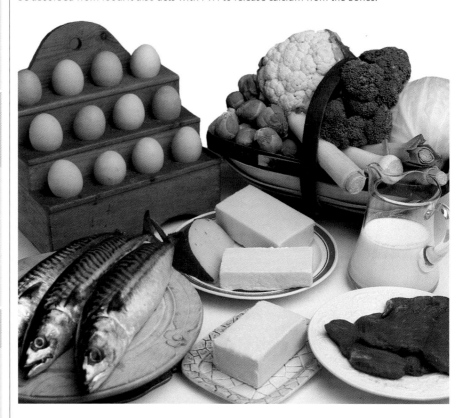

▲ *People need calcium to ensure, among other things, healthy bones and teeth. Calcium-rich foods include milk, cheese, eggs, meat, and vegetables.*

HOW THE BODY MAINTAINS A NORMAL CALCIUM BALANCE

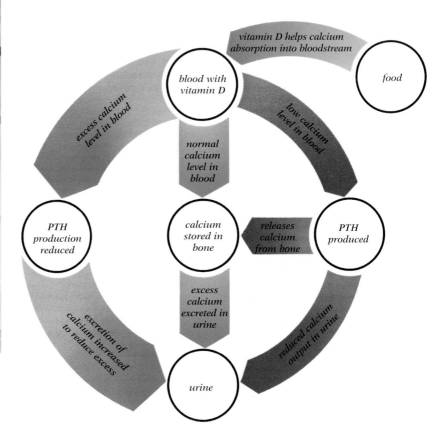

▲ *This child has rickets, a bone condition caused by a deficiency of calcium and vitamin D—the leg bones are soft, so the legs bow outward.*

▲ *Vitamin D is necessary for calcium to be absorbed from food. The level of calcium in the blood, which is controlled by PTH (parathyroid hormone), will be low if there is a lack of vitamin D. A lack of calcium in the blood causes PTH to be produced, and this encourages reduction of calcium stored in bones. Excess calcium in the blood reduces PTH production so that more calcium is excreted.*

Excessive calcium

If there is too much calcium in the body, vomiting and stomach pains may develop. Excess calcium may also be deposited in the kidneys and form renal stones. These are usually excreted naturally, but painfully.

Too much calcium could be the result of a parathyroid tumor secreting uncontrolled amounts of PTH, or it could be that a person has taken too many vitamin D pills.

In an emergency, calcium levels can be reduced by phosphate injections or pills. A parathyroid tumor needs surgery. If the cause is vitamin pills, the patient must stop taking them.

A lack of calcium

If there is too little calcium, a condition known as tetany occurs— this describes spasms of the muscles, especially in the hands, feet, and larynx. One cause is hysterical overbreathing, triggered by fear or emotion, which temporarily reduces available blood calcium. As the hysteria passes, the body returns to normal.

If the parathyroid glands have to be removed, because of a tumor, for example, PTH levels can drop and cause tetany. This can be treated by giving intravenous calcium and oral vitamin D.

Low calcium can also produce abnormal blood clotting and unbalanced heart rhythms. However, muscle spasms occur first, so treatment can prevent other problems from developing.

If left untreated for months, loss of calcium from bones causes rickets in children, which results in bone deformities. In elderly

people it causes osteoporosis (thinning bones). In both conditions, bones become weakened. Rickets still occurs today and can be helped by extra vitamin D. Many elderly women suffer from osteoporosis, largely because the loss of the anabolic steroid estrogen after menopause results in a progressive weakening of bones. The hormone calcitonin, given in pill form, is helpful to patients with osteoporosis.

Mother and baby

If a woman is pregnant or breast-feeding, her body loses calcium and vitamin D to the baby. Her intestine responds by absorbing more calcium and vitamin D from the food she eats. If she eats a balanced diet, there is no need for her to take calcium supplements. If a mother is bottle-feeding her baby, the formula milk should be made as instructed, so that there is no calcium problem.

See also: **Diet; Osteoporosis; Vitamin D**

Cancer

Of all the medical conditions known, the one that creates the most fear in people today is cancer. In fact, in many cases early diagnosis and continually improving forms of treatment can mean a complete cure.

Cancer is the result of disordered and disorganized cell growth. This can be fully understood only by looking at what happens in normal cells. The human body is made up of many different tissues—for example, skin, lung, and liver—in turn made up of millions of cells. These are all arranged in an orderly manner, each individual tissue having its own cellular structure. In addition, the appearance and shape of the cells of one organ differ from those of another. For example, a liver cell and skin cell look completely different.

In all tissues, cells are constantly being lost through general wear and tear. They are replaced by a process of cell division, occurring so that exactly the right number of cells are produced to replace those that are lost. A normal cell will divide in half to create two new cells, each identical to the original. If the body is injured, the rate of cell production speeds up automatically until the injury is healed, when it slows down again.

The cells of a cancer, however, divide and grow at their own speed, in an uncontrolled manner. They continue to do so indefinitely unless treatment is given. In time, the cancer cells increase in numbers until enough are present for the cancer to become visible as a growth.

In addition to growing too rapidly, cancer cells are unable to organize themselves properly, so the mass of tissue that forms is not like normal tissue. Cancer gets its nourishment parasitically from its host and serves no useful purpose in the body.

Cancers are classified according to the cell from which they originated. Those that arise from cells in the surface membranes of the body (the epithelial tissues), like the skin and the lining of the lungs and gastrointestinal tract, are called carcinomas. Those arising from structures deep inside the body, such as bone cartilage and muscle, are known as sarcomas. Carcinomas are much more common than sarcomas. This may be because the cells of the surface membranes need to divide more often in order to keep these membranes intact.

Benign and malignant tumors

Not all tumors are cancerous. Although tumor cells grow at their own speed, tumors can be benign or malignant. Benign tumors push aside normal tissues but do not grow into them. Malignant tumors (cancers), grow into surrounding tissue, a process called invasion. It is this clawlike process of abnormal cells permeating normal tissues that gives the name cancer—

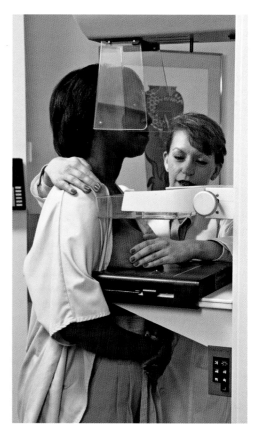

▶ *This patient is undergoing a mammogram, which is an X ray of the breast to screen for cancer and to investigate lumps in the breast.*

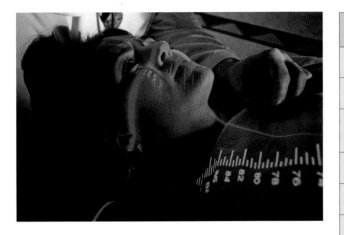

▲ *This woman is receiving laser radiation treatment, which damages the genetic material of cancer cells.*

from a zodiacal constellation, the crab. Its invasive properties enable unchecked cancer to spread through the body. The word malignant means "bad," while benign means "harmless." A benign tumor can look almost like normal tissue under the microscope, and it behaves accordingly, respecting its neighbors. It also grows more slowly than a malignant tumor. Although usually harmless, a benign tumor can be serious if it arises in an important part of the body, such as the brain cavity. An important difference between benign and malignant tumors is that the latter can seed themselves to start up in remote parts of the body (a process called metastasis); benign tumors never do this. Benign tumors should be removed, and surgery is nearly always curative.

Origin of cancer cells

Cancer cells develop from the body's own normal cells, and a single cancer cell is enough to start the growth of a tumor. However, the change to a cancer cell is a gradual one, taking place in stages over several years. With each stage the cell becomes slightly more abnormal in appearance and slightly less responsive to the body's control mechanisms. This process is usually unseen until a cancer develops, but in a few cases precancer can be recognized and treated. The best precancer known is seen in the uterine cervix, the neck of the womb, and this can be detected by a Pap smear.

How cancer spreads

The abnormal growth of a cancer is localized, at least at first, forming a mass around the original cells. However, the cancer usually invades normal tissues very early. If these tissues are important, life and health may be threatened.

The feature of cancer that accounts for most of its devastating effects is its ability to spread, or metastasize, to other parts of the body. Metastasis does not usually occur until the original collection of cells has grown to a fair size. Science does not yet fully understand the biological processes of metastasis, but evidence exists that single cancer cells, or small clumps, break off from the main cancer and are carried to other areas of the body by the blood or lymphatic system. Cancer cells carried by the blood are thought first to enter capillaries or very small veins or arteries. They travel until they come to a place where the blood vessels divide to form channels so small

that the cancer cells cannot easily get through. At that point they may lodge and begin to grow, producing a new cancer mass. The first place this is likely to occur is the liver, for most cancers of the gastrointestinal tract; or the lungs, for most cancers starting elsewhere in the body. This is because these organs are the first places where blood from other organs is filtered through a network of minute blood vessels. Thus, the lungs and liver are the most common sites of metastasis from blood-borne cancer cells. However, the cells can also pass through the liver and lungs to lodge in other regions of the body—often in the bones or structures of the head and trunk.

Normal lymph drainage begins in the peripheral lymphatic vessels, proceeding through a sequence of small structures called lymph nodes, and finally reaching one of the large central veins. These nodes, which serve as filters, contain many tiny channels through which the lymph and any cancer cells or other foreign matter must pass. Cancer cells that manage to pass through the lymph nodes and enter the bloodstream probably metastasize in the same way as cells that enter the blood directly.

Causes

The immune system is able to detect cells that have developed cancerous changes. Most of these cells are quickly attacked and destroyed by immune system cells. If it were not for this form of surveillance, cancer would be almost universal. There are, however, limits to the efficiency of the system. Cancer is most common in late middle age and old age. The increasing frequency of cancer in the Western world may, in part, be because people are living longer, but some cancers are associated with the Western way of life itself. Cancers due to smoking, for example, are still less common in the developing world. Nonetheless, the speed with which people are taking up smoking in these regions will ensure a high prevalence of cancers within a decade or two. The most common forms are lung, bowel, stomach, pancreas, and breast cancer. Despite developments in modern medicine, these cancers still account for many deaths in the United States each year. The most common cancers in children and young adults are leukemias, sarcomas, and kidney cancer. These cancers are rare, and their treatment has improved in recent years.

Questions and Answers

My uncle has had radiotherapy once and has now been told he has to have a second course of treatment. Is this safe?

Not if it is given to the same part of the body, unless it is a very small dose. However, the doctor will know how much radiotherapy a part of your uncle's body will tolerate. He or she will advise a second treatment only if it is safe. It is possible to give a full course of treatment to a different body part.

Can cancer ever be hereditary?

Not usually. There are a few cancers that run in families, but they are rare. Only if cancer is particularly common in your family is there any increased risk. If this is so, take better care of yourself, and report any persistent symptoms to your doctor.

I have been smoking up to 60 cigarettes a day and am worried about cancer. How many should I cut down to to be safe?

You are right to be worried. You do not say how many years you have been smoking, but it could be that you have damaged your lungs irreversibly—though this damage may not be cancerous. As far as cutting down is concerned, the advice can be summed up in two words—quit altogether!

I have read that cancer is sometimes stress-related. Also I have an aunt who literally willed herself to live against all odds. With cancer, can it ever be a case of mind over matter?

This is an interesting question. There are cases where the fear of getting cancer, often when one person in a family already has the disease, seems to bring it on in other members of the family. So perhaps fear does act as a trigger. In the same way, sheer determination has been known to get individuals out of the worst situations, as your aunt's case seems to indicate. The answer is that no one really knows for sure.

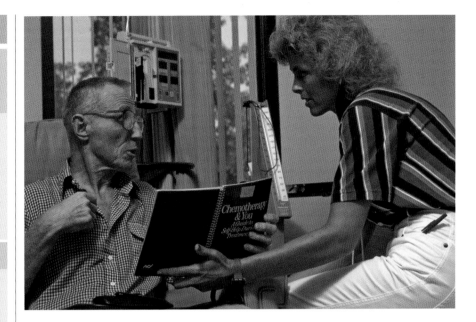

▲ *Chemotherapy, the use of cytotoxic drugs, may be a cancer treatment on its own or it may be combined with surgery, radiotherapy, or both.*

The cause of cancer is unknown, but two fundamental abnormalities are recognized. First, cancers are not subject to the normal influences that control cell growth. Second, the body will tolerate the presence of the cancer without rejecting it as a foreign invader. Environmental factors, such as chemical pollution and exposure to radiation, are thought to lead to cancer, but there are several other factors at work. Some cancers are known to be caused by viruses (oncoviruses) that can inject cancer-causing genes (oncogenes) into the DNA of normal cells.

Certain chemicals can also cause cells to become cancerous. These chemicals are irritants that may alter a cell's genetic structure and turn it into a cancer cell. Experiments have identified chemicals that cause cancer in animals (carcinogens). The best-known carcinogens are some of the 3,000 or so different chemicals present in tobacco smoke. However, despite research, it has not yet been possible to identify the carcinogens responsible for many common cancers. As no single theory explains all the facts about cancer, it seems probable that cancer has many causes, some of which are still unknown.

Pap smear

Cancer may be discovered because it causes symptoms, or it may be found by screening. The earlier a cancer is detected, the higher the chance of a cure. Much research has been done on developing screening examinations to detect cancer early. The greatest success has been the Pap test to detect carcinoma in the cervix. The test is effective, quick, simple, and inexpensive. A few cells are scraped off the cervix, put on a microscope slide, dyed, and examined. Any cancerous cells can sometimes be destroyed without having to remove the uterus. If this is not possible, surgical removal of the uterus at this stage results in complete cure of the carcinoma.

Cancer screening

Screening examinations of women without symptoms are also effective for the early detection of breast cancer, especially for women over the age of 50. A yearly combination of physical examination, study of medical history, and mammography—a special X-ray test—can reduce mortality from breast cancer in this age group by at least one-third.

Regular screening is also recommended as early as age 35 for women who have a mother or sister with this kind of cancer and for those who have already had breast cancer. In addition, two breast cancer genes, BRCA I and BRCA II, have now been identified. These occur in a small category of women whose tendency to breast cancer is significantly higher than normal. These women will also require close follow-up.

Two methods exist for detecting cancer of the colon and rectum before symptoms occur—careful medical examination and tests for small amounts of blood in the feces.

Doctors and others have also proposed screening for some other kinds of cancer, especially for persons known to be at high risk. However, it is currently felt that extensive screening of the general population is not advisable, because of the high costs of such tests, the low yield of unsuspected cancers, and the lack of evidence that survival rates would improve.

Diagnosis

It is no longer true that cancer is always fatal. There has been a vast improvement in the treatment of cancer in recent years, and many thousands of people are cured of the disease each year. However, a small cancer is easier to cure than a large one, so early diagnosis is vital and is helped by the prompt reporting of significant symptoms to a doctor. If the doctor suspects the possibility of cancer, he or she will refer the patient to a specialist.

The specialist will first confirm the diagnosis. This may initially involve X rays (such as a mammography) and scanning tests to show if there is a lump present. A part of the tissue will then be examined under the microscope. This can be done either by biopsy or by cytological examination. A biopsy involves a surgeon removing a small piece of the tumor, which is then sent to a pathologist for examination. This will determine whether the suspected tissue is cancerous or not. In a cytological examination, body fluids, such as mucus from the uterine cervix, are studied specifically for cancer cells.

The specialist will also carry out a thorough examination of the patient, taking particular care to check the lymph nodes adjacent to the tumor. He or she will also run blood tests to check liver and bone function and will arrange a chest X ray to look for evidence of spread into these sites. If the doctor suspects that cancer has spread to a particular part of the body, this area may also be scanned.

Various scanning techniques are used. In isotope scanning, a tiny amount of radioactive substance is injected into the body, and blood then carries it to the suspected organ or area of tissue. If the tissue contains a cancer, this will take up a different amount of isotope compared with the rest of the healthy tissue. The patient is then scanned with a special instrument that detects the radiation, and the cancer can be seen. Bones and the liver are the most common areas to be scanned in this way.

The doctor now has a detailed knowledge of the type of cancer involved and the stage of its development. Using this information, he or she can decide on the form of treatment that is most likely to be effective. The aim of all cancer treatment is to kill or remove every cancer cell. This is often possible.

Surgery

Cancer surgery aims at removing all of the cancer from the patient. It usually involves removing the visible growth with a wide margin of surrounding normal tissue to make sure every cell is taken. In addition, the surgeon will remove the draining lymph nodes and examine any adjacent structures. After removing the tumor, the surgeon will, where possible, reconstruct the patient's anatomy.

Nonetheless, patterns of surgery in breast cancer have changed in recent years to become more conservative. Research has shown that the long-term survival rate of women with small breast cancers

▲ *This poster emphasizes the dangers of smoking and reminds people that smoking is lethal.*

who undergo limited operations such as "lumpectomy" (in which only the discernible lump is removed), or breast-conserving surgery, is the same as in those who undergo complete breast removal.

There are some circumstances in which surgery is carried out without investigating the patient first. Obviously, when the patient is presented as an emergency, surgery is performed both to diagnose and to treat the patient.

There are also some situations when a biopsy and a cancer operation are carried out under the same anesthetic. For example, it used to be common practice to biopsy a breast lump, examine the tissue, and to then perform more extensive surgery if the lump was found to be malignant.

However, most breast biopsies are now done using a fine needle technique under local anesthetic. This leaves no scar and does not require hospital admission. It also permits the patient to participate in decisions about her treatment before surgery.

Radiotherapy

The aim of radiotherapy is to destroy the cancer with irradiation. Radiation damages the genetic material of cancer cells, so that they are unable to divide. Because they divide more rapidly than normal cells, cancer cells are more sensitive than normal cells to the damaging effects of radiation. Normal cells are also liable to be hair usually regrows within six months. Damage to other parts of the body is now rare, since the dosage that sensitive organs, such as the kidneys and lungs, will tolerate is known, and this dose is not exceeded.

Radiotherapy is used for localized tumors in addition to surgery. Some cancers—for example, some of the head and neck—can be cured by radiotherapy without surgery. In other cases, radiotherapy can be given either before or after an operation to increase the chances of success—as with breast cancer, for example.

Radioactive implants

In some circumstances it is actually possible to implant radioactive substances in the cancer. These give a very large dose to the cancer itself with only a small dose to the surrounding normal tissue. This form of treatment is ideal, as the damage to normal tissues is minimal. Unfortunately, it is possible only in accessible tumors, such as small cancers of the tongue and mouth and some that are gynecological in nature. Radiotherapy is also very good at relieving the symptoms of incurable cancer, particularly pain.

Chemotherapy

If a cancer is too widespread or metastases are present, it may not be possible to use radiotherapy effectively. Doctors can prescribe drug

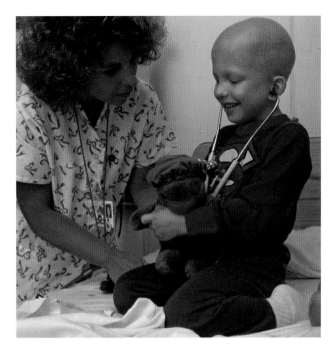

▲ *This nine-year-old girl is suffering from acute lymphoblastic leukemia (a cancer of the blood). Treatment includes a two-year course of chemotherapy, which has caused her hair to fall out.*

damaged by radiation, but it is the difference in the rate of reproduction between cancer cells and normal cells that makes radiotherapy both possible and valuable.

Radiotherapy is given in special rooms with thick floors, walls, ceilings, and windows to prevent radiation leaks. The patient lies on a special couch beneath the machine, and the machine is aimed at the tumor. Before treatment, the radiotherapist takes careful measurements of the position of the tumor to work out the best angle or combination of angles at which to set the machine. The staff leave the room before the machine is switched on. It is essential that the patient is in exactly the same position for every treatment. The treatment lasts only a few minutes and is painless—it is usually given daily for five to six weeks on an outpatient basis.

Side effects of radiotherapy can be kept to a minimum by careful medical supervision. Soreness of the skin is less of a problem today and may be avoided by infrequent washing of the treatment area. Soothing creams are also given to the patient. Sickness and diarrhea are problems only when the abdomen is treated, and they can usually be controlled with drugs. Loss of hair may occur if the head is treated, but

Symptoms of common cancers	
TYPE	**SYMPTOMS**
Breast cancer	Breast lump, bleeding from the nipple, inverted nipple, change in the shape of the breast.
Cancer of the larynx	Persistent hoarseness, spitting up blood.
Cancer of the esophagus (gullet)	Difficulty in swallowing, vomiting, loss of weight.
Cancer of the stomach	Difficulty in swallowing, vomiting, bringing up blood, loss of weight, indigestion.
Cancer of the bowel	Blood in the feces or from the rectum, a change of bowel habit—either constipation or diarrhea, or abdominal pain.
Cancer of the bladder	Blood in the urine.
Cancer of the prostate	Increased difficulty in passing urine; recurring urinary infections and back pain.
Cancer of the uterus or cervix	If menstruating, bleeding in between periods; if postmenopausal, vaginal bleeding. Offensive-smelling vaginal discharge, lower abdominal pain.
Cancer of the mouth and throat	Sore ulcer that refuses to heal; pain in ear or ears; difficulty in chewing or swallowing; dentures do not fit.
Leukemia	Tiredness, pallor, repeated infections, sore throat, bleeding from gums and nose, bruising.
Lung cancer	Persistent cough, spitting up blood, shortness of breath, chest pain, hoarseness.
Skin cancer	Sore skin that will not heal and continually bleeds.

Differences between benign and malignant tumors

TYPE OF GROWTH	BENIGN	MALIGNANT
	Pushes normal tissue aside.	Invades normal tissue.
Spread	Slight.	May form secondary growths.
Structure	Similar to normal growths.	May be disorganized.
Rate	Slow.	May be slow to rapid.
Outcome	Usually harmless.	May be fatal if untreated.
Treatment	Surgery is curative.	Surgery may not be curative.

Hormones are chemical messengers that circulate in the blood to control the growth and metabolism of tissue. If a cancer cell arises in a hormone-sensitive organ, such as the uterus (womb), it may continue to recognize and respond to hormonal messages. If the patient is then given an inhibitory hormone—one that tells the cells to stop dividing—the cancer will stop growing. This treatment is particularly useful in breast, uterine, and prostate cancers. Its great advantage is its freedom from unpleasant side effects.

treatment in this situation. The drugs combine with and damage the genetic material of cells so that they cannot divide properly. Historically, the earliest chemotherapeutic agents were developed from mustard gas. Doctors noticed that soldiers recovering from this poisoning had low blood counts. They quickly realized that the gas was interfering with the division of cells in the bone marrow, where blood is made. Nitrogen mustard (the active drug in mustard gas) was tried in cancer patients in an attempt to poison the cancer cells, and it proved successful. Many new, safer drugs have since been discovered, and effective combinations of drugs have been developed. Unfortunately, these drugs poison all dividing cells. The best way to minimize the damage to normal cells is to give fewer, larger doses of cytotoxic (cell poisoning) drugs over a short period of time. There is then a gap of a few weeks (usually three) before the next course of treatment. This allows normal cells to recover.

Side effects of cancer treatment

The possible side effects of cytotoxic drugs—or chemotherapy, as these are now called—include hair loss, nausea, and lowering of the blood count. Hair loss occurs with a few of the cytotoxic drugs, but the hair regrows when treatment stops. Nausea sometimes follows the injection of some cytotoxic drugs but usually lasts only a few hours. Drugs that combat nausea can be prescribed.

Alternatively, when nausea is severe, the patient may be admitted to a hospital and the treatment given under sedation. However, this is rarely necessary. The safe dosage for the various cytotoxic drugs is now known to doctors, so serious depression of the patient's blood count is now a much rarer occurrence than it used to be. However, the blood must be regularly tested both before and during drug treatment.

Chemotherapy is not used solely for solid-tissue tumors. It is also used to treat blood cancers, such as leukemia, as it has proved effective on bone marrow.

Other cancers, such as Hodgkin's disease, may respond better to a treatment like chemotherapy rather than to extensive radiotherapy. In some cases where the patient has tended to relapse after surgery or radiotherapy, chemotherapy is given even when there is no sign of cancer.

This treatment is called adjuvant chemotherapy and is being tried for breast cancer and childhood cancer. Although encouraging results have been obtained, it is still too early to advocate this kind of treatment for all cancer patients.

Blocking hormone action

Prostate cancers are usually encouraged by testosterone and can be effectively treated either by removal of the testosterone source (the testicles) or by the use of a drug such as bicalutamine (Casodex), which blocks the action of testosterone. Many breast cancers are encouraged by estrogen and can be helped, or possibly prevented, by the drug tamoxifen, which blocks the action of estrogens.

Combined treatment

Where more than one cancer therapy has been found to be effective, treatments may be combined. In some childhood tumors, for example, surgery is followed by local radiotherapy and then one year of chemotherapy. In head and neck cancer, chemotherapy is followed by local radiotherapy, and then any of the tumor that still remains is removed surgically. Much research is now being carried out to determine the best possible way of combining treatments.

Whole-body irradiation and bone-marrow transplantation

In recent years it has become possible to transplant bone marrow from one person to another. This specialized procedure requires that large doses of radiation be given to the recipient beforehand—an approach called whole-body irradiation. At present this treatment is generally used only for rare forms of anemia and leukemia. In the future, however, it may be possible to treat other forms of cancer in this way.

Outlook

Many cancers are curable if they are treated early enough, so regular screening is important for early diagnosis and treatment. Any persistent or unexplained symptoms must be reported to a doctor. Once the treatment has been completed, the doctor will regularly examine the original cancer site with care, and he or she will also investigate any new symptoms that appear. If the patient is still well and free of cancer five years later, there is room for cautious optimism.

Recent advances made in medical research, and subsequently treatment, are getting better all the time—as are the chances of surviving cancer.

See also: **Anemia; Leukemia; Smoking; Viruses; X rays**

Chicken pox

Children catch chicken pox so easily that it is almost a natural hazard of childhood. Fortunately, the illness does not last long and rarely has serious complications, so effective home nursing is a simple matter.

Questions and Answers

What is the best way to prevent scars forming from chicken pox? Both my older children scratched their spots, and it would be a shame if my daughter were to scar her face when she gets it.

Scarring occurs if the spots become infected or if the scabs are pulled off, taking fresh tissue with them and widening the area of damage. Preventing itching with calamine lotion or an antihistamine drug is helpful, but it does take willpower not to scratch. All you can do is explain what will happen if she picks the spots, and encourage her to resist the temptation.

Could my baby daughter get chicken pox, and if so, is it more serious than in an older child?

Babies seem to have some natural immunity to chicken pox, and few cases have ever been recorded. A baby could be seriously, but probably not fatally, ill with chicken pox—but any child under the age of two who develops a rash should be seen by a doctor.

My brother appears to have chicken pox for the second time. Is this possible?

It is unlikely. In general, chicken pox is a one-time-only infection. The first "attack" might have been scabies (severe itching and spots caused by a mite) or several gnat bites occurring together.

My daughter recently spent the day with a child who now has chicken pox. How soon will she come down with it?

Your daughter may show the first symptoms—headache and a vague illness—within 10 days, or it could take up to three weeks to develop. But she may not develop chicken pox at all—there is no certainty that she was infected.

Chicken pox—the medical name is varicella—is a highly infectious illness, easily recognized by the rash that it causes. It is generally considered a childhood illness. Babies are born with a natural ability (passed on by their mothers) to resist chicken pox, but this wears off by the time children are three or four years of age, leaving them vulnerable to infection.

The virus (germ) that causes chicken pox also causes shingles (which has similar symptoms, including a rash) in adults, so an adult with shingles can pass chicken pox on to a child. The virus is so infectious that many outbreaks of chicken pox occur, mainly in children between the ages of two and six. Outbreaks are strongest in the autumn and winter and appear to occur in three- or four-year cycles as the number of children who have never had the disease builds up.

Although slightly similar in appearance to smallpox, chicken pox has nothing else in common with the disease. Smallpox is much more serious, with a 40 percent death rate, and is caused by a completely different virus. It was eradicated more than 20 years ago.

How chicken pox is caught

Although the chicken pox virus is present and alive in the spots that form, it is transferred between people chiefly by droplet infection. Someone who already has the virus spreads clusters of it in the tiny droplets of water that are exhaled with every breath. When a child breathes in an infected droplet, the virus starts to multiply, and another case of chicken pox begins. The source is almost always another child. The illness is usually passed on before the skin spots appear, so the affected child is not suspected as a source—hence the rapid spread.

Symptoms

Once the virus enters the body, it needs an incubation, or breeding, period of between 10 days and three weeks to spread. The first a child will know of his or her illness will be a 24-hour period when there will be symptoms of a vague headache, a sick feeling, occasional slight fever, and sometimes a blotchy, red rash that fades. A parent may note that the child is pale. Within 24 hours the first spots appear, and the nature and position of these spots allow a diagnosis to be made. In very mild cases it can be difficult to distinguish chicken pox from gnat bites, but in a full-blown case, with hundreds of spots, the diagnosis is simple.

Spots appear on the face, in the throat, and on the trunk, only occasionally affecting the limbs. Each spot starts as a pink pimple, and within five or six hours becomes raised to form a tiny blister, or vesicle, containing clear fluid that is full of the virus. These teardrop spots, which are each at different stages of development, gradually become milky in color, forming a crust and finally a scab. The time from the appearance of a teardrop to the formation of a crust is about 24 hours. During this period the child may be agitated and uncomfortable, and run a temperature of 100° or 101°F (38°C).

Some children have only a few spots, while others may have several hundred. As soon as crusts form, the spots begin to itch, and this stage may last until the scabs drop off, leaving

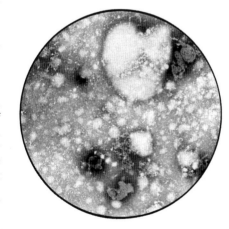

▲ *The chicken pox virus, enlarged about 8,000 times, is mainly transmitted through droplets of water in the breath.*

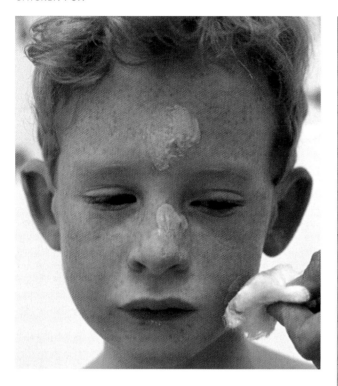

▲ *Chicken pox spots begin to itch as soon as the crusts form, and calamine lotion is a soothing, cooling treatment.*

Home care of a child

Reassure the child, allow him or her freedom, and do not insist on bed rest. Give mild painkillers for a sore throat or headache. The spots may look dramatic, but the child is rarely very sick.

Consult your doctor if the spots are very large, infected, or extremely painful (for instance, in the ear).

If the child is not hungry, cut down on food when temperature is high, but offer plenty of fluids.

Explain the need not to scratch, and suggest that the child might like to wear soft cotton gloves as a reminder.

Apply calamine lotion to reduce irritation, or ask the doctor for an antihistamine drug, which will have the same effect.

Make sure strict hygiene is observed—short nails, clean hands, and a daily bath at the scab stage.

Check with the school about isolation of the child. Usually a week is required from the appearance of the spots.

It can be reassuring for your child to ask another child with chicken pox to come to the house to play.

new skin after one or two weeks. Chicken pox spots come out in crops, which means that new ones appear every day for three or four days. When examining a child's skin, an adult will notice that the spots will be at different stages even in the same area.

In most cases the condition is mild, but in some cases the child is very sick and needs attentive home nursing.

Dangers

In children dangerous complications are rare, and most children with chicken pox feel well enough to play. Those who are taking steroid drugs or who are suffering from leukemia are the only ones likely to be seriously affected, and for them the condition can be fatal. In a small number of cases the virus can lead to a severe form of pneumonia.

Chicken pox can be dangerous in pregnant women, as it can affect the developing fetus, so a woman who has not had chicken pox should be vaccinated against it before becoming pregnant. In adults chicken pox pneumonia is fatal in more than 20 percent of cases.

Complications

The most common complications arise from infection of the spots, causing boils or other skin conditions. Similarly, spots near the eye may lead to infective conjunctivitis, commonly called pinkeye. In such cases treatment with antibiotics is needed.

Cases of arthritis and inflammation of the heart have followed chicken pox, but they are rare. The other danger arises when the virus attacks the nervous system and causes encephalitis (inflammation of the brain), as it may do on the fourth or tenth day after the rash appears. The patient becomes delirious, and intensive hospital treatment is needed. The chance of complete recovery is high.

Treatment

Children with a high temperature who feel unwell may prefer to stay in bed or lie downstairs to be with the family. Otherwise, there is no medical reason to enforce strict bed rest. Any pain from a sore throat or a headache is best relieved with a painkiller such as acetaminophen, or aspirin, in a child over 12. As there is no medical cure for the virus, the condition is left to take its natural course, and most children require no treatment at all.

Severe itching can be helped by applying calamine lotion, which has a cooling and anti-itching effect, or with an antihistamine drug. If any of the spots should become infected, they may take longer to heal, and antibiotics will be necessary.

Outlook

Most children who have had a mild case of chicken pox start losing their scabs after about 10 days and will be free of spots within about two weeks. If scabs have been scratched, the process takes a little longer. The scabs are not infectious and those that fall off do not leave a scar. Scabs that have been picked or have become infected are more likely to scar, so it is important to avoid scratching.

Chicken pox infection produces a lifelong immunity to the disease, but the virus remains in the body and can lead to shingles, which may develop later in a person's life.

A vaccine has now been developed for chicken pox, and this will probably become one of the standard set of childhood injections.

See also: **Blisters; Leukemia; Rashes; Vaccinations; Viruses**

Child abuse

Questions and Answers

I know my neighbor beats her son. I've seen terrible bruises on his face and arms. Whom should I contact?

A doctor or social worker will give practical help, and no one will know that it was you who contacted him or her. It would be better if you could offer some help yourself. Ask if you could look after the little boy; invite the mother in for coffee and get her to chat. Your friendship could make a lot of difference.

Will my child be taken away from me if it's discovered I've beaten her?

If you cooperate with the people who want to help you, and you manage to control your urges, then there is no danger that your child will be taken away. It is only as a last resort that children are placed in a foster home.

My husband has beaten our baby once or twice. Does he need help?

Yes, he does. To ignore his beating or to cover up for him can only be bad for the baby. Persuade him to see a doctor, who will refer him to someone who can help.

Sometimes I get really mad at my son. Will I end up beating him?

If you haven't done so before, the answer is probably no. Most abused babies are beaten in the first year of their life, and if you have managed to control your feelings so far, then you should be safe both now and in the future.

Can slapping develop into beating?

Physical violence to a child is never justified. If you find your child is driving you to distraction, get professional advice. Casual slapping can become a habit and can cross the line into child abuse.

Parents who abuse their children are likely to have suffered cruelty in childhood themselves, so they are emotionally damaged. How can they be helped—and what are the signs that a child is being abused?

"Child abuse" is a term used to describe the nonaccidental physical (including sexual) abuse of children by one or both parents or another adult, even though the children may be in all other respects well cared for and loved. Injuries can range from relatively minor to so serious that children die. Emotional abuse, in which children are taunted or told that they are not loved, or made to suffer mentally in other ways, often accompanies physical abuse, and the scars left from this can linger long after the body has healed.

Causes
Every parent has experienced helpless frustration in response to the nonstop crying of an infant who cannot be calmed. Most parents find that "something" stops them from hitting their child, but the lack of this internal psychological brake leads other parents to beat their children—not just once, but a number of times.

It is believed that as many as 20 percent of women experience difficulty in learning to become a mother. A small percentage of these go on to abuse their children, and the cause of this can be found far back in their own childhood.

Some child abusers of both sexes were beaten or sexually molested themselves as children, some are aggressive types with a pattern of physical violence in all their relationships, and others fall into neither group. Almost all were deprived of good parental care when they were children, so that they never learned to give and receive love and did not have a successful parent to model themselves on when the time came for them to raise their own children.

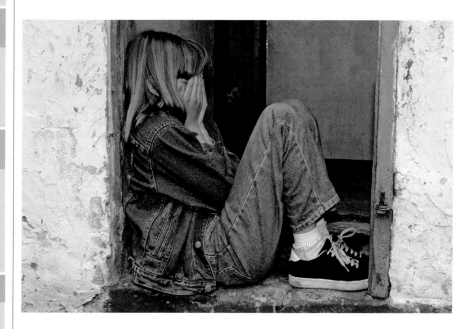

▲ *In 2008, the National Child Abuse and Neglect Data System recorded approximately 1,740 deaths related to child abuse and neglect. More than 3.7 million children were reported as victims of child abuse and neglect, and 758,289 cases of child maltreatment were identified; of these 71 percent were neglected, 16 percent were physically abused, 9 percent were sexually abused, and 7 percent were psychologically maltreated.*

Fewer than 10 percent of parents who abuse their children are severely psychologically ill, although half of the mothers who do so are classifiably neurotic and a third of fathers are said to have a gross personality defect. Many of them are depressed, passive, reclusive types who demand instant love from their children and fail to understand that for a long time babies are dependent and aware only of their own needs. Crying is interpreted as a sign that the baby does not love them, and the parents' feelings of anger and failure can trigger an attack. Other potential child abusers are obsessively clean and tidy, and a baby's natural soiling or a toddler's investigative messiness seem like deliberate naughtiness that must be punished. A mother who has had to give up her career or put it on hold to have a child may also feel strong resentment and frustration.

Isolation is another contributing factor. A young mother whose own parents live far away, and who does not have friends nearby, may find that her desires and fears center on her baby, and she does not have the natural safety valve of talking with a sympathetic listener. If her marriage is also difficult or unhappy, then the baby will be even more at risk. Child abusers may be shocked and horrified at the damage they have caused while in a rage. Even though they may realize that they are placing unrealistic demands on their children, not even self-disgust will stop them from doing it again.

Social background

Research reveals that most child abuse is reported among the poor and deprived and that the level of intelligence of the abusing parent

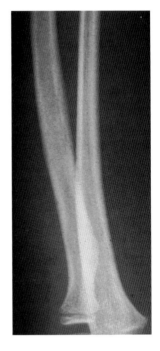

▶ *X ray showing child's forearm with a bent bone (right)—the result of a blow. A child's bones are soft and bend rather than break.*

is low. But statistics are compiled from cases that have come to the attention of the authorities— either from health visitors, social workers, hospitals, or the police— and experts are sure that the problem is more widespread.

Child abusers who are well-off are able to seek private treatment for their children. The more intelligent they are, and the higher their social class, the more easily they can deceive the authorities as to the true cause of their child's injuries. Doctors are also more disposed to believe the explanations of an articulate middle-class parent.

Some people also believe there is more chance that stepchildren or the children of single parents will be abused. But while these cases are represented in the statistics, most abuse occurs within normal family units. Another common supposition is that one child is singled out from a family group for beating. This is sometimes the case, but in most families where one child has been abused, other children suffer beatings too. One child may be be picked on at a particular time; and if the abusing parent is a good housekeeper, the clean, well-dressed appearance of the others makes them appear to be unharmed. Closer examination generally proves that, at different times, the others have also suffered unexplained injuries.

Anything is likely to trigger the violent rage of a harassed potential child abuser. However, some babies are more at risk: premature and underweight babies are in danger, because they need special care and patience and may be sickly and fretful, trying the patience of even the most well-meaning parent.

Emotional abuse

It is impossible to estimate the extent of emotional abuse when it occurs without physical injury. Parents who continually tell their children that they are clumsy, stupid, dishonest, unpleasant, or ugly do them great harm. The children begin to believe what is said of them, and it can affect their whole lives. If they are made to feel unloved, often they will unconsciously make themselves unlovable to other people, becoming antisocial. It is a vicious circle: a child's actions often make the parents feel that they are right, so they continue to hurt the child with words.

No physically abused child escapes an emotional battering either. Children who are hit repeatedly for real or imagined naughtiness live in fear. If physical contact means a blow as often as a hug, they may shrink from other people. Since it has been proved that children who are cuddled frequently tend to be mentally brighter, the implication for abused children is clear. Children who are beaten and then pampered by guilty parents will end up emotionally muddled and confused.

Preventing child abuse—A self-help guide

A baby has been crying all day and won't be comforted by her mother, or a toddler is aggravating his father. These are moments that any parent will recognize, when they feel themselves losing control and know they are in danger of lashing out. Punishment given in a blind rage can be dangerous—especially if the child is a baby.

Here are some suggestions that could help avert a crisis.

Work off aggression by working out at a gym. Spend time on the treadmill and lift some weights. The exercise may divert violent feelings.

Telephone someone and talk about any negative feelings.

Ask a neighbor or friend to watch the child for a while, and get out of the house. Walk and think until you feel calmer.

If getting out is not an option, go into a different room from the child. Go into the kitchen and make tea. Cry or shout. Giving angry feelings expression (without violence to the child) will make them go away faster.

When the feelings have passed, don't just hope that they will never occur again. Seek help from a doctor, nurse, or social worker. He or she will understand without being shocked and will offer practical aid and advice.

Symptoms

Identifying abused children is harder than it would seem. Most parents who abuse their children bring them for treatment voluntarily and are clearly distressed by the children's injuries. Usually, abused children are genuinely loved, the beating being performed in a rage by parents who have the emotional problems already mentioned. Some parents even have a partial memory blackout about the beating. They do not want to admit to themselves that they inflicted injuries on their own children, and they are often glib and convincing in explaining the "accident" that caused the injury. In other ways, the children may look well cared for, so the parent's explanation is often accepted. Alert doctors and teachers can spot the signs that indicate child abuse. Apart from the physical symptoms, a professional will notice if there is any delay in reporting an injury; even parents who bring their child in for treatment may wait a day or two before doing so. Another sign is the child's attitude: occasionally children may flinch from their parents, although some abused children are especially loving to their parents in an attempt to win their affection.

Actual injuries vary, but even when a reasonable excuse is given for the way in which the injuries happened, an examination can prove that the damage is inconsistent with, say, a fall downstairs or an accidental bang against a door frame. The most serious injuries are those to the face and head: fractured skulls or bruised and cut faces are often seen. Failure to thrive may be another sign. This is the term used for children who are underweight and not developing normally. Failure to thrive could indicate that they are neglected, but in the case of abused children, unhappiness could be the cause.

Children are abused in different ways, and the list makes unpleasant reading. Some are beaten on the head, punched, kicked, bitten, and thrown across a room or downstairs. Others are burned by cigarettes, thrown against fires, or even placed in ovens or boiling baths. Some parents confine themselves to shaking their children, believing that this does less harm—but young babies can suffer brain damage if shaken violently, even though their soft bones may sustain the shock of being thrown to the floor. Doctors look out for heavy bruising caused by tight gripping around the head or limbs while children are beaten or thrown. X rays can show old healed injuries or damage to internal organs.

Treatment

Physically curing abused children is the easiest part of the treatment, but it does not get to the root of the problem. According to some experts, severely abused children who are returned to their parents when the parents' problems have not been treated stand a 25 to 50 percent chance of being killed or permanently injured. Sixty percent will be abused again, and an even higher percentage will suffer minor attacks or emotional battering.

How can parents be treated to stop them from abusing their children? Certainly an increased knowledge of what to expect from their children at each stage of growth and development is a great help, along with practical aid with child-raising problems.

Doctors and social workers should recognize that sometimes the obvious nature of children's injuries is a cry for help from the parents, and it should be answered by offers of support rather than accusations and disgust. Above all, the best treatment enables the parents to relearn the art of loving and caring for their children, which is brought about by being loved and "mothered" themselves.

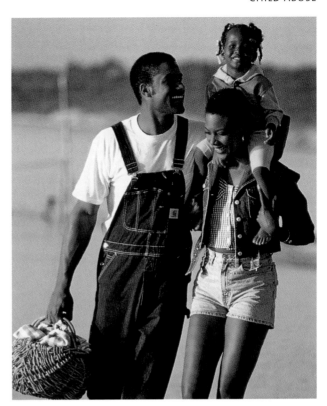

▲ *An abused child can be helped to recover physically and emotionally by being fostered in a loving home.*

The social worker or caring person involved should focus attention on the parent—even in the face of antisocial behavior.

It used to be thought that any kind of parent was better than none at all. However, it is now recognized that if parents repeatedly abuse a child, it is better for the child's physical and mental well-being if he or she is removed from home and placed in a loving, caring environment with foster parents.

Sexual abuse

Child abuse may also be of a sexual nature, and the damage can be done by family members or close family friends. The number of recognized cases has increased because doctors and teachers have learned to recognize the symptoms, but there is growing awareness that this serious problem has existed for many years, even though it may have been hidden inside the family.

Outlook

The problem of child abuse is becoming more widely acknowledged and understood. Whether children who have been physically and emotionally abused grow up to be disturbed depends entirely on how the problem is dealt with and at what stage of development. If the abuse stops and professional help is used to treat the physical and emotional scars, there is no reason why these children should not outgrow the terror of the experience.

> See also: **Depression; Fractures; Sexual abuse**

Child development

Human life from birth to age five involves a fascinating series of changes, as helpless infants gradually turn into sociable children who are ready to enter school. What progress can parents expect—and how can they help their children develop healthily and happily?

Children develop at different rates according to their inborn potential, although various factors such as their surroundings and how much attention they receive also influence their progress. The sequence of physical development, and of the acquisition of new skills, does not change, however—some children may be more advanced in some areas and slower in others, but the order in which they develop and learn is the same.

Birth to six months

Feeding: During the first three months of life babies get all the nutrients they need from milk, ideally breast milk. If they are bottle-fed, milk that has been specially prepared for infants should be bought and the formula carefully made up so that the feed is not too concentrated. Formula milk should be used until babies are a year old (using cow's milk before this can lead to an allergy to dairy products). Solid food should be introduced in tiny amounts beginning when the child is three or four months old. By the age of six months, babies will be eating three meals a day with a bottle- or breast-feeding at night. The solids should be finely mashed and the babies given rusks and cut-up vegetables and fruit to handle.

Crying: Crying is a baby's only method of communication. Parents find out by trial and error why their baby is crying and soon learn to interpret the cries. Small babies usually cry while being undressed or if roughly handled. From six weeks onward almost all babies will stop crying if they are cuddled. By the time they are six months old babies also cry because they are bored or lonely, but they will usually stop when picked up by their mother or father.

Physical development: During the first six months, babies learn to support their heads and to roll over by themselves. Eventually they will sit up with a little support, and if their hands are held, they will jump up and down on someone's lap. They also learn to coordinate hand and eye and are able to reach out and grasp objects with both hands. They are likely to cut their first teeth by six months.

Social development and play: From the start babies like to look at a human face, and enjoy the sound of a human voice, above all things. By four weeks they will be making cooing and gurgling noises, and at around six weeks the sounds will be phonetic and infants will "talk back" when spoken to.

The first smiles also come at about six weeks, and babies will smile in response to a smiling face and a human voice. As physical skills develop, they want interesting toys to look at and grasp, and they enjoy being talked to, held, and gently played with.

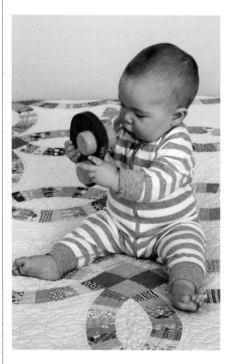

▲ *In the first six months a baby will learn to grasp objects with both hands.*

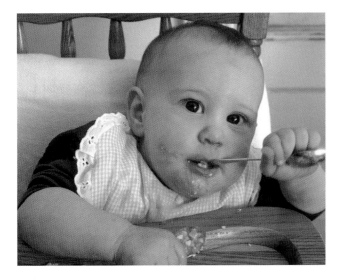

▲ *A baby has a strong will to do things without help—in time this infant will learn to feed himself without too much mess.*

Relationship with mother: By four months babies are usually more relaxed and happy with their mothers than with anyone else. Small babies treat their mother's body as an extension of their own and react with pleasure to the sound of her voice and to her face. They also rely on her for play and entertainment.

Six months to one year
During this period babies start to crawl. They are interested in everything but do not have enough coordination to be gentle with objects. Everything is put into the mouth—this is the way that small babies learn about the world.

Feeding: During this period babies can eat three meals a day at family mealtimes, supplemented by snacks in the morning and afternoon. Their digestive system is able to cope with the food that the family eats as long as it is minced or cut up. However, some mothers prefer to give their babies commercial foods.

Babies will also start to drink from cups and will want to feed themselves. Some babies will still need supplementary bottles, which should be of formula milk until the age of one year.

Crying: At this age babies cry mainly out of frustration and anger at not being able to do the things they want to do, and also from pain if they hurt themselves crawling or attempting to walk. They also cry when left alone—each time a parent leaves for any length of time, it is like a major separation.

Social development and play: Babies are less sociable with strangers than they were before and may be suspicious and really frightened of strangers at times. They need more things to play with now.

Physical development: Over these few months babies learn to sit up without support, and then to crawl. They start to pull themselves up to stand, and they may leave out the crawling stage altogether. Once standing, they may move around the room by holding onto furniture. They also become much more practiced at using their hands.

By the end of their first year, most babies will have cut their two upper front teeth, as well as the two lower ones and one molar.

Relationship with mother: Babies become increasingly attached to their mothers in a highly emotional way, and also become fond of other members of the family and pets. They need their mother's presence constantly, becoming highly disturbed when separated from her, although they will play happily by themselves as long as she is around. They also become unhappy when their mothers show disapproval, but their memory is so short that they are likely to do again the things they were told not to do minutes before—so punishment does no good at this stage.

One to two years
This is the stage between babyhood and childhood, and it can be frustrating for toddlers, who wish to do more than they are physically capable of, and tiring for mothers, since toddlers increasingly demand their own way.

Feeding: Most mothers understand the need for their children to have a good, mixed diet, but sometimes their preoccupation causes

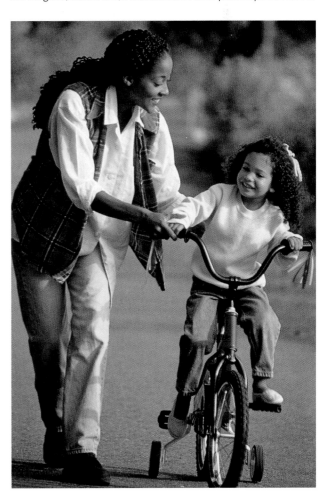

▲ *A child's attempts at learning a new skill are thrilling for a parent. Here a mother teaches her daughter to ride a bicycle.*

Questions and Answers

My one-year-old sister is very shy, even with close family friends. How can I help her?

It is natural for a baby of her age to be shy and dependent on family members. This is a stage that will pass in time, when she is ready to be more sociable. If you try to force her, then her fear of others will increase.

I frequently baby-sit for a two-year-old boy. How do I deal with his temper tantrums?

Tantrums are common in toddlers, and some children have tantrums until they are four years old. It would be more worrying if the child never expressed frustration or bad temper in this way.

Try to avoid frustration: suggest acceptable things to do rather than just saying "don't" when the child does something of which you disapprove. Allow him or her to express aggressive feelings in play. Don't lose your temper; a calm, reassuring attitude will soothe a child. Hold children so that they cannot hurt themselves, and never give in afterward—or they will believe that a tantrum is the way to get what they want.

How can I help my baby niece, who has colic?

Unfortunately, there is no absolute cure for colic. This condition is also called evening colic, because it tends to strike after the late-afternoon or early-evening feeding. It usually starts during the first two weeks of life and rarely lasts longer than nine weeks. It is distressing, for a colicky baby is not comforted even by being cuddled. You may just have to wait until the attacks pass.

My three-year-old son knows lots of words, but he can't make sentences yet. Is this normal?

Most children know about 800 words by age three, and it is at about this time that they start putting together sentences of four or five words.

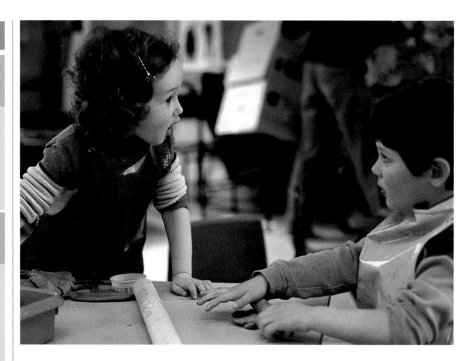

▲ *At nursery school children become used to playing with other children, cooperating and sharing their toys happily.*

feeding problems. Children themselves are a guide to whether they are eating enough of the right things—if they are healthy, growing, and energetic they are getting all the food they need.

Sleeping: Most toddlers of this age have trouble settling down for the night. All will cry when their mother leaves the room. The best solution may be to pop in every five minutes until they settle. Tuck them in with loving words, and say good night again. Children treated like this will not feel lonely and abandoned. They should not be allowed out of the crib, or getting out will become a difficult pattern to break.

Walking: Once toddlers have taken their first few steps, their ability to walk increases rapidly. By 16 months most can toddle well. By 20 months most can run and jump with both feet, but at this age they may prefer to be taken from place to place in a stroller or in their mother's arms.

Talking: The first words babies say are usually the names of loved ones and pets, then the words for favorite foods and drinks, followed by parts of the body, clothes, and everyday articles.

Social development and play: Because of their increased mobility, toddlers are into everything. They are extremely curious and experimental and want to copy what adults or other children do. Their imagination develops, and imaginative play also increases. They are still shy with strangers but may be pushy with other children.

Toilet training: Toilet training cannot begin until toddlers are aware that they have wet or soiled themselves. This can occur anytime between one year and 15 months, and toddlers will begin to indicate to their mother that they have a full diaper. Bladder control follows later—it is far harder for toddlers to "hold on" when they want to urinate. There is no use trying to train them to urinate in the potty if they are still wearing diapers, and they must be allowed the occasional accident. If mothers can remain calm and unemotional, toilet training is likely to be easier. Dirty diapers or pants are not naughty—they are unfortunate.

Relationship with mother: Toddlers are still very reliant on their mothers. They seek more protection and support than ever before, still feel great anxiety over any separation, and resent people who take up their mother's time. At the same time, they are seeking independence, and they resent their smallness and dependence on adults and the power that adults can wield; so they become increasingly negative and assertive, testing their own power against that of the adult world.

Tantrums are common at this age—and for the next year or so. Children are not being willful or naughty but are just reacting to a buildup of frustration that they are too young to control.

Two to five years

This preschool age sees children transformed from dependent babies into social human beings.

Toilet training: Some children will be able to use the potty efficiently by their second year. Others may be as old as three or well into their fourth year before they are completely potty-trained.

Physical development and play: Play is children's equivalent of work. Young children must have space to play and equipment to play with if they are to develop their physical skills. Developing physical skills also fosters self-confidence, independence, and self-reliance and assists emotional development. Fantasy games help social and emotional development.

▼ *By copying his father, this young child is learning to feed himself confidently using chopsticks.*

Social development: Social behavior with other children goes through three recognizable stages, though the transition is gradual and the stages do overlap. During the first stage children are indifferent or aloof with other infants, preferring to play alone. In the next stage they show hostility—they see other children as rivals and may be jealous. In the third stage children become friendly and cooperative, playing happily with other children and sharing toys.

Most children of three or older benefit from time spent at a nursery or child center. The range of equipment available is likely to be far greater there than at home, and a nursery encourages them to learn to do things for themselves that their mothers might do automatically at home. As they get to the stage of friendly cooperation with other children, they learn to give and take.

Relationship with mother: By the end of the first few years children have gone through the stage of being dependent on their mothers and have entered the resistant stage. This will go on into the third year, but as they become more mobile, physically capable, and self-reliant, the relationship should start to settle down. When children realize that their mothers always return after an absence, their separation anxiety decreases, and if they are otherwise confident, they will enjoy the occasional time away from home, perhaps with grandparents. The calmer and happier the first two years are, the more likely children are to become happy and sociable.

See also: **Nutrition**

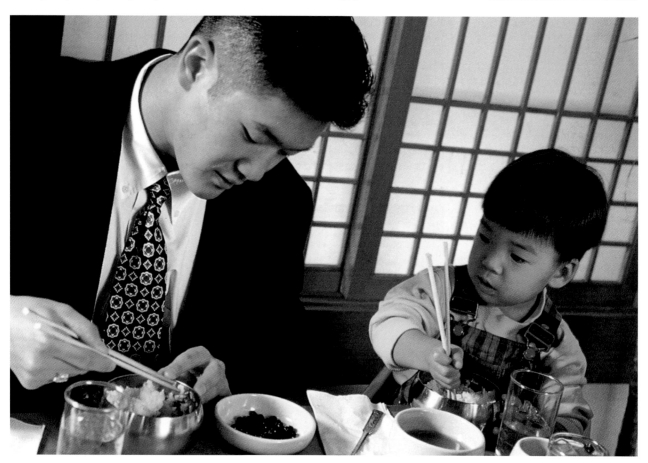

Cholesterol

A certain amount of cholesterol is essential to health, but too much can contribute to artery disease and heart attacks. Careful attention to diet and lifestyle will help to avoid potential problems.

Questions and Answers

Will a low-cholesterol diet help me avoid getting heart disease?

It might, but only when combined with other measures, such as quitting smoking (if you smoke), which causes the arteries to contract and so makes them more likely to clog. Other precautionary measures are controlling your weight, exercising regularly, and avoiding stress whenever possible.

Does a high level of blood cholesterol run in families? Several of my relations have had heart attacks. Is there any connection?

Yes, there are some well-known medical conditions in which abnormalities of the fats and cholesterol in the blood are inherited. People thus affected may need intensive treatment with both diet and drugs.

My son has always been teased about being fat. Does this mean he has a high blood cholesterol level?

Not necessarily. People who are very overweight consume more food than they need, storing the excess food energy in the form of fat. Their blood cholesterol, however, depends largely on the makeup of their diet, and your son may also be eating the wrong kinds of foods. Try to get him to cut out fast food, ice cream, cake, and candy, but remember that losing weight too quickly or eating too little could damage his health.

Are there any danger signs of a high cholesterol level?

Most people with yellowish deposits of cholesterol around the eyes, called xanthelasma, do not have raised blood cholesterol levels, but a check is justified. When this condition is present in young people, the cholesterol levels should always be checked.

Cholesterol is a fatty or oily substance that normally forms part of the wall around each cell in the body. It is also a basic building block of the steroid hormones, a major group of the body's chemical messengers. However, when cholesterol becomes lodged in the arterial walls, it can contribute to the condition called atherosclerosis, or hardening of the arteries, which causes heart attacks and strokes—a major cause of death in the Western world. The body usually makes sufficient cholesterol, but levels may be increased by extra amounts of animal fats and eggs in the diet.

People at risk

A number of factors contribute to the risk of arterial or heart disease. Smoking and a family history of these conditions are as important as the level of cholesterol in the blood. People in the United States get about 40 percent of their food energy from fats. Surveys of other groups of people who traditionally eat a less fatty diet suggest that if this figure were reduced to below 30 percent, cholesterol levels would probably be lowered. Such a reduction could be achieved by replacing fats with carbohydrates (starchy foods such as bread, potatoes, and rice). Also, fats of animal origin—the so-called saturated fats—seem to increase cholesterol levels, whereas unsaturated fats, such as sunflower, safflower, and corn oil, do not.

What happens in the body

Only a quarter of the cholesterol that circulates in the blood comes directly from the digestive tract, where it has been absorbed from food. Some of the circulating cholesterol returns to the liver, where it is broken down and secreted as bile by the gallbladder. Any excess may enter the arterial walls.

The body binds cholesterol with protein to form lipoproteins, of which there are two forms: a low-density (or lightweight) form called LDL and a heavy-density form called HDL. Relative to HDL, LDL is lightweight because it contains more fat; therefore, LDL floats. LDL deposits cholesterol in the walls of arteries, and can thus be regarded as the bad lipoprotein. HDL, on the other hand, seems to operate in reverse by mopping up loose cholesterol from the arteries and elsewhere in the body and carrying it back to the liver, where it is broken down in the bile and excreted. A greater proportion of HDL in the blood has beneficial effects. The only known way to increase HDL is through exercise. Although much research is being carried out into HDL and LDL, how they work is not yet known. However, it is clear that lowering the cholesterol level helps prevent heart attacks.

Altering the diet

Most experts agree that a sensible diet can help prevent heart attacks. Consumption of sugar, in many commercially made foods, should be reduced and consumption of poultry, fish, and vegetable protein increased. Carbohydrates are best eaten as bread, potatoes, rice, and beans. Red meat should be eaten only once every few days, and no more than four eggs per week should be eaten. Fats should be half of vegetable (polyunsaturated fats) and half of animal origin.

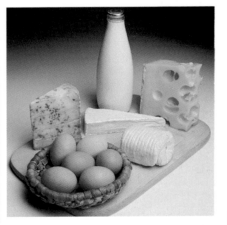

▲ *These foods contain large amounts of fat and should be eaten in moderation.*

See also: Diet; Dieting; Fats; Heart attack; Heart disease; Protein

Common cold

The common cold affects millions of people every year, particularly in the winter months. Although research continues, so far no cure for the common cold has ever been found.

Questions and Answers

I've often been tempted to try cold cures that I see in advertisements. Do these work?

There is no cure for a cold. Some commercial products contain antihistamines, which can reduce secretions and help you sleep. But a cold will always run its course.

My father always seems to have more colds in the summer than in the winter. Why is this?

He may have hay fever, which has symptoms similar to those of the cold virus. Such allergic reactions are usually seasonal, except when someone becomes allergic to material that is present in the air all year long, such as house dust. In such cases it can be difficult, without tests, to distinguish between an allergy and a cold.

Are there any special foods I can eat to protect myself from colds?

Some people feel that taking large amounts of vitamin C, contained in citrus fruits or ascorbic acid preparations, provides some protection—thus the old belief in honey-and-lemon mixture. However, experiments have not yet proved that this helps.

I've heard that you can get a cold by standing in a draft. Is this true?

No. But exposure to wet and miserable weather may lower your resistance, making it easier for the cold virus to gain entry.

What is the difference between a cold and the flu?

Flu involves a specific virus, whereas a cold involves many different viruses. Flu and colds both have upper respiratory symptoms, but flu symptoms are more severe.

The common cold is not one disease, but many. They all have similar symptoms, all of which are caused by viruses that are transmitted to other people by hand contact, coughing, or sneezing.

Causes

There are at least 150 types of viruses that are known to produce the common cold. Antibiotics are of no use in treatment, nor are there yet any effective antiviral drugs.

Not only is the body faced with a bewildering variety of viruses, but these viruses are always likely to undergo DNA mutations, and no practical solution has yet been found to this very complex problem.

People at risk

The sick, the elderly, and the undernourished are not as good as healthy people at fighting infection, and so they are more susceptible to the ravages of the common cold. Young children, whose immune system has not come into contact with so many viruses, can suffer 20 or more such infections each year—as often happens when children start school.

Symptoms

The symptoms of the common cold are well known. The first sign is a feeling of being under the weather, which lasts a few hours. This is usually characterized by aching joints and a cold, shivery feeling. The body temperature is commonly subnormal at this stage; within the next few days—and sometimes hours—the body temperature goes up. A person may have a sore throat and generally feel miserable. As the throat begins to clear, the eyes and nose begin to stream, and there are bouts of repeated sneezing. For most people the common cold is a relatively trivial illness, lasting only a few days.

Treatment

Unless complications like bronchitis develop, there is no need to call a doctor. The best plan is to make the patient as comfortable as possible. Acetaminophen or aspirin can help reduce a fever. Aspirin should not be given to children with viral infections—acetaminophen is safer.

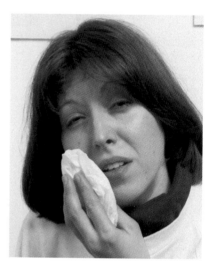

▼▲ *Colds are caused by many viruses, including the coronavirus (below), and the symptoms of a cold are very unpleasant (above). For most people, having a common cold is a trivial condition. However, it can be a serious matter for a person who suffers from bronchitis, especially if he or she is also a smoker.*

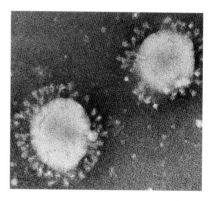

See also: Aspirin and analgesics; Fevers; Genetics; Infection and infectious diseases; Influenza; Sore throat; Viruses

Contraception

If I have an IUD (intrauterine device) fitted, how long will it take to start working?

An IUD is effective as soon as it is in place. However, for the first three months, you must check the string once a week, because this is the time the IUD is most likely to be expelled. If that happened, you would no longer be protected.

I am 21 and would like to have an IUD fitted, but I've heard it is not suitable for women who have not had children. Is this true?

IUDs are not a first-choice method of contraception for women who have not had children, because the uterus and cervix have not been stretched by having a baby. This makes it more difficult and more painful to insert an IUD, and there is more chance that the uterus will expel it. There is also a higher chance of side effects such as painful periods, bleeding, and pelvic inflammatory disease (PID).

I am pregnant and want to have an IUD fitted after the baby is born. I plan to breast-feed my baby. Do I need to have it fitted during this time?

Some doctors like to fit an IUD soon after the baby is born; others prefer to wait six to eight weeks. Ask your doctor, and if he or she wants you to wait six weeks, you must use other contraceptive measures in the meantime. Just because you are breast-feeding does not mean that you will not get pregnant.

Can using a condom really keep you from catching sexually transmitted diseases?

A condom does give a high level of protection to both the man and the woman, but it cannot be relied on to give total protection.

Some contraceptives prevent pregnancy by creating a barrier between the sperm and egg; others either stop the fertilized egg from developing or convince the woman's body that it is already pregnant. Couples should think carefully and ask for advice about what method is best for them.

For thousands of years people have been trying different ideas to prevent women from getting pregnant, ranging from putting crocodile dung into the vagina to standing up after intercourse.

Nowadays the reproductive system is better understood, and more reliable methods are available. The Pill, an oral contraceptive, is one of the best-known, but not every woman can use it. This article deals with the other effective contraceptive methods available.

Choosing a method of contraceptive can be confusing for a woman unless she knows how all of them work and what they do. Some methods are safer than others but may have side effects. Others are more difficult to use and have a higher failure rate. Some women are allergic to rubber and so are unable to use many forms of the diaphragm and condom. Others have heavy, painful periods, so an IUD (intrauterine device) would be unsuitable because it can accentuate menstrual pain and cause heavy bleeding.

A woman should ask her doctor which methods are most suitable. If she goes to a birth control clinic, the clinic should be advised of her medical history. Whichever type of contraceptive she chooses, she should make sure she understands exactly how it works before using it.

In certain countries the use of contraceptives is barred or discouraged for religious reasons. In these places the only method condoned is the rhythm method.

Spermicides
Spermicides contain chemicals that kill sperm. They also inhibit the movement of sperm up the vagina and through the cervical canal (the passage into the uterus). Spermicides are not reliable on their own, so they are usually used with a condom or a diaphragm. Either of these creates a barrier between the man's sperm and the woman's egg (the ovum). If sperm somehow escape contact with the spermicide, the barrier will prevent them from reaching and fertilizing the egg.

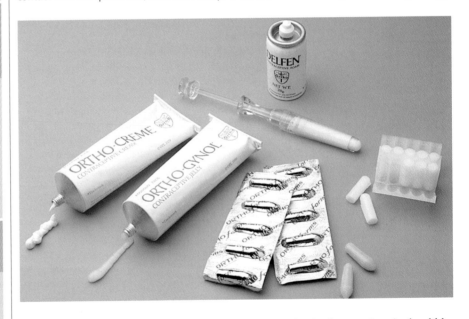

▲ *Spermicide, in the form of a cream, jelly, or pessary (vaginal suppository), should be used by the woman when she uses a diaphragm or when her partner uses a condom.*

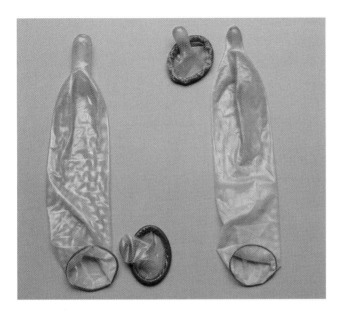

▲ *Condoms are tubes of fine rubber of varying thickness and texture that are unrolled to cover the erect penis.*

Spermicides are readily available from drugstores without a prescription and come in a variety of forms—pressure spray foams (which are the most reliable), tubes of cream and jelly, pessaries, and foaming tablets (which break up in the moist environment of the vagina and release chemicals). However, some spermicides have been found to be almost totally ineffective, and others can cause rubber to deteriorate. Before buying one it is wise to consult a birth control clinic to find out which brands are recommended.

The creams, foams, and jellies come with a syringelike applicator with a plunger. The woman fills the applicator with spermicide and puts it into her vagina, with the applicator tip as close to the cervix (the neck of the uterus) as possible to ensure that any sperm which get that far come into contact with the spermicide. The spermicide is released when she pushes the plunger down the applicator.

When to apply spermicide
Used with a diaphragm, spermicide can be applied up to an hour before intercourse. If a couple decides to use a spermicide on its own, they should apply it not more than 15 minutes before intercourse. However, this is not an effective method of contraception. If they have intercourse a second time, they should apply more spermicide, as there is enough in one application to deal with sperm from only one ejaculation. The woman should not wash away the spermicide sooner than six to eight hours after intercourse.

Pessaries or tablets should be put in place only two to five minutes before intercourse, because they are not effective for very long. The woman can use her finger to place the pessaries as high up in the vagina as possible.

Condoms
Known by a variety of names—including French letter, sheath, rubber, protective, and prophylactic—a condom is a tube of fine rubber that is closed at one end. In its package, it is rolled up so that it looks like a flat circle with a thick rim. It unrolls as it is pulled over

the erect penis. It can then catch all the semen that the penis ejaculates and stop it from reaching the uterus. In addition to being a method of contraception, condoms are also recommended as a barrier against AIDS.

The tip of the condom should be held between the forefinger and thumb of one hand while it is put on, because this keeps air out and allows some space for the ejaculatory fluid. This method also reduces the risk that the condom will burst.

The condom should be put on not only before the penis enters the vagina but before it even touches the woman's genitals. This is because semen can leak out of the penis throughout foreplay. One complaint about condoms is that the couple must stop foreplay to put the condom on. However, many couples overcome this problem by making it part of their foreplay.

There are lubricated condoms available; the lubrication prevents the condom from tearing when it enters the vagina. If this type is not being used, it is a good idea to use spermicide as a lubricant (petroleum jelly should not be used, as it destroys rubber). It is better to use a spermicide in any case, as an extra precaution, since it is always possible that a condom is faulty. When the penis is withdrawn from the vagina, either partner should hold the condom at the base of the penis so that the penis does not slip out and allow semen to escape.

Condoms are available in many countries in a choice of textures, sizes, and colors, without prescription, from drugstores and mail-order companies. They are the only method of contraception, apart from a vasectomy (surgery that permanently prevents the presence of sperm in the ejaculation), in which the man takes total responsibility. Condoms are 96 to 97 percent effective when used properly with a reliable spermicide.

The female condom is made of plastic and is less likely to burst than a conventional male condom. It offers excellent protection against both conception and infection, since it covers the whole of the vulva and vagina. However, it is not popular with many couples.

Diaphragms
A diaphragm is a round, dome-shaped contraceptive made of rubber or plastic. It is inserted into the vagina and covers the cervix, preventing any sperm from entering the uterus. There are three different types of diaphragms, but they all work on the same principle. Used correctly—with spermicide —they are 96 to 97 percent reliable.

The Dutch diaphragm is the largest type, varying from 2 to 4 inches (5 to 10 cm) across. It has a strong spring in the rim, and when it is in position, the front of the rim rests on a little ledge on the pubic bone and the back in a small crevice behind the neck of the uterus. Dutch diaphragms are the easiest to use and for this reason are the most popular. But they are not suitable for women who have poor pelvic tone, because these women's muscles are not strong enough to hold the diaphragm in place. Such women should be able to use another type of diaphragm.

The cervical diaphragm is much smaller than the Dutch diaphragm and looks like a thimble with a thickened rim. Some women find it more difficult to handle and insert, and men can sometimes feel it during intercourse because it is not as flat as the Dutch diaphragm.

Finally, the vault diaphragm is a cross between the previous two types. Unlike the others, it can be made of plastic, so women who are allergic to rubber can use it. Like the cervical diaphragm, the vault diaphragm can occasionally be felt by the man.

HOW TO INSERT A DIAPHRAGM

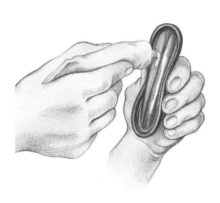

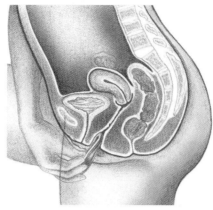

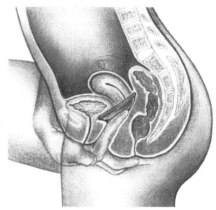

▲ *Place spermicide on both sides of the diaphragm and smear more around the rim. Squeeze into a cigar shape with the fingers.*

▲ *Squat or raise one leg, and after spreading the lips of the vagina, push the diaphragm deep into the vagina until it is in place.*

▲ *Be sure that you can feel the cervix through the diaphragm. Leave the diaphragm in place for at least six hours after the last ejaculation.*

Using a diaphragm

It is not possible to go to a drugstore and buy a diaphragm. A nurse or doctor must fit it to make sure it is the right size, as every woman is slightly different. A properly fitted diaphragm should stay in place during intercourse without causing discomfort to either the woman or her partner. If it is uncomfortable or if it moves, then either it has not been fitted correctly or it is not the right type of diaphragm for the woman concerned.

The couple should always use spermicide with a diaphragm, as a second line of defense, just in case any sperm get past. A spoonful of spermicidal jelly or cream should be squeezed onto both sides. Then more jelly or cream should be smeared all around the rim. To insert the diaphragm, the woman squeezes it into a cigar shape using the thumb and finger. She then uses one hand to spread the lips of the vagina while the other inserts the diaphragm. It is usually easier to insert if she squats down, as this shortens the length of the vagina.

The woman can check the position of her diaphragm by making sure she can feel the cervix through it. The doctor will show her how to do this when the diaphragm is fitted. If intercourse does not take place until more than an hour after insertion, she should apply more spermicide without removing the diaphragm. The woman should leave the diaphragm in place for at least six hours after intercourse, since sperm can live this long in the vagina. To remove a Dutch or vault diaphragm, hook a finger over the rim and pull. Cervical diaphragms have a string that can be pulled to remove them.

The woman should wash the diaphragm thoroughly in warm water after use and check it for any small holes, especially around the rim. If there is a fault, she should replace the diaphragm, using an alternative contraceptive method in the meantime. The diaphragm should be dried thoroughly and stored in the container provided, away from direct sunlight.

▶ *All varieties of diaphragm—cervical (top left), Dutch (right), and vault (bottom left)—are used with spermicide. If necessary, this can be reapplied with a special applicator (bottom right) when the diaphragm is in place.*

A diaphragm should be checked by the doctor at least once a year to make sure that it still fits correctly and does not need replacing. This annual check is especially important if the woman has recently had a baby, has gained or lost an excessive amount of weight, or has only just started to have an active sex life.

Benefits of a diaphragm

The most important benefit of the diaphragm is that it has virtually no side effects. Occasionally it may cause a slight vaginal irritation, and some women find that it brings on cystitis (inflammation of the bladder). These conditions are relatively minor, and after diagnosis

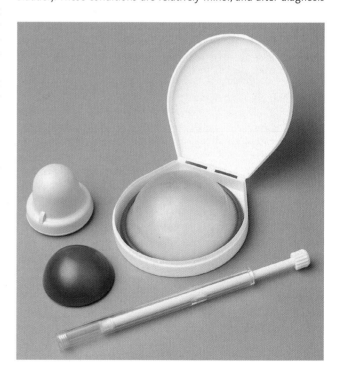

I have heard that there is a condom available which covers only the tip of the penis. Would this kind increase sensation for the man during intercourse?

This type of condom is often referred to as an American tip. However, it is not reliable as a means of contraception, even if used with spermicide, because it can easily slip off.

I like the idea of having a Dutch diaphragm because it has no side effects. But isn't it a messy method of contraception?

It all depends on how squeamish you are—some women do not like to use tampons, for instance. A diaphragm does involve using spermicide, so it is messier than an IUD. It also takes a conscious effort to use. On the other hand, there are fewer side effects. You really need to weigh the advantages and disadvantages.

I have just been fitted with a Dutch diaphragm, but the clinic said I must use a spermicide with it. I do not see why, provided the diaphragm is a good fit.

Even though the diaphragm is fitted for your size and has a strong spring to make sure it stays in place, sperm are tiny and there is always the possibility that they could swim around the edge of the diaphragm and into the uterus. However, if you use spermicide around the rim of the diaphragm and on the side nearest the uterus, it will kill any sperm that do get past.

Can I use a diaphragm during my period?

Yes. All that happens is that the diaphragm holds back the menstrual flow until it is removed. Keep it in for six hours after intercourse, and then use a pad or tampon as usual. Intercourse during a period can be less messy, and therefore more pleasant, if you do use a diaphragm.

by the doctor they can be treated easily and effectively. Nonetheless, a few women find that they cannot use any type of diaphragm. This may be because their muscles are too relaxed for it to stay in place. In addition, some young women may have a vaginal opening that is relatively small, and they have difficulty inserting a diaphragm. Other women find it too distasteful to use. Not all contraceptives are suitable for every woman. Doctors will help each woman to find one that is right for her.

Intrauterine devices

Intrauterine devices—commonly known as IUDs—work in a different way from condoms and diaphragms. They are inserted into the uterus and, rather than forming a barrier between the sperm and the egg, they prevent a fertilized egg from implanting in the uterus. Doctors are not sure exactly why IUDs work, but they are known to prevent the lining of the uterus from thickening—so the right environment for an egg to develop is not created. An IUD does not require any preparation before intercourse. The reliability rate of IUDs is 98 percent, slightly higher than that for diaphragms and condoms.

Internationally, and over the years, IUDs have been made in many shapes and sizes. Two IUDs that are available in the United States are the ParaGard and the Mirena. The ParaGard contains copper and can be left in place for 10 years. The Mirena is a hormone-releasing system placed in the uterus to prevent pregnancy for up to 5 years, although the system should be checked regularly as part of a regular annual exam. When using the Mirena, there is a risk of ectopic pregnancy (in which the fertilized egg lodges in the fallopian tube). The Progestasert, an earlier hormone-releasing IUD, had to be replaced every year and was discontinued in 2001.

Insertion of IUDs

Most IUDs are supplied to the doctor or clinic in sterilized packs with a fine plastic tube, about 0.08 inch (2 mm) in diameter, for insertion. An IUD is usually implanted during or just after menstruation, because the cervix is more relaxed at this time. The depth of the uterus is checked by passing a small probe through the neck of the cervix. This shows the doctor how deep to insert the IUD. The IUD is straightened out inside the tube, and the tube is inserted through the cervix. When the correct depth is reached, the tube is detached and the IUD springs back into shape inside the uterus. The whole process is simple and takes only a few minutes.

The insertion may be a little painful for some women, especially if they are nervous and tighten up their muscles. If there is any pain, however slight, after more than a few days, the woman should go back to see her doctor.

Disadvantages of IUDs

Some women may find that they have heavier periods than usual for the first two or three months after having an IUD fitted, and sometimes there may be slight spotting between periods, backache, or stomach cramps. These symptoms usually disappear after a couple of months, but anyone who is having a lot of pain should see her doctor.

Occasionally an IUD may be expelled from the body for no apparent reason other than that the woman's internal anatomy was unsuitable. If this does happen, it is usually within the first three months and can be during menstruation, when it may pass unnoticed. All IUDs have a fine nylon string attached that hangs down into the vagina, and it should be possible to feel this with a finger. If the string cannot be felt, or if it seems longer than usual, the woman should consult her doctor. She should use another method of contraception in the meantime.

After having an IUD fitted, the woman should check the string once a week for the first three months. After this she should check it once a month after menstruation, as this is the time the IUD is most likely to become dislodged. Some men complain that they can feel the string during intercourse. If this bothers them, a doctor can shorten the string. Tampons rarely get caught up in the string, but if the woman feels a sharp pain when she removes a tampon, she should check the string. Some types of IUD can be left in place for several years, but the woman should have

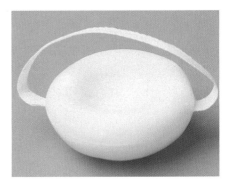

▲ *The vaginal sponge works a little like a diaphragm. The loop aids removal.*

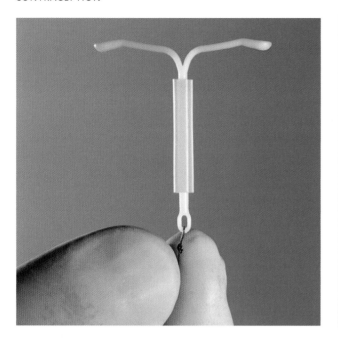

▲ *The Progestasert IUD (shown here) was developed in 1976 and discontinued in 2001. As with all IUDs, the fine plastic string at the bottom was designed to hang through the cervix into the vagina, making removal easy.*

a medical checkup at least once a year. A woman is unlikely to get pregnant with an IUD in place, but if she suspects she has conceived, she should see her doctor at once. The IUD must be removed, because it could cause a miscarriage.

Morning-after IUD

If a woman has had intercourse at the midpoint of her cycle—her most fertile time—without using any contraceptives, some doctors will fit an IUD afterward. This must be done within 72 hours of intercourse. It can be removed at the next menstruation. A better alternative may be the morning-after pill (postcoital contraception), although some people's religious beliefs prevent them using either of these methods as they may be considered a form of abortion.

Douching

It used to be thought that semen could be flushed out of the vagina with hot water or a mild solution that is hostile to sperm. Women used to insert a syringe with a rubber bulb at one end into the vagina and then squeeze out the contents. However, not only is this method totally unreliable, but it can also be dangerous—a dirty syringe can cause an infection.

Vaginal sponge

Usually made from polyurethane foam, the vaginal sponge fits over the cervix in the same way as a diaphragm. It is impregnated with spermicide that is released gradually over a 24-hour period. The sponge works in three ways: it blocks the entrance to the uterus, thereby preventing sperm from entering; it absorbs sperm; and the spermicide kills sperm on contact. The sponge must be left in place for at least six hours after ejaculation.

The rhythm method

The rhythm method of contraception relies on the fact that a woman is fertile for only a few days in each menstrual cycle. By determining which days these are, she can avoid pregnancy by avoiding intercourse on her fertile days.

The two or three days just after ovulation are the fertile days, so to avoid conception, no intercourse should take place during these days. Because sperm may live for 24 to 48 hours in the female reproductive tract, it is also wise to avoid intercourse for the few days before ovulation.

In order to determine when she will ovulate, a woman needs to become aware of, and to monitor, her temperature, the condition of the lower part of the uterus, and the production of fertile mucus (which keeps the sperm alive and guides them to the entrance of the uterus).

Although the rhythm method is better than using no contraception at all, it is not very reliable, and really should be used only if no other alternatives are possible.

New methods of contraception

The following are some of the new methods of contraception that are now available to women.

Depo-Provera shot: This is an injection of the female hormone progesterone, which is given about every three months. It works by inhibiting ovulation, and by preventing sperm from reaching the egg and the fertilized egg from implanting in the uterus. It is as reliable as the Pill (which is 99 percent-plus reliable), but because it does not contain estrogen, many of the dangers and side effects of the Pill are absent. It is especially good for women who have difficulty in remembering to take the Pill on a regular basis.

Lunelle shot: This is an injection of the hormones progesterone and estrogen, which is given about once a month. It is as reliable as Depo-Provera; its side effects and dangers are similar to those of the Pill.

NuvaRing contraceptive ring: This is a flexible ring about 2 inches (50 mm) in diameter that is impregnated with progesterone and estrogen and fits inside the vagina in the same way that a diaphragm does. It releases the hormones into the body in the quantities normally present during pregnancy, fooling the body into thinking it is pregnant so it does not release any eggs. The woman wears the ring for 21 days, then removes it to allow menstruation. After seven days she inserts a new ring, and the process is repeated. It is 99 percent reliable.

Ortho Evra patch: This is a skin patch about 1 3/4 square inches (18 mm²) worn on the buttocks, lower abdomen, or upper body, which releases estrogen and progesterone into the bloodstream. The woman replaces the patch with a new one once a week for three weeks, then removes it for a week to allow menstruation. The skin patch is 99 percent reliable, although it seems to be less effective for women who weigh more than 198 pounds (90 kg).

See also: **AIDS; Sexually transmitted diseases**

Counseling

Counseling is a way of helping people understand their problems and recognize and deal with their feelings. Through attentive listening and appropriate questioning, and sometimes by providing information, counselors enable people to find their own solutions to their problems.

Counseling is simply a formal way of having someone to talk to, but it is often more effective than just talking to a friend or relative. A trained counselor is able to listen in a more detached, unbiased, and honest way than someone who is involved in an individual's life, and the client has the reassurance that whatever is said is kept in complete confidence and will not be repeated.

Who counseling can help

An individual may feel that he or she would like to try counseling because of a specific problem in life, such as bullying, difficulties with other family members or the opposite sex, examination nerves, or just a general feeling of dissatisfaction or unhappiness. Counselors can also help at times of crisis: for example, the death of a loved one or rape.

Short-term counseling is sometimes provided when important decisions need to be made, such as whether to undergo a specific treatment at a hospital. In such cases the counselor will have specialized knowledge to help the person explore all the options. Counseling is also

What is the difference between counseling and psychotherapy?

Psychotherapists tend to treat deeper-seated problems than counselors, and they may delve into your distant past to find out about your childhood, or your internal world, and ask about your dreams and fantasies. In practice, however, there is considerable overlap between the two, and many counselors use psychotherapeutic techniques. Counseling can be short-term, and just one or two sessions can help you through a difficult time.

How can I be sure that nothing I say will be repeated elsewhere?

All counselors who belong to a professional body adhere to a strict code of ethics. This means that everything you say in a counseling session will be treated in confidence. However, if a counselor discovers that a murder or an act of terrorism has been committed, or is being planned, he or she must inform the police.

How do I find a good counselor?

Many schools, colleges, hospitals, and workplaces have counselors on the staff. Specialist bodies that deal with particular problems, such as drug and alcohol abuse, HIV/AIDS, interracial conflict, or family breakups usually have highly trained counselors. Private therapists can be found through your doctor, natural health centers, advertisements, or personal recommendations.

Is counseling expensive?

Counseling at school, college, or work may be free, but some organizations ask for voluntary contributions. Fees for private counseling vary; the most expensive is not always the best.

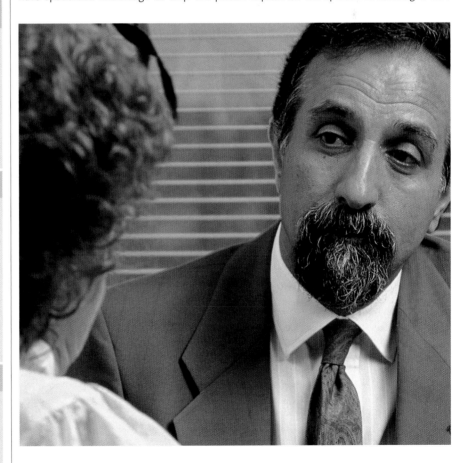

▲ *In a counseling session, client and counselor may sit quite close together. The counselor focuses his or her attention exclusively on the client and the client's problems.*

sometimes recommended for physical conditions that may have a psychological origin or be caused by stress, such as back pain or eating disorders. A person can be counseled alone, with a partner or other family members, or in a group.

Choosing a counselor

When counseling is provided as a service at a college, hospital, or workplace, it is not normally possible to choose a counselor. However, for long-term counseling it will usually be necessary to find a private therapist, and it is important to find the right person.

Counselors call the people that they see clients. Some counselors receive clients in their own homes; others have more formal premises elsewhere. Some will have a couch for the client to lie on; others, a comfortable chair to sit in. It is often up to the clients to decide what format suits them best and makes them feel relaxed. Some people prefer to keep a distance between themselves and their counselor; others prefer to be closer. The clients also need to decide what kind of counselor they will feel most comfortable with. Should he or she be the same sex—even the same race—a specialist, or someone used to dealing with more general problems?

Some counseling is done on the telephone. This is ideal for clients who want to preserve their anonymity, for people who are unable to travel, or when immediate support is vital—perhaps when someone is contemplating suicide.

Seeing a counselor

In long-term counseling, the first session is likely to be exploratory, with the client deciding whether this is someone he or she feels comfortable with, and the counselor assessing whether he or she can offer the kind of help the client needs. The client has nothing to lose at this stage by being honest and expressing any misgivings about the whole idea of counseling, about the counselor, or about anything else. The client may even find that this is the beginning of the unraveling process.

Counselors are trained to recognize serious mental problems, and if they think the client needs a different kind of therapy, they will say so immediately. On the other hand, a counselor would never dismiss a client's problems or concerns as trivial. This would go against the whole ethos of counseling.

At the first session the counselor will also give the client an idea of how many sessions he or she thinks may be needed. Sessions are usually weekly, and counseling may extend over a few weeks or a year or more. The client need not decide at the outset how long the counseling will last, and sessions are usually paid for one at a time.

What counseling is like

A counselor gives the client his or her complete attention. This in itself is therapeutic—how many people have the luxury in daily life of being properly listened to? In addition, this attention is uncritical. A counselor is there not to judge clients but to help them understand themselves. When someone else really listens, the client starts listening to him- or herself.

The counselor may prompt the client with questions, if he or she feels that this is necessary. These are not the sort of questions that friends ask, which are usually motivated by curiosity, but questions designed to help the client see things more clearly. They may be questions no one has ever asked before or questions the client has never asked him- or herself. In family therapy the counselor's

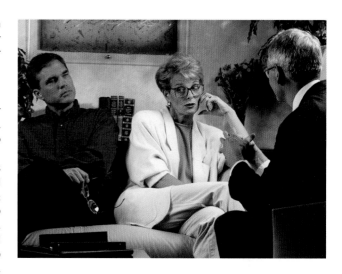

▲ *When partners are experiencing difficulties in their relationship, it can be helpful to discuss their differences with a third party who is a trained counselor.*

questions may induce family members to say things that other members of the family never knew they thought or felt. Another technique counselors use is "reflecting back" to clients the things the clients have said or feelings they have expressed or only hinted at. The counselor may say something like, "So, when this happens, you feel such and such, and this leads you to . . . ." This not only shows that the counselor has heard and taken in what a client has said but makes the clients feel that they are being taken seriously and that their feelings have been given validity.

Release of emotion

In the course of counseling, the client may experience strong emotions—perhaps unexpected ones—and the counselor will encourage the client to explore and release these emotions. Because the counselor is not involved in the emotions, it is safe for the client to feel them without any risk of upsetting anyone or provoking anger in anyone. In partner and group sessions, a counselor can act as a sort of referee, turning emotional conflicts into constructive events that offer insights into the relationships. Some counselors offer physical contact at these times—holding hands or hugging, for example—but this is a matter of personal style.

The aim of counseling is to increase a client's confidence and make him or her more at ease with life in general, and to enable the client to be more in control of his or her own life.

What can go wrong?

There may be a few counselors who are not as professional as they should be. Some of the problems that might be encountered are:

● Physical contact that oversteps the bounds of what is acceptable.

● Breaches of confidentiality.

● A counselor who tries to dominate the client. If this is happening, the client will tend to feel worse after a session rather than better.

● A counselor who spends too much time talking about him- or herself. A certain amount of self-revelation is permissible in a counselor—it shows sympathy for what the client is saying—but this should be relevant and kept to a minimum.

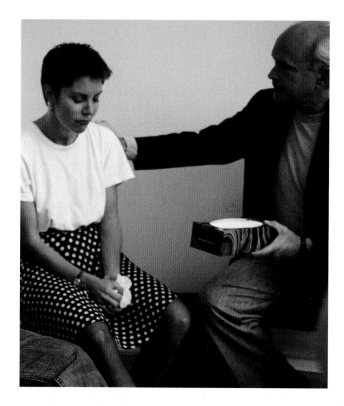

▲ *A client may find that strong and even surprising emotions emerge in him or her during a counseling session. However, counselors expect this to happen and are trained to sympathize with the client and to give him or her their support.*

● A counselor who wants too much social contact outside the sessions. Social contact changes the nature of the counseling relationship and is not usually a good idea.

When things go wrong

The first person a client should complain to is the counselor. Whether or not this is easy to do is in itself an indication of the health of the relationship between client and counselor. If the counselor works in an organization, such as a college, the client should discuss the problem with someone in authority. The professional organization the counselor belongs to can also be contacted. Serious offenses should be reported to the police, but it is wise in these circumstances to remember that it will be the client's word against the counselor's.

A bad experience should not be allowed to deter someone from finding another counselor. Most counselors are dedicated and skilled. However, dissatisfaction with the counselor may be a sign that the therapy is coming to an end.

Saying good-bye

The client is in charge of the course of the counseling and should always be the one to decide when to end it. Some people may need the support of a counselor all their lives, but this is highly unusual. The aim of counseling is to empower the client, not to make him or her dependent on another person, in this case the counselor. Some clinics allow only a limited number of sessions anyway. In short-term

---

Types of therapy

Cocounseling: In cocounseling, two people work together, taking turns as counselor and client. Both need to be trained to do this, but once trained, people can work in pairs to develop their own understanding of themselves, at the same time helping the other person.

Gestalt therapy: This is based on the belief that we all have an innate ability to function in a creative, positive, and healthy way but that social conditioning can impair this ability. The therapy uses techniques, such as reenacting arguments, to put you more in touch with your own emotions. It can be done either on your own or in a group.

Person (client)-centered therapy: This form of therapy aims to help people achieve their full potential. It is based on the belief that once people understand themselves better, they will be able to find their own way out of any difficulties they may have. The therapist relies less on theories and more on following what the client seems to want. The therapy was founded by U.S. psychologist Carl Rogers. Most counseling is based on person-centered therapy.

Psychiatry: The treatment of mental illness with drugs or surgery. Psychiatrists are medically trained.

Psychoanalysis: An intensive form of psychotherapy, often lasting several years, with several sessions a week.

Psychodynamic counseling: Counseling that uses psychotherapeutic techniques.

Psychology: The scientific study of the mind.

Transactional analysis: This was invented by Eric Berne, a Canadian doctor who believed that we have three ego states (ways of behaving): parent, adult, and child. Treatment aims to make people aware of which ego state they are in at any time and ultimately to express all three at once.

---

therapy the end will be in sight all through the counseling, and every counseling session will work toward this.

It is vital to finish counseling properly, so as not to undo what has been learned or devalue the whole process. There will be difficult emotions—anger that the counselor cannot help anymore, sorrow at the parting, fear that one cannot manage on one's own. All these emotions can be worked through in the final sessions.

Preparing to stop counseling can take several sessions. One way to prepare for an ending is to space counseling sessions more widely apart. The client can leave the door open at the final session: "I am leaving for now, but I can always come back if I need to." Some people return at times of stress throughout their lives.

See also: AIDS; Alcoholism; Anorexia and bulimia; Child abuse; Drug abuse; Family relationships

Cramp

Questions and Answers

My brother has to write a lot and suffers from writer's cramp. What is this, and is there a cure for it?

Writer's cramp is also known as professional or occupational cramp. It can affect people who use their hands for delicate work, such as musicians, seamstresses, and artists, as well as writers. The muscles of the fingers, and even the forearm, seize up, so that work with the affected hand is impossible. Usually the hand can be used normally for delicate work; thus the cramp is believed to be a psychological condition. It is not linked to an organic or bodily disease. The way to treat this form of cramp is to discover the underlying psychological cause and to treat that. Sometimes a rest from work is the best cure. In your brother's case, altering the way he holds his pen may help.

I suffer from cramps only on vacation in Mexico, although I exercise all through the year at home. Why does this happen?

If you exercise vigorously in a hot climate, for example by playing volleyball on the beach, you lose salt from your body with the sweat. It is this lack of salt that causes heat cramps. Try taking salt tablets while on vacation.

I am pregnant and frequently suffer from cramps in my legs at night, which keep me awake for a long time. Why is this?

Your muscles are under additional strain during the day owing to the unaccustomed weight of the developing baby. As a result, they go into spasm at night when you are lying down and relaxed. Ask your partner to massage your legs when the cramp occurs, since you will not be able to reach them comfortably. Once you have had your baby, it is likely that the attacks will disappear.

Almost everyone has experienced muscle cramps—unexpected and agonizing pain, usually in the backs of the legs. But cramps are not usually a sign that anything is seriously wrong, and can be relieved by self-massage.

A cramp is a painful and involuntary contraction of a muscle or group of muscles. Cramps in the limbs usually occur in the legs, affecting the muscles in the calf or the back of the thighs. They come on suddenly and without warning, sometimes when a person is deeply asleep. The muscle fibers contract into a hard knot, which may last from a few seconds to a few minutes.

Causes

Cramps can be caused by poor circulation, which results in an inadequate supply of blood reaching the muscles in the limbs. Exposure to cold can also bring on an attack and, when combined with exhaustion, is sometimes a cause of swimmer's cramp. Athletes with slight injuries to the muscles in their limbs may also suffer from cramping in an affected muscle. Heavy sweating, which leads to a severe loss of salt, can also induce cramps, as can eating just before exercise.

Symptoms

The cramped limb seizes up with a sharp local pain, and ordinary efforts to move and relax the muscle are useless. People who suffer from persistent cramps should check

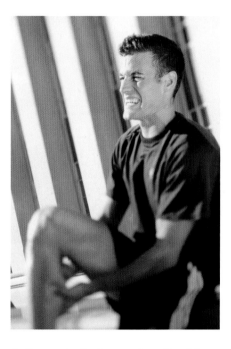

▲ *Cramps in the legs can be relieved by flexing the foot upward. Persistent leg cramps are often cured by pacing around the room for a while.*

with their doctor to be sure that it is not a symptom of a circulatory problem. A cramp in itself is unpleasant but not dangerous. However, someone suffering from cramps while swimming in deep water is in real danger. When engaging in any type of physical activity, a person should stop and deal with a cramp rather than attempting to continue with the exercise while suffering.

Treatment

Cramps caused by circulatory problems, such as artery disease, can be treated by vasodilator drugs, which a doctor can prescribe. These open the narrowed arteries, improving the flow of blood to the muscles. Cramps that are caused by artery disease usually occur later in life, and although drugs may alleviate the symptoms, they do not cure the hardened arteries. Young people and others involved in sports should avoid eating shortly before physical exertion. If a cramp has been brought on by loss of salt from the body, as happens after prolonged sweating, salt tablets taken with water will help to restore the balance in the body. An attack of cramps can be somewhat eased by massaging and manipulating the affected muscle. Most active people find that their cramp attacks are temporary. Pregnant women who suffer from cramps usually find that the attacks disappear after they give birth. Some people, especially the elderly, may get severe cramps at night. These night cramps can often be prevented with a type of quinine pill.

See also: **Exercise; Salt**

Depression

My son's girlfriend has died in a car accident. He is brokenhearted but won't let it show. Is it better to suppress grief or to let it out?

The take-it-like-a-man approach has no place in grief, in either sex—in every case it is better to let it out. The suppression of grief, advocated as a means of showing emotional strength, can lead to psychological problems later. The reason people advise this is that they are upset by the sight of natural grief in others—their motives are self-centered.

During family arguments, my teenage son has often said, "I'll just die, and then you'll be happy." Is there a real risk that he will commit suicide because he is depressed?

What your son may be asking is for you to tell him that you would be very unhappy if he died, because you love him even if you do occasionally argue. If he does seem to have more dark moods than most adolescents, watch out for other signs. Teenagers do not have to be as deeply depressed as adults do before they attempt suicide.

My friend takes prescribed drugs for her depression. Are they habit-forming?

Antidepressant drugs are not habit-forming but do have some undesirable side effects.

Is there any specific age when people are most likely to become depressed?

Depression can start at any age, although serious depression peaks at approximately age 60 for males and 55 for females. For milder cases of depression, the peak age is 50 for males and 45 for females.

Depression can be conquered—but the condition sometimes needs skilled medical and psychological help, in addition to support and understanding from both family and friends.

Many people feel down from time to time, but these feelings are usually passing phases. In defining where such moods end and actual depression begins, it should be remembered that depression is not a simple condition. It can show itself in various ways and have a number of causes. Neither does it respect sex or occupation, and it can strike at any time from the teens to middle age, when it claims the greatest number of victims.

Early warning signals

If a person suspects that a spouse, parent, child, or friend is suffering from depression, there are ways of detecting the signs of serious trouble. Perhaps the most significant fact is that the victim loses interest and enjoyment in every aspect of life. Such a change is quickly noticeable to other people. This can apply to work, school, the home, the family, food and drinks, hobbies, sports, and the desire for sex and may extend to personal appearance and hygiene.

Then the complaints may begin—about all kinds of physical problems, such as headaches, back pains, stomach troubles, tightening in the chest, dizziness, constipation, or blurred vision. Depressed people are also so apathetic that they are often unable to ask for professional help. Therefore, it is up to others to seek medical or psychiatric advice for them.

The many faces of depression

Not all the symptoms of depression are shown by every patient—two people behaving in completely different ways can both be considered depressed. What makes the picture even more complicated is that the condition can be accompanied by acute anxiety or may swing into a period of mania—a mood of almost forced gaiety, talkativeness, and compulsive activity, symptoms that lead to the term "manic-depressive."

In general depression, moods may vary from slight sadness to intense despair and a feeling of utter worthlessness. Strangely, people with this condition seldom talk of these feelings to their doctor; instead they may complain about small aches and pains, tiredness, or loss of weight. They may even find it difficult to speak to anyone; to them, other people may seem to chatter constantly. Compulsive chattering or virtual silence often occurs as a result of cognitive difficulties. Patients often complain of not being able to think clearly, concentrate, or make

▼ *This patient suffering from depression is curled in a typical posture.*

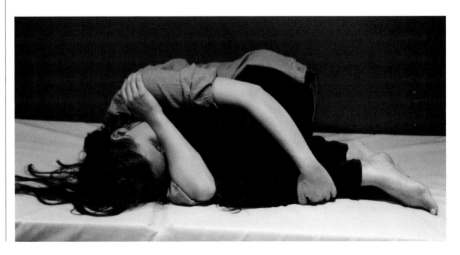

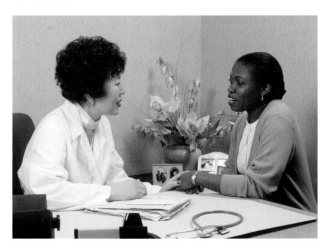

▲ *Someone who is depressed should first consult a doctor.*

decisions—they know that something is amiss. This ability to realize their own unhappy state, without being able to do anything about it, affects depressives in another way. They tend to be preoccupied with themselves and seem completely unable to count their blessings. Instead they magnify any mishap of the past and tend to blow it up into a major disaster, always regarding themselves as totally to blame for every misfortune. The habit of distorting events affects sleep patterns, which may already be disturbed by the illness itself. Depressives lie awake worrying about the past and the future. A vicious circle easily sets in, with worries about the inability to sleep added to all the others. As if all this were not enough, the depression itself can cause early-morning waking, so that the beginning of the day is the most miserable time of all. When depression is accompanied by anxiety, the sufferer is usually restless and talks in a nervous way; this is in marked contrast to the apathy of other depressives, who tend to conceal their worries.

Postpartum depression

The particular state arising in a small number of women soon after they have given birth is called postpartum depression. It was once thought of as little more than a mood caused by the exhaustion of labor and the unaccustomed strain of looking after the new arrival. However, it is now recognized as a definite illness; its symptoms include a surprising hostility toward the baby, with consequent feelings of guilt or indifference.

All this can cause serious neglect of the child and of the home, and a feeling of being unable to cope with the situation. The result is often a weakening of both marital and family relationships. In serious cases the condition may even lead to suicide.

There is evidence now that the real cause of all these problems is a disturbance of the mother's hormonal system, which is a side effect of pregnancy and birth. Treatment must always include the restoration of this hormone balance.

Heredity and environment

To some extent depression is thought to run in families; but this influence increases susceptibility to the condition, rather than actually producing it. In fact, there is nearly always a definite stressful event, or series of events, that precipitates the depressive

state. Another way in which these symptoms can be "transmitted" is that a parent who suffers from depression invariably acts out his or her condition to others in the household. Children then tend to copy this form of behavior later in life, if they themselves feel depressed. Because they have had such a role model, they adopt a type of depressive behavior much more easily than they would otherwise.

When there is no family history of depression, the condition is virtually always triggered by powerful patterns of outside events that affect the victim deeply. In such cases the chance of recovery from depression is somewhat better.

The effects of grief

Temporary, but very real, depression can be caused by bereavement. When a loved one dies, it is normal to express grief. To attempt to suppress this feeling because it is painful, because the bereaved person does not want to seem silly, or because the deceased person "wouldn't want me to be sad" is never helpful but rather tends to prolong the grieving period.

Besides the usual reactions of distress, there are often feelings of guilt, irritability, and lack of affection toward others. Sometimes there is an unnerving habit of taking on the personality traits or mannerisms of the dead person.

Mixed feelings

People in this state may also have problems in their relationships with other members of the family and with friends. They may show intense feelings of anger toward doctors, hospital authorities, or "uncaring" relatives. Alternatively there may be a complete lack of apparent signs of grief, accompanied by periods of restlessness and virtually pointless activity, which are justified as "keeping the mind busy" but which do nothing of the kind. In any of these situations, the bereaved person should be encouraged to let out his or her feelings of grief and to talk about the loss with friends, relatives, or even with a family doctor or therapist.

How to help with postpartum depression
Ask the doctor's advice: treatment may be needed to restore the mother's hormonal balance.
Psychotherapy might also be necessary, or even a stay in the hospital.
Take over care, or help with care, of the baby to allow the mother to rest and have undisturbed nights. The baby can be taken care of by the partner, a close relative, or even a professional helper, if necessary.
Help with, or take over, domestic chores such as cooking, shopping, laundry, and cleaning.
Be tolerant, understanding, and patient. The mother has very little control over her state of mind, and the more she is relieved of pressure and is given medical or psychological treatment, the more quickly she will be able to make a complete recovery.

INCIDENCE OF FIRST-CASE DEPRESSIVE ILLNESS IN THREE MAJOR HOSPITALS IN ONE YEAR

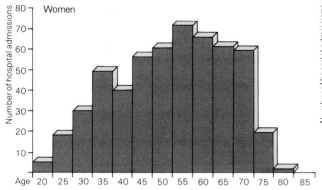

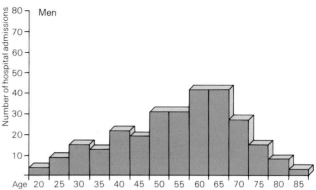

Treatment

Many people find it hard to appreciate the despair that a severely depressed person can experience. In fact, about one in six cases of severe depression results in suicide. It is thought that this rate would be even higher were it not for the fact that the sufferer is often too apathetic to go through with a suicide attempt. Modern antidepressant drugs play an important part in the management of depression. Indeed, they may be literally lifesaving. Patients need to know that most antidepressant drugs take from two to three weeks to have their full effect. During this period suicides are common.

There are several classes of antidepressants. Those most commonly used are the tricyclic drugs. This group includes drugs with sedative effects such as amitriptyline (Elavil, Enovil), doxepin (Adapin, Sinequan), and trimipramine (Surmontil). Nonsedative tricyclics include clomipramine (Anafranil), impiramine (Tofranil, Janimine), and nortriptyline (Aventyl, Pamelor). These drugs help patients to sleep and to stop losing weight. There is quickening of thought, speech, and activity, and a raising of mood. Anxiety may, however, persist. Tricyclic antidepressants may cause or worsen glaucoma, urinary retention, and prostate gland enlargement.

The selective serotonin and noradrenaline reuptake inhibitor drugs such as venlafaxine (Effexor) have some advantages over the tricyclics, and fewer side effects. Better tolerated are the selective serotonin reuptake inhibitors such as paroxetine (Paxil), citalopram (Celexa), fluoxetine (Prozac), and sertraline (Zoloft). Drugs of the Prozac class may cause nausea, diarrhea, insomnia, agitation, and sexual dysfunction. The monoamine oxidase inhibitor antidepressant drugs (MAOIs) such as tranylcypromine (Parnate) and phenelzine (Nardil) are less often used nowadays. They are helpful in the treatment of atypical depression with anxiety and complaints of physical symptoms and are often prescribed for patients who fail to respond adequately to tricyclic drugs, but they can cause dangerous reactions if taken with cheese, protein extracts such as Bovril or Oxo, yeast extracts like Marmite, flavored textured vegetable protein, or any alcohol drinks. Lithium salts are the mainstay of the treatment of the manic phase of manic-depressive illness and are very effective. However, the borderline between effectiveness and toxicity is narrow.

Psychological methods, such as self-assertion and learning to examine thoughts, in addition to behavioral therapy techniques, can work well. Even thinking about making the choice to use psychological methods has a certain power to lift depression.

Living with depression

Psychological treatment can help sufferers change their way of thinking about themselves and the world. But for those living with a depressed person, it is best not to expect too much too soon. What is needed is continual friendliness, interest, and support—even if these do not seem to be having much effect. Often, a positive approach is much appreciated by the depressed person, even if he or she cannot respond, and it will be remembered with gratitude later.

The technique of not doing too much at once also applies to relaxation. Vacations can lead to additional anxiety for the patient and should be reserved for the time when he or she is well on the road to recovery, when everyone concerned will benefit more.

Hospital treatment

In severe cases of depression, home care may be impossible and the patient may have to spend time in the hospital for care and therapy. Electroconvulsive therapy (ECT) may be given. Carefully controlled electrical discharges are passed through parts of the brain while the patient is anesthetized. The current induces a convulsion in the patient's brain and body. This is not felt, but it often produces an improvement in the patient's condition—as few as two or three treatments may induce a complete recovery. Although there may be temporary forgetfulness of recent events, many depressives believe that this is a small price to pay for the relief ECT provides. However, it is a technique that some doctors and psychiatrists question, since its results, in some cases, may be only short-term. Advances in drugs have resulted in a considerable reduction in the use of ECT.

Outlook

In spite of the large number of people who are afflicted with depressive illness, and the severity of some cases, the outlook is reasonably good. It has been estimated that of all those with a clearcut depressive illness, about 95 percent will probably recover and only 4 percent will remain in a state of chronic illness.

Of those who do recover, perhaps half may have another phase of depression at some time—but for most people the recovery rate is fairly high.

See also: **Headache; Heredity; Mental illness; Suicide**

Diabetes

If my son eats too much candy, is he likely to develop diabetes—either now or later in life?

No. If a child is going to get diabetes, it will be the type caused by failure to produce insulin (a hormone produced in the pancreas). Being overweight or eating sweet things has nothing to do with whether the insulin-producing cells in the pancreas are functioning properly or not.

Is there any age when diabetes is more likely to develop?

It can start at any age, but it is unusual in children under age five. If the disease does occur in early life, it is most likely to do so at puberty or in the late teens or early twenties. After that there is no particular age at which it is more or less likely.

My husband has been diagnosed as diabetic. I am afraid the illness may change his personality, by making him bad-tempered, for example. Am I right to worry about this?

Not really. Obviously diabetes, like any illness, can put the patient under strain, but it does not cause personality changes. There is certainly nothing to suggest that diabetic children develop inadequate personalities as they grow up because of their diabetes.

Is it safe for a diabetic person to drive a car or ride a motorcycle?

Usually. The only risk is that an insulin-controlled diabetic might suddenly lose consciousness because of hypoglycemia—a fall in the blood sugar level that can occur if the insulin dose gets out of balance. Diabetics have to declare that they suffer from the disorder when applying for a license to drive any sort of vehicle.

Diabetes and its symptoms have been recognized for hundreds of years. However, it is no longer feared as it was before treatment was discovered in the 1920s, and current research is constantly improving the outlook for diabetics.

Diabetes is a condition in which there is an abnormally high level of sugar in the blood. Affected people pass abnormally large quantities of urine as a result, developing an abnormal thirst and losing a great deal of weight.

In the 17th century, when diabetes was known as the "pissing evil," people noticed that the urine of most sufferers was particularly sweet. In a few cases, however, it was insipid—that is, it was not sweet. Diabetics of the first type had diabetes mellitus (mellitus means "like honey"), and this is the disease we know today as plain diabetes. The second type of the disease, diabetes insipidus, is extremely rare and results from a failure of the pituitary gland in the skull.

A common condition

Thousands of people in every country suffer from diabetes mellitus. In the United States, 2 to 4 percent of the population are diagnosed diabetics. One in 600 school children requires insulin.

Diabetes results from a failure in the production of insulin, one of the body's hormones or chemical messengers. Its job is to keep the blood's sugar content under control by directing it into the cells, where it can be put to its proper use—as fuel to produce energy. Without insulin the body's cells become starved of sugar, despite the high level in the blood.

How diabetes starts

In most diabetics, the lack of insulin is due to a failure of the part of the body responsible for producing insulin. This is the pancreas, and the failure is caused by the destruction of its

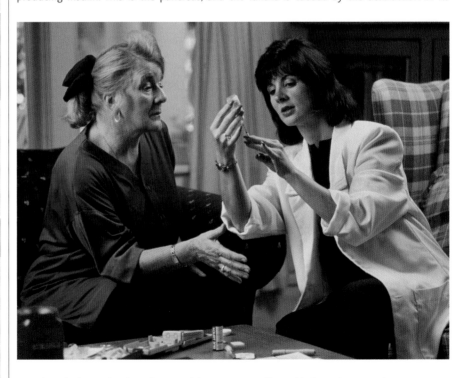

▲ *When diabetes develops later in life, patients will need help in learning how to measure their urine and blood sugar levels, and in administering insulin.*

How serious is diabetes?

The disease may be serious for two reasons. First, without insulin injections, the young diabetic simply continues to lose weight and may eventually lapse into a coma and die.

Second, diabetics can develop complications—in other words, additional complaints that are brought on as a result of their condition. Generally speaking, the better the level of blood sugar is controlled, the less likely complications are to occur.

The most serious complications concern the eyes and the kidneys and are caused by the effect of the disease on the blood vessels. It is usually possible to see changes to the blood vessels in the back of the eye of any long-standing diabetic; in very few cases, this worsens progressively to the extent that the patient eventually loses the sight of one or both eyes.

Diabetics may also develop abnormalities in their nerves that can lead to a loss of feeling in the hands and feet. Finally, the diabetic may develop artery trouble, which in turn causes strokes, arterial blockage with gangrene, and heart attacks. For this reason, anyone suffering from diabetes will be strongly encouraged not to smoke, since it is well known that smoking also increases the likelihood of arterial disease.

How insulin works

In general, the patient whose diabetes comes on early in life needs insulin, although a fair proportion of those whose diabetes starts later in life will also eventually need it. The hormone is given by injection, usually under the skin of the thigh. Diabetics are

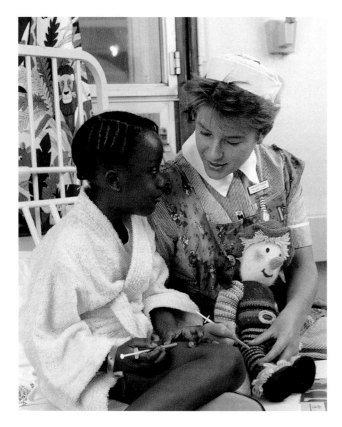

▲ *The treatment for juvenile diabetes is a strict diet combined with regular injections of insulin. Here a nurse shows a diabetic girl how to give herself an injection.*

insulin-producing cells. There is considerable evidence that this destruction is the result of an autoimmune process. The surfaces of these cells have been modified so that the immune system mistakenly identifies them as "foreign" and attacks and destroys them. There have been a few cases in which very early diabetes was cured when this mechanism was recognized and treated with immunosuppressive drugs.

The type of diabetes that develops suddenly, owing to a complete or serious failure of insulin, tends to afflict young people and children and is often called juvenile diabetes. It can be treated with injections of insulin from cattle or pigs, or with genetically engineered "human" insulin.

Most diabetics, however, suffer from what is called maturity-onset (type II) diabetes. In this case the pancreas does produce insulin, often in normal amounts, but the tissues of the body are insensitive to its action—and this condition produces the high blood sugar level.

The condition often coincides with being overweight and can be treated by dieting. Therefore, the diet is usually supplemented with tablets that stimulate the pancreas to produce more insulin.

However, this picture of two separate sorts of diabetes is too simple. In reality the two types tend to merge into each other. Some younger people, and even children, seem to have the maturity-onset type, and some elderly patients may require insulin to keep their blood sugar level down.

THE ROLE OF INSULIN

Insulin working normally

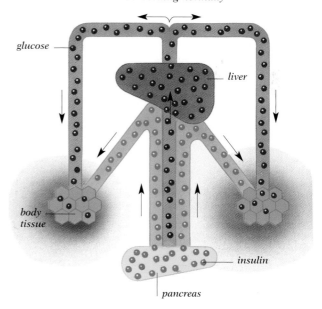

glucose

liver

body tissue

insulin

pancreas

▲ *When insulin is produced normally by the pancreas, it enables glucose—which body cells need to burn to produce energy—to be stored in the liver. Then, when the body cells need more energy, and therefore more glucose to make it, the glucose will be released from the liver, and insulin from the pancreas enables it to be used by the body cells.*

instructed how to draw insulin up into a syringe and give themselves the injections. This usually has to be done twice daily, and often different formulations of insulin are used to try to spread the total effect out over the course of the day.

Once a diabetic has taken insulin, his or her blood sugar level will start to fall, but this fall does not end the problem. Sometimes the sugar level falls too far as a result of taking the insulin. Sugar is an essential food, not only for the body's tissues in general but particularly for the brain. If the sugar falls too low, the brain ceases to function properly, and the patient becomes unconscious.

Diabetics can learn to recognize the early symptoms of a falling blood sugar level: shakiness, sweating, tingling around the mouth, and often a feeling of being rather muddled. The treatment for this condition, called hypoglycemia (which means low blood sugar), is to take some form of sugar by mouth immediately.

Balancing the insulin

Because of the risk of hypoglycemia, diabetics must balance their food intake with their insulin injections, so that the sugar level is kept near the normal range without too much soaring up and down. They must eat regular meals containing similar amounts of carbohydrates (foods that are broken down to sugar in the blood).

HOW LACK OF INSULIN CAUSES A DIABETIC COMA

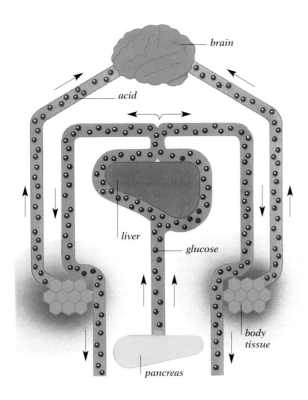

▲ *If there is no insulin, glucose cannot be stored or utilized. The result is a great deal of urine with a high glucose content. In place of the lost glucose, the cells produce energy by burning up fats, but these cannot be burned properly without glucose and therefore produce high acid in the blood. If the condition is untreated, a diabetic coma will result.*

All diabetics, whether insulin-treated or not, should avoid sugar itself or foods that contain sugar, such as jam, candy, cakes, and fruit drinks. (Sugar is absorbed rapidly in the stomach to produce brisk increases in the blood sugar level.)

The use of sugar to halt an attack of hypoglycemia is an exception to this general rule.

Measuring techniques

As well as carefully planned insulin injections and a regulated intake of carbohydrates, most diabetics use some measuring technique to keep a check on their blood sugar level. The traditional method is to measure the amount of sugar in the urine, which gives an idea of the amount of sugar in the blood.

However, diabetics are strongly advised to maintain control by frequent direct measurement of the blood sugar. This is done by using a pocket-size device that can accurately determine blood sugar levels in blood taken from a small prick in the finger.

What causes a coma?

Diabetics may suffer from two types of coma. A diabetic coma differs from a coma caused by hypoglycemia—when a low blood sugar level results in a loss of consciousness—in that the diabetic develops a high blood sugar level, which leads to complications.

The two conditions are different, although some people may confuse them. Hypoglycemia can develop in a matter of minutes and is easily stopped by taking sugar. A high blood sugar level, on the other hand, takes hours or even days to develop and may take hours to cure. As the sugar level rises, owing to lack of insulin, the cells are starved of fuel. They have to burn something to keep alive, and so they start burning fat instead. Used-up fat produces waste products called ketones, and the presence of excess ketones produces a high blood-acid level. If this is not corrected with insulin, coma and death can result.

The future for diabetics

Apart from research into the basic cause of the disease, there have been a number of helpful improvements in the treatment of diabetes.

Insulin is steadily becoming more highly purified, and thanks to the technique of genetic engineering, insulin that is identical to the insulin produced by the human pancreas can be used instead of the animal insulin that was used in the past.

New innovations

Techniques for taking insulin are, in addition, becoming more refined. The twice-daily injections may be replaced, for some diabetic patients, by a constant delivery of insulin from a special pump. This is worn, possibly on a belt, and is only about 6 inches (15 cm) in length. The insulin enters the blood by a needle that is inserted into the skin of the abdomen.

Finally, the treatment of eye problems caused by diabetes has also advanced tremendously in recent years. This improvement is due to the introduction of lasers that are able to treat some of the abnormalities that develop at the back of the eye.

See also: Glucose; Heart attack; Stroke; Sugars

Diet

Questions and Answers

I have always fed my daughter a proper diet, but suddenly she has become very thin, almost skeletal. I am afraid she is anorexic and is hiding her food. How could this have happened?

Anorexia nervosa is also known as the dieter's disease, but it is more complex than that. It almost always strikes young people between the ages of 11 and 30 (girls more than boys). A dramatic loss of weight is the most obvious sign; others include hypersensitivity about appearance, bouts of constipation that alternate with diarrhea, or sudden personality changes, such as withdrawal from friends. The anorexic may be secretly tortured by lack of self-esteem, confidence, and a true idea of self. He or she may fear maturity, making thinness seem desirable. Anorexics suffer from a defect of perception so that a painfully thin body may still appear fat. If you think your daughter is anorexic, you must take her to a doctor. Anorexia nervosa is a dangerous illness with a high mortality rate. Expert management is mandatory.

My son will refuse to eat when he is sick. Should I insist that he eats?

No, it is not necessary for him to eat solid foods when he is sick and may even be detrimental. Give him plenty of fluids instead. Weak tea or milk with some sugar will give him energy, and soups will provide nourishment. When he feels better, he will ask for solid foods again.

I suffer from eczema. Is it true that food allergies can cause this?

Yes. Research has shown that skin disorders may be caused by allergic reactions to some foods. Finding the causes involves tests to isolate possible reactions. Some clinics offer this service, or your doctor may be able to provide a plan for you to test yourself.

The body is like an engine, and food is the fuel it needs to keep running. Just as gasoline comes in different octanes, so foods have different energy-producing levels. How efficiently the body works depends on what is consumed.

The food a person eats is converted into energy and used by the body for its different functions. These include the obvious physical activities, such as walking or running, as well as the constant process of growth and repair of the body tissues. Throughout life, body tissues are continuously broken down and replaced by new cells to keep the person whole and in good working order.

Everyone must eat the right amount of food to fuel all these needs. If more food is consumed than is required, the excess will be stored in the body and lead to a person's becoming overweight.

Most foods have a chemical structure that is different from the body's, so they need to be changed into a form that the body can easily absorb. This absorption process is known as digestion.

Types of food

Food can be divided into three main types: carbohydrates, proteins, and fats. Carbohydrates and fats are used to fuel all the body's processes and functions; protein is used as building material for the body's tissues. Although the body can use both fats and protein as energy sources, and fats can be formed from other food sources, a minimum input of each of these groups is advisable.

Carbohydrates

Carbohydrates are commonly found in starch and sugar. Starch is present in all cereals and root vegetables, and sugar is found in its natural form in fruits or honey, or in a refined state in table sugar. Carbohydrates are found in greatest quantities in potatoes, breads, bananas, peas, corn,

▶ *Many of a child's favorite meals provide a large part of the dietary requirements for a full day, and will give him or her all the energy a rapidly growing body requires.*

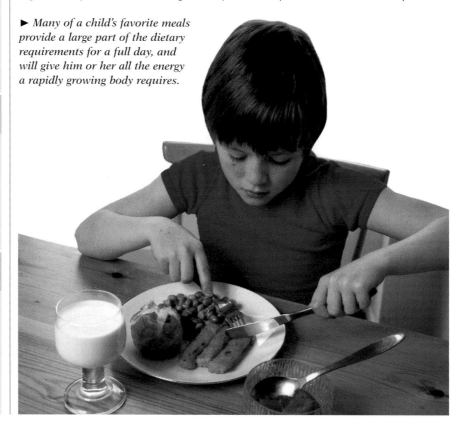

My baby is fatter than my friend's baby, who is the same age. Is it just puppy fat or should I put her on a diet?

Babies who are overfed become obese, and this is not normal. Ask your doctor if your baby is overweight. If the baby is, the doctor will probably suggest reducing the carbohydrate content of the diet and concentrating on protein foods. This means cutting out cereals, cakes, and sugar, reducing the amounts of potatoes and bread, and limiting milk intake to 1 pt. (0.5 l) a day.

I want to become a vegetarian but my friends say I won't get enough protein if I don't eat meat. Is this true?

It is perfectly possible to supply all the body's needs without eating meat, but you will need to make some adjustments to your diet. For example, it is not advisable to replace meat with more eggs and cheese. Some of your protein will have to be provided by nuts, beans, and cereals. You may need to take extra vitamin B12, as meat is by far the richest source of this.

My children will not eat any type of green vegetable. Is there any way I can ensure they get enough of the right vitamins in their diet?

Children who develop such a dislike usually grow out of it if you do not make it a big issue. Your children can get much of what they need from other foods. But if you are worried, ask your doctor about giving them a multivitamin and mineral supplement.

I want to lose weight, but I'm confused by all the different diets and their claims. What should I do?

A reducing diet allows for about 1,000 calories a day. It should include a variety of foods low in fat, and plenty of cooked or raw vegetables, fresh fruits, meats, and grain products. Try to avoid using salt and excess sugar. Drink alcohol in moderation, if at all.

beans and lentils, parsnips, rice, and yams. Sugar-rich foods include jams, cookies, chocolate, candy, and ice cream. These prepared products have high concentrations of refined sugar and should therefore be eaten in moderation.

Over half of an individual's dietary needs are met by carbohydrates, which are especially important for people doing heavy or strenuous physical work. Carbohydrates are converted to glucose (a form of sugar) in the body, and this fuels the muscles and the brain. It is the sole form of energy for the brain, which uses more than half of the daily supply.

Sugar levels

The amount of glucose in the blood is kept at constant levels under normal conditions. If too much carbohydrate is eaten, the excess is stored as glycogen in the liver and the muscles. When these have taken as much as they can hold, the excess is stored in the fat of the body.

If the level of sugar in the body becomes too high, insulin (a chemical manufactured by the pancreas) is released to make the liver absorb the excess from the blood. If the blood sugar level falls too low, the liver releases the stored glycogen and converts it back into glucose.

A diet that does not contain enough carbohydrates will lead to weakness and fatigue. To compensate for this, the body will instead convert fats into energy. However, the rapid burning of fats creates toxic by-products that make the blood too acidic. Carbohydrates are also important because they act to spare protein—that is, they are burned instead of protein, leaving the proteins to be used for bodybuilding.

Protein

Proteins are chemicals that form an essential part of every living cell. Muscles and bones, for instance, consist largely of protein. Proteins also go into the making of chromosomes (the gene carriers), enzymes (substances that activate almost all biochemical reactions), blood plasma (the liquid part of blood), and hemoglobin (the red-colored matter in blood).

In turn, proteins are made up of smaller units called amino acids. There are various types of protein, made of different arrangements of 20 or so amino acids. When protein is eaten, the digestive juices break it down into the amino acids. They are then carried in the bloodstream to various parts of the body and built up into new proteins as required.

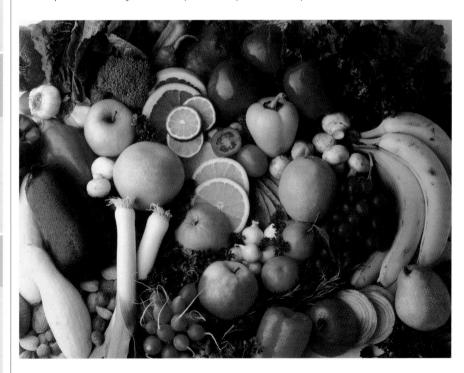

▲ *Fruit and vegetables are a rich source of vitamin C. People who do not eat enough vegetables may suffer from depression, swollen gums, pimples, and frequent infections.*

Any surplus protein is burned as fuel for energy. The body uses 0.9–1.4 ounces (25–40 g) a day, and this is the minimum amount that must be replaced to maintain the health of the tissues. A good rule of thumb is to eat 0.3 ounce (9.4 g) of protein for each 25 pounds (11.3 kg) of body weight daily.

Children, however, need more protein than adults—a baby requires five times as much per unit of weight, a young child two and a half times as much, and an adolescent one and a half times as much. Insufficient protein causes stunted growth and a weak body structure.

Sources of protein

Animal foods such as meat—especially organs such as the liver, kidneys, and heart—are very rich sources of protein. Lean meat should be chosen over fatty meat, and skin should be removed from poultry: these foods should be broiled, roasted, or boiled instead of fried. Fish, eggs, cheese, and milk are also good sources of protein, as are soybeans, nuts, and some pulses. Lentils and the seeds of pumpkin, squash, sunflower, and sesame are also rich in protein.

Complete and partial proteins

Complete proteins are those that have the same mixtures of amino acids as the body's proteins. They are found mostly in meats, fish, eggs, and dairy products.

Partial proteins, typically found in vegetables and cereals, lack one or another amino acid. Thus a vegetarian, for example, would have to eat more protein foods to make up the required amount of protein. Different vegetable proteins are missing different amino acids, and these can be combined to provide complete proteins.

In countries where animal foods are scarce or forbidden for religious reasons, many such food combinations have been developed. For instance, rice and beans are commonly eaten in Mexico. Also, a peanut butter sandwich, or bread and grilled cheese, is a good combination to make up complete proteins.

Fats

Fats provide nearly three times as much energy as other foods, so less of them are needed in the diet. In Western countries, people get about 40 percent of their overall energy from fats—a clear sign of prosperity. Fats may also add much taste and flavor to some foods and make certain types of foods easier to cook and process.

In the body, fat provides a layer of insulation beneath the skin and helps maintain an even temperature, especially in cold weather. It also serves as a cushion against minor injuries by absorbing the impact of blows or falls.

Types of fat

Fats are classified as saturated or unsaturated fats, according to their chemical structure. Saturated fats are found in the fat of animals, milk, butter, and some vegetable oils. Monounsaturated fats are found in olive oil, peanut oil, and fish oils. The polyunsaturated fats used in margarine and cooking oils come from soybean, corn, sunflower, cotton seed, and safflower plants.

Certain polyunsaturated fats are called essential fats, because the body cannot manufacture them and they are necessary in the diet. A lack of them can impair normal growth, making the skin dry and scaly. A diet high in polyunsaturated fats may help keep cholesterol levels low. However, too high a proportion of saturated fats in the diet may damage the arteries and lead to heart disease.

Consequently, most nutritionists recommend using mainly unsaturated fats. This goal is achieved by eating only lean meat, cooking with vegetable oils instead of butter or animal lard, and eating low-fat dairy products in moderation.

Vitamins

Apart from carbohydrates, proteins, and fats, the body must have vitamins and minerals. Vitamins are essential for normal growth and development, and because they cannot be manufactured in the body, they must be included in the diet. In certain cases they can be taken as supplements to the diet.

Vitamins are divided into fat-soluble and water-soluble types. The fat-soluble ones are vitamins A, D, E, and K; the water-soluble ones are vitamin C and the eight B vitamins. The body cannot store large amounts of water-soluble vitamins. They circulate in the blood, and any excess is eventually excreted in the urine.

In contrast, the fat-soluble vitamins are not excreted, and any excess is stored in the liver. An excess of vitamins A and D can be harmful, causing toxic symptoms in the system.

If there is a deficiency of water-soluble vitamins, it will become apparent within a

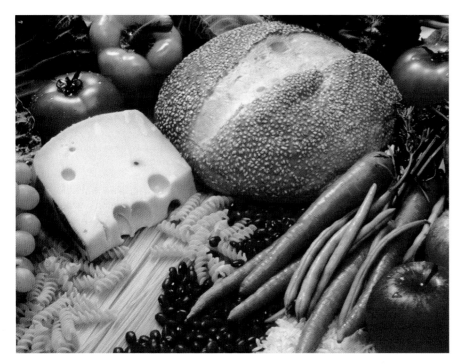

▲ *A good vegetarian diet: carbohydrates (bread, rice, pasta), vegetables (carrots, green beans), fruit (grapes, tomatoes, apples, peppers), pulses (dry beans), and dairy (cheese).*

Calories used in everyday activities

SEDENTARY OCCUPATIONS	CALORIES NEEDED OVER 24 HOURS	MODERATELY ACTIVE OCCUPATIONS	CALORIES NEEDED OVER 24 HOURS	ACTIVE OCCUPATIONS	CALORIES NEEDED OVER 24 HOURS
Office workers, truck drivers, doctors, journalists	Male: 2,500–2,700 Female: 1,700–2,200	Cleaners, plumbers, light-industry workers, mail deliverers, restaurant and waiting staff	Male: 2,700–3,200 Female: 2,000–2,400	Coal miners, construction workers, laborers, army recruits, athletes, firefighters	Male: 3,300–4,400 Female: 2,400–2,800

These figures are an average guide; they will vary according to age and weight.

matter of weeks. Reserves in the body are usually enough to prevent a deficiency for weeks, or even months, unless there is another irregularity in the body. In most developed countries, there is little cause to worry about vitamin deficiency—a good, mixed diet usually contains enough vitamins.

Minerals

Minerals are also essential for keeping the body healthy. They assist in many of the processes needed for normal nerve and muscle function and must be supplied frequently in the diet. The minerals that the body requires are calcium, phosphorus, iron, iodine, potassium, magnesium, fluorine, zinc, and copper. A balanced diet nearly always provides sufficient quantities of these, and as excess minerals may be harmful, it is not a good idea to take supplements except on a doctor's orders.

Roughage

Roughage, or dietary fiber, consists of the walls of plant cells that cannot be broken down by digestion and therefore pass through the stomach and intestine in solid form. Their use is to stimulate the action of the intestine, so that food passes through the digestive system. They also provide the bulk to make feces solid.

The best-known example of roughage is bran, which many people eat regularly as a natural method of relieving constipation. Vegetables, nuts, and cereals also contain fiber. Some fibers carry increased quantities of bile acids down the colon and help reduce the level of potentially harmful fats in the body.

African tribespeople who eat a low-fat, high-fiber diet rarely have diseases of the intestines and colon, appendicitis, or hemorrhoids, reinforcing the belief that these are diseases of Western civilization. The advent of modern food-processing techniques, some of which strip foods of many essential nutrients while adding unnecessary fats, sugar, and salt, have been key factors in the rise of these problems. High-fat, low-fiber fast food is a big culprit.

Energy

The food a person eats provides energy for the various activities of the body, from running fast to sitting and working in an office or repairing body tissue. The amount of energy needed (and therefore

Calories used in everyday activities

ACTIVITY	CALORIES USED PER HOUR
Sleeping	65
Standing still	110
Fast keyboarding	140
Walking slowly	200
Carpentry and painting	250
Swimming	500
Walking upstairs	1,100

THE FOOD GUIDE PYRAMID

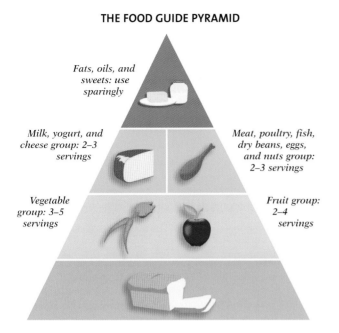

Fats, oils, and sweets: use sparingly

Milk, yogurt, and cheese group: 2–3 servings

Meat, poultry, fish, dry beans, eggs, and nuts group: 2–3 servings

Vegetable group: 3–5 servings

Fruit group: 2–4 servings

Whole-grain bread, cereal, rice, and pasta group: 6–11 servings

▲ *The original food guide pyramid emphasized the importance of eating more foods in the blue and yellow bands and fewer in the green and red bands.*

the amount of food) depends on how much energy is used. The energy from food is traditionally measured in calories, which are also referred to as kilocalories.

A balanced diet, food pyramids, and MyPlate

A balanced diet supplies all the necessary nutrients in quantities that suit a particular individual. The original food guide pyramid recommended that people should eat plenty of whole-grain foods, vegetables, and fruits and that they should eat fewer high-fat foods and high-sugar foods. In 2005, the U.S. Department of Agriculture (USDA) replaced the old food pyramid with MyPyramid, where the band for each food group was in proportion to the recommended daily allowance. The steps on the side of the MyPyramid image were intended to encourage exercise. The USDA replaced the MyPyramid system with the MyPlate guidelines in 2011. The MyPlate image represents the five basic food groups using a familiar mealtime place setting. The new system encourages people to balance calories by enjoying food but eating less of it and by avoiding oversized portions. MyPlate also emphasizes the importance of fruits and vegetables (with those two groups taking up half of the plate) and recommends that at least half of the grain allowance should be made up of whole grains. Detailed information related to MyPlate is available online (www.choosemyplate.gov), as is information on the *Dietary Guidelines for Americans, 2010* (www.cnpp.usda.gov/dietaryguidelines.htm).

Special diets and professional advice

Sometimes a diet has to be changed. For example, a pregnant woman has a higher need for some vitamins and minerals, but she should not increase her intake of fatty foods or foods with added sugars. Patients suffering from kidney disease may be put on a

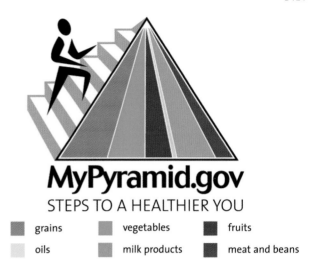

MyPyramid.gov
STEPS TO A HEALTHIER YOU

- grains
- oils
- vegetables
- milk products
- fruits
- meat and beans

▲ *The MyPyramid guidelines, which were introduced in 2005, highlighted the vital health benefits of making improvements in nutrition, physical activity, and lifestyle behavior.*

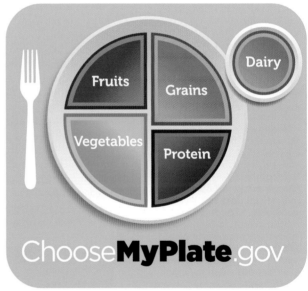

Fruits   Grains   Dairy

Vegetables   Protein

Choose**MyPlate**.gov

▲ *The U.S. Department of Agriculture introduced the MyPlate guidelines in 2011 to help people make better food choices and to remind people to eat healthfully.*

temporary protein-free diet. People suffering from gallbladder or liver disease will be put on a low-fat diet. High blood pressure, heart disease, and liver disease all call for low-salt diets. Any drastic change in diet should be undertaken only on the advice of a family doctor, a nutritionist, or a qualified health care practitioner.

See also: **Allergies; Anorexia and bulimia; Dieting; Fats; Glucose; Minerals; Nutrition; Obesity; Protein; Starch; Sugars; Vitamin A; Vitamin B; Vitamin C; Vitamin D; Vitamin E; Vitamin K; Weight**

Dieting

Questions and Answers

When I am dieting, is it OK to eat as much as I want of foods that are advertised as being "low-fat"?

No. Even if a product is advertised as having zero fat, it can still contain lots of calories. In fact, in a product that is fat-free, manufacturers have often replaced the fat with sugar. Always check the food's calorie content on the nutritional label.

Do you have any tips for losing weight healthily?

The following tips should help you lose weight and stay healthy:
• First, keep a food journal of everything you eat and drink for at least a month. This will allow you to see how much you are eating and when. It is then a good idea to see your doctor to obtain a correct, healthy caloric limit for your gender, weight, and height.
• Bearing your caloric limit in mind, eat a healthy diet that includes all the food groups, especially fresh fruit, vegetables, whole grains, and foods that are high in fiber.
• Never skip breakfast—it starts your day off right and allows your metabolism to begin burning fat.
• Avoid processed foods and foods that contain a lot of additives. Your body will have trouble breaking these down.
• Pay close attention to portion size; try putting less food on your plate when you serve a meal.
• Exercise at least three days each week for at least 30 minutes a day. If you are not used to exercise, start slowly and then gradually increase the amount of exercise you do. Exercise not only speeds up weight loss but will tone your body as you lose those pounds.
• Try to drink at least eight glasses of water each day.
• Try not to eat anything after eight o'clock in the evening.
• Remember, losing weight slowly and following a healthy diet and exercise program will help keep the weight off permanently.

There are different reasons why people diet, from attempting to lose weight to treating a disease or disorder that might benefit from a specific diet. It is advisable to get expert medical advice before embarking on a particular diet.

When people are dieting, they restrict themselves to a special diet—that is, to specific types of food and drink. Most people diet in order to lose weight; such a diet usually involves cutting down on food and drink that has a high fat or sugar content. Yet sometimes people are advised by a doctor or dietitian (a specialist in nutrition and diet) to go on a diet for medical reasons. However, the term "dieting" is most frequently used when people are restricting their intake of food and drink in order to lose weight.

When is it a good idea to lose weight?

Doctors will often advise patients who are seriously overweight or obese to go on a diet. Obesity, usually defined as being more than 30 percent above the ideal body weight, is reaching epidemic proportions in the United States and elsewhere in the Western world. Obesity, usually caused by eating too many calories (often in the form of fatty or sugar-rich foods) and not getting enough exercise, is a serious risk to health. Excess weight can put a strain on the heart, and fats and cholesterol will harm the arteries. Obese people are at risk of heart disease, high blood pressure, and dangerous levels of insulin in their blood, which can lead to diabetes.

The MyPlate system put forward in 2011 by the U.S. Department of Agriculture is designed to help people make better food choices. Detailed information related to MyPlate is available online (www.choosemyplate.gov), as is information on the *Dietary Guidelines for Americans, 2010* (www.cnpp.usda.gov/dietaryguidelines.htm).

How people gain and lose weight

While weight gain is a fact of life for many, actually losing weight—and maintaining that weight loss—often seems nearly impossible. This is because the human body at rest burns only about 12 calories per pound of body weight each day. A person who weighs 150 pounds (68 kg) will burn perhaps 1,800 calories each day, or 2,000 calories with moderate exercise.

Considering that an average fast-food meal of a burger sandwich, fries, and a drink contains more than 1,500 calories, it is easy to see how many people in the Western world could consume more calories each day than they use up. The body converts any excess calories and stores them

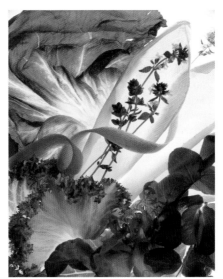

as fat. Even an extra 50 or 100 calories each day (just a cookie and a soft drink, say) will result in gradual weight gain. It is also easy to see how difficult it can be for people to lose excess weight. The only way to lose fat is to consume fewer calories each day than the body needs. For every 3,500 calories that the body burns up from its fat reserves, a person loses just 1 pound (0.45 kg) of body fat. The only way to lose weight, then, is to restrict the number of calories that the body takes in each day, or to exercise more, or both.

◄ *Salad ingredients—such as radicchio, endives, and watercress—are an excellent food source in many diets. Not only are they low in fat and calories, but they are rich in vitamin C and the mineral calcium, both of which are important nutrients for the health of the human body.*

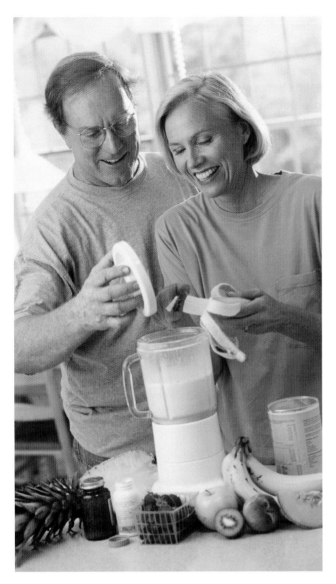

◄ *Many diets include healthy fruit drinks, to which vitamin, mineral, or protein supplements can be added. These drinks can be quickly and easily prepared with the help of a blender.*

supplements for the rest of their lives. Afterward, when the diet ends, most people usually return to their normal eating habits and the weight eventually comes back.

How to succeed

If a person is going to succeed in losing weight, and in keeping that weight off, there are a number of points that he or she should bear in mind. First the person should think about how many calories he or she normally consumes in a day and compare this with the number of calories that are actually needed. The person should then think about how he or she might go about bringing these two figures together. Although a faddish diet will reduce caloric intake in the short run, it is probably better for people to take a serious look at their eating habits. Cutting out all fried foods, such as potato chips, french fries, and fried chicken, and all sugar—cookies, candy, cake, etc.—is a good start. It may also a good idea to introduce healthy, filling foods that do not actually contain many calories, such as fresh fruit, vegetables, whole-grain bread, and brown rice.

Taking more exercise is also important because the more exercise a person takes, the more calories he or she will burn off in a day. Exercise will also, over time, improve the efficiency of a person's metabolism.

The dangers

It is important to bear in mind that some diets and weight control aids can be more dangerous than the excess weight they are seeking to address. Many fad diets, for example, involve eating only one particular type of food. Often such diets are not nutritionally sound and deprive the body of important vitamins and minerals. Rapid weight loss can also result in loss of muscle tissue; if that weight is then regained (as it often is), more fat and less muscle is replaced.

There are also many diet pills on the market. Although some of these work, they may be harmful. The active ingredients in many diet pills and supplements are ephedrines and caffeine. According to the Food and Drug Administration (FDA), products containing ephedrines have a stimulant effect on the central nervous system and the heart and have been known to cause heart attacks, seizures, and strokes. Side effects also include depression, nervousness, and insomnia. Ephedrines can be particularly dangerous when used in combination with caffeine.

People who are in the habit of dieting and who do not conduct their diets in a healthy way often experience a "yo-yo" pattern of weight loss followed by weight gain. This pattern lowers the metabolism, making it even easier to gain weight. Dieting can also become an obsession, particularly among young women and teenage girls, who may go on to develop eating disorders such as anorexia nervosa and bulimia. Although it is unhealthy to be seriously overweight, it can be much more dangerous to become obsessed with losing weight, dieting rigorously, and becoming too thin.

Is dieting the answer?

It is not just people who have been advised by their doctor who resort to dieting. People who are a little overweight often feel that they could benefit their health, body image, and self-esteem if they could only lose some weight. As a result, a huge proportion of the U.S. population is on some kind of a diet. There are many types of weight-loss diets, from long-standing traditional ones like the rice diet and the calorie-counting Weight Watchers diet to fad diets that tend to come and go, such as the grapefruit diet, the Scarsdale diet, the Hollywood "miracle" diet, the Atkins diet, etc. Yet whether a diet involves replacing meals with a drink supplement, cutting out particular food groups (carbohydrates, for example, as in the Atkins diet), or restricting oneself to just a few different foods, each works more or less in the same way—by restricting the intake of calories.

Most diets work only temporarily, however. This is because people usually stick to a particular dietary regimen for only a short period of time, often just a few weeks or months. Not many people are willing to keep to a mainly rice-based diet or to drink food

> **See also:** Anorexia and bulimia; Depression; Diet; Exercise; Fats; Heart disease; Minerals; Nutrition; Obesity; Stroke; Sugars; Weight

Dislocation

I dislocated my thumb recently. Is the joint likely to be loose now, and could it happen again?

Yes, there is a possibility that the joint will dislocate again. If the joint repeatedly discolates, a surgical operation may be needed to fix it.

A few months ago, my neighbor slipped on ice and dislocated her shoulder. She had it put back in place but has had a lot of aches and stiffness since then. Is there anything she can do about it?

Pain and stiffness after a dislocation are fairly common, so it is important to have adequate physiotherapy to keep the joint mobile. Aspirin may help relieve the pain, but occasionally, an injection of a steroid drug into the surrounding tissue is required.

I dislocated my right shoulder a few months ago. Now it dislocates easily and I have had to give up playing football. Is there anything I can do to strengthen the joint?

It is possible to have an operation to increase the strength of the joint if a shoulder is repeatedly dislocating. The Putti-Platt operation strengthens the front of the shoulder by building up the bone to make the socket deeper, making it more difficult for the bone to slip out. Healing takes about two months.

Could dislocating my hip cause arthritis when I am older?

If the dislocation was a central one, fracturing the pelvis and damaging surrounding tissue, this could increase your susceptibility to osteoarthritis (the arthritis that comes through wear and tear). Dislocation behind or in front of the pelvis, however, is unlikely to lead to arthritis.

Joints are the junction points between bones that enable the body to move. They can become dislocated, often as a result of accidents. However, this painful problem can usually be corrected easily.

A dislocated joint looks misshapen and cannot work properly. Movement is difficult, and there is considerable pain, especially if the bone presses on a nerve. The joints in the limbs, spine, hands, and feet can all be dislocated. However, some joints dislocate more easily than others. It all depends on the joint's stability, which in turn depends on the strength of the surrounding muscle and tendons (the tough, fibrous tissue that joins muscle to bone). The shoulder and finger joints are less stable and dislocate more frequently than hip joints, which are very stable.

If dislocation is suspected, the patient should be taken to a doctor immediately, as the correction should be done as soon as possible. After 24 hours, the tendons begin to shorten and the dislocation is more difficult to correct. Do not attempt correction without medical help. The most common dislocations are in the shoulders, hips, neck, elbows, and fingers.

The shoulder

The bone in the upper arm (humerus) and the shoulder blade (scapula) form the shoulder joint, which is a ball-and-socket joint, with the head of the arm bone forming the ball and the shoulder blade forming the socket. The socket has to be shallow for the enormous range of movement that the shoulder makes, and this means that the joint is unstable. The bone may slip out of the socket in one of four directions—forward, backward, up, or down—and these are known as anterior, posterior, superior, or inferior dislocations, respectively. About 90 percent of shoulder dislocations are anterior, occurring when the arm bone slips off the socket and lies in front of the acromium bone (the tip of the shoulder blade).

To get the joint back into place, the patient lies flat on his or her back on a bed. While an assistant holds the patient's body steady, the doctor stands at the foot of the bed and pulls down on the hand, twisting the arm inward while doing so. The joint slips back with a dull

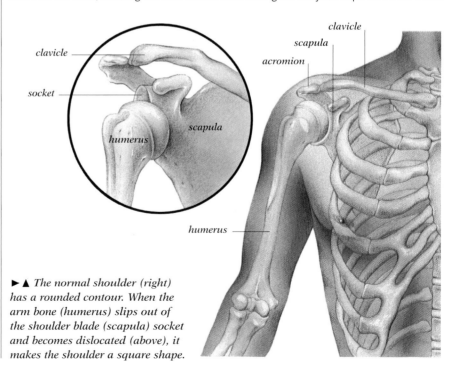

► ▲ *The normal shoulder (right) has a rounded contour. When the arm bone (humerus) slips out of the shoulder blade (scapula) socket and becomes dislocated (above), it makes the shoulder a square shape.*

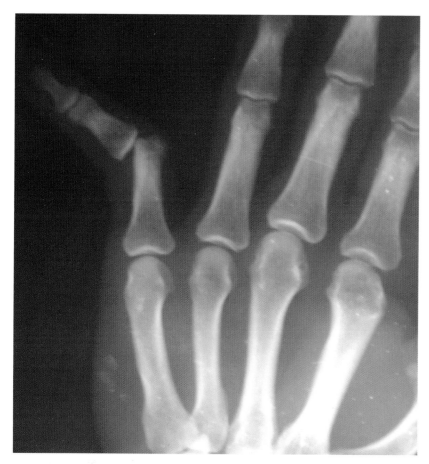

◄ This X ray shows a severe dislocation of the little finger. Dislocations are usually apparent from the symptoms, such as pain, deformity, swelling, and bruising. However, an X ray may be taken to check that the bones are not fractured.

difficult it is to correct, and if the child reaches the age of five with the condition undiagnosed, correction may be impossible. A midwife or pediatrician should always check the hips as a matter of routine at birth, by rolling the legs around in their sockets. If new parents are in doubt, they should ask if this has been done, since it could prevent problems later in life.

The neck

The bones of the neck are prone to dislocation because they have the least stable joints in the spinal column. A dislocation puts pressure on the spinal cord, which can result in paralysis of the arms and legs unless it is treated immediately. Most neck dislocations occur while people are playing active contact sports such as football.

A patient with neck dislocation is unable to get up and complains of numbness or paralysis in the legs or arms. This is a medical emergency, and more damage can be done if the patient is not handled correctly.

The golden rule is never to change the position of the head, and never allow the head to bend forward. Support the head, with a hand on each side of the face, while waiting for the ambulance and also on the journey to the hospital.

click, and immediately after this, the pain eases. Occasionally, the patient may be in so much discomfort that a general anesthetic is given before the procedure begins.

The hip

The hip is a ball-and-socket joint between the thighbone (femur) and the socket in the pelvis (acetabulum). It is a stable joint, and considerable force is needed to dislocate it. Most hip dislocations are the result of car accidents in which the knee has hit the dashboard.

Dislocation may occur in one of three directions—in front of the pelvic socket (anterior) or behind it (posterior), or the bone may have been driven through the socket, fracturing the pelvis at the same time (central dislocation). The posterior is the most common hip dislocation. In an anterior dislocation, the knee is turned outward; in a posterior dislocation, the knee is slightly bent and turned inward across the opposite leg. It is very difficult to move the leg, unless the thighbone has been fractured, and this difficulty is one way of diagnosing a dislocation. Hip dislocations are treated under a general anesthetic in the hospital.

Congenital hip dislocation

Occasionally, children are born with dislocated hips: this abnormality runs in families, affects girls more than boys, and is most common among Czechs, Slovaks, Chinese, and Navajo Native Americans. The deformity is easily corrected with splints if treatment is given within the first three months of life. The longer it is left untreated, the more

The elbow

Dislocation of an elbow usually results from a fall on an outstretched arm. The surrounding nerves and blood vessels may be damaged, and the injury is extremely painful. Correction under general anesthetic within 12 hours is essential. The patient can be made comfortable with a simple collar-and-cuff sling on the journey to the hospital.

The finger

If a finger is dislocated, it will look shorter than the others and it will swell up and become painful. The dislocation can be corrected by pulling the finger out in a straight line. A splint may be needed while the soft tissue is healing.

Outlook

The soft tissues around a dislocated joint may be damaged, and stiffness and pain may last for a few months. Physiotherapy may help to restore full movement. Generally, however, the long-term outlook is excellent.

See also: **Arthritis; Paralysis; Physical therapy**

Drug abuse

Questions and Answers

My son often appears dreamy, is losing weight, stays out late, and lies about where he has been. Could he be a heroin addict?

It is impossible to know whether your son is a drug addict without seeing him. However, the signs to look out for are poor appetite, slow and halting speech, uninterest in personal appearance, sudden and unexplained absences from home, long periods spent in his room, and uninterest in organized activities.

Check his clothing for blood spots and his arms for tracks made by the syringe, if possible. Look in his room for fully burned matches, teaspoons, small plastic or paper envelopes, and syringes. These are all part of the paraphernalia of taking heroin. If you find them, speak to your son and suggest to him that he seek professional help as soon as possible.

I heard that newborn babies whose mothers are drug addicts can suffer withdrawal symptoms. Is this true?

Yes. Doctors are familiar with this problem, but since babies have a metabolic system that is still developing, it is often difficult to treat them. The majority of addictions, however, normally start in the teenage years, peak in the second or third decade of life, and decline thereafter.

I am overweight, and my doctor has prescribed diet pills for me. Could I become addicted to them?

Tolerance to amphetamine-like diet pills is gradual, but you may become addicted to them psychologically. Not only will you get a high, but you will also want to keep taking them because you will be losing weight. These pills should be taken only under your doctor's guidance. If you feel you are becoming addicted to them tell your doctor, who may or may not wish you to continue taking them.

The abuse of many types of drugs is becoming an increasingly common problem, particularly among young people. It is essential for parents to recognize the signs of drug-taking, along with its effects and dangers.

A person is said to be addicted to a drug if he or she cannot stop taking it, either because of the need to experience its effects or because he or she feels terrible if the drug is not taken.

Only certain drugs, such as barbiturates and heroin, are truly addictive in the sense that they create both physical and mental dependency. With drugs such as LSD and crack, users may develop only a mental dependency but may still find it difficult to give them up.

What happens in addiction

Addictive drugs affect the nervous system, particularly the brain. If used in large quantities, they can become almost a part of the body's own chemistry. They often mimic a naturally occurring chemical in the body; for example, the opiates (the most powerfully addictive drugs) resemble endorphins, the brain's natural painkillers. An addictive drug also has a potent effect on key points in the pathways of the nerves. Whichever is the case, the more a drug becomes built in to the body's processes, the stronger the addiction becomes.

Another feature of drug addiction is called drug tolerance. This simply means that the body becomes so used to the drug it is receiving that increasingly large doses are needed.

Who is at risk?

There is no simple way to predict what type of person may be prone to drug abuse. Addiction occasionally results when seriously ill or badly injured people are on painkilling drugs longer than they should be: for example, after an accident at sea, when it has taken days to reach proper medical help. Sometimes addiction is a result of boredom, sometimes of pressure; some successful, high-powered professional people may be secretly dependent on drugs.

Social pressures

Fashion plays a large part in drug addiction, for drug-taking is, and always has been, done for pleasure, kicks, or thrills. Those who become addicts in this way may often be part of a

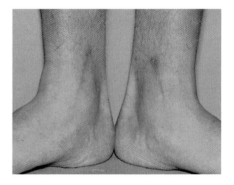

▲▼ The most obvious sign of a heroin or amphetamine addict is tracks near arteries on the arms or the legs, caused by repeated insertion of a hypodermic needle.

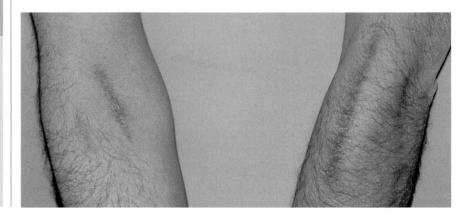

social group which believes that drug-taking is a technique to expand or improve the mind.

The sale of hard drugs, especially heroin and crack, to young people has become a major criminal industry in the United States and elsewhere. This lucrative illegal activity is not confined to deprived urban areas but occurs at every level of society. The trade is highly organized under the control of international gangs of criminals and is responsible for a large proportion of crime in Western countries. The principal weapon against this deadly trade is knowledge about drugs.

Inadequacies

Doctors generally agree that most addicts have personality problems. Many are drawn to tension-relieving drugs because they cannot handle the troubles of everyday life. Although a deprived or unsatisfactory home background can sometimes contribute to drug addiction, addicts may come from any social background and may be educated or not.

The dangers

Although some people may be quite heavily addicted to a drug as potent as heroin and still live apparently normal lives, it is more usual for addiction to bring an increasing spiral of disasters. Apart from deteriorating health, the addict suffers from a lack of direction and motivation, losing the urge to do anything except take the drug. In this state it is an easy step to losing one's job. Without money it may be difficult to purchase the expensive illegal supplies that are needed to satisfy the craving. From here the next step is often crime, especially thieving, to pay for the all-important doses.

Opiates

The most notorious of the addictive drugs are the opiates, so called because they are made from or chemically similar to opium. Opium comes from the seeds of the opium poppy plant, grown mainly in Asia.

Morphine is the opium extract most widely used in medicine, and of the several major opiates, the best-known is diamorphine, or heroin.

All the opiates are, to a greater or lesser extent, addictive, but heroin is the most often abused because it is the quickest-acting and most potent. It is also in relatively plentiful supply through illegal channels.

The opiates are excellent painkillers, with the essential and beneficial ability to make terrible injuries and the last stages of incurable illnesses bearable, possibly even comfortable. With carefully controlled quantities, given under medical supervision, there is minimal danger of addiction, and the relief from what may be excruciating pain undoubtedly justifies the risk.

Effects on the addict: The effects of the different opiates vary from person to person. In general the "high" achieved from a substantial dose of opiate goes through a number of phases, typically beginning with a warm feeling of peace, then often progressing to, or being combined with, sensations of nausea, disorientation, and drowsiness.

Detecting an addict: The heroin addict has skin damage at the points where he or she repeatedly inserts the needle to give the dose (the "fix") from a syringe. He or she is likely to suffer from loss of appetite, loss of weight, constipation, and loss of sex drive. The pupils of the eyes may be very tiny, about the size of pinpoints.

Withdrawal: The addict dreads withdrawal from the drug. It affects addicts in different ways but in general involves vomiting, abdominal pains, cramps in the limbs, general agitation, and collapse.

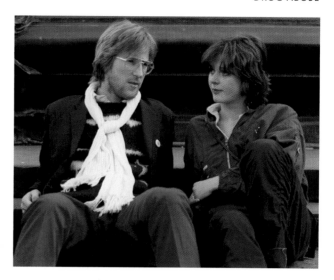

▲ *Young people are particularly likely to abuse drugs, owing to frustration with their lives and a need for companionship that the private world of drug-taking fulfills.*

Overdose: There is a constant risk of overdose in the addict. In a confused, irrational, or reckless state as a result of taking the drug, an addict may then accidentally or deliberately take a lethally large dose.

The outlook for an addict: Unless a hardened drug addict takes steps toward self-help, the chances of regaining normal health and lifestyle are not very good. Apart from the obvious danger of dying from an overdose, there are the risks of diseases connected with sharing the same needle. Ulceration, abscesses, hepatitis, and blood poisoning are common; meningitis, kidney disease, and tetanus are less so but must be considered. AIDS is also a serious risk.

A survey followed the histories of 108 known drug addicts. After seven years, 25 were off drugs altogether. Thirty-five were still receiving drugs, but in a clinic. Twenty-nine were possibly in the process of giving up their drug habit, and 19 were dead. These statistics illustrate how important it is to seek medical and psychological help from a doctor or a hospital clinic if a person is addicted to a drug.

Barbiturates

Abuse of barbiturates, which are essentially sedatives and sleeping pills, has on occasion caused as much physical suffering as misuse of opiates.

The danger associated with barbiturates is tolerance. Even those who use a barbiturate responsibly to help them go to sleep sometimes find that it begins to lose its effectiveness over time. When a heavy user stops taking barbiturates, there may be mental disturbances, which in turn lead to a further loss of sleep. It is for this reason that barbiturates, useful as they are in treating certain conditions such as epilepsy, are generally being prescribed less and less today.

People who abuse barbiturates often take them by injection. This usually causes elation and removal of inhibitions but leads to confusion, slower breathing, lack of coordination, and sometimes even unconsciousness.

Withdrawal symptoms start about a day after the addict stops taking the drug; these include disturbed sleep, anxiety, uncontrollable movements of the limbs, and even convulsions.

The most common dangerous drugs and their effects

NAME OF DRUG	FORM OF DRUG	METHOD OF USE	EFFECTS	DANGERS OF ABUSE
Alcohol	Fermented liquor such as wine and beer or distilled liquor such as gin and vodka	Social or private drinking	Small doses: relaxation, slight anesthetic effect, loss of inhibition, talkativeness. Large doses: memory loss, aggression, slurred speech, drowsiness.	Damages most body systems. Major cause of liver disease. Affects lifestyle, work, and family life, with increasing deterioration in health. Dangerous to drive a car.
Amphetamines (slang: speed, pep pills, uppers), such as Dexedrine, Methedrine, and Benzedrine	Capsules and tablets of different shapes and colors. Methedrine may be in liquid form.	Taken by mouth or, in the case of Methedrine, injected	Instant high, extra energy, elation at first, then rapid unconsciousness	Loss of appetite; aggression, skin problems, delusions of persecution, depression, exhaustion or fatigue, emotional or psychological problems, suicide
Barbiturates, such as Phenobarbital, Amobarbital, and Tuinal	Pills, capsules, and injections	Taken by mouth or injected	Relaxation, sleep; if injected, elation	Regular use ends in addiction. Withdrawal causes anxiety, disturbed sleep, uncontrolled limb movements, confusion, seizures, unconsciousness.
Cocaine (slang: coke, snow) and crack	White crystalline powder or small white marbles	Fine powder is sniffed (snorted) up the nose. Crack is smoked in a water pipe or regular pipe.	Strong feeling of exhilaration, extra energy, ability to concentrate, and the impression of being brilliantly lucid in conversation and thought	Long-term use can cause mental dependence; Circulatory problems and damage to membranes of nose and lungs. Use during pregnancy causes addicted, underweight babies.
Ecstasy (methylene dioxine methamphetamine)	Pure ecstasy (MDA) is white. Tablets come in various colors.	Taken by mouth	Roughly a combination of the effects of LSD and amphetamines	Can cause dehydration, coma, and death. May also precipitate a persistent state of paranoid psychosis.
Glue or other products such as dry-cleaning fluid	Often straight from the container, but user may try to concentrate dose by making a small tent from a plastic bag	Inhalation	Short-lived buzz or confused state of mind	Not physically addictive, but people who try it may suffer serious damage to the health, including brain, liver, and heart damage.
Heroin (slang: H, horse, junk)	White powder when pure; sold on the streets, it is often impure, ranging in color from white to brown	Injected or inhaled (snorted). Injecting into the skin is not as dangerous as injecting into a vein (mainlining).	Dramatic, pleasurable high, but also some nausea and drowsiness	Regular use ends in addiction. Withdrawal effects are particularly unpleasant. Tolerance develops rapidly.
LSD (slang: acid; scientific name: lysergic acid diethylamide)	Variety of colored tablets; sometimes in liquid form	Taken by mouth or, if liquid, on a sugar lump; tiny doses	Dramatically altered mental state (a trip) with strange hallucinations, grossly altered vision, and delusions (false beliefs as to physical powers); can last up to 18 hours	Not physically addictive, but the trip may be nightmarish. Impure LSD may be physically harmful. Disturbed behavior may cause physical harm to user: for example, trying to fly from upstairs windows.
Marijuana (slang: dope, pot, hash, grass). It is made from the Indian hemp plant.	Two forms: dried, crumbled leaves or resin. The first is often called grass; the second is often called hash.	Grass smoked as cigarettes; resin may be smoked mixed with cigarette tobacco; both forms smoked in pipes and cooked in food	Mild intoxication (being "stoned"); extra sensitivity to music, pictures, touch; loss of recent memory; sedative effect after a few hours. Large doses may cause hallucinations.	Much debated; not physically addictive, but effect on lifestyle can be a marked lethargy and lack of motivation

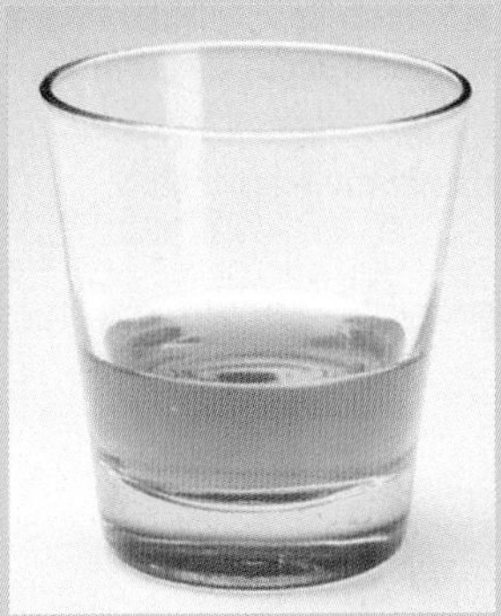

Alcohol

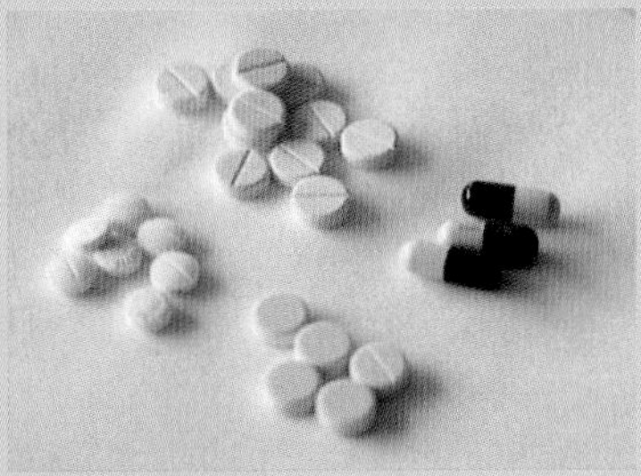

Amphetamines

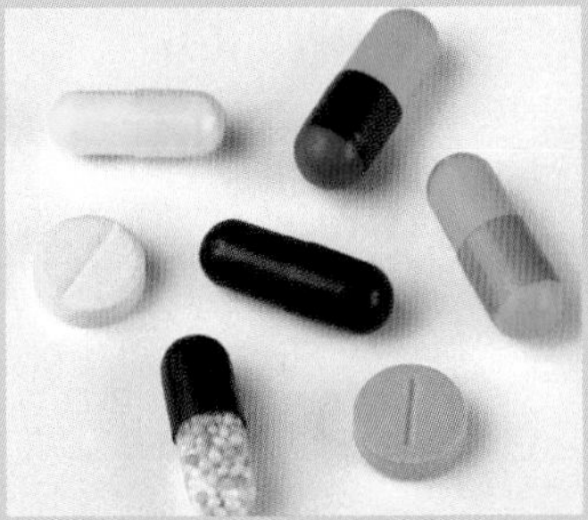

Barbiturates

Cocaine

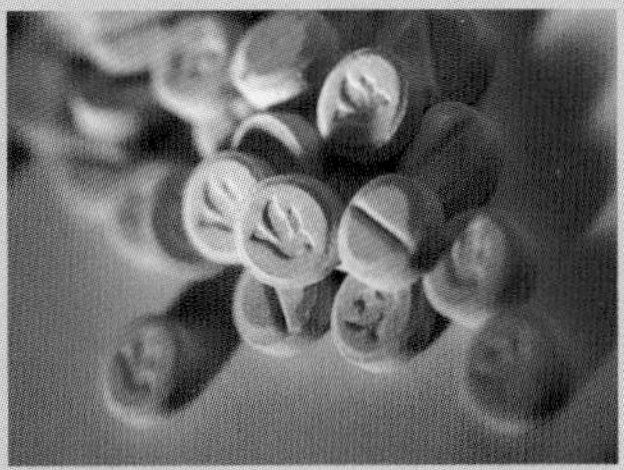

Ecstasy

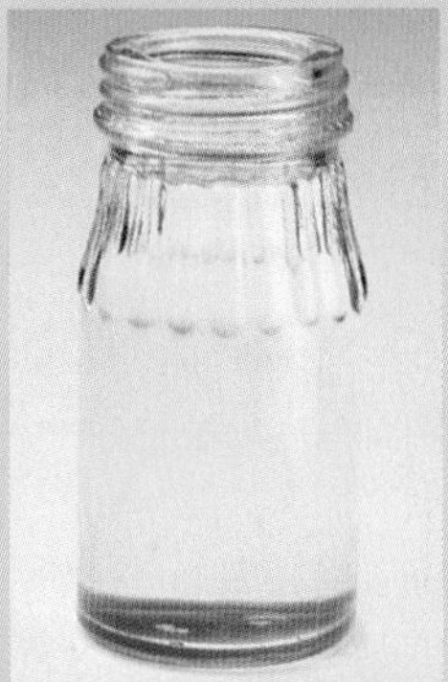

Dry-cleaning fluid

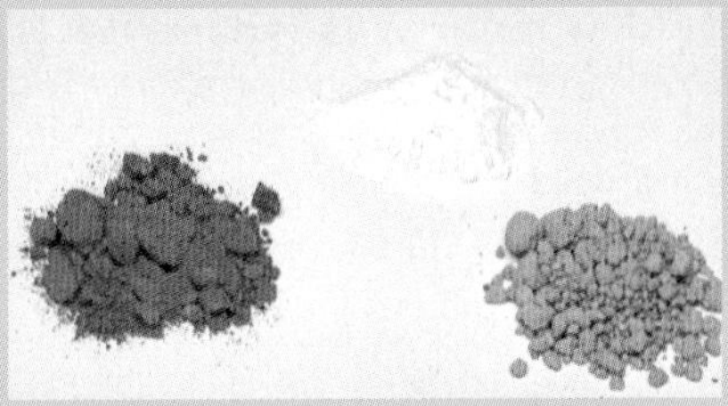

Heroin

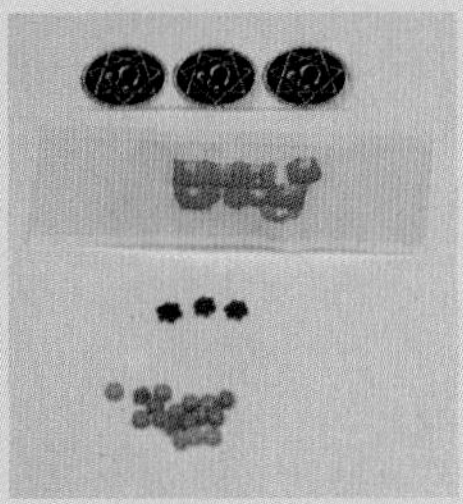

LSD

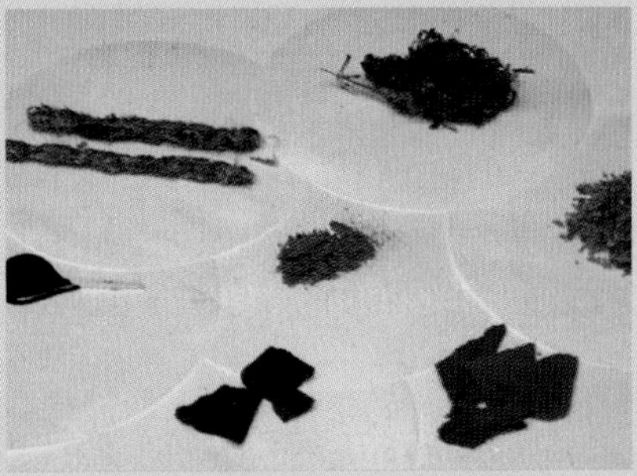

Marijuana

Cocaine and crack

The illegal use of cocaine and its derivative, crack, has become more common. Cocaine makes its users feel energetic and lively. Mental dependency is common, but cocaine is not thought to be physically addictive.

Stimulants

Stimulant drugs have the opposite effect from barbiturates and other depressants and are generally referred to as amphetamines. They make the user more alert and less susceptible to tiredness, and lift the mood. Tolerance can develop rapidly.

The amphetamine abuser may take the drug by injection to produce a feeling of elation, but this gives way to depression, feelings of persecution, and hallucinations. Although there are no physical withdrawal effects, ceasing to take amphetamines may give the addict psychological problems, including severe agitation and depression.

Drugs that distort the senses

Some drugs, although not addictive in the strict sense, distort the senses, and people may develop a mental dependence on them. In addition, they carry special physical dangers.

Marijuana stays in the body for an especially long time after being taken and usually causes lethargy in the user.

Another drug that distorts the senses, LSD (lysergic acid diethylamide), is potentially dangerous because some people react to it in disturbed ways, becoming violent, experiencing feelings of persecution, or developing strange and possibly disastrous beliefs, such as that they can fly.

The drug ecstasy is widely used by young people who find it an aid to energy at dance parties, also called "raves." Some tragic deaths have resulted from the use of this drug, which can cause a dangerous rise in body temperature and dehydration. If too much water is drunk too quickly it can cause a fatal buildup of water in the brain.

Inhalants, cigarettes, and alcohol

From time to time glue-sniffing and similar activities become popular, especially among teenagers. A variety of substances are used to produce a "kick": dry-cleaning fluid, paints, sprays, and petroleum-fuel products. They give a disappointing, short-lived high that is typically a fuzzy or confused state. Like the sense-distorting drugs, inhalants are not actually addictive, but their physical effects can be devastating. Accompanying or soon after the so-called high there is likely to be slurred speech, stupor, and a general state of confusion. Damage to the heart, liver, and brain is a real danger.

A survey of drug abuse would not be complete without cigarettes and alcohol, which are potent addictive drugs that cause widespread health and social problems.

See also: **Alcoholism; Personality; Smoking**

Environmental hazards

There are two main types of environmental hazards, those that occur naturally and those created or made worse by human activities. The air people breathe, the water they drink, and the food they eat can all be potentially harmful.

Questions and Answers

Can I get skin cancer from too much exposure to the sun?

Yes. Too much exposure to the sun is dangerous. Rates of skin cancer have risen in the United States, because people try to tan too rapidly and allow areas of skin to burn and peel. If you want to tan, do it slowly, and gradually increase your exposure. Apply sunscreen to exposed areas of the body. In Australia the depletion of the ozone layer has led to an increase in skin cancer, because people are exposed to more of the sun's ultraviolet radiation.

Is it safe to drink water directly from a faucet?

In many parts of the world faucet water is not sterilized and may contain *Escherichia coli* bacteria, *Shigella* bacteria, and the bacteria that cause typhus and cholera. Someone drinking the water might contract gastroenteritis or something more serious. In the United States, Canada, and many other countries, drinking water is chlorinated, so such health threats are likely to have been eradicated.

Other problems may occur if you ingest too much lead from water in old pipes or faucets (faucets made after 1997 contain less lead). If in doubt, run the water for 1 minute before use, use cold water for cooking, and drink bottled water instead.

Is there such a thing as indoor air pollution?

Yes. If they are badly constructed or fitted, materials used in building construction and fixtures can give off dangerous airborne chemicals. Fiberglass dust, carpet adhesives, wall insulation, plywood, and formaldehyde from insulation are in this category. Noxious fumes from materials may cause eye irritation, nausea, headaches, dizziness, and drowsiness.

Environmental hazards are not new—people have always lived with natural threats such as volcanic eruptions, earthquakes, floods, fires, and extreme weather conditions. As long ago as 79 C.E., for example, the eruption of the volcano Vesuvius famously destroyed the Roman cities of Herculaneum and Pompeii. It is also likely that early peoples suffered the consequences of natural radiation that emanated from certain volcanic rocks.

Artificial environmental hazards, on the other hand, are relatively recent. Many date only from the 19th century, when a growing world population and rapid industrialization meant that human activity could have an impact not only on the local environment but on a whole region or even a whole country. Such hazards include air pollution such as smog, water degradation, insanitary living conditions caused by overcrowding, and toxins in the food supply.

In the later 20th century many nations began taking steps to attempt to regulate the causes of such hazards. In many countries, however, legislation remains nonexistent or only patchily effective; meanwhile, of course, no legislation can

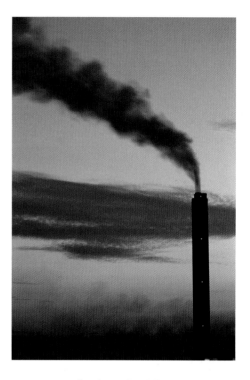

▲ *Factories that burn fossil fuels are a major source of air pollution, including smog.*

prevent natural hazards such as earthquakes or droughts. In such disasters authorities can be prepared only to ameliorate the worst effects and take care of any survivors.

Air pollution

Among the earliest and most obvious artificial environmental hazards was air pollution, which became a noticeable problem in the 19th century in the cities of North America and Europe, when people began routinely burning coal and other fossil fuels in factories and houses. Fires produced smoke that contained potentially harmful chemicals, such as sulfur dioxide, which could become concentrated during certain weather conditions. They caused smog—blanketing clouds of smoke and gas—that could create or exacerbate respiratory problems, particularly in cities. Sometimes the results could be fatal: acute bronchitis and asthma were the main culprits, and children and older adults were the prime victims. Other effects of smog included eye, nose, and throat irritation; shortness of breath; headache; and tiredness.

In the 20th century clean air legislation in many countries, including the United States, reduced the worst effects of fossil-fuel smog. By the century's end, however, there was another type of severe air pollution. This was a photochemical smog, dubbed Los Angeles smog, caused by emissions from vehicles and power plants. Hydrocarbons and nitrogen dioxide in the emissions react in strong sunlight to convert oxygen into ozone—a colorless, toxic gas that causes unpleasant symptoms ranging from headache to nausea, itching eyes, and coughing fits. Chemicals in the smog can cause anemia and damage to the heart, the brain, the lungs, and the

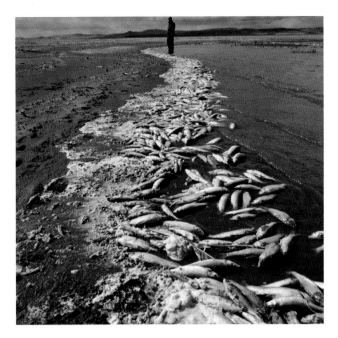

▲ *Toxic waste in water can have a devastating effect on fish.*

blood. The worst photochemical smog occurs in Mexico City. Despite attempts by governments to limit vehicle emissions, poor air quality remains a health hazard in many cities.

Other harmful air pollution continues to be caused by the burning of large tracts of forest in some parts of the world. Sulfur dioxide from burning fossil fuels also mixes with water in the atmosphere to form mild hydrochloric acid. When this falls as acid rain, it can destroy forests and other vegetation; as acid fog it triggers coughing, wheezing, bronchitis, and asthma attacks in people.

Chemical factories emit a wide range of pollutants into the air, including highly toxic substances such as benzene, mercury, and arsenic. These chemicals tend to collect slowly in the fatty tissues of the body. Their damaging nature may not be known about for years after exposure, but chemical pollution of the atmosphere has been linked to birth defects such as spina bifida and heart abnormalities. One of the most horrific incidents occurred in 1984, when an explosion at the Union Carbide pesticide factory in Bhopal, India, released 44 tons (40 t) of methyl isocyanate. Up to 10,000 people died, and more than 10 times that number were injured. At the start of the 21st century many thousands still bear afflictions caused by the gas, the most prevalent of which is cervical cancer in women.

The American Cancer Society has estimated that 25 percent of Americans will develop some form of cancer, and the World Health Organization has estimated that environmental factors cause 60 to 80 percent of all cancers.

Ozone depletion

While it can be dangerous for people to breathe ozone gas, its presence higher in the Earth's atmosphere is vital for human well-being because it forms a protective layer that absorbs much of the harmful ultraviolet radiation from the sun. Scientists discovered that chlorofluorocarbons (CFCs) in aerosol sprays and refrigerators were damaging the ozone layer, and were worried when they noticed that

a hole was forming in the ozone over Antarctica. Although controls on the use of CFCs have slowed the reduction of the ozone layer, it is still diminishing and may continue to diminish for several years. The depletion was linked to an increase in skin cancer in the southern hemisphere, so doctors advise people to protect their skin with clothing or sunscreen when outside.

Water pollution

When toxic chemicals from factories drain into rivers and the sea, they can remain in the food cycle for hundreds of years. They can accumulate in fish, and those who eat the fish unknowingly ingest the chemicals. When Japanese companies released mercury into the Pacific Ocean, mercury built up in the environment, poisoned the fish, and ultimately killed 52 villagers in Minamata. Many people were ill, and birth defects still affect the village's newborn.

In many parts of the world, raw sewage is discharged into rivers and the sea; and in regions where water filtration is poorly developed, contaminants may enter drinking water. If the bacteria and viruses in human effluent are ingested, gastrointestinal illness and hepatitis may result. Even in the United States, where water cleansing programs are among the best in the world, toxins can enter the supply. An increased incidence of leukemia in Woburn, Massachusetts, in the 1970s was thought to be linked to high levels of dangerous chemicals carried into the town's wells in groundwater from a waste disposal site.

Other examples of waterborne hazards include nitrates washed off farmland into rivers and lakes, and oil spills from tankers at sea or from disasters such as the explosion of an oil rig in the Gulf of Mexico in 2010.

Nuclear radiation

People living in some parts of the world are exposed to low levels of naturally occurring radiation from elements present in rocks. However, the development of a nuclear energy program in some countries from the 1950s on created a potential for exposure to larger, even lethal doses. Despite strict safety controls, accidents have occurred. The worst peacetime incident occurred in April 1986, when a nuclear reactor exploded at Chernobyl, Ukraine. Apart from those who died in the explosion, the instances of thyroid cancer reported in local children tripled in subsequent years. Birth defects and health problems in those exposed to the radiation are likely to persist for decades.

Food hazards

Even the food people eat can threaten their health. If food has not been kept in sanitary conditions or has not been thoroughly cooked it may be infected by microbes that cause salmonella infections, botulism, and cholera. If pesticides such as DDT and polychlorinated biphenyls (PCBs), or other chemicals, are used carelessly to treat food, they can accumulate inside the body, causing headaches, fatigue, burning skin and eyes, vomiting, and convulsions. There are strict controls regarding the use of these chemicals, but only in some parts of the world. Other hazards come from flavor- or color-enhancing additives, which may cause burning, dizziness, and nausea; and some cancers may originate from the use of dyes and nitrites.

> See also: **Anemia; Birth defects; Cancer; Hepatitis; Hygiene; Leukemia**

Exercise

I am considering using a toning machine, the type that gives you small electric shocks. Would it be as effective as taking exercise?

No. The machines do not provide the same benefit as exercise because they do not increase the body's workload. Your muscles will be stimulated to expand and contract rapidly, but this will not make them use up many more calories or make the heart and lungs increase their output. The machines encourage you to be lazy about exercise, and there is not much evidence that they will make you thinner, either.

Is it normal to feel stiff in the neck and shoulders after jogging?

No. It simply shows that you are not using your arms and shoulders properly. It is fairly common for muscles to get tense in the early stages of a new activity and for you not to notice stiffness until afterward. Try to jog with your shoulders relaxed, and let your arms swing loosely at your side.

Why do I get stomach cramps if I swim too soon after a light meal?

After eating, the stomach and intestines need extra blood to aid digestion. The muscles also need more blood for swimming. If they do not receive enough, they are deprived of oxygen and go into spasms. Thus it is best to take a half-hour rest after a light meal so that the stomach can empty itself.

Will some types of exercise give me large, unfeminine muscles?

No. Women have less muscle than men, and exercise simply firms and tones the muscles you already have. Sometimes women athletes develop rather masculine proportions, but only as a result of long and strenuous training.

Not only does exercise increase people's stamina and improve their health and appearance, but it also affects the way they feel and allows them to enjoy everyday activities more fully. If a person walks up five flights of stairs and is out of breath by the fourth, he or she is unfit.

Good health is not just the absence of disease; it is a state of vitality in which all the parts of the body work efficiently and respond easily to a person's needs. Regular exercise is an essential element of good health. It helps to build and maintain a degree of physical fitness that enables people to perform all their daily activities safely and enjoyably.

How much exercise do people need?

The amount of exercise people need to keep fit varies considerably. It depends on factors such as diet, the type of work a person does, normal body weight, metabolic rate, and how well that person handles various forms of stress.

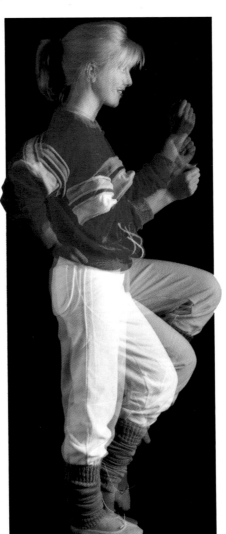

Walking, jogging, swimming, cycling, and games such as tennis and squash are ideal forms of exercise for keeping the whole body in shape. Other types, such as yoga and calisthenics (from the Greek, meaning "beauty and strength"), exercise specific areas of the body or are used as part of an overall program.

Some people do more exercise than they need to keep the body working properly. This type of training usually involves increasing muscle bulk and strength and developing the capacity of the lungs and heart. It is vital for any strenuous sporting activity but unnecessary for normal pursuits.

Why exercise?

Being physically fit is not just a question of muscular strength. Someone who is badly out of shape may have an impaired digestion, lowered mental alertness, and shortness of breath, all of which can be improved by exercise. People's state of mind may also be affected by exercise or the lack of it, since being fitter usually means being happier too. The immediate effect of exercise is improved muscle tone. Even when the muscles are at rest, a certain amount of tension remains, ensuring that the body is ready to respond to any demands.

Occasional bouts of exercise are not the answer. The cumulative effects of regular

◄ *Walking in place improves a person's overall cardiovascular fitness and helps to keep the whole body trim. It is a simple way of exercising because it can be done anywhere.*

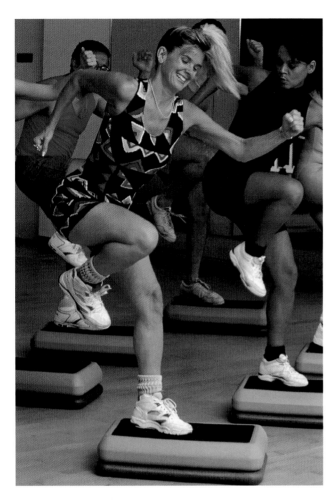

◄ *It is important to have proper instruction before undertaking any strenuous exercise such as step aerobics. The teacher should take class members through preliminary exercises that warm up the muscles, and they should avoid any overexertion that could cause injury.*

exercise on the heart and lungs are well known. The right exercise program will strengthen the muscles and increase the ability of the heart and lungs to supply oxygen to the tissues.

Exercise has been shown to reduce high blood pressure and is recognized as important in treating some heart conditions. Many cardiovascular disorders are caused or aggravated by atherosclerosis, a condition in which deposits left on the walls of the arteries make them harder and thicker and progressively reduce the blood supply. Exercise increases the force and speed of blood circulation, making arteriosclerosis less likely.

Exercise is also a valuable part of any overall plan to lose weight. During increased muscular activity the body's need for carbohydrates as a source of energy increases dramatically. If the intake of food is reduced, the body has to rely on stores of fat to meet this need, with a resulting loss of weight. If enough exercise is built into a regular weight-reducing program, the need for dietary restrictions will be less severe.

Who needs exercise?

As a general rule planned exercise is good for everyone except very young children and people suffering from serious illnesses or disabilities. However, the degree of exercise will vary according to a person's age, sex, and state of health.

Children up to the age of six do not need special exercise. Their natural play is enough, and too much activity can exhaust them.

For school-age children a planned exercise program is often part of the curriculum. Some children take naturally to an exercise routine, while those who dislike such a program are usually unfit to start with and embarrassed by their poor performance. They should be encouraged to enjoy exercise for its own sake because it is essential to ensure the proper development of muscles, bones, and ligaments in normal growth.

▼ *Exercising in water is an excellent way to stay in shape. It is particularly useful for pregnant women or anyone recovering from an injury, because the water supports the body and helps prevent unnecessary strain.*

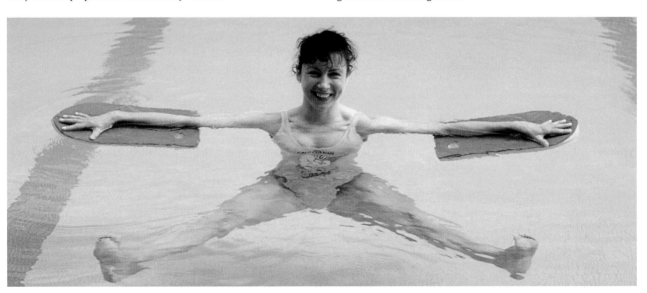

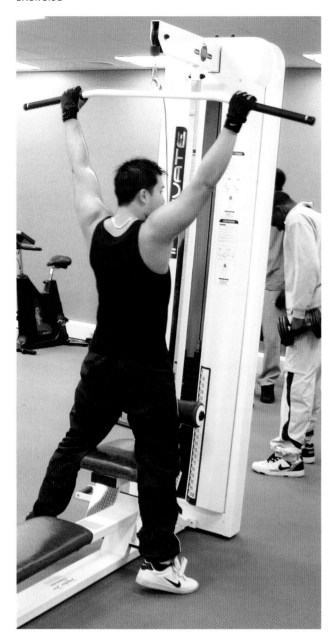

◄ *Weight-training equipment can be used to exercise and tone specific muscle groups, but bear in mind that weight-training alone will not improve overall cardiovascular fitness—it needs to be combined with regular aerobic exercise such as walking, jogging, or swimming.*

excessive back pain. There is usually a positive effect on the child's prenatal development too, with a reduced risk of circulatory or cardiac complications for the mother. Exercise tones the muscles before and after the birth and enables the new mother to regain her figure as quickly as possible.

Exercise also helps to smooth out the emotional ups and downs of menopause in later years.

Exercising at the same time every day may help to boost willpower. To create a routine, people should choose a regular time when they know they will be free. Exercising in the morning shakes off sluggishness. Lunchtime has advantages for dieters; it reduces the time available for eating and drinking and also reduces the appetite (research shows that appetite increases initially but is then reduced for several hours). Exercising after work helps to relieve tension and stress. The main thing is to find the time of day that is most suitable, and then to stick to it as much as possible.

A period of vigorous exercise each day will help both sexes reduce tension, and increase mental clarity and alertness, by improving the oxygen supply to the brain. Such exercise may be particularly beneficial for men, since they are statistically at a much greater risk from stress-induced health problems.

Saving exercise for the weekends can be dangerous, especially for middle-aged and older men. The only way a body can be kept in good condition is through regular, steady training, at least every other day.

When to take exercise

There are certain times when exercise can be especially valuable. For many women the greatest physical test is becoming a mother, and exercises designed to tone the abdomen and back muscles will enable them to go through pregnancy more easily and avoid

When not to exercise

There are times when exercise is unwise. During illness the body needs rest to recover, and activity may only aggravate the condition. Never exercise while suffering from a cold, an acute infection, or the flu. Vigorous activity will simply add to the feeling of exhaustion. A fever requires rest in bed to allow the body to cool down, so people should never try to exercise when they have one.

Women who suffer from menstrual cramps may prefer not to exercise at this time, but they may find that gentle relaxation exercises alleviate the pain.

Tiredness can be due to both fatigue and lethargy. If the body is really exhausted, it needs to recover and build up its reserves. However, if the problem is lethargy caused by too little exercise or

Types of exercise

TYPE	EFFECT	USES
Isotonic (exercises that make muscles lengthen and shorten)	Develops muscle strength: muscles shorten, tension remains constant. Stimulates heart, lungs, and circulation.	Spot training for lifting weights, rowing, and push-ups.
Isometric (exercises with muscles in state of contraction)	Develops muscle strength: muscles operate against a fixed object. Does not shorten muscles, does not place load on heart, blood flow is not increased dramatically.	Needs to be combined with running, swimming, or some other vigorous exercise to be beneficial overall. Can be practiced at a desk or in a car to relieve tension in specific muscles or for limited spot training.
Calisthenic (gymnastic exercises to achieve bodily health)	Helps build real endurance by encouraging the body to take in more oxygen, which is used by muscles; better gauge of fitness than muscular strength.	Training for all competitive sports that require endurance, from athletics to football. Used in fitness routines: toe touching, push-ups, knee bends. When weather is bad, indoor skipping with a rope and running in place.
Yoga (posture and breathing exercises)	Increases flexibility in joints of spine, arms, and legs. Tones muscles, ligaments, and tendons. Improves circulation and relaxation.	Good for people who prefer a quiet and more thoughtful method of exercise that affects all physical, mental, and emotional aspects of life.

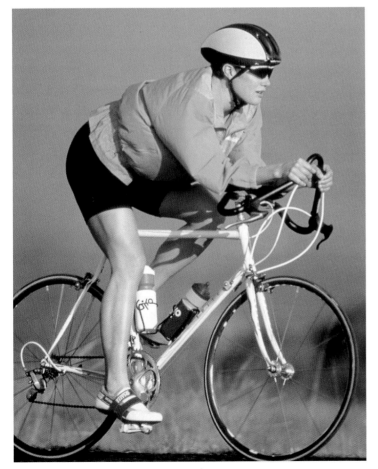

◄ *Cycling is a simple and healthy form of exercise that can be enjoyed throughout much of the year.*

too much eating and drinking, a brisk but mild activity such as swimming would be suitable.

It is important that people do not exert themselves too much, especially if they are unfit. The first signs of trouble include tightness and pain in the chest, severe breathlessness, dizziness or light-headedness, nausea, and a loss of muscle control. If one or a combination of these symptoms occurs, they should stop exercising at once.

The pulse rate should be checked at the wrist five minutes after exercising. If it is more than 120 beats a minute, the person is overdoing it. Ten minutes later it should be down to only 80 beats a minute.

Forms of exercise

The main forms of exercise are isotonics, isometrics, calisthenics, and yoga, which vary in their method and effects. People should choose the ones that suit them best, and it is helpful if they have clear objectives in mind. Are they exercising to maintain a basic level of good health? Or do they wish to train for a particular sport?

The most important thing is to choose a form of exercise that they find enjoyable. They will inevitably have to suffer a little in the beginning, but this will soon pass and they will feel the benefits.

See also: Diet; Dieting; Physical fitness; Weight

Family relationships

Why is it that so many marriages fail and end in divorce nowadays? Were people prepared to work harder at relationships in the past?

There are many reasons for the high rate of divorce. Some people blame it on the ease with which people can now get divorced, since many countries have legislated "quickie" and no-fault divorces. Other factors include women's changing role in society. Fifty years ago women who left their husbands often faced poverty and the possibility of losing custody of their children. Today women have more equality with men and more financial independence, so if they are unhappy in a marriage they are more likely to file for divorce. In addition, society no longer sees divorce as being shameful, as it did in the past; and there is an increasing view that children suffer more in a family that fights and argues than they do when their parents separate.

My friend was sexually abused by her father. Not only did it destroy her relationship with him, but her mother and sister refused to believe her and will have nothing to do with her. Is this common in cases of incest?

Yes. This tragic scenario shows the strong interdependent structure that exists in the family. What happens between one family member and another affects the entire group. Since the lives of family members are so close-knit, such an incident will compel the members to take sides. Denial of incest within a family is common. People want to see their families and homes as havens safe from such dangers and have difficulty accepting that such events could happen. They may prefer to deny that incest occurred rather than admit that they did nothing to stop it, but most psychologists tell victims and their families to focus responsibility on the abuser.

When most people in the Western world think of the word "family," they think of the nuclear family: a mother, a father, and their children. However, this concept of what makes up a family bears little resemblance to an increasing number of modern families in the United States and elsewhere in the world.

A family comprising a happily married man and woman and their dependent children does not necessarily provide a stress- or conflict-free situation; many families today face complexities and sources of tension that were almost unheard of 50 or even 20 years ago. In the United States, a number of trends have resulted in the nuclear family's becoming the exception rather than the rule.

One of the primary reasons for this change is the increasing participation of women in the workforce in the United States, Europe, and elsewhere in the West. Until the late 1960s the vast majority of women remained at home after they were married and had children. Today women make up close to half of the labor force and many return to their jobs after having a baby—or, at least initially, to part-time work. Legislation provides for maternity leave and pay, and ensures that employers keep a woman's job open for her return over a set period of time.

In many cases women are happy to return to work, although many have little choice in the matter—often a family is unable to survive on a single wage. This trend makes a considerable difference to the family in terms of male and female roles, and the decisions parents have to make about the care of their children while both partners are at work.

▲ *Games provide a structured activity in which families can interact and in which parents can teach children concentration, participation, skills, and the rules of fair play.*

Separation, divorce, and single parents

A second trend is the increasing prevalence of divorce and remarriage. In the United States today nearly half of all first marriages will end in divorce for the under-45 age group, up from around one-third in the mid-1970s. Although many of these couples will go on to remarry, another half of those will divorce again.

Separations and divorces, along with the forming of new families, result in more complex relationships. In addition to mothers, fathers, and children, families often now include new partners (the boyfriend or girlfriend of a divorced or separated mother or father), stepmothers, stepfathers, and stepchildren. If and when men and women have children with a new partner, there are also half brothers and half sisters.

One consequence of the frequent breakdown of marriages is an increasing number of single parents (usually women). In 2007, according to the U.S. Census Bureau, there were 13.7 million single parents in the United States, and those parents were responsible for 21.8 million children (26 percent of children under 21 years of age).

I have been suffering from low-level, flulike symptoms off and on for about two years, a condition that has coincided with problems in my marriage. My doctor now says my symptoms could be psychosomatic. What can I do?

It sounds as if you are suffering from stress, which can cause physical symptoms such as the ones you describe. If you and your partner have been trying to work through your problems without outside help up until now, it may be time to undergo some kind of therapy. Seeing a relationship counselor as a couple, or perhaps attending group therapy, could help you resolve your difficulties. This, in time, could lead to an improvement in your health.

What is it that attracts two people to each other to form a couple? Is it true that opposites attract?

Sometimes. For example, you will often find a person who appears strong and assertive on the surface married to someone quieter and more passive. Most psychologists, however, believe that we are usually attracted to people from a background similar to our own, particularly in terms of our experiences as a child. As a result, both people in the partnership may be similarly open and talkative about their deepest feelings or, by the same token, similarly reserved, shutting out and refusing to talk about certain emotions or experiences.

I am the single mom of a 10-year-old boy and fear that he will be affected by the lack of a strong male role model in his life. Should I worry and if so, what should I do?

It is true that both boys and girls benefit from strong role models of the same sex. Make sure that your son spends time with any grandfathers or uncles he might have, or the fathers of his friends. Encourage him to join youth or sports groups where male adults are present, and perhaps find out how he would feel about attending an all-male school.

Other problems

A trend that could add to the problems of people facing relationship breakdowns and those who are bringing up children alone is that people are increasingly likely to have moved away from their families and the area in which they grew up. Often they do so to be near a source of employment, to be with a partner, or maybe because they wish to live somewhere different, in a larger town or city, say. The result is that families frequently find themselves removed from the network of grandparents, aunts, uncles, cousins, and so on that in the past provided so much support, both practical (child care, for example) and emotional.

Other trends that have resulted in many families' no longer conforming to the nuclear-family model include the frequent adoption of children, sometimes from overseas; the possibility that a couple might resort to IVF using donated sperm or eggs to have children; or that a couple might pay another woman to have a child for them.

The rights of natural parents (particularly mothers) in comparison with the rights of parents who have actually brought up a child (or who have paid a donor to help them have a child) are becoming not only a legal but also an ethical minefield in many parts of the world.

Families today may also consist of a single-sex couple, either homosexual men or women, living together. Increasingly, such couples now have the choice of having children, through donor insemination, adoption, surrogacy, or sometimes just an arrangement between friends.

Families and health

The connection between physical and mental health has long been recognized, particularly by practitioners of alternative, holistic health therapies, such as homeopathy, massage, and acupuncture. Modern medicine, even when it does not recognize such therapies as valid treatments in themselves, is giving increasing credence to this connection. People's mental attitude can make a huge difference not only to how quickly they recover from some physical illnesses and disease, but also to whether or not they develop the conditions in the first place.

Regardless of the makeup of their family, people's relationships within that family also have a great influence on their mental and physical health. A woman or man living with a physically abusive or violent partner, for example, does not suffer just the physical trauma of that abuse. She or he is also more likely to suffer from low self-esteem, depression, stress, and nervous disorders.

To a lesser degree, the trauma of a divorce will be stressful for all those concerned. Stress, in turn, can lead to a number of other conditions, including flulike symptoms, anxiety and panic attacks, skin conditions such as eczema and psoriasis, asthma, eating disorders such as anorexia nervosa and bulimia, digestive disorders such as irritable bowel syndrome and diverticulitis, and drug abuse or alcoholism.

"Healthy" family relationships

Many of the problems people face as adults are really childhood difficulties that they failed to resolve when they were young. According to therapists, every person has a "front"—the personality and characteristics that he or she projects to the outside world (the store window, as it were)—and a "screen," behind which he or she hides and protects certain feelings and experiences. Psychologists such as Freud referred to this screening of emotions as "repression" and to the feelings that were being screened as the "unconscious."

Many psychologists today talk about the existence of many different kinds of partnerships and marriages. These types of partnerships are classified according to the roles that each partner adopts, the side of his or her personality that each is projecting (for example, the assertive, dominant side), and the kind of things that each partner is screening (for example, the needy, childlike side). Most therapists agree that successful or "healthy" relationships tend to be those between people who have fewer repressed emotions and who are willing to admit those feelings to one another, help bring them out into the open, and talk about them. The most angry, argumentative, and violent (emotionally or physically) relationships, on the other hand, tend to be those between people who have a lot of screened-off feelings and who are unable to admit and talk about those feelings.

Therapists have also found that any kind of change—be it bad or good—can produce tension. Among the most stressful changes are the death of a spouse or close family member, a divorce or marital separation, a prison term, personal injury or illness, and getting fired from a job. However, almost as stressful, and in some cases more so, can be the good changes, such as marriage or a

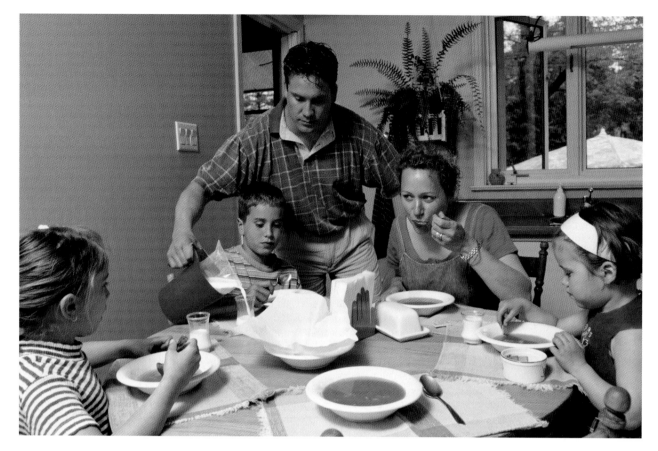

▲ *Family meals at the dinner table provide an excellent opportunity for family members to interact by engaging in conversations about their daily thoughts and experiences.*

marital reconciliation, retirement, pregnancy, changing a job, and the arrival of a new baby. A "healthy" family will be good at adjusting to these kinds of changes, and will therefore be less stressed by them.

Child development

Most of an adult's attitudes and characteristics come from his or her original family experiences and relationships as a child. Similarly, a child's relationships with the mother, father, siblings, and other family members have a strong effect on his or her development and health. While few would dispute that children need to be brought up in a stable, secure, loving environment if they are to thrive, other issues are not so clear.

Mother and child relationship

The effect of a child's relationship with his or her mother has long been debated among psychiatrists, psychologists, therapists, and others. Crucial issues include the amount of empathy and emotional contact a mother has with her child, whether or not she is over-protective, the establishment of clear boundaries, and if and when she decides to (or has to) return to work. Fathers, too, have started to come under increasing scrutiny. Will a father who is strict produce a well-disciplined, polite child or spur his son or daughter on to greater rebellion as a teenager? Absent fathers, too, are under the spotlight,

sometimes blamed for their children's underachievement at school or for their children's later criminal activity.

The most extreme examples of how a child is molded by his or her family experiences occur in cases of physical or sexual abuse. Modern psychiatry has found that adults who were abused, physically and sexually, as children not only find it hard to form relationships later in life but are more likely to suffer from depression, anxiety, nervous disorders, and sometimes serious mental illness.

Outlook for modern families

Although some people look back on the era of the nuclear family as a golden age, family relationships have never been easy or conflict-free. That there seem to be more stresses, tensions, and dangers within families today is at least in part due to the fact that people tend to be more open about their problems and relationships than they were in the past.

It is likely that families will continue to change and develop, and that relationships will become more complex. This is not necessarily a bad thing. What is important is that people find ways to deal with these complexities and to communicate with one another, so that a family provides the best possible environment for its adult and child members regardless of its makeup.

> *See also:* **Alcoholism; Child development; Depression; Drug abuse; Mental illness; Sexual abuse; Stress**

Fats

Fats are foods with a bad reputation; they have been linked with heart disease, obesity, and other threats to health. What are fats, what does the body do with them, and are they really necessary?

Questions and Answers

Does eating fat make you fat?

It can, depending on how much you eat. Weight for weight, fat provides nearly three times as many energy units or calories as carbohydrates or proteins. Fats are often eaten in a pure form (such as butter or margarine), so they can easily add too many calories to your diet, making you overweight.

Are fats essential in a person's diet?

Yes, fats perform vital functions in the human body. Fats provide the body with energy, produce vitamin D and hormones, carry vitamins throughout the body, insulate the body by keeping it warm, protect internal organs from physical damage, and form cell membranes.

My doctor has told me to eat fewer eggs to cut down on cholesterol. Why should I reduce the number of eggs when they do not contain much fat?

Most of the cholesterol we eat is in the saturated fats of animal-based foods, yet some other foods, such as eggs, are high in cholesterol though they contain very little fat.

Is it healthier to eat broiled meat rather than fried meat?

Yes, but it also depends on what meat you eat. It is better to broil fatty meat such as bacon, but there is less fat in fried chicken than in the same weight of broiled bacon.

I seem to have difficulty digesting fats. Is there something wrong?

There may be something wrong with the way your liver is making or releasing bile, a substance essential to fat digestion. Visit your doctor as soon as possible so he or she can investigate the problem.

Fats are one of the three substances, alongside proteins and carbohydrates, that make up the bulk of the human diet. Fats are important for other reasons, too. They make food more palatable; think of the difference between dry and buttered toast, or salad with and without salad dressing. They are also the most energy-rich of all foods. For example, 3½ ounces (99 g) of bread supplies about 250 calories. The same weight of butter, which is 80 percent pure fat, provides 720 calories.

What are fats?

About 90 percent of the fats people eat are known as neutral fats. They are made up of two chemicals—fatty acids and glycerol—which are both formed from carbon, hydrogen, and oxygen. Fatty acids and glycerol form molecules called triglycerides.

These fats can be either saturated or unsaturated, depending on the structure of the fatty acids. Fatty acids consist of chains of linked carbon atoms, with hydrogen atoms linked to each carbon atom. Any carbon atom can link to four other atoms and is thus said to be capable of making four bonds. A carbon atom in a fatty-acid chain will use two of its bonds to link to adjacent carbon atoms. If it is also linked to two hydrogen atoms, so that the four bonds are used up, it is said to be saturated. However, if it links to only one hydrogen atom, there will be a spare bond, and a double bond will form between it and the next carbon atom. In this case it is said to be unsaturated. So fatty acids with only single bonds between the carbon atoms are saturated fatty acids, and those with one or more double bonds are unsaturated. Most saturated fats are solid at room temperature, and unsaturated fats are liquid. This happens because most saturated fats are from warm-blooded animals, whose fat is just about liquid at their body temperature, which is above that of their surroundings. Unsaturated fats tend to be from fish and plants that are adapted for life at much lower temperatures.

What fat is best?

Saturated fats have a bad reputation because of their association with cholesterol, which makes up 10 percent of the fat people eat. It is not a true fat, because its structure is different from that of fat, but it is usually found with saturated fat. This means that the more saturated fat people eat, the more cholesterol they eat.

The body needs cholesterol for a range of functions, from maintaining brain tissues to making sex hormones, but the body can make all

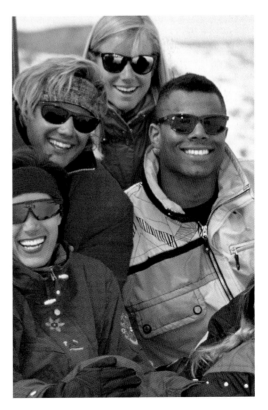

▶ *In freezing, wintry weather the body needs insulation against the cold. The body can get this from fat and from warm clothing.*

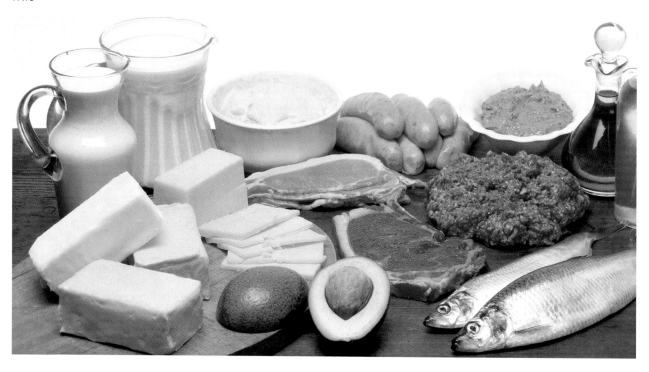

▲ *These foods all contain fat. Some, such as that in meat and cheese, is saturated, and some, such as that in fish and avocado, is unsaturated.*

A guide to high-fat foods

FOODS CONTAINING SATURATED FATS

Food	Percentage of fat
Lard	100
Coconut oil	100
Butter	80
Fried bacon	67
Double cream	48
Cheddar cheese	33.5
Broiled steak	32.5
Broiled pork sausage	23
Stewed ground beef	20
Milk (whole)	3.6

FOODS CONTAINING UNSATURATED FATS

Food	Percentage of fat
Olive oil	100
Margarine	100
Peanut butter	48.5
Broiled herring	13
Broiled mackerel	10
Avocado	8
Ice cream (made with vegetable fat)	8

Note: Some foods contain a mixture of saturated and unsaturated fats; for example, mayonnaise is 79 percent mixed fats and french fries are around 20 percent, depending on the cooking oil used.

the cholesterol it needs in the liver. The extra cholesterol taken in when saturated fat is eaten seems to interfere with the body's cholesterol-controlling mechanism, and the bloodstream becomes flooded with it. Surplus cholesterol, combined with other fats, becomes deposited on the walls of the blood vessels and can lead to arterial and heart disease. This is why doctors recommend changing from eating saturated fats that are high in cholesterol to unsaturated ones low in cholesterol.

How the body uses fats

Fats make up part of the wall surrounding every body cell. The body uses fats to insulate it against cold, to store reserve energy, to absorb shock around bones and organs, to insulate nerve cables, to lubricate skin, and to help transport vitamins.

The digestive system breaks down fats into fatty acids and glycerol. The fatty acids are then broken down further to release energy for immediate use. Any excess is reconverted to triglycerides and stored in the cells under the skin and around the internal organs. The glycerol is converted into glycogen, which is either broken down at once to release energy or stored in the liver until it is needed. Once the liver's glycogen storage system is full, the glycogen is changed into fat and stored in the body cells. If an excess of fat is stored there, it makes a person overweight. That is why it is important not to eat more than is needed.

Burning up fats

Hormones from the thyroid, adrenal, and pituitary glands control the rate at which the body burns up fats for energy. At times of stress or during intense physical activity, the hormones adrenaline and noradrenaline have a rapid effect on the rate of fat breakdown, increasing the amount of fatty acids in the blood by as much as 15 times, and pushing up the cholesterol level. If the fatty acids are burned up in exercise, they do no harm; but if they remain in the body, they can, with the cholesterol, lead to a fatty buildup in the arteries. This is one reason why exercise is a good way of dealing with stress.

See also: **Cholesterol; Diet; Protein; Weight**

Fevers

Questions and Answers

Is it important to bundle up and keep warm when you have a fever?

You should not allow yourself to get too cold. On the other hand, there is no need to pile on the blankets or heat the room to oven temperature. With plenty of rest, your body should recover.

When I have a fever, I shiver one minute and sweat the next. Why is this?

In a fever, the temperature swings up and down much more than usual. When it is on its way up, people get shivering chills, which may cause uncontrollable shaking attacks, called rigors. As the temperature starts to fall again, there is a lot of sweating.

Can a fever keep returning?

Yes. The best-known example is the fever that accompanies malaria, a disease transmitted by mosquitoes. Malaria can continue years after people have left the tropics. It can also recur years later. Fevers may also recur with other chronic infections.

Do fevers cause lasting damage?

Not usually. Any damage after a feverish illness usually results from the disease itself, rather than from the fever. However, a very high fever, if not controlled, can cause permanent brain damage.

I've been told that you shouldn't exercise when you've got a fever. Is exercise really harmful?

This is sensible advice. When your temperature begins to rise, the infection is becoming established. The infection is likely to become more widespread if you exercise strenuously at this point.

A fever is not an illness: it is a raised body temperature and is usually a sign of some form of infection. In a majority of cases, plenty of fluids and rest in bed will aid recovery.

Most fevers are due to infections by bacteria or by a virus and often coincide with a cough, a cold, or a sore throat. However, fevers can be caused by inflammation anywhere in the body.

The body temperature is generally kept within fairly close limits by the hypothalamus, the brain region concerned with the control of many of the body's automatic functions. If the body temperature rises too much, the body sweats to lose heat. If the temperature drops too low, heat is made in the body by activity of the muscles, which burn glucose fuel and so create heat. If someone becomes very cold, the muscle activity increases greatly and he or she starts to shiver.

Normal body temperature

The normal body temperature—98.6°F (37°C)—is only an average value; it is not uncommon for healthy people to have temperatures anywhere between 96° and 99°F (35.6°–37.2°C). Body temperature normally goes up through the day, starting at about 4:00 A.M. and reaching a peak about 6:00 P.M., and the variation may be 2–3°F (1–1.7°C).

High temperatures

Very high temperatures can be fatal. A body temperature over 106°F (41.1°C) can cause a convulsion in an adult, and permanent brain damage may occur if the temperature rises to 108°F (42.2°C). However, temperatures as high as this are extremely rare. In most cases, a high temperature can be brought down simply by sponging the patient's body with tepid water and by giving medication, such as acetaminophen.

The exact reason why people develop a raised temperature with infections and other causes of inflammation is not well understood. The white blood cells, which are an essential part of the body's defense system, produce a substance called pyrogen. This acts upon the

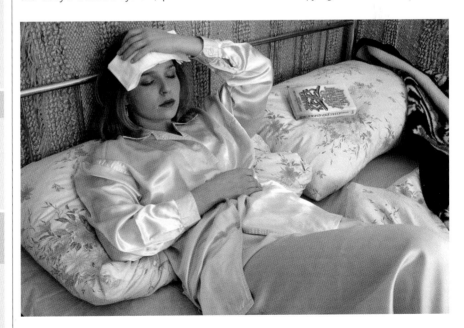

▲ *Viral infections, such as influenza, commonly cause fevers. The best treatment in such a case is to rest and drink plenty of fluids until the fever passes.*

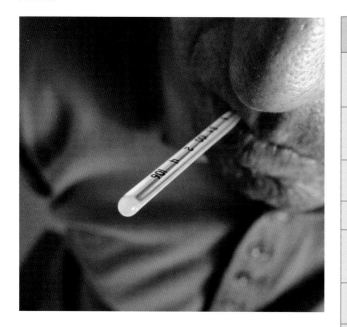

▲ *When a person has a fever, his or her temperature may rise and fall, causing both shivering and sweating.*

hypothalamus, causing a person's body temperature to rise. Some drugs, such as acetaminophen and aspirin, act to bring about a reduction in high temperatures by blocking messages sent out by the hypothalamus. Children should not be given aspirin.

Causes of fevers

The most common causes of fevers are viral infections such as influenza, which are usually associated with colds or sore throats. Specific antiviral treatment is inappropriate for most infections of this type—the only thing to do is rest until the fever passes.

Almost all other fevers in temperate parts of the world are caused by bacteria, which cause infections of the respiratory passages, the urinary tract, or the intestines and bowels. Bacteria also cause more serious infections, such as tuberculosis and typhoid fever, and collections of pus—abscesses—that are accompanied by fever. Bacterial infections are treated with antibiotics.

In the tropics, there are many feverish diseases caused by parasites slightly larger than bacteria, called protozoa; a common example is malaria. Finally, there are rare fevers that may result from unusual forms of tumors or from drugs.

Children with fevers

A child can produce quite a high temperature with a very minor infection. As a result, temperature alone is not a particularly good guide to a child's health. A better guide is whether he or she seems to be generally ill. Symptoms such as loss of appetite, vomiting, and lethargic behavior are much more important signs of illness than the degree of fever that the child is suffering.

The most common viral infections that cause fevers in children are usually accompanied by a cold, coughing, or a sore throat. Children are also likely to catch childhood illnesses that cause fevers, such as measles, rubella, mumps, chicken pox, and whooping cough.

What to do in cases of fever

Take the patient's temperature, but don't become a slave to the thermometer. The patient's general condition is a better guide to health than his or her exact temperature.

Rest. Do not go to work or school. Drink plenty of fluids— they are much more important than food, especially for young children, who may be in danger from dehydration.

Keep children with a mild fever indoors and occupied. There is no need to insist that they go to bed.

Use warm but lightweight bedclothes.

Use acetaminophen to bring the patient's fever down. This is particularly important when a child has a very high temperature, to avoid the risk of convulsions.

If a feverish child has a convulsion, do not leave him or her alone at any time. Call the doctor once the convulsion is over.

Do not take a child who has been in contact with an infection and has developed a temperature to the doctor's office—it is likely to spread infection. Call the doctor and ask for advice.

Spreading illnesses

The belief some parents have that it is a good thing for children to catch childhood illnesses and get them over with is sensible in some cases. Mumps is certainly more unpleasant in adults than in children. However, measles and whooping cough are unpleasant at any age, and both can be fatal in babies and very young children. As the risks of vaccination are less than the risks involved in having these illnesses, doctors recommend that children be vaccinated against such childhood diseases.

Children with fevers do not have to be kept in bed. Nor is it necessary to force them to eat solid food. However, it is important for feverish children to drink as much as possible. The danger of dehydration is particularly great in babies and very young children who are suffering a high temperature.

Convulsions

Children tend to develop convulsions with very high temperatures, such as those above 103°F (39.4°C). This mainly happens to children between the ages of one and three and is rare after the age of five. A child can be given acetaminophen to bring his or her temperature down and to avoid the risk of a convulsion. Parents should never give aspirin to a child with a fever, because of the possibility that he or she may develop Reye's syndrome. This is a dangerous condition that can cause liver inflammation and brain damage.

See also: **Antibiotics; Aspirin and analgesics; Bacteria; Chicken pox; Common cold; Infection and infectious diseases; Influenza; Measles; Mumps; Rubella; Sore throat; Vaccinations; Viruses; Whooping cough**

Food poisoning

Most people have suffered from the effects of food poisoning at some time in their lives. In the majority of cases, the symptoms subside and disappear as quickly and dramatically as they appeared.

"Food poisoning" refers to a number of different illnesses caused by eating foods contaminated with bacteria, toxins, or chemicals. Although symptoms often disappear quite quickly, in other cases food poisoning can be extremely serious.

Causes
Food can be contaminated by infective bacteria or viruses; sometimes the bacteria produce toxins (poisonous proteins) that are absorbed into the body. Chemicals such as DDT (now banned in the United States) and other agricultural sprays that have not been washed off food may also cause food poisoning. It may also be caused by eating poisonous mushrooms or sewage-contaminated mussels, which produce toxins that affect the human nervous system.

Symptoms
Food poisoning almost always produces vomiting, abdominal pain, and diarrhea, and occasionally fever and other symptoms. The time between eating the infected food and the onset of the symptoms is an excellent clue as to their cause. With the exception of poisoning that occurs slowly as a direct result of eating insecticides, food poisoning almost always appears quickly and dramatically. The symptoms usually occur so suddenly that the sufferer automatically thinks back to his or her last meal.

Dangers
In most cases the sufferer recovers from a bout of food poisoning in 24 hours. However, in some severe cases dehydration can result from the diarrhea, and people who become severely ill may need hospital treatment.

Botulism is an extremely serious form of food poisoning, caused by improperly canned or badly preserved food. The toxin that causes it is thought to be the most potent poison known—an antitoxin must be administered swiftly to counteract its effects. Intensive nursing is also needed. If it is left untreated, botulism can cause death.

If contaminated food is eaten by a large number of people, as in a school or hotel, an epidemic may occur. Therefore, all cases of food poisoning should be reported to health officials.

Treatment
Once the source of the food poisoning has been discovered, the treatment can be given accordingly. This can range from supportive measures given in the home to intensive nursing in the hospital.

In most cases the patient will be in pain, will vomit, and may also have frequent diarrhea. Vomiting and diarrhea may help to get rid of

How to prevent specific types of poisoning

Salmonella: Maintain strict personal hygiene. Isolate infected individuals until three stool specimens are clear of bacteria.

Staphylococcal: Treat all infected spots and infected areas on the body. Never prepare food if you have a septic spot.

Botulism: Do not eat canned or bottled foods that do not look or smell right, or that have a layer of fungus growing on top. When cooking outdoors, keep soil and compost away from food.

Chemicals: Fruits and vegetables sprayed with insecticides should be washed thoroughly.

Mushrooms: Familiarize yourself with edible and poisonous mushrooms. If in doubt, do not eat them.

Mussels: Avoid mussels gathered near sewage outlets and those in rusty or red water. (Mussels that cause food poisoning color the water red.) Never eat mussels that stay closed after boiling.

Questions and Answers

Someone told me that if I don't defrost a frozen chicken completely before I cook it, I could get food poisoning. Is this true?

Yes. This is because with a chicken there is always the possibility that germs might have been transferred to the meat from the guts when they were removed. When the chicken is cooked from a partially defrosted state, only the outside will get warm and the inside may remain raw. Salmonella and other bacteria breed very quickly in this warm medium. To be on the safe side, make sure you defrost poultry and meats completely before cooking them. Also, make sure that the chicken is cooked thoroughly before serving it.

How can you tell food poisoning from a severe attack of vomiting and diarrhea?

There are two clues to food poisoning. First, more than one person is usually affected, so the source of the food poisoning can be easily identified. Second, the symptoms often appear within a few hours of eating the food and are very dramatic: profuse diarrhea and vomiting, accompanied by severe abdominal pains that may make you double up. If you are in doubt, contact your doctor.

My father told me that he recently had ptomaine poisoning. Is this the same as food poisoning?

Contrary to popular opinion, ptomaine poisoning is not food poisoning—in fact, ptomaine poisoning is a myth.
Food poisoning is not caused by eating bad or decomposed food, although this was originally thought to be the case. When food rots or decomposes, substances called ptomaines are formed, but they are not harmful to health. Bad food tastes bad but does little actual harm.
Contamination is the key cause of food poisoning. Chances are that your father ate contaminated food and what he suffered from was, in fact, food poisoning.

How to prevent food poisoning

Maintain scrupulous personal hygiene. Always wash your hands before eating and after using the toilet.

Keep all perishable foods refrigerated.

Wash all vegetables and fruits before eating them.

Make sure you defrost meat and poultry completely before cooking, and then cook them thoroughly.

Never refreeze foods that have been defrosted, since they may have picked up germs at room temperature.

If you reheat food, make sure it is hot and cooked through to the middle.

Never eat foods that smell of, or that look as if they have been exposed to, insects or mice.

Keep all insecticides and weed killers locked away.

Use only those pesticides you know well in the garden.

Never eat unknown fruits or vegetables that are growing wild.

When in doubt, throw out any food that may be contaminated. This includes food in a dented or rusted can, or preserved food with fungus on top.

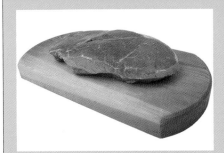

▲ *Raw meat can harbor bacteria.*

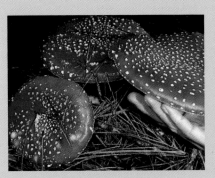

▲ *Don't eat wild mushrooms.*

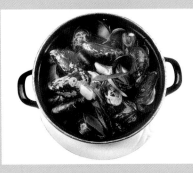

▲ *Avoid eating mussels that do not open.*

the cause of the poisoning. The patient's caregiver should call a doctor if they are severe. The patient should be reassured, as he or she is likely to be distressed. A vomit receptacle should also be placed within reach and cleaned every time the patient has vomited. If possible the person caring for the patient should place a portable toilet near his or her bed. Alternatively, the caregiver can seat the patient in the bathroom, keeping the patient wrapped up and warm, and supporting him or her if necessary.

The patient should be offered frequent sips of water, even if he or she continues to vomit. This will help prevent dehydration. The caregiver should not give any food; the chances are that the patient will not even want to think about it. When the patient feels better, he or she can be given light meals. With this type of food poisoning, the patient is often completely well within 24 hours of the onset of symptoms with no aftereffects.

If the cause of the food poisoning is infective bacteria, treatment should be started at home. Sometimes a doctor might need to prescribe antibiotics or sulfonamides. Patients should be isolated at home and not be allowed to return to work until they have had three stool specimens that are free of bacteria.

Causes and treatment of food poisoning

CAUSE	TIME INTERVAL	SYMPTOMS	TREATMENT
Infective bacteria in food Includes salmonella, dysentery, and paratyphoid bacteria. Comes from uncooked or undercooked food, or food that has been only partially defrosted before cooking.	12–48 hours	Abdominal pain, vomiting, diarrhea (occasionally with blood), excess mucus, and a fever. Serious dehydration may result.	Rest in bed; drink plenty of fluids. Call doctor as antibiotics or sulfonamides may be needed. Keep patient isolated at home.
Poisons (toxins) produced by bacteria in food **Staphylococcal** Bacteria are not destroyed by cooking, or are spread by infected person handling food.	1–6 hours	Excessive salivation, nausea, vomiting, abdominal pain, collapse, low body temperature.	Rest in bed. If vomiting occurs do not give food, only small sips of water with light meals thereafter. Usually cured within a few hours, but if symptoms get worse, call doctor since fluids may have to be given intravenously.
Botulism *Clostridium botulinum* bacteria. Eating improperly canned or badly preserved food.	30 minutes– 36 hours	Dramatic onset of generalized paralysis. Voice change, double vision, squint, muscle weakness. Sometimes cramps and diarrhea. Difficulty in breathing and swallowing.	Hospital treatment needed urgently. Stomach washed out. Support on ventilator in intensive care unit. Botulism antitoxin administered if caught in early stages.
Chemicals in food Irritant chemicals eaten mistakenly; or from the action of acid on cooking containers.	10 minutes– 2 hours	Sickness, abdominal pain, diarrhea. Sore mouth and metallic taste to food.	Call doctor, who may give chelating agents (substances that can engulf metallic compounds) for dangerous chemicals. In less severe cases simply withdraw poison and give supportive treatment.
Insecticides in food Agricultural sprays not washed off of fruits and vegetables.	2–12 days	Early muscular paralysis, sometimes delayed as poison builds up.	Same as above.
Mushroom poisoning Eating poisonous mushrooms (for example, *Amanita muscaria*—red toadstool with white spots).	2 hours–3 days	Vomiting, abdominal pain. Symptoms depend on type of mushroom eaten (can lead to diarrhea, and damage to the nervous system, blood cells, or liver).	Rest in bed; attention to diet. Call doctor. Careful observation of function of liver, which may be damaged. Antidote in some cases.
Mussel poisoning Eating sewage-contaminated mussels or mussels that have not opened after cooking.	2 hours–3 days	Weakness, unsteadiness, and headache with vomiting.	Rest in bed; drink plenty of fluids. Call doctor.

Patients suspected to be suffering from botulism must be admitted to the hospital immediately. A botulism antitoxin must be administered in the early stages, and the patient's stomach washed out. Patients who are seriously ill will have to be supported on a ventilator in an intensive care unit. If they survive the acute stage, the outlook is good, and most will make a full recovery.

When complex chemicals or insecticides are involved, it may be necessary to give chelating agents—substances that attract the foreign material, become attached to it, and make it harmless. If there has been gradual long-term chemical poisoning, the source of the poison must be traced and avoided in the future. The patient should be given supportive treatment. The outlook depends very much on the individual case.

With mushroom poisoning an antidote may be given, depending on the type of mushroom involved. The patient should rest in bed and have a bland diet. There is a possibility that the liver may have been damaged, so its function will have to be closely observed, possibly in a hospital.

With mussel poisoning, home treatment measures should be taken swiftly to avert dehydration. The outlook is good, but the patient needs to rest in bed and take fluids. If the symptoms persist, the doctor should be called.

See also: **Bacteria; Hygiene; Infection and infectious diseases; Poisoning; Staphylococcus; Viruses**

Fractures

Many people will fracture, or break, a bone in their body at some time in their life. The power of the human body to heal itself is so great that in most cases the patient will experience a complete recovery.

The word "fracture," when applied to a bone, means that it is broken, but there are several different kinds of fractures. The fracture may be a crack that runs only partway across the bone; this is called a greenstick fracture. If the bone breaks right through but does not pierce the skin, it is known as a simple fracture. If part of the bone is driven through the skin, it is called a compound fracture. If the fracture is so bad that the bone is broken into several small pieces, it is known as a comminuted (crushed) fracture; and if the break occurs as a result of a disease of the bone, the fracture is described as pathological.

The greenstick fracture gets its name from the way in which a willow sapling breaks along its outer edge if it is bent too far. Very young and supple bones sustain this type of injury, and it is found mainly in infants and children.

Compound fractures are always more serious than simple fractures (those in which the skin is not broken), because of the greatly increased risk of infection. Both simple and compound fractures may be comminuted, and these are by far the most difficult to knit together again.

When bones are excessively weak owing to a condition called osteoporosis, found mainly in older people or where there is a tumor of the bone, pathological fractures may occur spontaneously with only minimal or even no force being applied.

Causes

A great deal of force is needed to break a healthy bone, but its susceptibility to fracture also depends upon other factors, such as its location in the body, its thickness, and the circumstances in which force was applied. The limbs, for example, are much more prone to damage than the pelvis.

The long bones of the limbs are very resistant to force applied along their length but are much more likely to break if the same force is applied across the length. These long bones are not of uniform thickness, and they tend to break at their narrowest point. The three types of break that occur most frequently are fractures of the wrist, hip, and ankle.

The most common injury to the wrist is caused by a fall on an outstretched hand (which is used automatically in an attempt to break the fall). This results in a fracture of the lower end of the large bone of the forearm (the radius). The broken lower end is displaced backward so that the forearm bends upward before it reaches the hand. When the resulting deformity is viewed from the side, it looks like a dinner fork. This is called Colles' fracture and can happen to people of all ages.

Fractures of the hip occur almost exclusively in older people. The injury results from a sideways fall, and the fracture takes place across the upper part of the thighbone

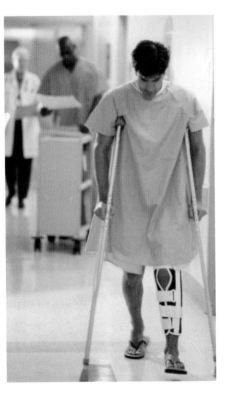

▲ *Crutches are used in cases of leg or foot fractures to ease pressure on the affected part while walking. Undue pressure could cause pain or misalignment of bones.*

COMMON TYPES OF FRACTURE

SIMPLE FRACTURE

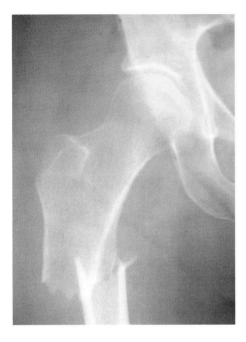

▲ *The X ray above shows a simple fracture of the neck of the femur near the pelvic socket in a 60-year-old woman. To hold the two parts together and enable the bone to heal, a nail and screws were used to attach a metal plate to the bone.*
▶ *In a comminuted fracture (right), the bone shatters into small pieces.*

COMMINUTED FRACTURE

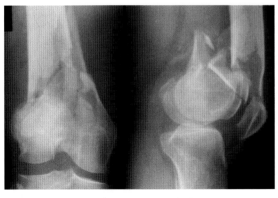

▲ *The X ray above shows a femur (thighbone) fractured above the knee, seen from the front (above left), and the side (above right). Treatment involves operating to remove fragments, joining the bone ends with a metal plate, and immobilizing the limb in plaster.*

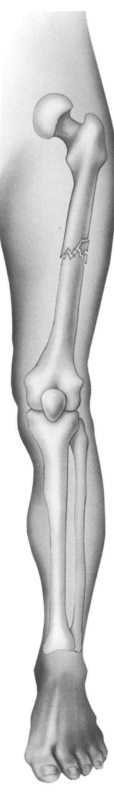

Recognizing a fracture
If the answer to these questions is yes, get medical help immediately:
Does the injured limb hurt?
Does it look abnormal?
Is it unable to bear weight?
Do the bones grate?

(femur) at its narrowest point, just behind the joint with the pelvis. This is a medical emergency, because the victim is unable to walk and may be in severe pain. Any elderly person who has suffered a fall at home and is then unable to get up needs to be taken to the hospital by ambulance for an immediate X ray.

The injury caused by a twisting motion of the ankle (with the full weight of the body above) is a mixture of a fracture of the bones of the lower end of the leg combined with tearing of the ligaments of the ankle. This is called Pott's fracture and can easily happen to a woman wearing high heels if her ankle twists as she is walking or running.

Symptoms

Whatever the cause of the fracture, the symptoms are similar: the victim is in pain, the limb may be in an unnatural position and cannot be used, and there may be signs of shock (sweating and pallor) owing to internal bleeding from the ruptured blood vessels. If the bone is moved, the fractured ends may grind together (producing a creaking sound called crepitus). Doctors can feel this by placing a hand over the fracture site. Although pain is usually present, if the bones are not displaced at all, other signs may not be apparent. An X ray is therefore necessary to check the diagnosis and the extent of the damage to the bone.

Although fractures of weight-bearing bones such as the leg are generally fairly obvious because the victim finds it impossible to walk, a fracture elsewhere—for example, of the ribs or hand—may pass unnoticed. Fractures in young children are also harder to spot because they cannot always explain clearly where it hurts. It is also possible for the elderly to break fragile bones without much force being applied.

After I broke my femur, friends told me I'll probably get arthritis years from now as a result. Is this really true?

The vast majority of fractures, provided that they are treated quickly, do not lead to any harmful aftereffects. If there has been a delay or complication in treating a fracture involving a joint, then the injured joint may wear out faster than it would normally, and in such cases arthritis could develop later in life.

Is it possible to break a bone and not know it?

Most bones are broken as a result of some definite accident, and the resulting pain, swelling, and change of shape in the part concerned make it clear that the injury is serious. The smaller bones in the body, however, can be broken as a result of undue stress without the patient's being aware of it. This sometimes happens with the small bones of the hands or feet. For example, a fall on an outstretched hand that is not sufficient to break the arm can fracture one of the metacarpal bones in the hand without there being much to show for it. Similarly, the so-called march fracture of the foot sometimes occurs in soldiers, following a long period of marching. Such fractures heal without treatment.

I've heard that bones can chip and not break. Would it be dangerous to have one of these chips floating around inside the body?

A bone may chip or crack when the force of an injury is not sufficient to break it entirely. The damage often is revealed only when the part is X-rayed. Usually no special treatment is necessary for this kind of injury, and the chip or crack simply joins up with the bone again. There is no danger that loose chips of bone will move freely around the body, but occasionally a chip may float near the break but not join. If the site is near a joint, movement may cause pain, and the chip may have to be removed.

GREENSTICK FRACTURE

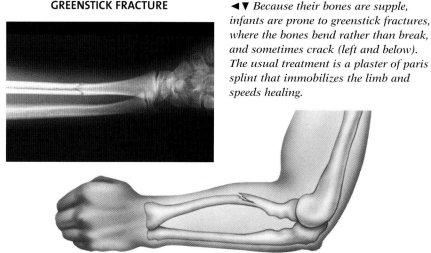

◄▼ *Because their bones are supple, infants are prone to greenstick fractures, where the bones bend rather than break, and sometimes crack (left and below). The usual treatment is a plaster of paris splint that immobilizes the limb and speeds healing.*

COMPOUND FRACTURE

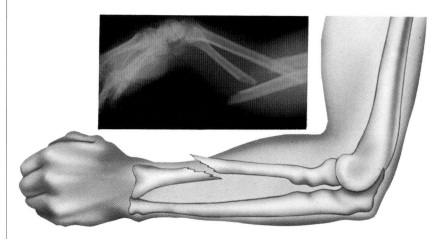

▲ *In a compound fracture the broken bone pierces the skin. The limb will be operated on to remove damaged tissue and bone fragments and to realign the bone ends; the limb will then be set in a plaster cast. With an upper arm or leg, the bone may also be secured by a metal plate.*

SKULL FRACTURE

► *In treating a skull fracture (see arrow in circle, right), the patient is first observed for any signs of brain damage. If internal bleeding is causing pressure on the brain, an operation will be necessary. A steel or plastic plate may be used to replace shattered bone that was removed during the operation.*

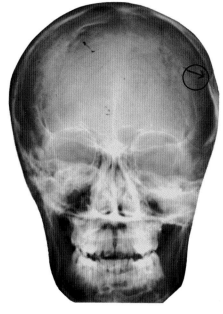

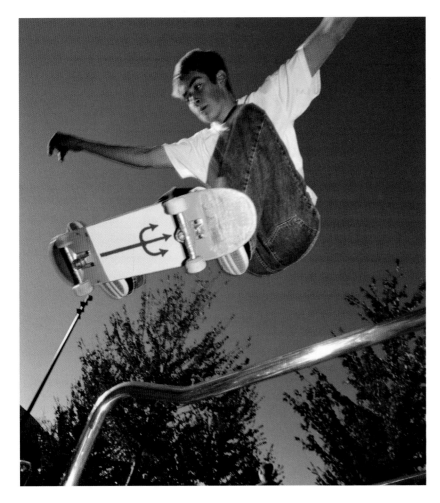

DO
Do call 911 for an ambulance.
Do reassure the patient.
Do make the patient comfortable.
Do handle the patient with care, moving him or her only if necessary.

DON'T
Don't get excited or panicky.
Don't move the patient, unless you must.
Don't give the patient anything by mouth (in case an anesthetic has to be given when the bone is set).
Don't leave the patient alone while you send for help.
Don't sit the patient upright (especially in cases of spinal injury).
Don't try to do things in a hurry.
Don't try to realign the fracture yourself; you could cause further damage.

▲ *Fractures commonly occur in people who engage in demanding leisure sports such as skateboarding, skiing, and snowboarding, and who do not wear protective gear.*

Dangers

The chief danger from a fracture is shock due to bleeding and pain. This can be a potentially life-threatening complication. Bone is nourished by a rich blood supply, and the bigger the bone that breaks, the greater the loss of blood. For example, an automobile accident victim who suffered a fracture of the pelvis and two fractures of the leg could lose up to 7 pints (3 l) of blood in a short time, often without any external blood loss. This is why if a broken bone is suspected, anyone administering first aid should call for medical help or the Emergency Medical Services. Medical treatment deals with bleeding and shock and relieves pain before the fracture itself is repaired.

Fractures of certain bones must be treated cautiously because of the risk of damage to tissues underneath. Fractures of the skull, for example, may be complicated by damage to the brain from increased pressure owing to bleeding. Whenever a fractured skull is suspected, the patient is admitted to the hospital as a precaution and is kept under observation for at least 12 hours. The most obvious warning sign of possible brain damage is an increase in drowsiness after the injury.

A fracture of the lower part of the rib cage on the right side could be complicated by a rupture of the spleen, and on the left side by a rupture of the liver. In each case shock can develop owing to loss of blood, and it is vital that the situation is dealt with immediately.

Fractures of the pelvis can damage the bladder or urethra. Any fracture of the spine needs particularly skillful handling by a surgeon to avoid damage to the spinal cord and paralysis.

Fractures of the limbs, although very painful, are not particularly dangerous, providing that the loss of blood has been controlled. Damage to the blood supply to the bone sometimes occurs, however, with the result that the fracture does not heal. This can sometimes happen when one of the small bones in the hand or foot is damaged.

Young bones may stop growing if the line of the fracture runs across the growing end. The result of this is that the affected limb does not reach the same size as the one on the other side. Clearly, this problem affects children only. The growing end of the bone is always close to the joint, so a fracture at the joint is more serious than a fracture through the shaft of the bone.

Treatment

The immediate treatment may have to be a blood transfusion if the patient has lost a lot of blood. Drugs may also be given to relieve the pain. Then the fracture is repaired. In cases where there has been no

Questions and Answers

Why do some people end up with one leg noticeably shorter than the other after a break has healed?

In badly comminuted fractures (when the bone has fragmented) there may be a little shortening, but in most cases there is no change in bone length. However, if a child's bone is broken at the growing end, the affected limb may not reach its full size.

My neighbor's little boy is always breaking his bones. She says he is accident-prone. Can this be true?

Active children inevitably run a greater risk of injury, as any teacher will tell you. A person who breaks bones repeatedly may have an inherited bone disease, however, especially if these fractures occur when the child is very young. Your neighbor would be wise to seek her doctor's advice.

Is it possible for a bone to heal by itself without any form of treatment whatsoever?

Bone possesses remarkable healing powers, and a fracture may heal without any outside help at all. The result may not be as strong or as straight as before, but full use of the limb does return, and so a failure to diagnose a fracture will not necessarily result in a complete disaster. Obviously, however, the outlook is far better if a fracture receives prompt medical attention.

I am planning my first skiing vacation, and I am terrified of breaking my leg. Since this seems to happen to so many skiers, I wonder if there is anything I can do to avoid it?

Yes, there are several things you can do. You can make sure that you are physically fit before you go. Start toning up your muscles for a few weeks before you leave. Jogging, in-line skating, and bicycle exercises are very good for the leg muscles. Better still, take a ski class, which will certainly save you from a few unnecessary falls.

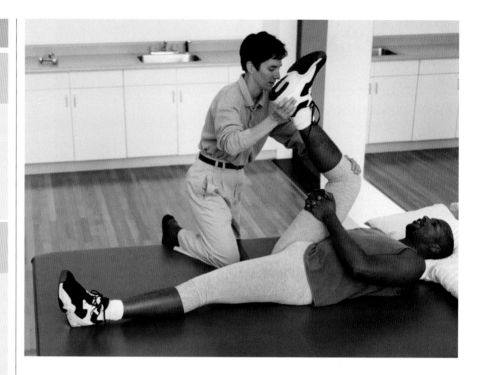

▲ *Because the surrounding muscles waste away from disuse while the fractured limb is in a cast, it is a good idea, when the cast is removed, to do exercises that stretch and strengthen the limb to get the muscles working properly again.*

displacement of bones, the fractured ends do not need to be realigned. In other cases, especially fractures of the leg, muscle spasms can pull the bone ends past one another and a force needs to be applied in the opposite direction to correct this; this is called traction.

Badly comminuted fractures or spiral-shaped breaks may be impossible to bring together, and in these cases the bone ends are joined with a metal plate screwed along the side.

After realignment the bone ends must be held in the correct position while healing takes place. This is done by using a plaster cast, which is worn for a variable period of time depending on the type and position of the fracture. Because it has to bear the body's weight, a fractured leg usually has to be kept in plaster for at least 12 weeks. Non-weight-bearing injuries, such as those of the arm, need be immobilized for only six weeks, or even less in children. Some fractures, such as fractures of the ribs, need no immobilization whatsoever.

Recovery period

The speed at which healing of the fracture takes place depends upon the blood supply at the fracture site. Age does not matter. The body heals just as fast in a person of 80 as it does in a child of eight. If a screw has been inserted, a simple supporting cast is all that is needed, and weight can be placed on the limb again as soon as the pain and swelling have subsided.

People often forget that the muscles waste away a little after a period of disuse, but the surrounding muscles should be strong and provide good support, thereby strengthening the area. Patients are thus encouraged to do active exercises at an early stage. This is painful at first but gets easier with each day. Isometrics, which are exercises that contract the muscles without any movement of the affected limb, are particularly useful. Physical therapy, in general, can help strengthen muscles that have become weak and is important in speeding patients on their road to recovery.

Bones possess remarkable healing powers, and a fracture may mend completely without any sort of treatment.

> **See also:** Arthritis; Osteoporosis; Physical therapy; Shock; X rays

Genetics

Genes are the means by which parents pass on physical characteristics, and some mental characteristics, to their children. In turn the next generation passes them on to its children. If people have any worries about transmitting unhealthy genes, a genetic counselor can offer advice.

Most of the body's features, from the size of the toes to the color of the eyes, are determined from the moment of conception by chemical information supplied by each parent. This information is held in threadlike structures called chromosomes in the nucleus of each cell.

Each chromosome has rows of genes along its length. Each of these genes carries the instructions for an enzyme that brings about a particular characteristic. A single gene is a length of the chemical deoxyribonucleic acid (DNA), which is shaped like a twisted ladder known as the double helix. The outer, longitudinal parts of the DNA molecule each consist of a chain of alternate sugar and phosphate units. The sugar is called deoxyribose. Lying like rungs between the outer parts, and attached at each end to a sugar molecule, are linked pairs of molecules

HOW BLOND HAIR IS INHERITED

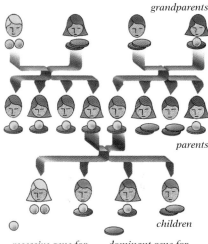

grandparents

parents

children

○ *recessive gene for blond hair*

⬭ *dominant gene for brown hair*

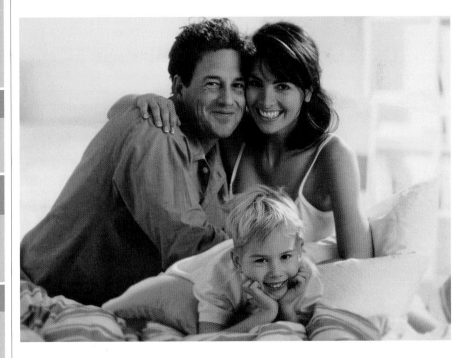

▲ *Two brown-haired parents may have a blond child if they have both inherited a recessive gene for blond hair. Siblings may have blond or brown hair.*

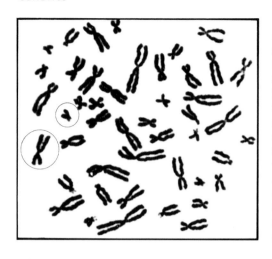

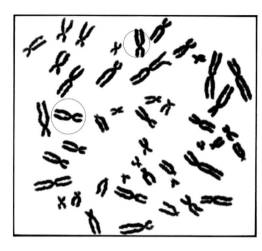

◄► Geneticists can distinguish male from female chromosomes by the unique pairs: XY—male (left) and XX—female (right). Every normal human cell has 46 chromosomes, except female egg and male sperm cells, which each contain 23. During fertilization each chromosome in the egg cell matches its partner from the sperm cell.

called bases. There are just four bases in the DNA ladder: adenine (A), thymine (T), guanine (G), and cytosine (C). The sequence of bases along the sugar-phosphate chains is called the genetic code. The code is divided into lengths called genes, each of which provides information for the construction of a single protein, which is usually an enzyme. During protein synthesis in the cell, the two vertical posts of the DNA ladder break apart. The exposed bases form a carrier substance known as messenger ribonucleic acid (mRNA). This is in the form of a single strand of split DNA, but it contains the base uracil (U) in place of thymine (T). The vital function of mRNA is to organize the manufacture of proteins, (the biochemical molecules that are essential to every bodily action); it does so by directing the stringing together of smaller units called amino acids.

What can go wrong

A wide range of genetic alterations (mutations) or other mistakes can occur. On the one hand, it is possible to inherit a gene that makes a single abnormal protein. At the other extreme, a whole block of genes can be lost on inheritance, as when a piece of chromosome is missing, or an extra chromosome can be gained. However, survival is impossible if an entire chromosome is missing.

Problems are most common at the time when an egg or sperm is formed. Almost all of the body's cells have 46 chromosomes, organized in 23 pairs. Eggs and sperm, however, are specialized cells called gametes and contain only 23 chromosomes, or half the usual number. This is because the father's sperm and mother's egg must recombine to make a cell with a total of 46 chromosomes when fertilization takes place. When an egg or sperm is produced, only one of each chromosome pair is included. This halving process is called meiosis. Sometimes pieces of chromosomes may break off and get lost when this happens.

Alternatively, an extra chromosome or piece of chromosome may be donated at the time that meiosis takes place. The best-known example of this is the condition called Down syndrome, which results from inheriting an additional chromosome in the 21st chromosome pair.

Many of these mistakes result in miscarriage long before a pregnancy comes to term because the fetus is too malformed to develop. If the child lives after birth, however, nothing can be done to treat the abnormality. It is locked in the genetic code and may therefore be passed on to the sufferer's children.

Where to turn for help

Couples at risk are usually referred to a genetic counselor by their family doctor. A genetic counselor is a specialist in human genetics and statistics. Genetic counseling may also be one of the functions of a hospital team including an obstetrician, a social worker, and a pediatrician as well as a genetics expert. It helps people understand how genetics is involved in certain disorders. It involves estimating the risk of a disorder that may arise if a couple have children, or the chance that a further baby will be affected by a disorder which has already occurred in an older child.

A couple may receive genetic counseling if one or each of them has a relative with a serious health problem, a child with a serious disease or deformity, or a family history of ill health. One of the couple may have an inherited disease, or the two may be worried because they are blood relatives. The first thing a genetic counselor will do is draw up a detailed family tree of both the man and the woman, if possible going back at least three generations. This involves drawing on hospital and public records as well as family information. Sometimes family trees are very difficult to compile, either because a family has become widely scattered or because records have been lost or never kept. It may also be hard to make the family tree completely accurate in medical terms, because of the great advances in medical knowledge in the past century.

The counselor then has to figure out the chance that the couple will have a child with an inherited disease. The ease or difficulty of this part of the task depends very much on the type of disorder, the way it has been passed on in previous generations, and the family relationship, if any, between the couple.

Genetic counseling will also have to consider the frequency of a particular disease in the community as a whole, because this affects the statistical analysis. In addition, the counselor may want to obtain information from medical tests on any abnormal children already born to a couple, to find out whether the abnormality fits into a hereditary pattern or stems from another cause.

Dominant and recessive genes

The easiest genetic diseases to assess in terms of risk are those that have a simple path of inheritance. Such diseases are called dominant or recessive, depending on the way the genes controlling them are expressed. It is not only certain illnesses that result from dominant or recessive genes; characteristics such as hair and eye color follow a

Questions and Answers

My son is epileptic. I would like to have another baby, but would a second child also be affected?

Except in one rare form, or when it accompanies other inherited diseases, epilepsy is not usually passed on genetically.

If you have serious worries about having another baby, or if there is a history of epilepsy in your own or your husband's family, ask your doctor to arrange an appointment for you to see a genetic counselor. The counselor will be able to assess the risk that the problem will recur. You and your husband can then decide whether or not to have another baby.

My husband was adopted and does not know his real parents. He is worried that they may have had some genetic disorder. Is there any way he can find out?

If you and your husband are worried about this, ask your doctor to refer you for genetic counseling. It may be possible to test your husband's blood to find out if he has the genes for an abnormality without actually showing them. The tests are by no means comprehensive but may help set your minds at rest.

I am engaged to my second cousin but am doubtful about whether or not we should get married, because I have read that marriage between cousins can result in abnormal babies. What should I do to find out about it?

Ask your doctor to arrange an appointment for you to receive genetic counseling. This will involve compiling a detailed family tree and analyzing the medical history of your relatives. The counselor will then be able to see if there are any patterns of inherited disease in your family. He or she will also be able to give you some statistics on the chances of you and your cousin having abnormal children.

It is probable, however, that you and your cousin come from a healthy family and have no cause to worry.

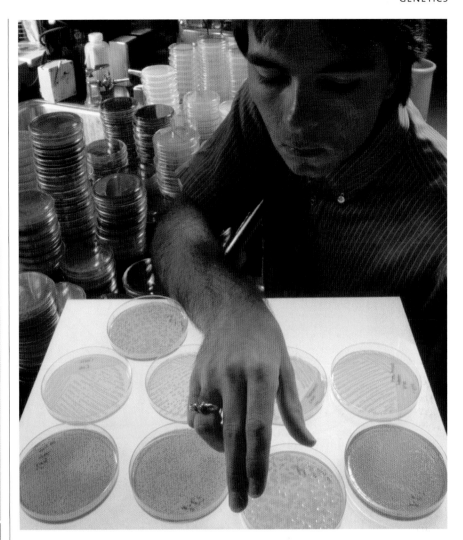

▲ *A doctor at the University of Illinois studies genetic clues for cystic fibrosis.*

similar complicated pattern. One example of a disease known to be caused by a dominant gene is an inherited form of cataract (clouding of the lens of the eye). If a child inherits a normal gene from one parent but an abnormal, cataract-causing gene from the other, the abnormal gene will show itself, even though it is present only once.

Other examples of inherited disorders caused by dominant genes include a form of dwarfism in which the head and trunk are normal in size but the limbs are very short; spina bifida, a serious spinal abnormality; brachydactyly, a disorder that affects the way the fingers develop; Huntington's chorea, a disease of the nervous system in which nerve cells in areas of the brain are gradually lost; and some types of muscular dystrophy.

Phenylketonuria (a severe disorder of the metabolism, which, if not treated early, is associated with serious mental defects) is an example of a disease caused by a recessive gene. In the case of phenylketonuria, a child must inherit the gene for the condition from both parents to suffer from the disease. A child who inherits only one gene for phenylketonuria from one parent will not be affected.

More diseases are caused by recessive genes. Among the better-known diseases that are caused by inheritance of two recessive genes is albinism. In this condition there is a complete lack of pigment in the skin and hair (which are white), and in the eyes (which are pink and may have severe vision defects). Other diseases caused by recessive genes are certain types of deafness and blindness; cystic fibrosis, a disease that causes abnormal secretions of mucus; and metabolic disorders, including galactosemia, in which the body cannot break down galactose, the sugar in milk.

Dominant and recessive diseases

If one partner is known to have a dominant inherited disorder but the other does not, then the risk that the disorder will be passed on is one in two. The chance is one in four if one of the parents is known to have a recessive disorder. Matters are complicated in the case of recessive traits, because both the parents are more likely to be carrying the same recessive gene, which may be combined in their children. Establishing the odds is especially relevant when first and second cousins marry, because the more closely two people are related, the greater the chance that they will both have inherited a recessive gene from the same grandparent or great-grandparent.

With some inherited diseases the sex of the individual affected is also important. The hereditary disease called hemophilia (which affects the blood-clotting process and leads to excessive bleeding) is passed on by recessive inheritance and almost always affects boys. The gene for hemophilia is carried on the male X chromosome, one of the two chromosomes that together determine the gender of a

▼ *DNA molecules in the cell nucleus make up the chromosomes, which are divided into genes: the blueprint of each human. DNA has a backbone with groups of chemical bases (codons) along it. Each codon contains instructions such as "message starts here." To work, this information must move to the outer cytoplasm, so the instructions cause the DNA to split into two, the single bases forming two types of RNA: messenger (mRNA) and transfer (tRNA). Each tRNA picks up one of 20 amino acids (the building blocks of protein from which the body is made). A ribosome (cell translator) picks up messages from the mRNA, duplicates it, and ensures that the matching tRNA codon is translated.*

THE PROCESS FUNDAMENTAL TO LIFE—THE MAKING OF A PROTEIN

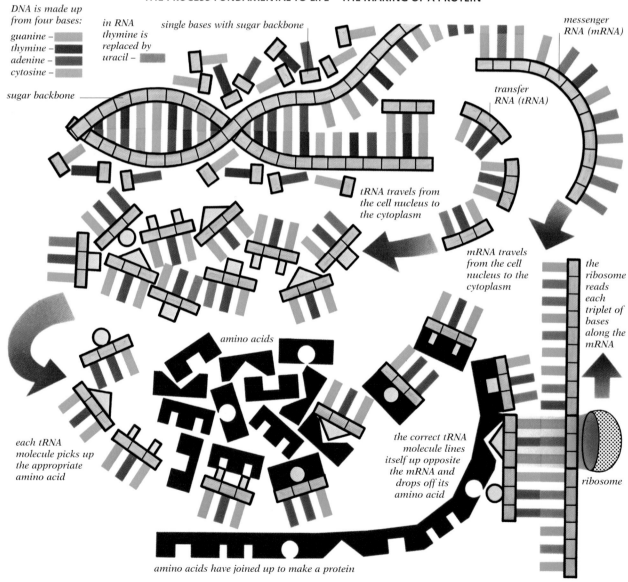

DNA is made up from four bases:

guanine –
thymine –
adenine –
cytosine –

in RNA thymine is replaced by uracil –

sugar backbone

single bases with sugar backbone

messenger RNA (mRNA)

transfer RNA (tRNA)

tRNA travels from the cell nucleus to the cytoplasm

mRNA travels from the cell nucleus to the cytoplasm

the ribosome reads each triplet of bases along the mRNA

each tRNA molecule picks up the appropriate amino acid

amino acids

the correct tRNA molecule lines itself up opposite the mRNA and drops off its amino acid

ribosome

amino acids have joined up to make a protein

Hints for a healthy baby

To give your child the best possible chance in life:

Try and have your children early rather than late in life.

Avoid taking drugs during pregnancy.

Do not smoke during pregnancy.

Avoid alcohol during pregnancy.

Consider amniocentesis if your doctor recommends having it. This is a test performed during pregnancy to check that the fetus is normal and healthy.

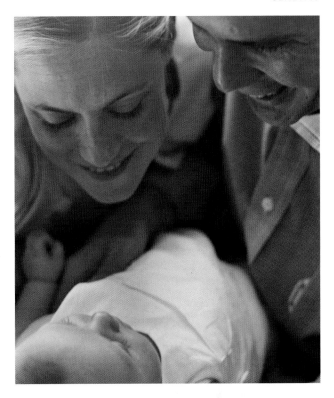

▲ *Genetic counseling can help an older mother and her partner to decide whether to risk having a baby.*

baby. If a woman has inherited an X chromosome with the hemophilia gene from her father, she will be a carrier of the condition. But it is extremely unlikely that she will inherit the gene-carrying chromosome from her mother, too, and so develop hemophilia. Females have two sex chromosomes, designated XX. Males have one X and one small Y chromosome. A female carrier, however, has the gene on half of her X chromosomes and so has a 50-50 chance of passing it to her sons, who will inherit an X from her and a Y chromosome from their father. A male who has inherited the gene from his mother is bound to develop hemophilia, because the Y chromosome cannot cancel out the gene.

Several other types of inherited diseases, including harelip, cleft palate, and some forms of allergy, are more common in boys than in girls. It is often hard to calculate the odds, because some genetic disorders result from a defect in more than one gene, or from the interaction of genes and other factors.

Estimating the odds

Genetic counseling uses a combination of knowledge about the family history of an inherited disorder and the disorder's general occurrence to make predictions.

To illustrate how a counselor can predict the likelihood of inheriting a disorder, consider the case of a normal daughter, Mary, who has an albino father. The chance that Mary will carry the albino gene is two in three. Mary's husband John has no family history of albinism. Therefore, given the frequency of the albino gene in the general population, the counselor knows that John's chance of carrying an albino gene is one in 70. Even if both Mary and John carry the albino gene, there is only a one-in-four chance that these genes will combine in any children they have.

All these possibilities are multiplied together: 2/3 x 1/70 x 1/4. The answer found is that Mary and John's risk of having an albino child is only one in 420. The genes responsible for albinism are recessive, so there is a three-in-four chance that two albino parents will have normal offspring.

Decision making and genetic counseling

Good genetic counseling involves more than mere statistics. The psychological as well as the medical needs of the patients or prospective parents must also be taken into account. The likelihood that a baby may be born with a genetic disease is only one factor in the parents' decision to go ahead with a pregnancy. Parents should not be afraid to express their fears to a genetic counselor, even if these fears later prove unfounded. They should not be alarmed by the questions the counselor will ask, which will explore their attitude toward such matters as contraception and abortion, as well as their feelings about the possible risks they are taking. The more the counselor knows about how the couple feel, the better able he or she will be to advise them.

Amniocentesis

If someone has a higher than average risk, one possible route is to opt for a test such as amniocentesis, which is carried out during pregnancy. A sample of the fluid in the uterus is removed and analyzed for genetic abnormalities. If the test shows that the fetus is abnormal, an abortion can be performed. Some women feel that abortion is morally wrong and may prefer not to risk having children in the first place. Amniocentesis is often recommended for older mothers because they have a greater risk of having a child with Down syndrome, but some women are uneasy about the idea of aborting a baby who has a good chance of survival. If a person is worried about passing on a hereditary disease, it is best for him or her to ask a doctor to recommend a suitable genetic counselor.

See also: **Birth defects; Hemophilia; Heredity; Personality**

Glucose

The human body is able to break down many kinds of food into glucose, which provides it with energy. As a result, people do not need the refined sugar and candies that are often part of their diet.

Every cell in the human body needs energy to stay alive, and glucose provides the basic fuel that the body burns. Glucose and fructose are the two most important examples of a group of sugar compounds found in various foods, including fruit (fructose) and milk (lactose). These compounds are all changed to glucose when absorbed into the body.

Ordinary white sugar is actually sucrose, which is glucose combined with fructose. Sucrose provides sweetness and supplies energy, but it has also been blamed for all kinds of physical ills.

The various sugars are all made from the same three chemical elements—carbon, hydrogen, and oxygen. The only difference between them is that the hydrogen and oxygen atoms are arranged on a carbon backbone in slightly different patterns. Therefore, the process of changing them into glucose is a fairly simple one. The chemical structure gives the name "carbohydrates" to all the foods that are based on sugar molecules.

Breaking down starch

One task of the digestive system is to break down starch-based carbohydrates, such as potatoes and bread, into individual sugar molecules. This process begins in the mouth, where the saliva contains a starch-splitting enzyme called amylase. More amylase is mixed with food when it has passed down through the stomach into the intestine. Amylase breaks the starch down into pairs of sugar molecules, which are then split by another series of enzymes in the small intestine so that only individual sugar molecules are absorbed. Finally, the sugars are all carried to the liver by the bloodstream. The liver changes fructose and other similar compounds into glucose.

How glucose produces energy

The body has many mechanisms that make sure there is an adequate level of glucose in the bloodstream to supply its needs. These mechanisms work by switching on or off the release of glucose that is stored in the liver. Glucose is stored as a compound called glycogen, which is a loose-knit mesh of glucose molecules. Glycogen is also stored in the muscles.

When glucose is released into the blood, it is taken in by the cells. A hormone called insulin is essential for this process. Insulin is produced by the pancreas from areas of tissue called the

▼ *Glucose is stored in the liver and the muscles until it is needed to produce energy.*

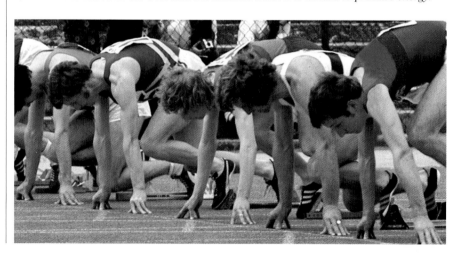

HOW THE BODY USES GLUCOSE

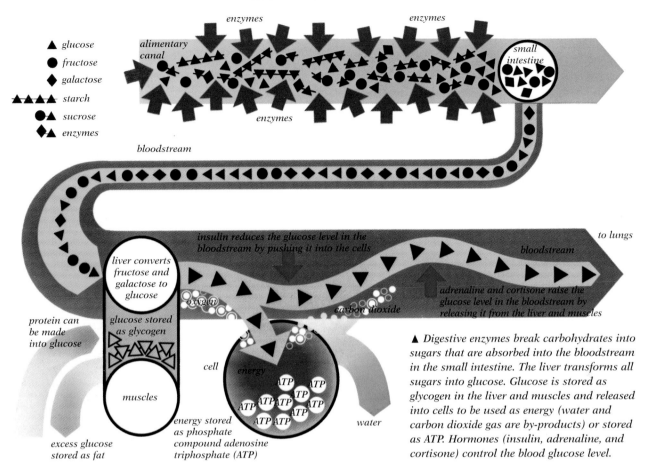

▲ *glucose*
● *fructose*
◆ *galactose*
▲▲▲▲ *starch*
●▲ *sucrose*
◆▲ *enzymes*

enzymes

alimentary canal

enzymes

small intestine

enzymes

bloodstream

insulin reduces the glucose level in the bloodstream by pushing it into the cells

to lungs

bloodstream

liver converts fructose and galactose to glucose

oxygen

carbon dioxide

adrenaline and cortisone raise the glucose level in the bloodstream by releasing it from the liver and muscles

protein can be made into glucose

glucose stored as glycogen

cell

energy

muscles

ATP ATP TP ATP ATP ATP ATP ATP ATP ATP

water

excess glucose stored as fat

energy stored as phosphate compound adenosine triphosphate (ATP)

▲ *Digestive enzymes break carbohydrates into sugars that are absorbed into the bloodstream in the small intestine. The liver transforms all sugars into glucose. Glucose is stored as glycogen in the liver and muscles and released into cells to be used as energy (water and carbon dioxide gas are by-products) or stored as ATP. Hormones (insulin, adrenaline, and cortisone) control the blood glucose level.*

islets of Langerhans. Unlike amylase, insulin is secreted into the blood, not into the intestine.

Inside the cells the glucose is burned with oxygen to produce energy plus two waste products—carbon dioxide gas and water. The carbon dioxide is carried in the blood to the lungs, where it is excreted into the air as a person breathes out. The water rejoins the rest of the water in the body.

The energy made by burning glucose is stored in each cell, where it is used to provide power for the chemical reactions on which the cell depends. The cells do this by creating high-energy phosphate compounds that are broken down to release the energy. These phosphate compounds (the most common has the chemical name adenosine triphosphate or ATP) are a little like a battery that can be used and recharged at will to supply small amounts of energy as they are needed. Burning glucose is equivalent to recharging it.

Emergency sources of energy

The stores of glucose-producing glycogen in the body are not very large. If they run down because an individual has not been eating enough—as happens when someone is on a diet or is fasting—the body will need to draw on other sources of energy.

The body has two alternative sources. It may start to convert protein, the main structural compound of the body, into glucose. Alternatively, it may start to burn fat in the tissues instead of glucose. The fat provides just as good a source of energy as glucose, but as it is burned it produces extra waste products, called ketones.

Control of glucose levels

The level of glucose in the blood needs to be kept within certain limits if a person is to stay healthy. Too high a level of blood glucose is a feature of diabetes, the condition caused by insulin deficiency. If the glucose level falls too low, the result is hypoglycemia—the brain can no longer function properly and the person loses consciousness.

The blood glucose level is kept constant by balancing the effects of various hormones. Insulin lowers the level of glucose in the blood by enabling cells to use it. It is counteracted by other hormones, all of which push blood glucose up by releasing glucose from the liver. The most important of these are adrenaline and cortisone. Growth hormone also increases the glucose in the blood.

Although increased blood sugar is a symptom that something is seriously wrong, a healthy person can cope with a short-term increase in glucose—for example, after eating a quantity of candy. However, eating too much sugar on a regular basis may be harmful and should be avoided.

See also: **Diabetes; Diet; Nutrition; Sugars**

Hamstring injuries

The hamstring muscles are at the backs of the thighs. Although these muscles are prone to injury, particularly in athletes, prompt treatment can restore them to health.

The hamstring muscles are a group of three muscles that form the back of the thigh (ham area). They span the thighbone and join the ischial part of the pelvis with the upper end of the tibia.

The purpose of the hamstring muscles is to bend the leg at the knee. They also help to tilt the trunk backward when a person is stooping, and the individual muscles help to twist the leg in or out by rotation of the knee. They are extremely important in walking and running, and they support the knee joint by acting as muscular braces at the back.

In medieval times, "hamstringing" a person (cutting the tendons of the muscles) was a barbaric punishment that left him or her lame for life.

Injuries

Hamstring injuries are common, especially among athletes, mainly because the muscles are very long and thin. When they contract, the shortening takes place over a relatively small area. A sudden contraction during stretching can cause damage, and a blow to the contracted muscle can bruise the hamstring muscles. A person can even injure the hamstring muscles by standing up suddenly from a half-bending or reaching position.

However, two main types of injury are the most common. The first type is a sheering blow to the contracted hamstring muscle, such as a person might get from a kick or a fall. This type of injury will bruise and tear an area of muscle.

The second type of injury occurs when an overstretched muscle contracts and tears, either because it has not been prepared for action by suitable warm-up exercises or because the muscle itself has become very tired.

These injuries usually take place in the body of the muscle, but sudden, unusual strain on an unprepared muscle can also tear part of the muscle from the bone. This could happen as a result of an apparently simple action, such as swinging a leg over a bicycle.

Symptoms

Sprinters and football players often get hamstring injuries because of the stretching effect of long strides. Injuries occur most commonly in the last quarter of the game when a player is tired. The first sign is often an aching pain in the back of the thigh. Continuing to play after the pain has begun causes further damage, and in many cases the muscle eventually goes into a cramplike spasm. In severe strains the pain is shooting and intense, and the leg starts to

HAMSTRING MUSCLES

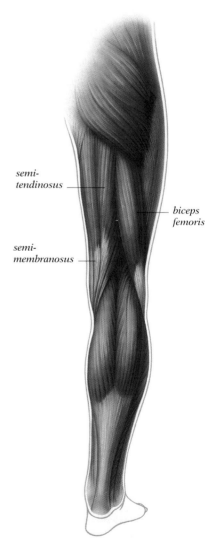

semi-
tendinosus

biceps
femoris

semi-
membranosus

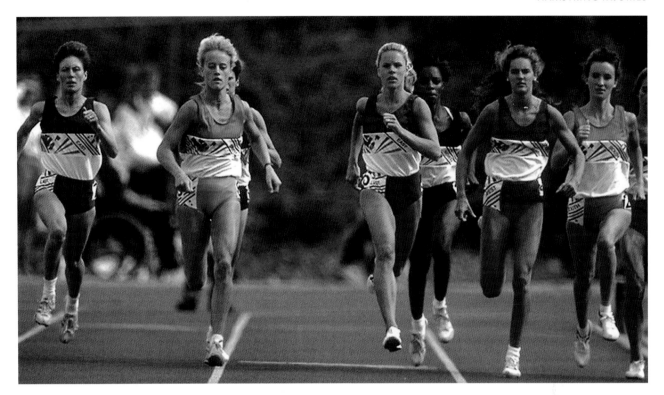

▲ *It is essential to warm up before running if the hamstrings are to be prevented from tearing or from other injury.*

cramp immediately. Bleeding into the muscle causes swelling, and the area becomes extremely tender.

Although it is often easy to recognize a hamstring injury, diagnosis becomes more difficult as the injury gets closer to the knee. Sometimes an injury in this area is actually an acute cartilage injury or a ruptured blood vessel. Even if a person is positive that he or she has a hamstring injury, it is still worth seeking medical advice.

Treatment

In a hamstring injury the muscle is usually torn and bruised and may be bleeding internally. Prompt treatment will shorten the recovery time dramatically.

There are a number of treatment stages. First, when injury occurs the person should stop putting strain on the leg immediately. It may be tempting to continue playing or running, but this will only make the damage worse. The injury should be bandaged with a compression bandage and the leg raised; this stops any bleeding. The bandage should then be removed and an ice pack applied for about 25 minutes. This reduces the swelling and inflammation. The patient should rest completely for 24 hours before the follow-up treatment.

The next stage of treatment is given by a physical therapist or a doctor. Hamstring injuries are sometimes treated by ultrasound—very high-frequency sound waves that provide micromassage. The unit consists of a box plugged into the electric supply and a head that looks a little like a microphone. The physical therapist places the head over the injured part, in close contact with the skin. The patient feels little or no sensation from the treatment, which is given for about 15 minutes a day or sometimes more often.

Heat and conventional massage also help to disperse blood clots and prevent fibrosis and internal scarring in the area. Another technique used by the physical therapist is passive stretching—moving the leg gradually and slowly straining it, thus allowing the muscle to go back to its original shape.

People with severe hamstring injuries need both crutches and painkillers, and these injuries can take from several weeks to three months to heal. The chances of recovery are excellent, and the patient should regain a complete range of pain-free movement.

Prevention

Adequate warming up before strenuous physical activity is essential if people are to avoid hamstring injuries. This means gradually putting the muscles through a range of stretching movements.

Before exercising, a person should first stretch gently, without bouncing or straining. It does not matter if he or she is unable to touch the toes, for example. The important thing is to stretch the muscles. Next, the person should gradually increase the speed of his or her activity. After two or three minutes of stretching, the body will be fully warmed up and the hamstring muscles should be protected against injury.

While playing or running, athletes should try to avoid becoming unduly tired because fatigue increases the risk of hamstring injuries. If a slight pain develops at the back of the knee, the athlete should come off the field and try a gentle massage or put on a support bandage. He or she should repeat the warm-up exercises. If the pain continues, the athlete should stop playing and seek medical treatment.

See also: **Bruises; Cramp; Exercise; Physical therapy; Sports medicine; Sprains**

Hay fever

Hay fever results from an allergy to inhaled dusts, the most common of which is grass pollen. About 10 percent of the population in the Western world is affected. There is no complete cure for this unpleasant affliction, but the symptoms can be relieved.

Questions and Answers

I am a hay fever sufferer and so is my husband. Will our children inherit the condition?

People with hay fever have an underlying genetic state called atopy. Such people are more likely to develop asthma, eczema, or hay fever. Look out for these conditions in your children.

I am severely affected by hay fever. What can I do to prevent an attack during exams this summer?

To avoid hay fever for a short time when ordinary treatments do not control the symptoms, some doctors will give a small dose of steroids by injection. Ask your doctor's advice.

My pills for hay fever make me feel very sleepy all the time. Is there something else I could take?

Most of the early antihistamine drugs caused drowsiness, but you can ask your doctor to prescribe one of the many nonsedating antihistamines now available.

Why is the pollen count important to hay fever sufferers?

If you are pollen-sensitive your symptoms will be worse if the pollen count is high. This usually occurs after a hot, dry spell, when there is little wind. The pollen count is usually low after a heavy rainstorm or thundershower.

I am 17 and I've had hay fever for several years. Will I grow out of it, or will I always suffer from it?

It is hard to say. It is very common for young people with all types of allergies to get better as they pass through their teens and early adult life. However, occasionally the symptoms may return later. The reason for this is not known.

Hay fever is misnamed; it is not caused by hay and it does not include fever among its symptoms. Instead there is profuse watery discharge from the nose and eyes, as well as irritation and sneezing. The correct name is seasonal allergic rhinitis (rhinitis is inflammation of the nose lining). The parts of the body that are affected by hay fever are those most commonly exposed to allergy-causing dusts: the eyes, the nose, the sinuses, and the upper part of the throat.

Causes

While the most common cause of hay fever is an allergy to grass or tree pollens, identical symptoms may result from inhaling other dusts, such as fungal spores, animal hair and scurf (skin particles), and house mite droppings.

When hay fever symptoms are seasonal, the timing of their appearance depends on the sort of dust that causes an allergic reaction in the sufferer. The first pollens to appear each year are tree pollens, which can cause hay fever in early spring, depending on how severe the winter has been. Pollen from trees is a powerful allergen (a substance that causes allergic reactions) and frequently causes hay fever. Later in the season, typically in midsummer, grass pollens appear for a short season; they are then followed by ragweed pollen.

Fungal spores are abundant in the air from midsummer until late fall. They are the most likely allergens in the fall. Other agents that are present in the air throughout the year may also cause problems from time to time and seem to result in seasonal symptoms.

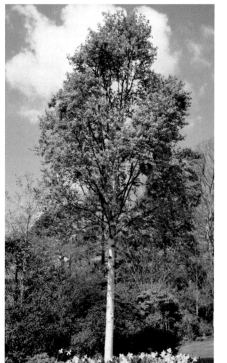

How hay fever develops

Hay fever develops because of an error in the body's own defense mechanism, the immune system. Normally, the immune system can distinguish between a harmless organism, such as pollen, and a dangerous infectious organism. In an allergic person, however, the immune system treats pollens and other allergens as if they were dangerous, and the white blood cells, whose function it is to fight infection, start forming an antibody to neutralize the intruder.

The antibody attaches itself to cells, named mast cells, which contain a number of chemicals; the most important is histamine. The antibody tries to neutralize the allergen, and in so doing upsets the structure of the mast cell, which disintegrates and releases the histamine and other chemicals. Some people, called atopic individuals, make a large quantity of antibodies to these common

◄ *Some tree pollens, such as silver birch pollen, are powerful allergens and can cause hay fever early in the spring in some people.*

dusts, and they tend to develop childhood eczema and asthma in addition to hay fever. The condition tends to run in families.

Symptoms

The release of histamine and other chemicals from the mast cells causes the blood vessels to increase in diameter, and the mucous cells in both the nose and the sinuses begin to generate more mucus. As a result, the eyes itch and run, and the nose and sinuses become blocked and cause feelings of stuffiness and heaviness in the head. The throat becomes sore, and the sufferer feels generally unwell.

Sneezing is very common first thing in the morning; the sufferer may sneeze repeatedly between getting up and eating breakfast. If asthma is associated with hay fever, the sufferer usually suffers the worst symptoms at night.

Treatments

By far the best way to reduce allergic rhinitis is to avoid the cause of the allergy. If the cause is a family pet, the pet should be groomed regularly and kept in its own quarters. House dust and mites are more difficult to avoid, but a person can wear a mask while cleaning. Carpets and bedding should be vacuumed frequently.

It is impossible to stay completely away from tree and grass pollens. However, an air conditioner may help prevent pollen from entering a home; and vacations can be taken by the sea, where there are fewer pollen-producing plants around. If it is impossible to avoid allergens completely, there are three possible methods of treatment available to hay fever sufferers.

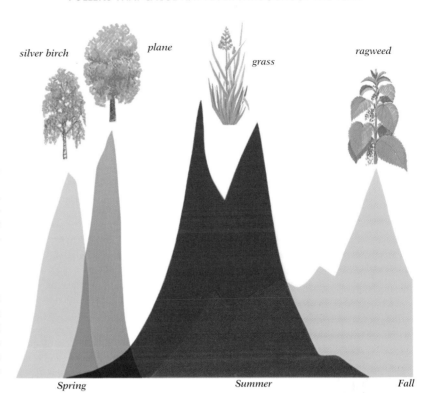

POLLENS THAT CAUSE HAY FEVER THROUGHOUT THE YEAR

silver birch *plane* *grass* *ragweed*

Spring *Summer* *Fall*

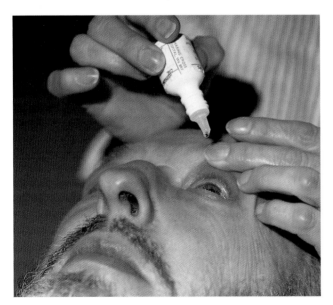

▲ *Eyedrops given three times a day help prevent the release of histamine, which causes watery eyes and a running nose.*

Local treatment

Medicines may be sprayed in the nose or inhaled, or eyedrops can be applied to the eyes. A solution of sodium cromogycate is made up to treat the eyes and nose. This prevents the mast cells from releasing histamine. It usually has to be taken three times a day throughout the hay fever season. Alternatively, an inhaler that supplies a very low dose of steroids can be used in the nose only. Both these medicines stop the symptoms from developing but offer little relief once symptoms have developed.

General treatment

Antihistamines may be of some help in hay fever, but many cause sleepiness, which some people find inconvenient. However, there are plenty of effective antihistamines that do not cause drowsiness. Steroid injections bring relief, but because of their side effects they are not used unless the symptoms are really incapacitating.

Desensitizing injections

A course of desensitization treatment is given as a set of injections early in the year. The vaccine may be tailored to fit the particular patient's allergy, but the only really effective vaccine is against grass pollen. If the vaccine gives good protection, the course can be repeated year after year.

It is not effective for everybody, however, and allergic reactions to the vaccine may occur. The vaccine contains a minute dose of pollen, so the doctor may ask the patient to wait for 15 or 20 minutes after an injection to ensure that no allergic reaction occurs.

See also: Allergies

157

Headache

Questions and Answers

I get bad headaches a week before my period starts. Is there any preventive treatment I could take?

Premenstrual headaches are common, but their cause is not fully understood. Some doctors believe they are caused by excess fluid stored in the body before a period starts. Others believe they are the effect of hormone levels. Sometimes a diuretic drug (which removes the excess fluid from your body) will help relieve this type of headache, and your doctor may advise you to try one.

My father had a terrible headache when he was on vacation last year, and recently he had another attack. Should he see a doctor?

A really bad headache in someone who does not usually suffer from headaches can be a serious sign of trouble inside the skull. The other more likely possibility is that he is getting migraines. He should certainly see a doctor; a simple examination can determine the cause of the headaches.

My baby boy is very anxious and cries a lot. Is there a way to tell if he is suffering from a headache?

Tiny babies cannot give a clear indication of where their pain is. The usual telltale sign is fretful crying that doesn't stop even when the baby is lifted up and cuddled. Unless there is an obvious and safe explanation, any baby who cries continually should be seen by a doctor.

Doctors routinely look down the throats and in the ears of babies to check for infection, because middle ear infections are a common cause of headaches and pains in children.

Symptoms described by older children can be unreliable because many children have not yet figured out their own anatomy. Therefore a headache can mean anything from a toothache to a stomachache.

A headache is a common symptom of a variety of conditions. How can a person tell what sort of a headache he or she is suffering from, and what should be done to relieve it?

Every person experiences headaches at some time or other, and all home medicine chests contain mild painkillers. Simple factors such as excessive noise at a concert, or a chronic cough, lack of sleep, or tension can cause a headache in an otherwise healthy person.

A headache is also a common symptom of more serious conditions, such as nose, throat, and ear infections; high blood pressure; damaged blood vessels; or a brain tumor. If a headache persists, recurs, is very severe, or is accompanied by other symptoms, the sufferer should see a doctor.

Common causes

The brain itself cannot feel pain, but the tiny nerve endings near the arteries and veins that supply the brain and scalp are very sensitive to changes of pressure. All sorts of conditions, such as tension and fatigue, can affect the pressure and result in a headache, but exactly why it happens is not known. The sensation of pain is also transmitted to the brain by substances called prostaglandins from nerve endings in the skin, the eyes, the ears, and the nose.

The most common cause of recurrent headaches is tension in the scalp muscles. The headaches are usually mild and clear up quickly with the help of ibuprofen, an anti inflammatory drug, or painkillers such as aspirin and acetaminophen. Aspirin should not be given to children under 12, however, because of the risk of Reye's syndrome, which is often fatal.

Migraine: This is an intense type of headache that is caused when the blood vessels on one side of the brain contract and then dilate. Some people are far more susceptible than others to this type of headache, and all sorts of things can trigger an attack. The headache is usually preceded by a severe feeling of nausea and there may be a 20-minute period in which there is loss of vision in an expanding area of the fields of vision of both eyes. This area has a scintillating margin.

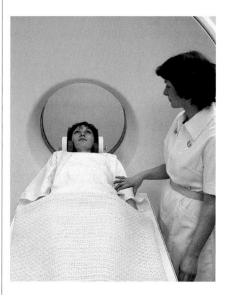

▲ *A magnetic resonance imaging (MRI) scan linked to a computer produces pictures of areas within the brain, and can indicate any abnormal areas that might be causing headaches.*

Sinuses and teeth: An inflammation in either or both of these locations can cause headaches as well as produce tender areas at the site of the trouble.

Faulty eyesight: This is a common cause of headaches that occur in the region of the brow, especially after close work such as sewing. They may be accompanied by a feeling of grittiness in the eye.

Poisons: Headaches with high temperatures are usually caused by the toxic (poisonous) products made by viruses. Other toxic substances can also cause headaches. Alcohol and tobacco in excess may lead to a headache. Foul air from gasoline fumes, lead poisoning, carbon monoxide poisoning, and lack of ventilation all cause chronic, mild headaches. Even stomach upsets can result in headaches.

Neuralgia: This is a pain that originates in a nerve. When it happens in nerves supplying the head or face, a headache is acute and may be set off by the touch of a brush or comb.

More serious cases

Brain tumors can cause persistent headaches, usually accompanied by other symptoms such

Common causes of headaches and their treatment

CAUSE	SYMPTOMS	TREATMENT
Tension	Recurrent, intermittent headache, moderately severe, mostly at the front of the head	Headache relieved if patient relaxes. May benefit from tranquilizers.
Migraine	Throbbing headache starting often from one eye, sometimes spreading to both sides. Occasional numbness and tingling on one side or temporary loss of vision in an area with a sparkling edge. Often with nausea or vomiting.	See your doctor to make sure there is no serious medical condition. Take antimigraine drugs. Avoid triggers that cause migraine, such as noise, tension, and certain foods.
Sinusitis	Dull, severe headache at the front of the face. May be puslike nasal discharge. Pain worse in cold weather and on bending down.	Decongestant drugs such as ephedrine. Antibiotics in persistent cases. Sinus wash and drainage may be necessary in chronic cases.
High blood pressure (hypertension)	Throbbing, recurrent headaches, often worse in mornings and on stooping. Front of head or temples usually affected. Often accompanied by giddiness.	Urgent medical attention required. Treatment with drugs to bring down and control blood pressure. Drugs will probably need to be taken indefinitely.
Fever	Any fever will produce a headache. It is often severe.	Treatment will be given for the cause of the fever. Aspirin for those over 12.
Neuralgia (pain in a nerve)	Extremely painful, sharp, shooting pains, usually in the upper head or face	Drugs can control neuralgia in the majority of cases
Eyestrain	Moderate or severe headache behind or above one or both eyes	An eye test will show whether the patient needs to wear glasses

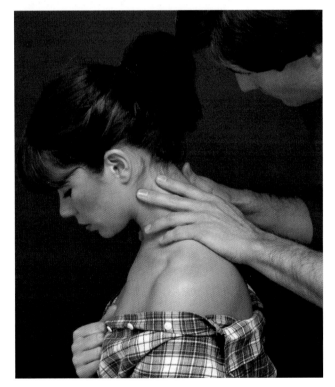

▲ *Tension headaches are often worse at the end of the day. A massage of the neck muscles is one way of relieving the headache by helping the sufferer to relax.*

as vomiting. Careful investigation is needed to locate the tumor's source and plan treatment.

High blood pressure does not cause headaches unless it reaches a dangerous stage at which there is a risk of a major stroke, and urgent medical attention is required if life is to be saved. With proper checks of the blood pressure this stage should never be reached.

Meningitis is an inflammation of the meninges, the tissue layers covering the brain and spinal cord, and separating them from their bony casing. The patient develops a severe headache, a stiff neck, and a dislike of light (photophobia). Treatment is usually by means of drugs for bacterial infections and rest.

If blood vessels supplying the brain are damaged from an accident, blood may leak into the space between the skull and the brain tissue, causing a blood clot. A severe headache may be the first sign of this. The condition may correct itself, or surgery may be required.

Diagnosis and treatment

The exact site and nature of the pain help trace its cause, so the patient should tell the doctor as much as possible about when the headache started, how it developed, and the frequency and duration of attacks. The doctor will usually examine the eyes and take the patient's blood pressure. If the diagnosis is still in doubt, the patient may go to a neurologist for a CT scan—a series of X rays that produce a computerized picture of the brain.

Acetaminophen or aspirin usually cures headache by reducing the production of the prostaglandins, which transmit pain. Treatment for other headaches depends on the cause; most can be cured.

See also: **Aspirin and analgesics; Fevers; Poisoning**

Heart attack

Questions and Answers

Is there anything I can do to prevent a heart attack in later life?

One thing that will definitely reduce the risk if you are a smoker is to stop smoking. Smoking significantly accelerates the pace of atherosclerosis (hardening and thickening of the artery walls), which is the cause of coronary artery disease, and it is thus a main factor in heart attacks. There is also strong evidence that if you eat less of the foods that contain saturated fats, you can reduce the risk that your coronary arteries will become narrowed by cholesterol deposits. Exercise in the form of running, cycling, and swimming may also help, but you should check with your doctor before you undertake very strenuous aerobic exercise such as jogging or uphill cycling.

I have recently had a heart attack. Will I be able to go back to the active and enjoyable sex life that I used to have before the attack?

Yes, you will. However, you should not engage in very strenuous activity immediately. Your doctor or the hospital will give you guidelines about exertion when you leave the hospital. It is usual to suggest to people that they should build up to their previous level of activity over a period of about four to six weeks.

My father, who has always been very active, has just had a heart attack. Does this mean that he will have to slow down now?

Not necessarily, unless he has been told to do so by his doctor. Your father should avoid sudden bursts of activity, however, and build up to any exertion more gradually than he did before, in the way that professional athletes do. He should be particularly careful in cold weather—keeping warm and gradually warming up for physical activity at his normal level.

A heart attack is the most common serious illness in the developed world. Many patients make an excellent recovery, but leading a healthy life in the first place can prevent some heart attacks.

The heart is a muscular bag that acts as a pump to maintain the circulation of the blood to all parts of the body. It consists mainly of a special type of muscle that contracts rhythmically and continuously throughout life. When the blood supply to this vital organ is obstructed, the heart cannot work properly and the result is a heart attack.

The normal action of the heart

The heart contains a four-valve system that ensures that blood is directed through the lungs (where it picks up oxygen) and then distributed through the arteries to all other parts of the body, including the brain, muscles, liver, and intestines (where it picks up essential fuel and bodybuilding materials). Blood depleted of oxygen and fuel returns from all these parts to the heart by way of the veins.

Because the heart muscle works constantly, it consumes a lot of energy and requires an uninterrupted supply of glucose and oxygen. This is provided by the coronary arteries—the first two branches of the main artery (the

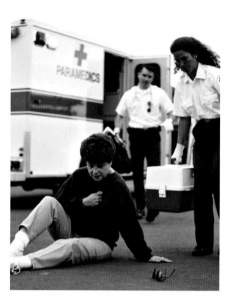

▲ *A woman suffering from a suspected heart attack is attended by paramedics before they transport her to the hospital.*

aorta) that emerge from the heart. The coronary arteries branch repeatedly and spread over the surface of the heart like a crown; thus the name coronary, from the Latin *corona*, or "crown." The left coronary artery branches into two almost immediately, so for all practical purposes doctors often consider that there are three coronary arteries. A large quantity of blood passes through these vital arteries and returns to the circulation through veins that open into one of the chambers on the right side of the heart. This blood carries glucose and oxygen to all parts of the constantly moving heart muscle so that it can continue to contract (beat) 60 to 80 times a minute.

What can go wrong

The coronary arteries are particularly susceptible to the dangerous and very common disease atherosclerosis, often described as the number one killer in the Western world. In atherosclerosis the artery lining develops local deposits of raised areas of deteriorated tissue, cholesterol, and other fats called atheromatous plaques, or atheroma, which narrow the arteries. They do not directly cause heart attacks but may limit the amount of work the heart can do. If the heart pump has to work harder than its fuel supply will allow during physical exertion, substances accumulate in the muscle that cause the pain of angina pectoris (a crushing, suffocating pain in the chest).

Blood will not clot within a healthy artery, because the normal lining is smooth and does not encourage stickiness. However, if the lining has been roughened by atheroma and the blood is able to come into contact with tissue material in the plaque, it may produce the series of biochemical events through which blood forms a clot. Such a clot that forms on top of an atheromatous plaque is called a coronary thrombosis. It will narrow the artery further and may block it altogether. In this case the part of the heart muscle supplied by the artery or arterial branch will be completely deprived of its blood supply. The significance of such an event depends on the size of the artery that has been blocked. If it is a small peripheral branch, only a small part of the heart muscle will be affected, and recovery is likely. If it is a whole artery or one of the major branches, however, so much muscle volume is involved that the whole heart may be unable to continue to contract and death will occur rapidly.

About half of all people who die from a coronary occlusion (obstruction) do so within three or four hours, and if a large artery is involved death may occur immediately.

A heart attack is a continuous process. Interruption of the blood supply is the first stage. As the blood supply to the heart muscle (myocardial cells) is stopped, the patient feels pain. The affected cells die; and if the blood supply is not restored, that area of muscle will die and be replaced over some weeks with fibrous scar tissue. This can weaken the heart if a large area of muscle has been affected.

The people most at risk from a heart attack are smokers, people who eat a lot of fat, people under stress, diabetics, and those with a

family history of heart attacks. Heart attacks occur most often in middle-aged men. They are unusual in women before menopause and in men under 35.

Warning signs

Sometimes the first heart attack is totally unexpected, but often there is a warning sign—the development of angina. Angina is a pain in the central chest that occurs during exertion or excitement and lasts a few minutes. Often the pain spreads to the arms, shoulders, and neck. Anyone who develops angina or who has attacks that are increasing in frequency or in length should see a doctor.

Symptoms of an attack

Symptoms of a heart attack are more severe than those of angina. Angina pain always settles quickly when the patient rests, but symptoms of a heart attack continue for at least half an hour. The main symptoms are:

- severe pain or sense of pressure in the center of the chest, often spreading through to the back, up into the neck, or down either arm
- physical collapse
- sweating
- a terrifying conviction that one is going to die
- extreme restlessness
- nausea and sometimes vomiting
- sometimes shortness of breath
- weak, irregular pulse, and sometimes a very slow pulse.

HOW ARTERIES BECOME BLOCKED

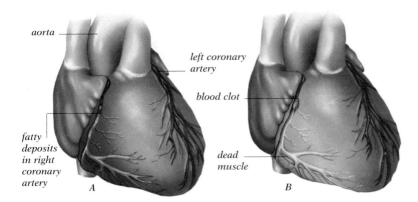

aorta

left coronary artery

blood clot

fatty deposits in right coronary artery

dead muscle

A

B

▲ A: Fatty deposits have caused a partial blockage, restricting blood flow. B: A blood clot (thrombosis) has now caused a total blockage in the narrowed artery, cutting blood supply to some of the heart muscle so that an area of muscle dies.

▲ Gentle exercise helps victims of heart attacks to build up slowly to the normal level of physical activity that they enjoyed before the attack.

What to do if someone has a heart attack

Phone the patient's doctor, who will either come to you or have you call 911. If you cannot reach the doctor, call 911 immediately.

The patient should rest, either sitting in a chair or lying down. He or she should not walk around.

Give the patient an aspirin tablet. If the patient regularly suffers from angina and takes nitroglycerin tablets, it is also worth having him or her take one of these tablets to see if it brings relief.

Stay with the patient until the emergency services arrive. If the patient becomes unconscious with loss of pulse and of breathing, mouth-to-mouth resuscitation and cardiac massage should be given. Continue until medical help arrives.

Caution: Do not try resuscitation or massage without first consulting a doctor, unless you are trained to do so.

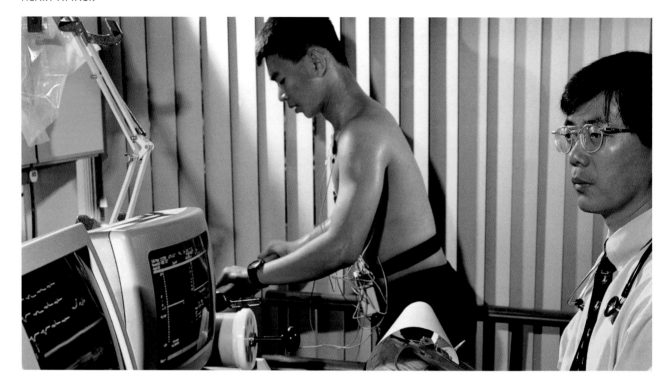

▲ *The doctor watches an ECG machine that is monitoring a patient's heartbeat to check the effects of physical exertion on his heart after his recovery from a recent heart attack.*

It is not widely understood that severe pain is not necessarily a feature of a heart attack. In some cases pain is absent. Because of this up to 20 percent of mild coronaries are not recognized as such. They may be mistaken for heartburn, gallbladder problems, or indigestion. Repeated "silent" coronary attacks can progressively damage the heart and may eventually lead to heart failure.

Because of the risk of sudden death, a person with a coronary thrombosis should be taken to the hospital immediately. Never delay on the assumption that it might be a minor upset, such as a chest infection or indigestion. Many people who could be saved die because no one realizes that their condition is life-threatening. Emergency treatment with drugs to dissolve the blood clot can save a life.

A small dose of aspirin may be valuable, because this can prevent a clot that has begun to form from developing further. Many men who are at risk of coronary heart disease take a small dose of aspirin every day as a precautionary routine, but this should never be done without consulting a doctor.

A person who suffers from an attack of pain that he or she thinks might be a heart attack should see a doctor but should not be too alarmed, since some other conditions have similar symptoms, such as indigestion, chest infection, gallbladder problems, or the washing back of the acid contents of the stomach into the esophagus.

Diagnosis and treatment

Most cases of heart attacks are clearly diagnosed from the patient's appearance, an electrocardiogram (ECG) that shows the characteristic electrical changes in the heart, and the level of cardiac enzymes in the blood. These enzymes are chemical substances released from the heart muscle as it dies.

The priority for any doctor treating a patient who has had a heart attack is to relieve the pain. This is normally done with an injection of morphine, which is repeated when necessary.

The next priority is to prevent complications. The first two and a half hours after the onset of a heart attack are critical because half of all deaths owing to heart attacks occur then. These are caused by severe disturbances of the heart rhythm, which may become very slow or irregular. Drugs are used to treat these problems, but it is important to get the patient to a hospital as soon as possible so that the required treatment may be given at the earliest opportunity.

Coronary care units and rehabilitation

Once in the hospital, the patient is admitted to the coronary care unit, where special equipment is used to monitor the heart rhythm until the condition stabilizes. Drugs may also be given to improve the circulation and to limit the extent of damage to the heart muscle. Periodic checks on the level of heart enzymes in the blood are also carried out.

In some countries low-risk patients are managed at home by their family physician, but this approach is rarely taken in the United States.

Patients admitted to a coronary care unit will probably spend a day or two there receiving specialist treatment before they are transferred to a general ward. They are not usually kept in bed for longer than a few days, and if there are no complications, they will be sent home in about a week.

Patients should build up to their normal level of activity gradually. In a few cases there may be severe damage to the heart muscle; these patients usually take a little longer to recover full physical activity.

See also: Aspirin and analgesics; Exercise; Fats; Glucose; Heart disease; Pain; Stroke

Heart disease

Heart disease is very common and may result from a number of causes. However, advances in the techniques of investigation, treatment, and heart surgery have done a great deal to help sufferers.

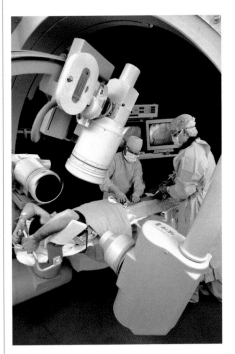

▲ *Cardiac catheterization involves passing tubes into the patient's heart through the arteries or veins. It is often carried out to evaluate heart disease.*

The heart is vital to life and must work continuously; hence it is very prone to a number of diseases. The majority of people with heart problems suffer the arterial disease atherosclerosis, but there are also other types of heart disease.

The heart valves

The heart depends on four valves to keep blood flowing in the right direction. Diseases of the valves used to be common, often occurring as a result of rheumatic fever in children. However, valve disease has become less common because of improvements in standards of living and hygiene.

Most valve problems arise from abnormalities in structure that have been present since birth. The inlet and outlet valves (mitral and aortic valves) of the left ventricle, the main pumping chamber of the heart, cause the most trouble.

There are two things that may go wrong with a valve. It may become permanently narrowed and impede the forward flow of the blood, a condition that is called stenosis; or it may leak and allow backward flow, a condition that is called regurgitation or incompetence. Stenosis and incompetence often occur together.

Usually people with minor abnormalities of the heart valves have no problems. However, there is a small risk of suffering from a condition known as infective endocarditis.

This happens when an infecting bacterium becomes lodged on the valves and starts to grow there, usually after rheumatic fever or some other febrile (fever-causing) disease. The heart valves are actually made of fibrous tissue with no blood supply of their own, so the organism finds it easy to become established in them. The body's defense system is also less effective, because the valves have no blood supply to provide infection-fighting white blood cells.

Congenital heart disease

The reason the heart is so prone to structural abnormalities is that its development in the womb is very complicated. During the early weeks of pregnancy, it evolves in the fetus from a single, straight tube into a four-chambered pump with two separate circulation systems. This is a complex process that can occasionally go wrong.

Sometimes a baby is born with holes in the partition between the two atria or the two ventricles of its heart. These are called atrial and ventricular septal defects. If the blood flow to the lungs is insufficient, the blood never becomes enriched with oxygen, and the result is a condition called cyanosis, "cyan" referring to the blue-green color of the baby's skin. Modern heart surgery has advanced so much in recent years that it is now standard practice to operate on tiny babies suffering from this condition.

Treatment of heart diseases

DISEASE/PROBLEM	CAUSES	SYMPTOMS	TREATMENT
Coronary artery disease	Results from hardening or blocking of the coronary arteries with atheroma (fatty deposits).	Angina pain. May cause a heart attack and heart failure.	Treatment is with drugs or by surgery to improve the heart's blood supply and end the pain. Diuretics remove excess fluid from lungs and tissues.
Heart failure	May result from almost any form of heart disease.	Breathlessness on exertion due to fluid in the lungs. Swelling of the ankles.	May be treated with diuretics or with drugs to increase the strength of the heartbeat.
Valve disease	Sometimes caused by rheumatic fever. May be congenital (present from birth).	The symptoms of heart failure. Aortic valve problems often cause angina because heart wall thickens. Fainting can also occur with aortic stenosis (blocked outlet valve) when there is insufficient blood in the circulation. Mitral (inlet) valve problems usually cause palpitations.	When the symptoms are sufficiently bad, treatment is surgical widening with a finger or valve replacement. Otherwise, drugs are used to control the symptoms. An operation is often necessary for marked aortic stenosis.
Cardiomyopathy (a) congestive	In most cases the cause is not known; occasionally, alcohol, metal poisoning, and hormonal conditions are the cause.	Heart failure, problems with heart block (slow heartbeat), and possibly palpitations. Valves may become leaky.	Symptoms are treated with drugs; sometimes a pacemaker is necessary.
(b) hypertrophic	Cause unknown; may run in families.	Angina and occasionally fainting attacks due to obstruction of left ventricle's outflow.	Drugs may relieve the obstruction; occasionally an operation may be necessary.
Endocarditis	Always happens as a result of preexisting heart problem, usually an abnormal valve. Wall of the heart becomes infected and lesioned.	Fever, heart failure, and general ill health.	Antibiotics. Badly damaged valves may need surgery.
Palpitations	(a) In normal hearts may be caused by anxiety and by overactivity of the thyroid gland. (b) There may be abnormalities in heart structure. (c) May occur after heart attacks.	In most cases there is a sense that the heart is stopping momentarily (extrasystoles). Sensation of rapid heartbeat with dizziness or fainting if insufficient blood reaches the brain.	Drugs are used to suppress the abnormal heart rhythm.
Heart block (very slow heartbeat)	(a) A degenerative disease of the heart. (b) May be complication of heart attack.	Dizziness and fainting.	Pacemaker.

Inadequate pumping

Sometimes there are problems if the force of the pumping is inadequate, because the power of the muscular walls of the left ventricle starts to fail. The usual reason for this is coronary artery disease, when there is an insufficient blood supply to the heart itself.

Cardiomyopathy

Congestive cardiomyopathy is a heart muscle disease that causes the muscle to become weak and flabby so that the heart grows larger and larger as the muscle wall dilates under the strain. In most cases the cause of congestive cardiomyopathy is not known. Occasionally the heart muscle thickens and obstructs the flow of blood out of the left ventricle. Called hypertrophic cardiomyopathy, this condition is one of the few heart diseases that run in families.

Heart rhythm disorders

The electrical conducting system of the heart is responsible for making sure that each part contracts in its proper sequence. There are three classes of rhythm disorders: (1) the heart may beat irregularly, or it may beat (2) too quickly or (3) too slowly.

Any of these disorders may cause dizziness and even loss of consciousness because of an inadequate supply of blood to the brain. With a slow heartbeat, called a heart block, the heart beats so slowly that not much of the blood flows forward. When the

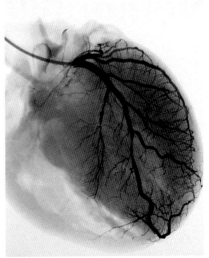

▲ *In a coronary angiogram (above) dye is injected into the bloodstream so that any narrowing of the arteries can be seen on an X ray.*

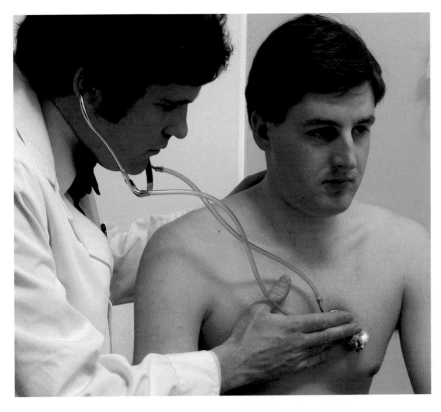

◄ *The doctor (left) is listening to heart sounds to detect any murmurs.*

heart is beating very fast, it does not have time to fill properly between beats. As before, the result is a much reduced rate of blood flow.

When the dizziness and fainting are due to fast rather than slow beating, there are often palpitations—an uncomfortable sensation of the heart beating. Heart rhythm disorders can happen as a result of other heart diseases, or they may occur on their own.

Diagnosis of rhythm disorders

An ECG (electrocardiogram) can diagnose the cause of symptoms. An advance in this field is the 24-hour ECG recording, which uses a small tape recorder (Holter machine) that the patient wears for a day. The results are then analyzed on a machine that speeds up the playback by about 60 times. Newer advances include electrophysiological studies that use tiny electrodes on the heart to measure its current.

Abnormal heart rhythms can sometimes be treated by electrical destruction (ablation) of the areas of muscle where the defects arise. Slow heart rates are treated with pacemakers and fast rates are treated with drugs.

Symptoms of heart disease

Heart disease causes pain (angina) when the heart is starved of oxygen (although indigestion can also produce angina-like pain). The other main symptom is heart (cardiac) failure. When the left ventricle fails to pump blood adequately, fluid accumulates in the lungs. This can cause breathlessness, particularly during exercise.

Chronic (long-term) heart failure usually involves both ventricles so that there is fluid in the tissues as well as in the lungs. This causes swelling of the ankles. The treatment for edema includes diuretics,

drugs that cause much of the excess fluid to be excreted through the kidneys, thus reducing the swelling.

Diagnosis and further tests

Fluid on the lungs can be heard through a stethoscope as crackling with each breath, and fluid around the ankles is obvious because of the uncomfortable swelling it causes. However, the key to diagnosis is examination of the heart itself. The doctor will feel the patient's pulse for irregularities and measure its rate; he or she will also feel the chest wall. The heart becomes enlarged before heart failure, and its beat becomes unduly forceful if the wall of the ventricle is thicker than normal; this can be felt through the chest wall.

The doctor also listens to the sounds of the valve closing during different phases of the heartbeat, and for murmurs. Murmurs are caused by the turbulent flow of blood through the heart. If a valve is obstructed or leaking, it will cause a murmur.

Further investigations may include an ECG and a chest X ray. Alternatively, a test may be performed using an echocardiogram, which uses sound waves, or ultrasound, to build a picture of the heart valves and detect any potential problems.

An examination may also be carried out using cardiac catheterization. This is an X-ray procedure where tubes (catheters) are passed into the heart through the arteries or veins. The tubes measure the pressure and blood gases in the heart chambers. X-ray dye may be injected into the tube to outline one of the heart's chambers and reveal any abnormalities.

Catheterization can help evaluate heart disease, is used in the diagnosis of coronary artery disease, and must be done before surgery.

> *See also:* **Heart attack; X rays**

Hemophilia

Hemophilia is a hereditary disease in which the blood fails to clot, and so bleeding cannot be stopped without medical attention. Sufferers can lead a normal life provided that they are vigilant.

Hemophilia is an inherited disease in which one of the essential factors needed to make blood coagulate is missing. As a result, bleeding fails to stop when a blood vessel has been damaged, sometimes because of a slight injury or, with internal bleeding, without any obvious cause. Hemophilia mainly affects males and is known for its prevalence among some royal families.

Cause

Hemophilia is caused by an abnormal gene. Genes are inherited and carry information that determines a person's physical makeup. In this case the gene is part of the X chromosome that is the female sex chromosome carried by men. The X chromosome contains thousands of genes, one of which should ordinarily make a blood-clotting factor called factor VIII. The lack of this factor causes hemophilia A; the lack of factor IX causes hemophilia B.

Blood clotting is a complicated series of chemical reactions that run in a chain involving a domino effect. The reaction starts with a special factor in the blood called the Hageman factor,

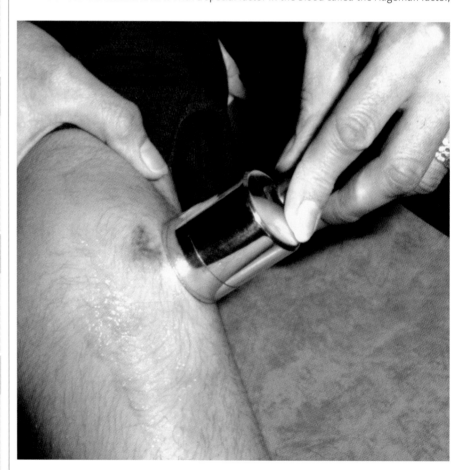

▲ *A hemophiliac receives ultrasound therapy to disperse fluid buildup after suffering bleeding into the knee joint.*

TRANSMISSION OF HEMOPHILIA

▼ *By a carrier mother*

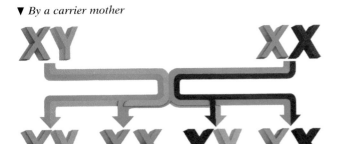

▼ *By a hemophiliac father*

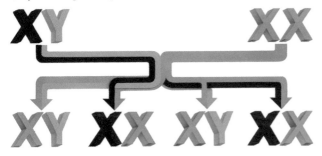

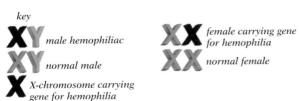

key

XY *male hemophiliac*

XY *normal male*

X *X-chromosome carrying gene for hemophilia*

XX *female carrying gene for hemophilia*

XX *normal female*

On the other hand, there is a genetic possibility that female carriers will transmit the disease to half of their sons. Half of their daughters, meanwhile, will be carriers.

For females to develop hemophilia they must inherit an abnormal gene both from a hemophiliac father and a carrier mother. However, this is an extremely rare occurrence, since unions between two such people seldom take place—particularly since genetic counseling is now more widely available to alert people to the risks.

Symptoms

The symptoms of hemophilia often appear early in an individual's life. Babies affected by the disease bruise easily. As they grow older, they develop more worrying symptoms, the most troublesome being bleeding into the joints (hemarthrosis). The result is severe pain, and ultimately the affected joint becomes deformed. After repeated injuries of this type, the patient will become crippled. Large weight-bearing joints are usually affected, most especially the knees and the ankles.

Mild hemophilia is often discovered after a tooth extraction, when the dentist finds it difficult to stop the patient's bleeding. Diagnosis is made by a measurement of the amount of factor VIII in the patient's blood. The severity of the disease depends on the level of factor VIII present: in some instances it may be only mildly lower than usual, but in others there may be no factor VIII at all, and this lack can cause serious bleeding problems.

Dangers

Bleeding may occur after even trivial injuries, despite there being no break or bruising over the skin. Bleeding into the abdomen can mimic other illnesses, including appendicitis. In severe cases the patient can become an invalid or have a massive fatal hemorrhage. It is dangerous for hemophiliacs to take aspirin as a painkiller, because it is an anticoagulant.

Treatment and outlook

If hemophiliacs are injured, they will require immediate supervision at a hospital. The severity of their bleeding depends on how much factor VIII they have; this in turn will determine the amount of factor VIII they will need to receive.

In the early 1980s, many hemophiliacs were accidentally infected with hepatitis C and with the HIV virus, after being given infected plasma concentrates. Today, all donated blood is checked thoroughly. It is now also possible to extract factor VIII from donated blood and gather it in one pool. It can then be given to the patient as an intravenous injection or a transfusion.

Bleeding into the joints is painful, but it can be controlled by injection or transfusion. The injured joint must also be exercised passively, usually with the help of a physical therapist. Bleeding from soft tissues may take longer to stanch, and the treatment may need to be continued for days with repeated blood transfusions.

Hemophilia cannot be cured, but if sufferers are careful they can expect to live relatively normal lives.

See also: **AIDS; Aspirin and analgesics; Bruises; Genetics; Heredity; Physical therapy**

otherwise known as factor XII. Factor XII then activates factor XI, then factor X, and so on down to factor I. The final step in the clotting process is the reaction of prothrombin, an enzyme, with the protein fibrinogen, to form sticky fibrin strands. They form a mesh across a wound to trap blood cells and form a clot. Each factor in the chain is determined by a particular gene on a certain chromosome, so if the gene is missing, the reaction fails to take place properly and the blood fails to clot.

How hemophilia is inherited

For males to develop hemophilia, the abnormal gene forming a part of the female sex chromosome must be inherited from a female carrier. A female has two X chromosomes and a male has an X and a Y (male) chromosome; this means that for a fetus to be a male it must have inherited a Y chromosome from the father and an X from the mother.

If the father has hemophilia, this would be carried on his X chromosome. Consequently, hemophilia can never be transmitted to a son by his father but will always be inherited by a daughter, since a daughter inherits one X chromosome from her father and one from her mother. Therefore the son of a male hemophiliac will be unaffected and will not transmit the disease; however, all of a male hemophiliac's daughters will be carriers.

Hepatitis

My brother has just gone to sea. He now writes that he wants to get a tattoo when he reaches the next port. Is there any risk?

You are probably referring to the risk of contracting hepatitis or HIV. This is purely a question of hygiene. No matter how competent the tattooist, it is still possible to be infected with a hepatitis virus or HIV from an unsterile needle.

There is no central regulatory body for tattooists, nor is there a code of professional practice that would protect the public. Although attempts have been made to organize a professional body, at the moment people must use common sense and not patronize tattooists' premises that look unhygienic.

I would like to go on the Pill but have had hepatitis. People tell me that I will not be allowed to take the Pill. Is there a reason for this?

Medical opinions vary on this point, but most doctors agree that if you have had liver damage from hepatitis you should never use this means of contraception. The reason is that the Pill contains powerful chemicals that could cause further damage to your liver if they did not pass through it very quickly; the result could be complete liver failure. You should use other forms of contraception rather than run this risk.

I am five months' pregnant and have just been told that I have hepatitis. Does this mean that my baby will catch it from me?

Your baby may also develop hepatitis and may have the virus in its blood when it is born. However, both of you can be treated with an injection of gamma globulin, which is given shortly after the child is born, to deal with the infection.

Although hepatitis—inflammation of the liver—can be a serious illness, many people make a complete recovery. However, it is advisable for anyone who has had hepatitis to give up alcohol for at least six months after an attack.

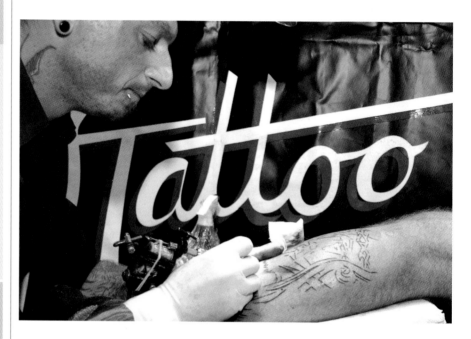

▲ *Tattooing must be carried out using sterile needles if the individual receiving the tattoo is to avoid the risk of hepatitis (and HIV) infection.*

Hepatitis is a highly infectious viral disease involving inflammation of the liver. The viruses are transmitted in blood, feces, or saliva. It is a disease that affects people of all ages but tends to occur more in the young and among those whose work involves handling contaminated material.

Causes

There are two viruses that are chiefly responsible, known as hepatitis A (formerly called infectious hepatitis) and hepatitis B (serum hepatitis). A third kind of virus that resembles hepatitis B in its transmission occurs in the absence of either the A or B virus. This is called hepatitis non-A, non-B (or hepatitis C).

Another agent (cause), called delta hepatitis, has also been discovered. This virus (hepatitis D) cannot cause disease on its own, but if it is acquired together with hepatitis B, or if it is superimposed on a hepatitis B carrier, it causes a virulent form of liver infection. Other less common viruses that can cause hepatitis are known as hepatitis E and hepatitis F.

Transmission

Hepatitis A is usually transmitted by food or water that has been contaminated, although this virus can also be transmitted in infected blood. The disease is infectious only in the incubation stage, and it is not transmitted by carriers. Outbreaks happen from time to time in areas with overcrowded housing and poor sanitation.

Hepatitis B takes longer to incubate, sometimes several months. Although it may be transmitted in the same way as hepatitis A, the B virus is more often transmitted in infected blood, either from hypodermic needles or as a result of a transfusion of infected blood or plasma. Disposable needles and blood screening tests have made this virtually unknown in Western

My friend is a heavy drinker. Is he in danger of getting hepatitis?

People who drink heavily do suffer more from chronic hepatitis or from cirrhosis of the liver, which could result in death from liver damage. The message is clear—persuade him to cut down.

My baby had jaundice soon after he was born. Might he go on to develop hepatitis?

No, this is unlikely. Young babies sometimes develop jaundice through the destruction of red blood cells that are no longer needed. It is rarely due to inflammation of the liver, as in hepatitis. However, hospitals watch out for symptoms of jaundice in newborn infants so that treatment can be given if necessary.

My mother is being treated for infectious hepatitis at home. Must we take special precautions?

During the infectious stage you should cook her food in separate pots and use different utensils; you should also take extra care with personal hygiene. However, your mother will stop being infectious soon after the jaundice begins to disappear.

I have read that you cannot be a blood donor if you have had hepatitis. Is this true?

Yes. The organisms that cause this disease can go on living in your blood long after you have recovered. If this blood were given to others, they could be infected with the disease.

My teenage daughter had glandular fever and has now developed jaundice. Why is this?

People with glandular fever sometimes develop jaundice that is due to hepatitis. This also happens in other viral diseases; numerous viruses can cause liver inflammation.

hospitals. However, about 40 percent of heroin addicts are carriers of the B virus, and transmission still occurs through the use of unsterile tattoo needles and razor blades.

If a pregnant woman contracts hepatitis B, the virus can infect her unborn child by crossing the placenta and so getting into the fetal bloodstream. Hepatitis B can also be spread by sexual contact.

A group of people especially at risk are members of hospital staffs, particularly those whose work involves handling blood on a regular basis in operating rooms or renal dialysis units (where sick patients are treated on kidney machines).

Symptoms

The majority of infections with either the A or B virus are mild and may even pass unnoticed. However, both viruses leave chemical evidence in the blood after an infection, and signs of this can be found in blood tests.

When the disease is severe enough to cause sufficient inflammation of the liver to block the drainage of bile, the sufferer becomes jaundiced. When this happens the skin and the whites of

HOW HEPATITIS AFFECTS THE LIVER

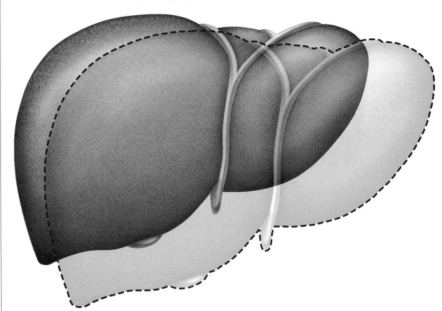

▲ *When the liver becomes inflamed by hepatitis, its size increases greatly. The colored liver (above) is of normal size. The dotted line and shaded area shows a liver enlarged by hepatitis. When examining a patient with hepatitis, the doctor can feel the liver extending below the rib cage.*

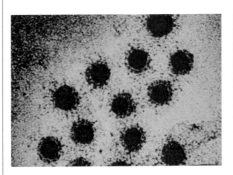

▲ *The magnified photograph shows several hepatitis A viruses.*

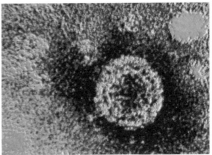

▲ *The structure of the hepatitis B virus is shown above.*

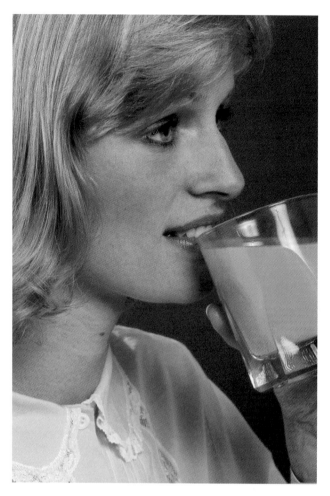

▲ *Abstinence from alcohol is essential for at least six months after an attack of hepatitis.*

the eyes develop a yellowish tinge. This is caused when bile pigments made by the liver enter the circulation instead of being eliminated through the intestine.

Jaundice may occur fairly rapidly after an infection by hepatitis A but is usually slower if the illness is due to hepatitis B.

Very often the victim feels unwell for some time beforehand, rejecting food and losing any desire to smoke (if he or she was formerly a smoker). Pain is felt high in the abdomen on the right side. There may be arthritic-type pains in the joints, and also a rash. While the jaundice is most marked, the patient feels sick and frequently vomits. The jaundice does not usually last for more than two weeks, and recovery takes place within six weeks or so.

In a few cases of hepatitis B or C, the virus is not eliminated and the patient becomes a carrier. Some of these patients develop chronic inflammation of the liver, which progresses to cirrhosis. This does not occur in hepatitis A, since there is no carrier state.

Diagnosis

Doctors can diagnose hepatitis easily if typical symptoms are present; these can be confirmed by blood tests. After a person has had a hepatitis A infection, the antibodies made against it can be detected in his or her blood. Hepatitis B is more complex and therefore more difficult to detect. During infection a portion of the virus called surface antigen can be found in the blood. When the patient has overcome the infection, antibodies to this virus antigen appear. If no antibody is made, this indicates that the patient is still carrying the virus. If the doctor suspects that a virus carrier is developing chronic liver disease, blood tests for chemicals leaking from damaged liver cells will be done. If the tests show any abnormality, a liver biopsy is performed and a minute sample of tissue is examined under a microscope.

Dangers

Until the recent increase in liver disease produced by alcoholism, viral hepatitis was the most common cause of cirrhosis of the liver, which can be fatal. Some people with viral hepatitis make a complete recovery, but others fail to eliminate the virus from the body; they become chronic carriers and may infect others.

In many parts of the developing world, the combination of hepatitis B and aflatoxin from fungus on nuts and grain is a potent cause of primary liver cancer—a condition that is rare in the West.

Treatment

It is not necessary to admit all hepatitis sufferers to the hospital—only those who become extremely unwell or who are at risk, such as expectant mothers, diabetics, or the elderly.

Both while the liver is inflamed and while it is recovering, its cells will be sensitive to all kinds of drugs. The sufferer should not take any medicines at this time. It is particularly important for him or her to avoid alcohol, which has a poisonous effect on the liver.

Whether the patient is being treated in the hospital or at home, it is essential to reduce the chances of cross-infection by using separate cooking and eating utensils for the patient and being careful about hygiene. There has been a certain amount of argument as to the importance of complete rest in bed. Some doctors feel that the later complications (cirrhosis or chronic hepatitis) can be avoided, provided that the patient rests as much as possible while jaundiced. There are no dietary restrictions, but the patient should eat properly.

People who are exposed to infection by hepatitis or who intend to live cheaply on walking or camping vacations in areas such as southern Europe, India, or Africa can be protected against hepatitis A by an injection of gamma globulin. Vaccination against hepatitis B is also available, but it is recommended only for groups at very high risk. Accidental exposure to hepatitis B can be treated with hyperimmune globulin, given within a week of exposure to the virus. Infants born to mothers with hepatitis can also be protected in the same way if they are injected within a week of birth.

Outlook

The majority of hepatitis attacks are mild and are followed by complete recovery. Hepatitis can recur, but in such cases it is rarely caused by the same type of virus. It is, however, possible for patients who are carriers to suffer a relapse. If a person has had hepatitis the best advice is never to drink alcohol again. Failing that, he or she should abstain from all alcoholic drinks for at least six months.

See also: Infection and infectious diseases; Sexually transmitted diseases; Vaccinations; Viruses

Heredity

Questions and Answers

My parents were overweight, and I am too. Why do heavy parents often have heavy children?

Being overweight seems to be a problem that is both inherited and caused by environment. Overweight parents tend to have heavy children, not just because the children are overfed or encouraged to eat fattening foods, but also because they inherit certain physical and chemical tendencies.

I suffer from dyslexia, and I think my son may have the same problem. Is dyslexia inherited?

Yes. Dyslexia is sometimes called word blindness, and it causes severe problems with reading. The disability can be inherited, so if a parent suffers from it, there is a risk that it will be passed on to the children. Given early and expert treatment, most children with dyslexia can learn to read. In fact, many inherited problems can be overcome with suitable treatment.

My mother went through menopause early—at the age of 43. Will I be the same?

It is likely. The length of a woman's reproductive life (the years when she may bear children) does tend to be inherited. It is not understood exactly how this happens, but it is thought that many different genes are involved, which regulate such mechanisms as egg release and hormone production.

My husband is a twin. Are our children likely to be twins?

No. This tendency is inherited only through females. If there are no twins in your family tree, you are unlikely to have them. If you are over 35, your chance of having twins is increased.

Everyone knows that children resemble their parents, grandparents, brothers, and sisters to some extent, but just how far is it possible to predict the way they will turn out? Some of the answers are provided by the study of heredity.

Every time a person says "it runs in the family" or "she has her mother's eyes," he or she is talking about heredity. In scientific terminology this is known as genetics, which is the study of heredity in general and of genes in particular. Genes can be described as biochemical codes. Genes are tiny; they are much too small to be seen even under an electron microscope. Research has shown that they are carried on the chromosomes (tiny threadlike structures within all human cells which can be seen under a very powerful microscope).

Everyone has 46 chromosomes arranged in 23 pairs. One member of each pair comes from the father's sperm, the other from the mother's egg. Together these structures make up a complete chemical blueprint for a person's entire lifetime.

Simple forms of heredity

The pairing of chromosomes is a significant factor in the way heredity works, because each pair contains similar genes, and the most simple form of heredity can be traced to the operation of single pairs of genes. Genes acting in this way can occur in two different forms: one will be dominant, the other recessive. Dominant genes are distinguished by the tendency to display their characteristics in the physical makeup of a person, even if they are present on only one of the pair. A pair of similar recessive genes, with one gene inherited from each parent, must be present if that characteristic is to become obvious in an individual.

Geneticists have identified various dominant and recessive genes. For example, the gene for curly hair is dominant, so if a child inherits it from the father, and also inherits a gene for straight hair (which is recessive) from the mother, the curly-hair gene will dominate and the child will have curly hair. In practical terms this does not mean that parents can predict whether their child will inherit the father's curly hair. The actual passing on of genes is a random occurrence, and the

▼ *Children of racially mixed parents will reflect characteristics of both parents.*

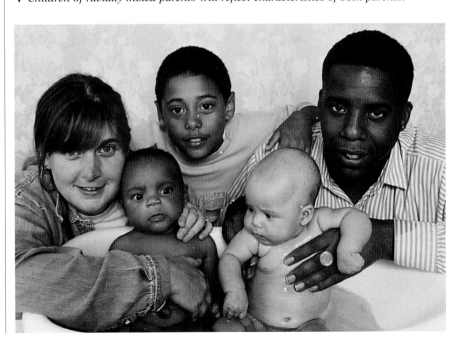

171

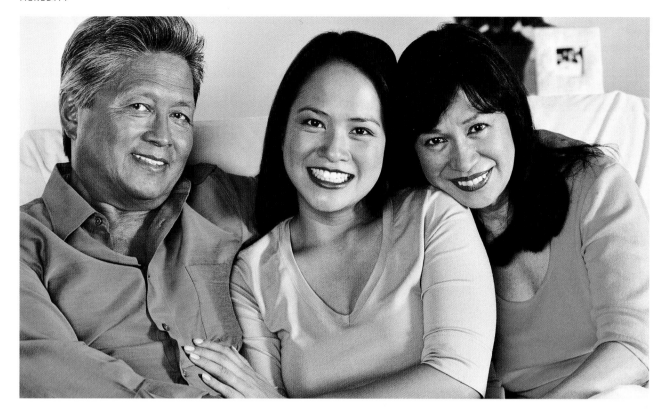

▲ *The strong family resemblance between the daughter and mother, and similarities between the daughter and father, are caused by inheriting genes from both parents.*

curly-haired dominant trait has a slightly better than even chance of being transferred. However, the principle does help us in a general way, making it clear that we cannot count on a child's having straight hair (if that is preferred) if one partner is curly-haired and the other is straight-haired.

Normality

One form of heredity, known as single-factor inheritance or normality, is relatively simple and tells us some important and reassuring things about how our children will turn out in terms of their general health and makeup. This is because the majority of healthy characteristics are governed by dominant genes. So, as one might expect, most babies born to healthy mothers are themselves healthy. Just a few hereditary diseases are inherited on dominant genes, but recessive genes can cause many more, including albinism, which is a lack of pigment, or coloring, and some types of deafness. Recessive genes, by nature, can be carried by a human all through life without the characteristics they convey actually showing up. Also, there is nothing to stop them from being passed on to the next generation and, if the circumstances are right, showing up there. However, there are complications even in single-factor inheritance.

Other types of heredity

There are several other ways in which genes can work. These vary in complexity. Perhaps one of the most interesting is the polygene system, which governs such characteristics as skin color, height, and probably intelligence. Polygenes can be thought of as groups of genes working together. The rules of dominance apply to each gene in the group, and the effect of the genes is cumulative; they build up to produce an overall effect.

So although it is impossible to lay down a general rule, it is fair to say that tallness or shortness tends to run in families because the polygene for height contains more tall or short genes in some families than others. If a taller-than-average man has children by a shorter-than-average woman, the geneticist would expect them to be closer to the average height than either parent. In a similar way, the polygenes governing skin color produce a whole range of complexions among the races of the world, ranging from very dark to extremely pale.

Mixed genes

Children born to parents of completely different skin colors—say, a pale Caucasian and a dark African—will tend to be intermediate between their parents, although because the darker-skin genes are dominant over the pale-skin genes, such a child would tend to be darker than the exact halfway shade. However, there is no simple pattern of inheritance for either dark or pale skin. At least four pairs of genes are involved in determining skin color, so the genes of remote ancestors of a different race will be greatly diluted.

Nature or nurture

Intelligence is the most argued-over aspect of the whole subject. The only certain fact is that intelligence is both inherited and affected by a child's environment—that is, the atmosphere and conditions in which a child is raised and then lives during adult life. The reason why certain talents, such as musical ability, tend to run

▶ *In this family, dominant genes have produced some obvious inherited features, like the father's eyes and the mother's nose.*

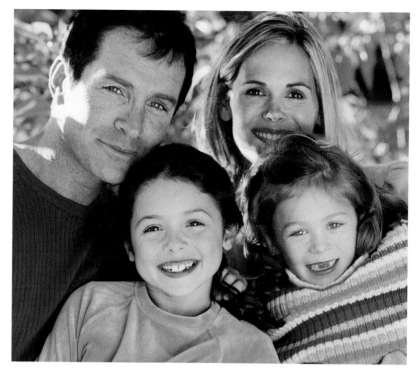

in families to such an extent cannot be exactly explained. No one knows how much of it is inherited and how much occurs as a result of being brought up in an environment where music is part of family life. The same applies to acting ability, sports skills, literary ability, and other talents.

Environment may also act as the trigger for an inherited physical characteristic. For example, two people may be born with a tendency to tan easily, which requires a concentration of pigment-producing cells known as melanocytes in the skin. However, if one of them stays indoors for most of the time, his or her skin is unlikely to tan, while the other, doing an outdoor job, will quickly develop a tan.

Penetrance

The question of heredity is further complicated because genes show their strength not only in terms of dominance over other genes, but by the degree to which they penetrate; geneticists call this penetrance. Penetrance may be weak or strong. For example, the fixed flexion of the fingers known as camptodactyly is produced by a dominant gene and can thus show up by being inherited in the single-factor method. However, the degree to which a person suffers from it will vary from severe stiffness in several fingers (full penetrance) to stiffness in just one finger (partial penetrance). Geneticists also suspect that longevity (the length of life) is determined by genes, possibly by polygenes. On the other hand, they recognize that however long a person's genes have programmed him or her to live, their effect can be counteracted by an unhealthy lifestyle, such as smoking, drinking, or overeating.

These various principles of heredity are only tiny corners of an extremely complex jigsaw. Most geneticists are concerned with trying to unravel the way diseases and abnormalities are inherited. Doctors now believe that most body traits are determined as described by the polygene theory.

THEORIES ABOUT EYE COLOR

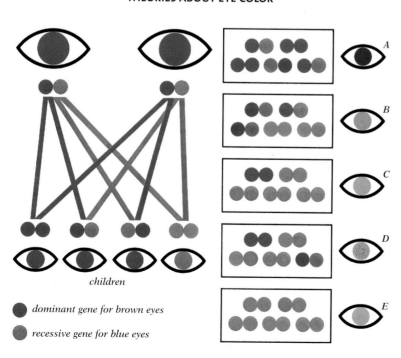

children

● dominant gene for brown eyes

● recessive gene for blue eyes

◀ *According to the single-factor theory of heredity, children of brown-eyed parents will have pure brown or pure blue eyes. So how are color variations explained? The polygene theory suggests that several pairs of genes determine color. Parents with blue eyes will have children with blue eyes (E), but the eye color of children whose parents have other eye colors cannot be predicted because the greater number of genes and the ways in which they can interact (A, B, C, and D) produce a greater potential for color variation.*

See also: **Counseling; Genetics**

Hernia

Hernias are protrusions of an organ through a weakened muscle wall. Sometimes they cause no discomfort at all, but when they do require treatment, they can be cured with complete success.

Questions and Answers

Does a hernia hurt? My uncle has a hernia but he is not in pain.

Hernias do not usually hurt, except when they first occur—for example, during heavy lifting. Afterward they may be a bit uncomfortable but are usually not painful. If a hernia does hurt, it may be strangulating because its blood supply is cut off; medical advice should be sought.

Can a tendency toward hernias run in families?

Yes, but there is no definite hereditary link. Members of some families tend to do the same types of jobs—for example, those involving heavy labor, which are more likely to cause a hernia.

Is a big hernia more serious than a small one?

No, it may be the other way around. Some very small hernias, such as femoral hernias in the groin, may be so small they can be detected only by touch, especially in an overweight person, but they often strangulate.

My mother has a hernia in the wound left after a hysterectomy, but the doctors say that it does not need repair. Is this right?

Probably. Most incisional hernias have a wide neck, so there is very little chance of strangulation. Also, they can be difficult to repair satisfactorily. A surgical belt may be enough to control them.

I have just had a hernia operation. When can I go back to work?

That depends on your job. If you have a desk job, go back after about 10 days. If your work involves heavy lifting, stay away for six weeks to three months.

A hernia occurs when an organ (usually the intestine) protrudes through the muscle or tissue that usually contains it. It can be external—so that it shows as a lump on the surface of the abdomen or in the groin—or internal, like a hiatal hernia, caused by a weakness in the diaphragm.

Common types of hernia

The most common types of hernia occur in the groin and are called inguinal or femoral hernias, depending on the site of the weakness. They can also occur in the diaphragm (hiatal hernias); near the navel (umbilical hernias); in the upper part of the abdomen in the midline (ventral hernias); and through weakness in the posterior (back) wall of the abdomen, when they are usually not visible as lumps.

Hernias that develop at an operation site where the muscles have failed to heal properly are called incisional hernias.

What is a hernia?

A hernia usually consists of a sac made of peritoneum (the thin membrane lining the abdominal cavity) that protrudes through a weakness in the muscular wall of the abdomen. If it is an external hernia, the sac will be covered with a layer of fat and skin.

The sac contains either part of an intra-abdominal organ, usually a loop of small intestine, or part of the omentum, the fatty membrane that covers the intestines. The omentum often fills the sac completely, preventing other structures from entering it, and this helps to prevent the complications that may result from the presence of a hernia.

Causes

Hernias are common, and various conditions may cause them. People may be born with a particular weakness in the muscle wall that makes them prone to develop a hernia. This may mean that a hernia develops in infancy, or later in life, owing to heavy lifting, for example. Anything that weakens or strains the muscle wall until it ruptures can cause a hernia. This includes coughing and straining to lift heavy objects.

A common type of hernia is an inguinal hernia in the groin, which occurs more often in men than women. In men part of the intestine protrudes into the inguinal canal (the passage through which the testicle descends to the scrotum early in a boy's life).

Women are more prone to develop a hiatal hernia (in which the upper part of the stomach moves upward into the chest through a weakness in the diaphragm); this can be related to the increase in intra-abdominal pressure during pregnancy.

▲ *An X ray of a hiatus hernia. The junction of the esophagus and the stomach becomes weakened and part of the stomach moves into the chest cavity.*

TYPES OF HERNIA

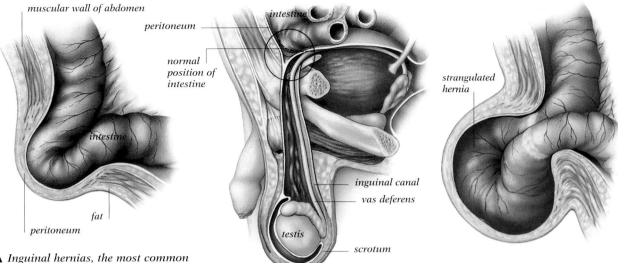

▲ Inguinal hernias, the most common type of hernia, occur more often in men than in women. In men the hernia is usually located at the point where the inguinal canal meets the peritoneum. The soft lump that develops in the groin bulges when the patient coughs and disappears completely when the man lies down.

▲ When the testes descend into the scrotum, they may drag on the peritoneum and weaken it so that it sags downward slightly into the groin. Later a hernia may develop at this weak point.

▲ A strangulated hernia is dangerous and could cause death. When the blood supply to the contents of the hernia is cut off, it swells and may eventually become gangrenous. If this happens, gangrene may be followed by perforation and peritonitis.

Symptoms

An inguinal hernia caused by heavy lifting will often occur suddenly; the patient may describe a feeling of something giving way, accompanied by some pain. This usually lasts for only a short time, and the patient then notices a lump in the groin. This lump is usually soft, bulges when he or she coughs, and goes away completely when he or she lies down.

If the hernia gets very large, it may extend down into the scrotum in a man, but hernias can become large before they cause many symptoms. If the patient's job involves a lot of heavy lifting, the hernia may become uncomfortable all the time and prevent him or her from working. Sometimes a hernia develops so slowly that the first thing the patient notices is a lump in the groin.

A hiatal hernia, because it bulges into the chest, is never seen or felt as a lump, but it causes symptoms by its effect on the junction between the esophagus and the stomach. There is a ring of muscle at the lower end of the esophagus, just at the point where it joins the stomach, which relaxes to allow swallowed food to pass into the stomach but tightens to prevent food from going back up the esophagus. When a hiatal hernia is present, the effect of the ring of muscle is lost, and food and acid can pass freely out of the stomach and up into the esophagus. Because the lining of the esophagus is not designed to withstand acid, it becomes damaged and inflamed. The condition is known as reflux esophagitis.

The symptoms of this type of hernia are burning pain behind the sternum (breastbone), which is made worse by bending down or lying flat. If the esophagus is severely damaged over a number of years, it may become narrowed and make swallowing difficult. Hiatal hernias are very common, especially after middle age. Many people may have a small hiatal hernia of which they are unaware, and which causes them no harm whatsoever.

Dangers

If strangulation occurs, a hernia becomes extremely serious and potentially life-threatening. This condition occurs when the punctured muscle wall surrounding the protruding herniated intestine tightens. The muscle squeezes the contents of the hernial sac, cutting off its blood supply. First the veins are obstructed. This causes the contents to swell, putting further pressure on the arteries, and eventually this can lead to gangrene of the contents. If the hernia contains part of the intestine, gangrene of the intestine may develop followed by perforation and peritonitis.

The hernia, formerly soft and perhaps only uncomfortable, becomes tense and tender, and does not go away when the patient lies down. If the intestine is strangulated, the patient may develop symptoms of intestinal obstruction—vomiting, abdominal pain, distension, and constipation. If this happens, emergency surgery is needed to free the strangulated intestine and repair the hernia. If it is left for more than a few hours, the intestine may become irreparably damaged, so that part of it will have to be removed and the two ends joined together again.

Of course, if strangulation occurs in one of the rare internal hernias, there will be no lump to feel and the patient will become ill because of an intestinal obstruction. The hernia that most commonly strangulates is a femoral hernia, followed by inguinal and umbilical hernias. Hiatal hernias can strangulate, but because the chest cavity is large they rarely do so.

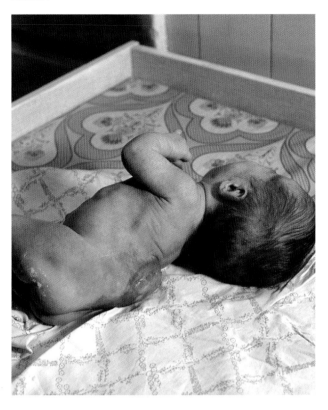

▲ *A two-month-old baby girl suffering from a birth defect as a result of the Chernobyl disaster in Ukraine. The baby has a hernia of the backbone.*

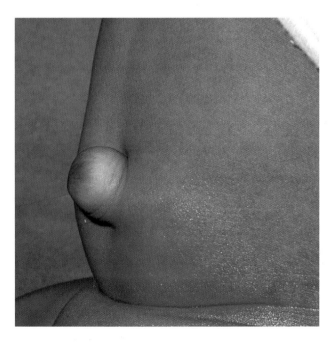

▲ *An umbilical hernia (at the navel) is common in babies. The swelling flattens easily; if it does not, consult a doctor. A paraumbilical hernia (near the navel) occurs in women.*

Treatment

If there is a recognizable predisposition to suffering from a hernia, such as obesity, constipation, a cough, or difficulty in urinating, this should be treated first. Most hiatal hernias can be treated without resorting to surgery. Weight loss is probably the most important measure of the severity of the hernia. To deal with the symptoms, it is helpful to avoid bending, use several pillows at night, avoid drinking just before bedtime, and take regular antacids to neutralize the stomach acids.

Surgery is contemplated only after these measures have failed and if the symptoms are very severe. Surgery can be performed, through either the upper part of the abdomen or the chest wall, to repair the weakness in the diaphragm. Nowadays, however, it is quite rare to have to operate on a hiatal hernia.

Treatment for inguinal hernias involves either wearing a truss or surgical repair. A truss is a special belt with an extra strap that passes between the legs to prevent it from riding up. It has a specially designed pad that presses on the area of the hernia, preventing it from bulging out. It can be uncomfortable to wear and can also be dangerous, because it may allow the hernia (which contains part of the intestines) to bulge and then press on the neck of the herniated intestinal sac, making strangulation more likely. This will usually happen if the hernia has not been fully pushed back before the truss is put on.

By far the best form of treatment for an inguinal hernia is surgery. This may be performed in order to prevent strangulation in the future, because the hernia is uncomfortable and is preventing the patient from working, or because there is strangulation, in which case emergency surgery would be done.

The surgery is very simple and is generally performed under a general anesthetic. However, it can be performed under a local anesthetic if the patient is thin and the hernia is small, or if the patient is unfit for a general anesthetic. The thin sac of peritoneum is carefully removed and tied off at the neck, after all its contents have been returned to the abdominal cavity. In a child this is all that would be done, but in an adult the defect in the muscle wall of the abdomen is repaired. Usually a strong, nonsoluble thread such as nylon is used and the defect is stitched. When the scar tissue has formed around the stitches, usually about three months after the operation, the area should be as strong as normal.

Postoperative recovery

After an operation for a hernia, it takes some time for the muscle wall around the region of the hernia to be repaired and to become strong again. The length of time this takes varies, but it is probably around three months. After this time there is no reason why a person who has had a hernia repair should not lead a completely normal life. This includes even doing a job that requires heavy lifting.

A hernia operation does not guarantee that there will never be a recurrence of the hernia. However, the chances of a recurrence are small; if it does happen, a second operation can be performed. If a hernia does return, the person should consult his or her doctor.

See also: **Pain**

Hygiene

My daughter is allergic to some soaps. How can she keep clean?

She should try a nonperfumed, mild soap. Allergies can be caused by an additive, such as scent in the soap, rather than the soap itself. If this does not work, your doctor can prescribe a cleansing cream that contains no soap.

My child is being taught personal hygiene at school, but isn't this my responsibility?

Yes, it is, but schools also have a responsibility to pupils whose parents do not bother to educate their children in this way. It might help to have a chat with your child's teacher so that you can compare notes about the points you stress to your child.

My neighbor says I should separate raw meat and cooked food. Is this true?

Yes. Any bacteria on raw meat may be transferred to your hands. If you then handle food such as bread, cakes, or salad ingredients before you wash your hands, you could contaminate them with bacteria. Cooking the meat kills bacteria, but your bread, cake, or lettuce will be eaten as they are. Also, flies could transfer bacteria from raw meat to other foods if they are left next to each other. Your neighbor's suggestion is a sensible precaution to stop the spread of bacteria.

I know that people should wash their hands after using the toilet, but just how important is it to do this every time?

It is important enough to insist that it becomes a regular routine for every member of your family from an early age. Bacteria can be transmitted to the hands from even the smallest trace of feces.

Hygiene is the means by which people can maintain good health and lessen the risk of infection. Learning and practicing the basic rules of hygiene are essential for protecting the health of each member of the family.

Possibly the greatest advance in standards of hygiene in most developed countries was the introduction of safe water supplies and sewage systems during the 19th century. Medical historians think that this did even more to combat the spread of infectious diseases than the great advances in vaccination.

However, many countries are still without a safe water supply for the majority of the population. Diseases spread through contaminated water remain a fact of life for countless people, however dedicated they are to keeping their homes clean. Cholera and typhoid are probably the most serious of the diseases associated with unsanitary living conditions.

Even those people who do have access to clean and sanitary water cannot relax their standards. Dangerous germs, such as bacteria, can be found in the most modern of homes if the basic rules of hygiene are not respected. Homes with young children need particularly high standards, because children are exposed to an abundance of germs.

A healthy life

Keeping the home clean is just the beginning. Hygiene extends to every aspect of life. As with many health precautions, the benefits of hygiene can be reduced to nothing if a person drinks excessively or smokes. A healthy, balanced diet also helps to keep the body free of disease, and regular exercise, combined with relaxation, will reinforce the good effects of all the other basic efforts to maintain health.

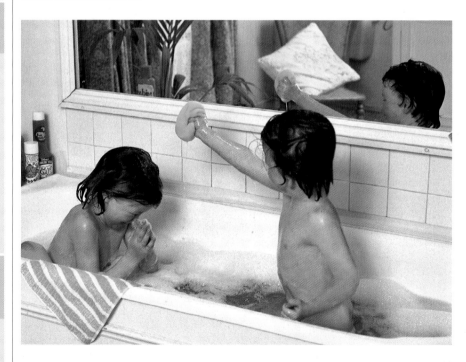

▲ *Once young children are over any fears they may have had about bathing, and are old enough to do so without close supervision, parents should let them enjoy themselves in the bath as much as possible. If children can link bath time with fun and games, it will be easier to teach them the basics of personal hygiene.*

Personal hygiene

Clothing should always be kept clean. Underwear should be changed every day, and clothes should never be worn once they become dirty. It is important to make sure that clothes fit well—which means not too tightly. This applies particularly to shoes, because if they are badly fitting, they can cause foot problems that last for the rest of the wearer's life.

Corns, bunions, and ingrown toenails are usually caused by very tight shoes, and high heels can create back problems. The basic rule in buying shoes should be comfort, not fashion, although wearing uncomfortable shoes for a short time is unlikely to cause damage. Such principles can be difficult to explain to the teenager who is determined always to wear the highest of heels or the most pointed toes, dismissing healthy footwear as uncool.

Modern shoe stores offer a wide range of styles, and it is now much easier to find comfortable stylish shoes. A majority of people, not only the young, wear sneakers. Provided they fit properly, such shoes are both safe and comfortable. If young people are unwilling to accept comfortable shoes, their parents may want to remind them of the thousands of people who need frequent, often painful, treatment by podiatrists, a result of having been slaves to fashion as young adults.

The right fabrics

Although modern advances in clothing technology have made washing and fabric care easier, it is now clear that synthetic fibers can be unhealthy—especially for women, because they can lead to vaginal infections. Natural fibers, such as wool or cotton, are porous, whereas artificial fibers tend to leave the body hot and clammy—an ideal environment for bacteria. Women should always choose cotton underpants, particularly for wearing with nylon stockings. Those who are prone to vaginal infections may find that such infections cease if they stop wearing tights altogether; stockings with an open or cotton gusset can also help.

Washing

Keeping the body clean is vitally important. The hair should be washed at least once a week, and probably twice or more in city environments. Aside from the more obvious benefits, this will help to prevent head lice infestation, a much more common problem than many people realize. The lice are usually caught from other human carriers rather than from dirty or unhygienic surroundings. If children or their parents get head lice, the scalp will feel irritated, and scratching can spread infection to new sites. Special lotions and shampoos are available over the counter to deal with the problem.

Dandruff (loose flakes of skin from the scalp) can be helped by regular washing with an antidandruff shampoo.

Ears should be gently washed with warm water to remove wax. Any large buildup of wax should be dealt with only by a doctor, because the ear is a delicate organ that should never be poked or scraped with any rigid object.

Blemishes

Pimples and acne are common complaints among teenagers. Acne is not caused by dirty habits, but anyone who suffers in this way should be especially scrupulous about general cleanliness because the pimples can be a symptom of infection, which aggravates the

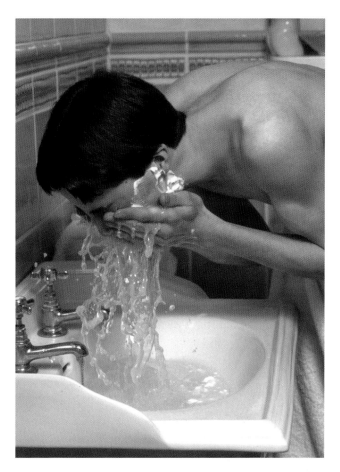

▲ *Although acne and pimples are not caused by poor hygiene, teenagers with such conditions should pay particular attention to cleanliness.*

condition. A helpful approach is to keep reminding the teenager that the skin will almost certainly clear after a few years. Mild acne can be improved by washing with a gentle, nonperfumed cleanser. Serious cases require medical advice.

Acne sufferers should avoid makeup and wearing wool next to the skin. The pimples should not be picked, because picking can spread infection and cause scarring. The hair should be kept well washed and brushed back from the face.

Commonsense precautions

A person should always cover his or her nose and mouth when coughing or sneezing, to prevent the thousands of germ-bearing droplets from spreading onto other people or food. Teeth should be brushed at least twice a day, preferably after every meal, for three minutes. An electric toothbrush will automatically provide the correct and most efficient movement of the brush head.

People should always wash their hands after using the toilet. Bacteria from the feces can be transmitted through toilet paper onto the hands.

Nails should always be kept clean because bacteria can be harbored underneath them. Feet should be washed daily and dried carefully between the toes. If all these practices are followed

Questions and Answers

Where do food-poisoning germs live? I want to know which places I should clean most regularly.

The bacteria that cause food poisoning live in house dust, on the human skin, on raw meat, and even in cracks in tabletops. They can also be picked up from dishcloths and cloth napkins, or from kitchen equipment such as wooden spoons.

From this it should be clear that the only foolproof approach is to ensure overall cleanliness in your kitchen. Dust and wipe regularly. Wash your hands and wrists before preparing food. Use clean dishcloths. Wash all cooking implements and dishes thoroughly. Cook meat as soon as possible after buying it. Unfreeze meat fully before cooking it; cooking kills bacteria, but they can survive in a partially frozen area.

Some of the local children have foot infections, and I'm worried that my son will catch one. How can I prevent this?

There are two main infectious foot conditions—athlete's foot (in its mild form, split skin and soreness between the toes) and warts on the sole of the foot. The trouble with these infections is that they are usually caught when people go barefoot, typically in changing rooms. For this reason, there is not much you can do to keep your son from catching them.

If there is an epidemic of athlete's foot among your son's friends, try to persuade him to stay away from the swimming pool for a while. If he does catch athlete's foot, this may indicate that he is vulnerable to the fungus that causes it. With this in mind you could give him a suitable antifungal powder (available from drugstores) to use every day in his shoes and socks. Plantar warts are much less common, and people usually do not worry about them until they happen.

If a family member does have a foot infection, you should make sure that he or she uses a separate towel and bath mat and does not walk around the house in bare feet.

regularly, the body will stay clean and fresh. Some people may wish to use a deodorant on the underarms, but this is usually unnecessary if daily washing takes place.

The genital area needs to be washed with soap and warm water at least once a day. However, douching for women is not necessary, because the vagina has its own delicate self-cleaning mechanism, which can be disturbed by harsh douching or vaginal deodorants. This can lead to vaginal infection and abnormal discharges. If a woman is worried about a discharge and thinks she may have an infection, she should see a doctor. Tampons and sanitary napkins should be changed at least three times a day; tampons should be used only during menstruation.

Men should thoroughly clean the penis, including under the foreskin, and wash the genital area before sexual intercourse.

Cystitis

Urinary infections, particularly cystitis (a painful inflammation of the bladder interior; are often caused when bacteria from the anus are transmitted to the urethral opening. A woman should wipe herself from front to back after using the toilet and keep the whole genital area very clean.

Hygiene and the baby

If a baby is bottle-fed, all bottles, nipples, and spoons should be kept sterilized. There are special sterilizing units on sale for this purpose.

If terry-cloth diapers are used instead of the disposable variety, they need to be soaked for an hour in a solution of cold water and a diaper cleaning agent. They should then be washed on the hottest setting of the washing machine. If no washing machine is available, the diapers should be boiled for 15 minutes and then washed in the hottest possible water (use rubber gloves).

Food

People should eat food within 24 hours of any "sell by" date, and food that seems even slightly suspicious should be thrown away. This also applies to bulging, swollen cans of any type of food, though not to dented cans.

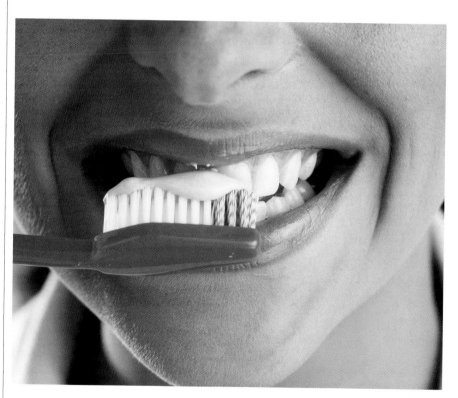

▲ *Dental hygiene involves brushing the teeth thoroughly at least twice a day; using floss to clean between the teeth can also prevent the buildup of bacteria that cause decay.*

Hygiene in the kitchen

DO

Do wash hands before touching food, and make sure that any cut or sore is covered by an adhesive bandage.

Do keep food covered and away from flies. Use a fly spray if flies are a nuisance.

Do wash all salad ingredients very thoroughly.

Do wash saucepans thoroughly.

Do use liners in kitchen wastebaskets and trash cans.

Do soak dishcloths, mops, and floor cloths in a solution of bleach once a week.

Do use clean cloths for drying dishes.

Do use paper towels for mopping up.

DON'T

Don't keep the trash can near the kitchen door; this encourages flies to make trips between it and any food left out in the kitchen.

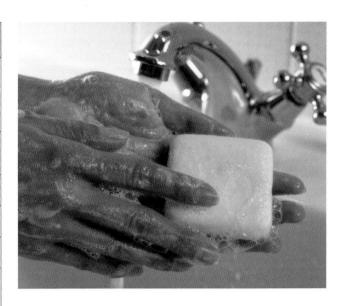

▲ *Washing the hands after using the toilet, before meals, and before touching or preparing food is important in preventing the spread of harmful bacteria and disease.*

Precooked meats—pies, ham, or luncheon meat, for example—should be covered and refrigerated immediately. Any food cooked at home should be quickly cooled and refrigerated if it is not to be eaten at once. Frozen meat, particularly poultry, should be thawed thoroughly before cooking, because salmonellosis (a severe kind of food poisoning caused by the salmonella bacteria) can be caught from meat that has not been cooked properly.

Salad ingredients should be washed under running water, and fruit should be washed or peeled before being eaten.

A refrigerator is an important aid to hygiene. However, people need to remember that it does not kill germs—it only stops them from multiplying; refrigerated food will go bad eventually.

Pets

Animals can be a source of infection. All pets should be kept healthy, because some animal illnesses can be passed on to humans. Cats and dogs, for example, can infect humans with ringworm, which is a fungus infection; it is also possible to catch roundworm from dogs.

Any bite or scratch caused by an animal should be held under running water immediately and then dabbed with an antiseptic. If the animal was wild, the person should carefully note its behavior and go to the doctor immediately. If a child is scratched or bitten, he or she should be taken to a doctor if there is any fever or inflammation; children must be kept away from sick animals.

Vermin such as rats or mice, along with other kinds of infestations, are best dealt with by the local public health department. Vermin droppings can contaminate food, so anyone who observes mice droppings in the kitchen, say, should take action right away.

On vacation

Going abroad may require a person to take extra precautions, although most Western countries now have high public health standards. Traveler's diarrhea—usually taken to mean any kind of

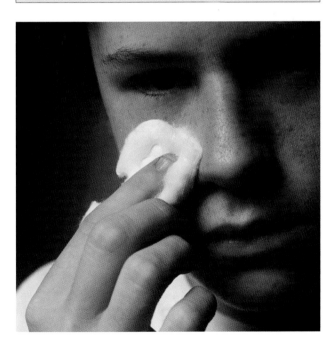

▲ *Facial cleansing can prevent a teenager's skin pores from becoming blocked; a regular cleansing regime will help cut down the number of pimples he or she suffers.*

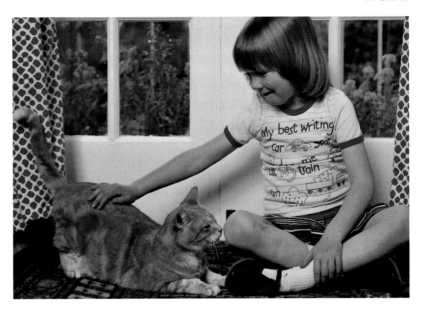

▶ *Household pets are not a health hazard as long as they are clean, healthy, and kept free of fleas and worms.*

diarrhea caught abroad—is often a result of fecal contamination of food, so travelers should select only clean restaurants. Travelers should also drink bottled water if there is any doubt about the cleanliness of the water supply, and they must always make sure that water for babies is boiled before being drunk. People should not eat in restaurants that look unhygienic.

If a person is on a camping vacation and does not have access to a refrigerator, he or she should always eat fresh or cooked meat the day it is bought. Care needs to be taken when disposing of trash; the camper should burn it if there are no trash cans on the campsite.

Travelers should make sure they are immunized according to the regulations for any country they visit: for example, against cholera and typhoid.

Learning about hygiene

Children learn best by example, so it is pointless for parents to tell a child to observe rules that they themselves do not bother with. Parents should explain why the rules are important. Certain rules should be followed from an early age, particularly the washing of hands before meals and after defecating. Children should have a daily bath, but if this is not possible, parents should make sure that there is daily washing of the hands, face, feet, and genitals.

Hygiene in the bathroom
DO
Do keep everything scrupulously clean. All surfaces, handles, and faucets should be washed with a powerful cleaner or bleach at least once a week.
Do clean the toilet bowl, sink, and faucets at least once a day if someone in the family has a stomach upset or is suffering from diarrhea.
Do make sure everyone in the family has his or her own washcloth and towel. If family members have a foot infection (such as athlete's foot), make them use a separate bath mat and wear slippers as soon as they step out of the bath.
DON'T
Don't leave leaking outlet pipes to drip, or delay before calling the plumber if the bath or sink outlet smells foul.
Don't allow children to neglect washing their hands after using the toilet.

Hygiene and the community

However hygiene-conscious a person is, he or she may still be at risk of infection if the local water and sewage systems are not properly maintained. Simple plumbing problems within the home, such as a leaking toilet cistern, can be solved easily by a plumber, but if something goes wrong with the drains or external sewage pipes, then the person should call in the public health department. His or her house may be connected to the town's water supply, which is usually the responsibility of the local public health department.

People who live in private rented accommodation will need to arrange with their landlord for repairs of internal plumbing or improvement of unhygienic conditions in the kitchen or bathroom. New homes as well as old ones can be affected by condensation or mold (each a potential health risk).

People also have the right to report stores or restaurants that they believe fall below public health standards. Although there are frequent spot-checks of such places and the rules governing them are strict, public health inspectors cannot be everywhere at once.

If a person sees suspicious-looking food on sale, or if a store is selling food later than its "sell by" date, he or she should report it to the local inspector.

Keeping hygiene in perspective

In spite of all this, people should not turn the home into a battle-ground in the campaign against bacteria. The rules of hygiene should not take over or interfere with family life. Even the most hygienic person is bound to catch an infectious disease now and then.

In addition, current immunilogical research is producing more and more evidence that too much hygiene early in life prevents healthy maturation of T cells and may encourage the development of atopic disorders such as asthma and eczema in children.

See also: Acne and pimples; Bacteria; Food poisoning; Immunization; Infection and infectious diseases; Lice; Rabies; Ringworm

Immunization

Immunization increases human resistance to certain infectious diseases by adding to the body's natural supply of protective antibodies. It is useful to be aware of the types of immunization available and when to take them.

Infection with rubella (German measles) during the first three months of pregnancy often results in an abnormal baby. This is because the rubella virus crosses the placenta and invades the baby's tissues. The main strategy in the United States has been to immunize all children, regardless of sex, to prevent epidemics and thus reduce the risk of exposing pregnant women to rubella. Women of childbearing age are handled individually and immunized if necessary, but never if they are already pregnant or likely to be.

Immunization may be done either by injecting an antibody that has been made outside the patient directly into him or her (passive immunization) or by injecting an inactive form of the germ into the patient, thereby provoking an antibody response against further infection (active immunization). After passive immunization, protection against infection is immediate and gradually diminishes over the next three to four weeks. After active immunization, complete immunity does not develop for a month or so but in some instances is lifelong.

Passive immunization

Passive immunization is used frequently only in the prevention of tetanus (lockjaw). It is given to people who are seriously exposed to the risk of developing the disease, for example, from a cut made by a garden rake. The object of the treatment is to supply the patient with an antibody that has been derived from another source. Horses have been used as reservoirs for this type of antibody since 1894, but more and more use is being made of human immunoglobulin (IgG). This has many advantages over horse globulin, the most important being that patients no longer have the allergic reaction to horse serum itself that was so common a few years ago. The disease caused by horse serum (known as serum sickness) developed within 36 to 48 hours of an injection and was characterized by a fever, aching joints, a rash, and sometimes the appearance of protein in the urine.

It is important to remember that passive immunization, although it provides protection immediately after the injection is given, does not last long and in no way protects the patient against the possibility of subsequent infection. For this reason the antitetanus serum (passive

This is done to get the utmost antibody response; it is the level of IgG antibody that is so important. After the first injection at three months, little change in antibody level occurs. After a second dose, however, there is a large increase, and after the third an even bigger one. Subsequent injections of the tetanus toxoid throughout a person's life will result in very large increases in antibody response, so the injections are used as boosters.

Yes, but this happens only when a live, as opposed to a dead, virus is used. For example, the first form of smallpox vaccination discovered in Turkey more than 300 years ago could itself cause smallpox. Later forms, however, were much safer. The virus used in the measles vaccination can cause a type of inflammation of the brain that may result in permanent damage to the patient. However, these side effects are very rare, and the odds are much in favor of vaccination.

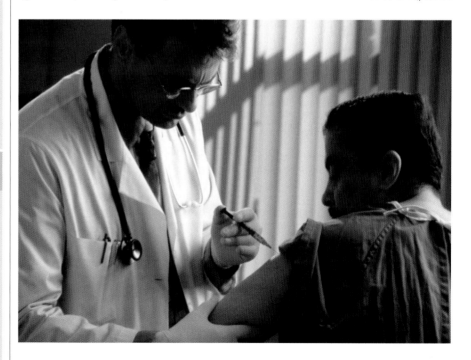

▲ *Influenza vaccines are prepared each year to match the prevailing virus strain. The vaccine is recommended for people at high risk, such as diabetics or the elderly.*

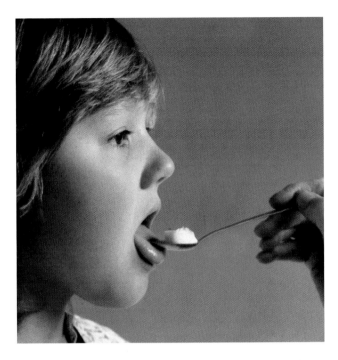

▲ *Polio vaccine can be given orally. In rare cases, oral polio vaccine has caused vaccine-associated paralytic poliomyelitis.*

immunization) is followed by an injection of tetanus toxoid (active immunization), unless the last injection of toxoid was given less than 10 years previously. (A toxoid is a harmful substance treated to destroy its harmful qualities but able to make antibodies when it is used in an injection form.) Passive immunization is used for a number of other diseases such as diphtheria, botulism, and rabies, but these are rare.

Active immunization

The earliest forms of protection against disease by immunization were practiced in Turkey over three centuries ago against poxvirus variolae, which caused the dreaded smallpox. The process was known as variolation and was first introduced into England in 1721. Inoculation was effected by scratching the skin of the patient with pus from the ulcers on the skin of a sufferer, thereby transmitting the infection. The disease transmitted in this way was usually less severe, and the patient survived infection to live with a permanent immunity to smallpox.

A much safer form of inoculation by injection of cowpox germs was introduced by an English country doctor, Edward Jenner, in the early 19th century. He noticed that farm laborers who suffered a mild disease known as cowpox—for it was from cows that the disease was contracted—developed a surprising resistance to smallpox. He reasoned that the cowpox germ was sufficiently similar in structure to the deadly smallpox germ for the antibody-producing system of the body to be fooled into making globulins that would kill both smallpox and cowpox germs. Jenner's method was so successful that the variolation method was banned in England in 1840.

The widespread use of smallpox vaccination has led to one of the great success stories of medicine; the last time smallpox was seen as a natural infection was in 1975. Since then there have been only two

cases, both in England and both the result of accidents in laboratories where strains of smallpox virus were kept for reference purposes. Since the disease has been wiped out, there is no further need for vaccination, and a certificate of vaccination is no longer necessary for people who travel abroad.

The principles of immunization by vaccination are now widely applied to a variety of infectious diseases. The injected material that is used to raise the antibody response and provide protection may be living or dead. In certain cases only a portion of it may be injected, for example, a protein derived from its cell wall. The live vaccines are made less vigorous by being grown in the laboratory for generations or by being grown in animals. The process by which the vigor of the vaccine is blunted is called attenuation. Live attenuated vaccines cause mild illnesses in the patient to whom they are given, and they are infectious.

Considering vaccinations

The decision to use vaccinations involves balancing the risks of the side effects of vaccination itself against the risks of suffering from the disease. Measles, for example, causes severe illness in one in every 15 patients, while the live and attenuated vaccine offers good protection and causes only a mild illness, sometimes with a rash, in 10 percent of patients. Mumps does not usually produce a severe illness and a vaccine is not as important as for other diseases.

Geographical location is also important. For example, it is not necessary to vaccinate against yellow fever or cholera in western Europe or Australasia, where both diseases are very rare.

Before long it should be possible to vaccinate against such diseases as HIV, melanoma, Lyme disease, anthrax, Ebola fever, eczema, psoriasis, and even smoking and some forms of cancer.

Diseases prevented by vaccination

The following diseases are most commonly prevented by vaccination.

Diphtheria, tetanus, whooping cough: Vaccines are prepared from dead bacteria and given mixed together as a single injection known as the triple vaccine. The first is given at the age of four months. The second and third doses are given at age six months and 12 months; a fourth dose is given at 15 to 18 months, and a final dose at four to six years. Thus full protection is provided at stages in the child's life at which he or she is most likely to encounter infection.

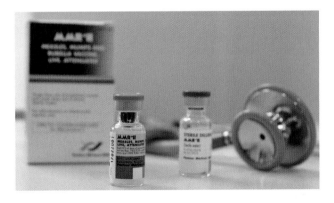

▲ *The triple vaccine (MMR) to immunize for measles, mumps, and rubella is given in two doses. The first dose is given at 12 to 15 months; the second dose is given at four to six years.*

Questions and Answers

Why doesn't the body become immune to some diseases?

There may be a number of reasons for this, the most important being that the infecting germ is capable of changing its structure, or that it may exist in many different forms. For example, the polio virus exists in three forms, and natural infection with one does not lead to immunity against the other two. The common cold is caused by about 200 different viruses, and it is very difficult to produce a vaccine against all of these.

Are flu shots truly effective against flu epidemics?

There is a good deal of evidence to suggest that people who have been vaccinated against influenza are less likely to get it and that if they do, their illness is less severe than in unvaccinated people. At the present time influenza is still regarded as a fairly trivial disease in healthy people; but for those who are elderly or sick, especially those with severe bronchitis, it is wise to have a flu injection before the start of winter.

To travel abroad do I need to get a vaccination against smallpox?

Smallpox was wiped out in 1975. There are now very few countries in the world that insist on a vaccination certificate. The last two cases of smallpox have both been in England—a country that does not require routine smallpox vaccination—and they resulted from laboratory accidents.

Does my child have to be vaccinated against tuberculosis?

No. There is no compulsion to have this vaccination, known as the BCG vaccine. In the United States the approach to controlling tuberculosis (TB) is to identify, by testing their skin, people who have been infected, but the use of BCG vaccine is no longer routinely recommended, despite the recent rise in the occurrence of TB.

Childhood vaccinations and immunizations

DISEASE	VACCINE	DOSE	AGE AND INTERVAL
Hepatitis B	Hep B	3	If mother hepatitis B-positive: 12 hours after birth plus hepatitis B immune globulin (HBIG), second dose at 1–2 months, third at 6 months. If mother hepatitis B-negative: first dose at 1–4 months, second at least 1 month later, third at least 4 months from first and after 6 months old.
Polio	Inactivated poliovirus vaccine (IPV); oral poliovirus vaccine (OPV)	4 / 2	First dose of IPV at 2 months old, second dose at 4 months old, third at 12–18 months old, fourth at 4–6 years; or After two doses of IPV at 2 months old and 4 months old, first dose of OPV at 4–6 months old, second dose at 4–6 years
Hemophilus influenza b (a cause of meningitis)	Hib	4	First dose at 2 months old, second dose at 4 months old, third at 6 months old, fourth at 12 months old
Diphtheria, tetanus, and pertussis (whooping cough)	Triple vaccine DTaP (or DTP)	5	First dose at 4 months old, second dose at 6 months old, third at 12 months old, fourth at 15 months old, fifth at 4–6 years
Measles, mumps, and rubella	Triple vaccine (MMR)	2	First dose at 12–15 months old, second dose at 4–6 years
Chicken pox	Varicella	1	At 12–18 months old

Polio: Polio vaccine is given either by injection as the inactivated poliovirus vaccine (IPV) or by mouth as the oral poliovirus vaccine (OPV). IPV is a killed, or dead, virus, whereas OPV combines a mixture of three types of live attenuated virus. Both vaccines give good protection against the three types of naturally occurring polio virus. However, since the OPV virus is live, in rare cases it has been known to cause vaccine-associated paralytic poliomyelitis (VAPP). In 2000 the Centers for Disease Control and Prevention (CDC) recommended that OPV not be given routinely and that only IPV be given. Outbreaks of polio still sometimes occur in Western countries, and it is wise to revaccinate during these outbreaks.

Rubella (German measles): Infection with German measles in the first three months of pregnancy frequently results in the birth of an abnormal baby. Immunization should be given before childbearing age to all girls who have not already contracted the disease; this gives them lifelong immunity.

Tuberculosis: Many people acquire a degree of immunity to tuberculosis naturally by early, inapparent, and harmless infection. For those who do not, it has, in the past, been the practice to confer partial immunity with Bacille Calmette-Guerin (BCG) vaccine. Immunity can be tested by using a skin sensitivity test called the Mantoux reaction test. BCG is now rarely used in the United States, and there is currently no legal requirement for the vaccination. In recent years, however, the prevalence of tuberculosis has risen again to an extent that is causing concern.

Meningitis: Hib conjugate vaccine (also called HbCV) gives protection against infection by hemophilus influenza type b, which is the leading cause of bacterial meningitis. It is given in four doses, ideally at two, four, six, and 12 months of age.

See also: Antibiotics; Infection and infectious diseases; Measles; Mumps; Rabies; Rubella; Tetanus; Tuberculosis; Vaccinations

Infection and infectious diseases

Questions and Answers

Is there any difference between an infectious and a contagious disease?

A contagious disease is one that is caught by touching an infectious person, but people use the word "contagious" to mean infectious.

I heard that you can catch some forms of cancer. Is this true?

No, you cannot catch cancer from another person. However, viruses may be involved in the irregular division of cells that is the basic abnormality in cancer. For instance, in African children the Epstein-Barr virus causes Burkitt's lymphoma. Viruses may also be involved in producing cancer of the cervix.

Are childhood diseases more severe in adults?

Generally, yes, although this does not apply to all childhood illnesses. It is especially true of mumps, which can cause severe inflammation of the testes in men; and chicken pox, which can cause severe pneumonia.

Is it possible to have a disease without knowing it?

Yes. Some people may be exposed to an infection and gain immunity to it without developing the full-blown symptoms of the disease. This is a subclinical infection, and it seems to occur in young children with mumps, and in many people with rubella (German measles).

Can I catch diseases from animals?

Yes. Birds, dogs, and insects carry infections that can be transmitted to humans, but only people who work with animals are at high risk.

Infectious diseases caused by microorganisms were once the most common cause of death. Improved sanitation, housing, and hygiene, and the use of vaccines, antibiotics, and other drugs have greatly reduced mortality rates.

Infections occur when an infecting organism invades the body, and they can range from minor ailments—such as colds and the flu—to illnesses that are invariably fatal, such as rabies. An infection may be localized, affecting only a small area of the body (an abscess, for example) or a single system (the way that pneumonia affects the lungs), or it may be generalized, affecting a greater part of the body, as in septicemia.

Causes

The tiny organisms that cause infections are too small to be seen with the naked eye; they are therefore called microorganisms. Most infections are caused by two different types of microorganism—the virus and the bacterium.

A virus consists of an outer shell of protein with a core of genetic material (DNA or RNA). When this genetic material infects a cell, it instructs the cell to make other viruses, and in this way the virus reproduces itself. Thus viruses are not really complete organisms, since they are unable to maintain a separate existence outside the cells of another living entity. Many viruses infect humans, and there are also viruses that infect animals, plants, and even bacteria.

In contrast, bacteria are single-cell organisms that can exist quite happily away from other living things. Many types live in the soil and do not cause any infections, and others commonly live in or on the body. For example, many bacteria inhabit the colon, where they do no harm and may even be helpful, preventing the growth of other, more dangerous bacteria. These are called commensal (literally, "eating with") bacteria. Of those bacteria that cause infections, some may enter body cells during the course of the infection, whereas others remain outside.

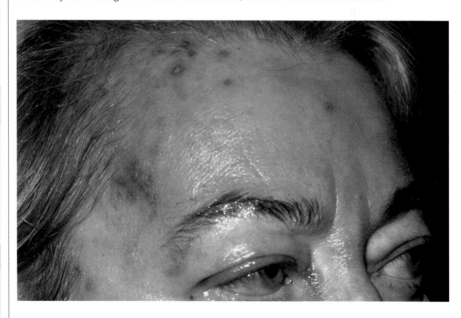

▲ *The lesions of shingles are the result of a renewed outbreak of varicella-zoster virus infection—the first time around, the virus causes chicken pox.*

185

I seem to catch one infection after another. Could there be something wrong with the way my body copes with infection?

People vary in their ability to fight off infections, but if you have had one, your resistance is lowered and you are more likely to catch another. So even if you do seem to have nasty runs of infections, you are probably quite normal in the way you respond to them.

Viral infections also tend to leave the way open for further infection by a bacterium. This is why some people with diseases such as chronic bronchitis take antibiotics at the first sign of any cold. Although the antibiotics do not help to treat the cold, they may stop it from spreading to the chest as a bacterial infection.

Could I catch AIDS from someone at work or socially?

The virus that causes AIDS is not infectious in that it cannot be caught as a result of someone's coughing or sneezing, or by using the same cup or toilet. Neither has shaking hands or hugging been found to be a source of infection. Do not, however, share items that could carry blood, such as razors or toothbrushes; and if you are looking after an infected person, cover cuts on your own skin with a waterproof dressing and avoid contact with the patient's blood or any other body fluid.

I can't stand having colds or the flu. Why can't scientists develop a vaccine against them?

Many different viruses cause the common cold, so even if a vaccine were to be successful against one sort, it would not protect against all the others.

Influenza has the capacity to change the way it appears to the body's immune system, so if you have the flu one year, you will not necessarily be immune the next year. The makers of a flu vaccine have to try to predict which strain is likely to be present in any year and to produce a vaccine against that one.

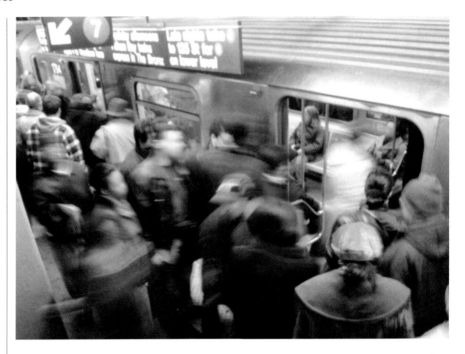

▲ *People should try to avoid coughing or sneezing in crowds if they have a cold, because they may infect others by releasing infectious droplets into the air.*

A third type of infective microorganism is the protozoan, which is a larger single-cell organism. Malaria is caused by a protozoan called plasmodium.

A further class of infecting organisms are the fungi. Fungal diseases include thrush (candidiasis); athlete's foot (tinea pedis); other similar fungal infections of the skin, such as ringworm (tinea corporis), jock itch (tinea cruris), and kerion or scalp tinea (tinea capitis); and the lung infection histoplasmosis. Internal fungal infections are uncommon except in people with severe immunodeficiency disorders, such as those with AIDS, those with congenital immune deficiencies, and those who have received immunosuppressive treatment after organ grafting. In these people, internal fungal infections frequently occur.

How infections begin

Once a microorganism has entered the body, it reproduces itself using the plentifully available supply of nutrient substances as its food source. Viruses, which usually spread through the body via the bloodstream, go one stage further by using the chemical building apparatus of the cells to build new viruses. The symptoms of the disease usually start as the cells release a second wave of viruses. In contrast, a bacterium reproduces simply by splitting in two.

Microorganisms can cause disease in a number of different ways, but only if they interfere sufficiently with normal body processes. Potentially dangerous organisms may be present in considerable numbers without causing enough change in the body to produce symptoms. In these cases the people infected may be carriers of the disease.

One of the most important properties of disease-causing microorganisms is invasiveness, or the ability to make their way across tissue planes into new areas. They are able to do this because they produce chemical activators called enzymes. One of these enzymes, called hyaluronidase, breaks down hyaluronic acid, the substance that glues together the cells of connective tissue. Thus organisms that synthesize this enzyme can spread rapidly through body tissues. Other bacterial enzymes can break down the protein collagen, an important structural protein in the body, and this breakdown also enables bacteria to spread rapidly. Other bacteria produce enzymes that dissolve blood clots by breaking down the fibrin of which the clots are made, and some produce enzymes that destroy red blood cells and various tissue cells.

The principal way in which microorganisms cause disease is by producing poisonous substances called toxins. Most of these are endotoxins—they are released when the

HOW INFECTIONS OCCUR

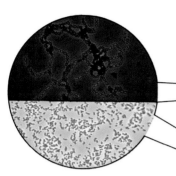

The throat infection bacterium and pneumonia bacterium are transmitted by droplet infection and cause inflammation of the throat and lungs.

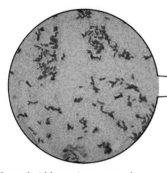

The typhoid bacterium enters the intestines through infected water or food and causes a generalized illness.

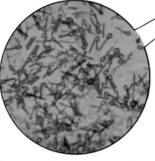

The tetanus bacterium enters through a skin wound. By producing a toxin, it causes a generalized illness that particularly affects the nervous system.

An infection arises when bacteria, viruses, protozoa, or fungi enter the body, establish themselves, and multiply. The point of entry varies according to the type of invading organism, the manner of transmission, and the suitability of the site for breeding.

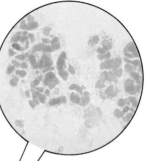

The typhus rickettsia, carried by a louse, tick, or flea bite, produces a rash and a generalized illness.

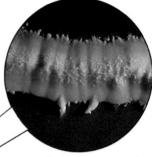

A yeast infection is transmitted by sexual contact or contracted from infected towels and induces a vaginal discharge.

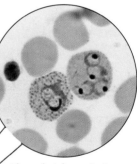

The malarial parasite is contracted from an infected mosquito bite and multiplies in the blood cells, producing a fever.

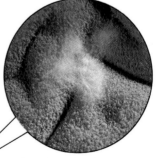

The athlete's foot fungus is picked up from infected ground or towels and causes itchy, peeling skin.

Infectious diseases and their treatment

DISEASE	CAUSE	HOW TRANSFERRED	IMMUNIZATION	SYMPTOMS	TREATMENT
AIDS	Virus	Contact with infected blood, sexual intercourse	No	Resistance to infection reduced	Antiviral drugs, HIV protease inhibitors
Chicken pox	Virus	Person to person	Yes	Rash	Antiviral drugs
Common cold	Virus (many types)	Person to person	No	Runny nose	None
Diphtheria	Bacterium	Person to person	Yes	Obstructed throat, localized paralysis	Antibiotics
Gonorrhea	Bacterium	Sexual intercourse	No	Genital discharge	Antibiotics
Hepatitis	Virus (at least 3 types)	May be via skin, via infected food, or by sexual transmission	Available for type A and type B	Jaundice	Antiviral drugs. Chronic hepatitis B can be treated with an interferon
Influenza	Virus (many types give flulike illness)	Person to person	Yes, but not 100 percent effective	Cold, sore throat, muscle aches	Amantadine
Legionnaires' disease	Bacterium	Air-conditioning or water systems	No	Pneumonia, general ill health	Antibiotics
Malaria	Protozoa (3 types)	Mosquito bite	No	Fever	Antimalarial drugs
Measles	Virus	Person to person	Yes	Runny nose and eyes, rash, ill health	None
Meningitis	Virus (many types) or meningococcus (bacterium)	Person to person	For meningitis caused by hemophilus	Neck pain, pain on looking at light, drowsiness	Nursing care for viral, antibiotics for bacterial
Mumps	Virus	Person to person	No	Swollen glands	None
Pneumonia	Bronchopneumonia (usually bacterial, may be viral)	Person to person	No	Cough	Antibiotics
	Lobar pneumonia (bacterial)	Person to person	Yes, for patients at risk	Cough and chest pain	Antibiotics
Ringworm	Fungus	Person to person (contact required)	No	Skin rash	Antifungal drugs applied to skin
SARS	Virus	Person to person	No	Fever, body aches, dry cough	None
Syphilis	Bacterium	Sexual intercourse	No	Many symptoms, often years later	Penicillin
Tetanus	Bacterium (disease caused by poison)	Soil infection of wounds	Yes	Lockjaw and other spasms	Antitoxin; respirator support if necessary
Tuberculosis	Bacterium	Person to person, by infected phlegm	Yes (varying effectiveness)	Cough with blood (affects lungs)	Special antibiotics
Typhoid	Bacterium	Infected food or water	Yes	Fever, headache, and later diarrhea	Antibiotics
Typhus	Rickettsia (different types)	By lice, ticks, or fleas	No	Fever, rash	Antibiotics and tetracycline
Yeast infection	Fungus	Sexual intercourse or from infected towels	No	Irritating white genital discharge	Antifungal drugs

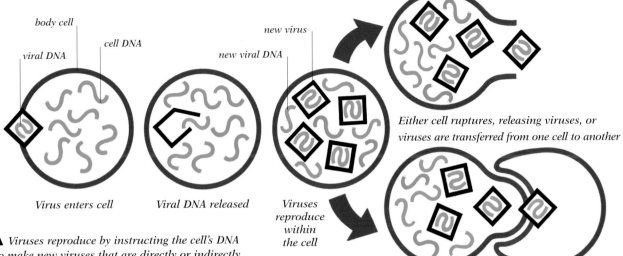

▲ Viruses reproduce by instructing the cell's DNA to make new viruses that are directly or indirectly transferred to other cells.

body cell

viral DNA

cell DNA

new virus

new viral DNA

Virus enters cell

Viral DNA released

Viruses reproduce within the cell

Either cell ruptures, releasing viruses, or viruses are transferred from one cell to another

microorganism dies and its cell membrane ruptures, and they operate only at the site of the colonies of organisms. Others are called exotoxins because they may be carried in the bloodstream to remote parts of the body. This is the case with diphtheria: the bacteria remain in the throat but produce exotoxins that can severely damage the nervous system, the heart, and various other organs. Bacterial toxins that damage the intestine, such as those that cause cholera and typhoid, are called enterotoxins.

Bacterial toxins act in various ways, all of them damaging. They can interfere with vital processes in the cells and lead to cell death; interfere with the body's synthesis of proteins; block transmission of nerve impulses and hence cause paralysis; damage the lining of blood vessels so that they lose so much fluid that the heart cannot maintain the circulation (shock); interfere with the action of vital body enzymes; cause red blood cells to rupture; and produce severe inflammation of various tissues, especially the lining of the intestine. Bacterial toxins are among the most poisonous substances known, and even in minute quantities they can cause serious illness and death. For instance, it has been estimated that 0.035 ounce (1 g) of botulinum toxin could kill more than 200 million people—nearly the entire population of the United States.

The damaging effects of viruses differ from those of bacteria. Viruses do not produce toxins but can kill cells by multiplying so vigorously within them that the sheer bulk of viral material bursts the cells; by coding for "fusion proteins," which cause cells to join together to form highly abnormal giant cells; and by forming new markers on the surface of cells that label those cells as foreign and cause the normal processes of the immune system to attack and destroy them.

Infectious organisms and disease

Many infectious organisms tend to infect only one organ. For instance, the hepatitis virus lodges in the liver; the pneumococcus bacterium causes pneumonia in the lungs; and the meningococcus bacterium, which causes meningitis, results in an inflammation of the meninges covering the brain. Why organisms show this preference is unknown.

Other organisms may produce disease in any system by circulating in the blood and settling in organs far away from the point of entry. For example, the staphylococcus bacterium can multiply and produce an abscess (a pus-containing cavity surrounded by inflamed tissue).

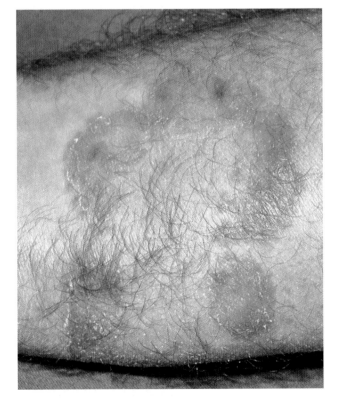

▲ Fungal infections of the skin, such as ringworm, cause redness and itching. Internal fungal infections are uncommon.

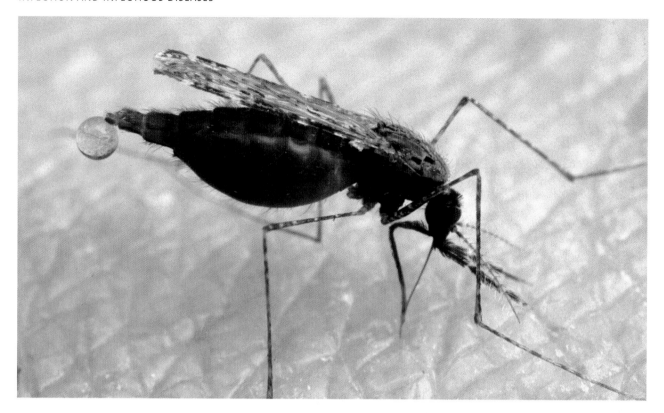

▲ *Mosquitoes transmit malaria by piercing human skin with their proboscis, allowing the protozoan that causes the disease to enter the bloodstream.*

Finally, the toxins produced by bacteria may poison particular areas of the body: tetanus produces a toxin that affects the nervous system, and cholera produces a toxin that causes severe diarrhea.

How the body defends itself

The primary barrier against infection is the skin, and most infectious organisms enter the body either through a break in the skin or by entering the respiratory tract or the alimentary (digestive) tract. Once inside the body, the organism may be consumed by a phagocytic cell—a type of white blood cell (although there are similar cells in other tissues) that swallows up and destroys viruses and bacteria. In some cases both the organism and the phagocyte die, leading to the production of pus, which is simply an accumulation of dead organisms and phagocytes. The activity and effectiveness of phagocytes depend on the health of the immune system, the body's complex defense system, but this will not work properly if AIDS is present.

The immune system combats invasion by foreign organisms in three main ways. First, it produces an inflammatory reaction. Second, it produces antibodies: protein molecules that travel in blood and tissues and bind to the surface of specific organisms, making it easier for the phagocytic cells to attack. Antibodies may also prevent organisms from being effective; for example, they may stop viruses from entering cells. Finally, antibodies may trigger a system that breaks down invading cells. The third method is called cell-mediated immunity. The cells of this system, T lymphocytes, come from the lymphatic system and may be specially primed to kill particular organisms. They may also produce substances that help phagocytes attack infecting organisms.

Immune response

In many diseases, a large part of the problem results from the interaction between the infecting organism and the body's defense mechanism. For example, in pneumonia, the production of large amounts of phlegm is often the leading symptom of the disease, although it is really a result of the immune response. Similarly, the lung destruction that may follow from tuberculosis is primarily caused by the immune response rather than the disease itself.

Treatment

One of medicine's major contributions to health has been the development of vaccines. Vaccines contain substances that cause the immune system to react to a specific disease without producing the disease itself. Most vaccines use dead bacteria or viruses that have the same cell wall structure as the live organism and so cause antibody production.

Antibiotics have also made a huge difference in the treatment of infection. These drugs are toxic to bacteria but not to human cells, and they often act by interfering with the bacterial cell wall, which has a different structure from human cell walls. They are ineffective against viruses and some protozoa, so other types of drugs must be used in such cases.

> *See also:* **Antibiotics; Bacteria; Pneumonia; Ringworm; Tetanus; Tuberculosis; Viruses**

Influenza

Influenza is one of the most common illnesses and one of the most infectious. What can be done to guard against catching flu and to keep attacks to a minimum?

Influenza, commonly known as "flu," often occurs in epidemics: many people catch it at once. This usually happens in the winter, but people can get flu at any time of the year.

Cause

The virus that causes influenza has an unusual characteristic; it is always changing its appearance to fool the body's defense mechanisms. The virus changes every year by a process called drift, and this results in outbreaks of flu. Every 30 to 40 years a bigger change, known as shift, takes place, during which a different virus appears and causes a worldwide epidemic, or pandemic. Occasionally, the flu virus changes to a form that resembles a former virus; when this happens, people who were infected by the first virus are immune to the second one because they have memory cells that recognize and destroy the invader.

Influenza is transmitted from person to person by coughing and sneezing. Droplets of secretions containing the virus from the infected person are breathed in by someone who is not infected, and this person starts to have the symptoms from one to three days later.

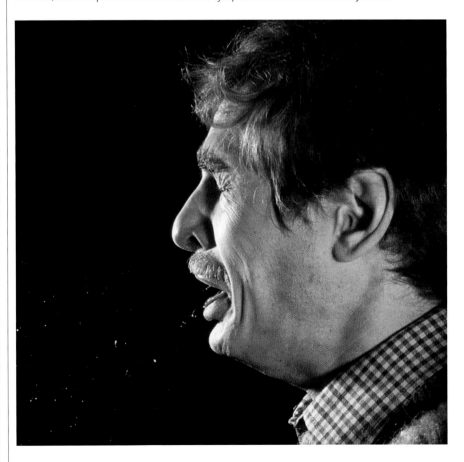

▲ *When a person infected with the influenza virus sneezes, water is expelled from the nose and spreads in tiny droplets, which may be breathed in by anyone in the vicinity.*

191

If you get flu
Go to bed and keep warm.
Drink plenty of fluids; fluids are much more important than food. Drinks containing sugar provide some energy.
Take one or two acetaminophen pills every four hours to relieve aches and lower temperature.
Be careful to cough and sneeze into a handkerchief to limit the spread of infection.
When your temperature returns to normal, get up; but take things easy for a few days.
If your fever lasts more than three to four days or is higher than 102°F (39°C), ask your doctor for advice.

The role of animals in the spread of influenza is not well known. Although domestic pets do not carry the disease, there is some evidence that farm animals—for example, horses, hens, and pigs—can develop an illness similar to influenza. The pig is thought to act as a potential carrier of swine influenza, which caused a pandemic between 1918 and 1919.

Scientists have studied antibodies in the blood of people born from the 1850s onward. They found that the influenza epidemics of 1889–1890, 1918–1919, 1946–1947, 1957, and 1968 were all variants of one virus, the A virus—the first to be discovered. (There are three main types of viruses, A, B, and C.)

The ability of influenza viruses from different species to swap genetic material and form new, deadly viruses has led to past influenza pandemics. In 2009, a virus containing genes from swine, birds, and humans became the first pandemic of the 21st century with predictions that it could infect as much as one-third of the world's human population.

Early in 2009, human cases of infection with a novel H1N1 influenza virus were identified in Mexico. This new virus had a unique combination of human, swine, and avian (bird) genes, an assortment that was quite different from past circulating influenza strains. Because of the presence of swine flu genes, this influenza virus was initially referred to as "swine flu." By April, this new type A influenza virus reached the United States and within several weeks became so widespread that the World Health Organization declared that a pandemic was underway as the virus continued to spread in significant numbers from person to person around the world.

Symptoms
Flu symptoms come on suddenly, with shivering and generalized aching in the arms, legs, and back. The patient may have a headache, aching eyes, a sore or dry throat, and sometimes a cough and a runny nose. Occasionally there may also be the symptoms of a stomach upset, with vomiting and diarrhea. The body temperature at this point is above normal, usually between 101°F (38.4°C) and 102°F (39°C). The symptoms and fever continue for two to five days and leave the patient feeling tired and weak. After the symptoms have

subsided, he or she may also feel depressed and fatigued. A sufferer should be reassured that this feeling is quite normal after flu and may last a few weeks. The cough may also persist for one to two weeks after the other symptoms have disappeared.

If a patient with flu is examined by a doctor when he or she is ill, there is usually little sign of illness, except for a fever and an inflamed throat. These are the classic signs of flu. If a patient has some immunity, he or she may often have a milder illness with fewer symptoms and only a small rise in temperature.

The difference in immunity explains why some people get a worse case of the disease than others, and why some people who have been in very close contact with an infected person may not feel ill at all. People become immune once they have had influenza because their body's defense mechanism recognizes the virus when it reappears and so prevents it from multiplying. However, this recognition does not happen if the flu virus has altered its appearance.

Complications
Influenza can strike all age groups, but the elderly, babies, young children, those with reduced immunity, and those who have heart or lung problems are particularly prone to complications of the flu. The most common complication is a chest infection. This can vary from a mild cough to pneumonia. Sometimes the virus itself causes this, but more commonly another opportunistic germ enters the body, which has been weakened by flu, and infects the chest. Older people and those who already have chest trouble are more likely to develop a chest infection after an attack of the flu.

If the flu patient has a severe cough, is producing green or yellow phlegm, has chest pains, or feels breathless, it is best to call the doctor. People who have other things wrong with them—for example, chest trouble, heart disease, or kidney problems—should let their doctor know if they catch the flu, because he or she may want to give them an antibiotic to prevent complications. If an attack of flu seems prolonged and the patient is not making normal progress, the patient should see a doctor.

In rare cases the influenza virus can cause severe pneumonia, or pneumonia can be caused by another germ, which invades the body when it is already undermined by the flu. In very severe cases of the flu virus itself, the heart or brain can be affected.

Treatment and prevention
The drugs amantadine, tamiflu, and zanamivir are effective against influenza if given within the first 24 to 48 hours. However, because the flu virus is always changing, drugs do not always work, which is why antiviral medications are not substitutes for the vaccine.

Vaccination
Although the flu virus changes, vaccination is still useful, especially in communities such as schools, factories, and retirement or nursing homes. It is also used to prevent flu in people who are elderly or likely to develop serious complications because of another illness, such as chest trouble. The flu injection is given in a single dose in the fall. It usually has no side effects, but it can make the arm sore or cause a slight rise in temperature that may last for up to 24 hours.

See also: Fevers; Infection and infectious diseases; Pneumonia; Vaccinations; Viruses

Iron

Questions and Answers

Do you lose iron if you give blood regularly?

Yes. If you give blood once every three months, you lose about twice as much iron as normal, but a good mixed diet will replace the loss.

Is it true that spinach contains a lot of iron?

Spinach contains about 4 mg of iron per 3.5 oz. (100 g) of spinach, which is a moderate amount. Unrefined flour and dried peas and beans contain more iron than most green vegetables, as does meat. The iron in meat is also more easily absorbed by the intestine than the iron in vegetables.

After my doctor gave me iron pills my feces turned an odd black color. Is this normal?

Yes. Black feces are a common side effect of taking iron supplements. Iron may also cause diarrhea and constipation, but generally any side effects are minimal.

Should I take iron pills while I am having a period?

No. A mixed diet should provide adequate iron, even for women who are having a period or who are pregnant, except occasionally during the last four months of pregnancy. However, vegetarian women may find it necessary to take iron supplements during their reproductive years.

Is it true that iron pills are dangerous for children?

It is unusual for children to suffer from anemia due to iron deficiency, but they can be given iron under medical supervision. However, iron pills can poison children if an overdose is taken, so they should be kept well out of children's reach.

Just as iron plays a vital role in industry, its presence in the body is essential for good health. Various problems can arise when a deficiency occurs, but the right diet and iron supplements can restore the balance.

The body contains about 0.1 ounce (3–4 g) of the chemical element iron. This cannot be produced in the body, so, to stay healthy, people must eat some foods containing iron.

Seventy percent of the iron in the body is found in the red blood cells that circulate in the bloodstream, with a further small amount in the bone marrow. In the red blood cells, iron is an essential ingredient of hemoglobin, which is responsible for the vital activity of carrying oxygen from the lungs to the body tissues. Iron also gives blood its red coloring. Another 20 percent of the iron is stored in the liver and the spleen, much of it in the form of ferritin—an iron-containing protein. A small amount of the body's iron is not concerned with the manufacture of hemoglobin but is involved in other important cellular functions, and many of the enzymes that regulate a normal cell's activity depend upon it.

Iron deficiency

Anemia is a blood disorder involving the red blood cells, and anemia caused by iron deficiency is one of the most common deficiency disorders in women, although it rarely occurs in healthy men. This is because women lose iron regularly in the blood shed during menstruation, and tend not to take enough iron in their diet to replace it. The condition may result in tiredness, breathlessness, and a general feeling of ill health.

Iron deficiency anemia in children, men, or postmenopausal women suggests that there is a problem elsewhere. For instance, there may be a slow-bleeding duodenal ulcer or hemorrhoids or, particularly in children, some disease causing abnormal iron absorption from food in the intestine.

Iron deficiency can also cause ridges and brittleness in the nails—which may become spoon-shaped in severe cases—soreness at the corners of the mouth, and thinning of the lining of the esophagus and stomach, in turn causing indigestion.

Iron loss

The main cause of iron loss is through bleeding. However, since iron is also widely distributed in the tissues, the shedding of cells from surfaces such as the skin and the lining of the intestine

▼ *Egg yolks and spinach are both good sources of dietary iron.*

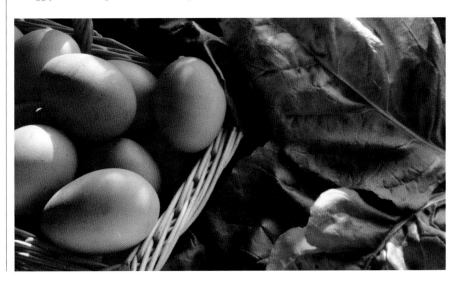

Foods containing iron

The recommended iron intake is 10 mg per day for children and adults; a doctor may prescribe iron supplements for women during pregnancy and for iron deficiency anemia.

Iron levels are given in milligrams per 3.5 oz. (100 g) of food, but these levels are subject to variation, particularly in the vegetables, because of the variable amount of iron in the soil.

Food	Iron level
Liver	6.0–14.10
Beef	2.0–4.5
Eggs	2.0–3.0
Milk	0.1–4.5
Lentils	1.9–14.0
Unrefined wheat flour	3.0
Refined wheat flour	0.7–1.5
Parsley	8.0
Spinach	4.0 approx.
Other green vegetables	very variable
Lettuce	0.8
Potatoes and root vegetables	0.3–2.0

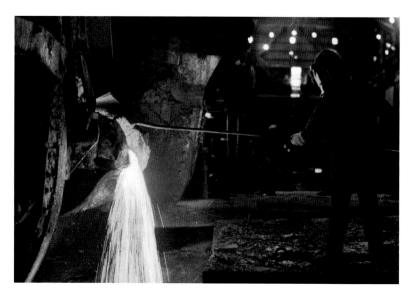

▲ *The iron used in industry is the same basic chemical element as the iron found in the body. When metals are combined with other chemicals they produce salts, and such salt is the form in which iron is absorbed into the body. This type of iron is known biologically as ferrous salts. The best source of iron in the food that people eat is red meat, particularly liver.*

also leads to iron loss. The total amount lost in this way is about 1 mg per day, and since the normal iron stores in the body are reasonably large, it would take a healthy man about three years to develop iron deficiency anemia. In women, however, menstrual bleeding amounts to a further loss of about 1 mg per day, so, at this time, women normally lose about twice as much iron as men.

Iron loss in a woman is also increased during pregnancy, when the developing fetus and the placenta absorb much of her iron stores. Her total daily iron requirement is almost double that of other women during the reproductive years.

This requirement is particularly high during the last four months of pregnancy, when a great deal of iron goes into building the blood volume of the baby ready for birth. During these four months up to 7.5 mg of iron is required per day. For this reason iron supplements are frequently prescribed, although usually not until after the fourteenth week of pregnancy, since iron pills can disturb the intestine, causing either constipation or diarrhea, occasionally nausea, and in some cases, vomiting.

Iron absorption

Iron is absorbed from the small intestine. The usual rate of absorption is about 1 mg per day, and this balances normal losses. The fact that iron loss and iron absorption are set in this critical balance, however, explains why it is relatively easy for a person to have an iron deficiency, and therefore why this is a relatively common complaint.

Iron in food is found mainly in red meat, particularly liver. There is also a considerable amount in lentils and in unrefined wheat flour. Purified white flour contains less iron, although iron is artificially added to flour and to many breakfast cereals.

Only about 10 percent of the iron people eat is absorbed by the body, although this proportion may be higher when there is an iron deficiency. People should ingest about 10 mg of iron per day, since the normal loss is about 1 mg. Menstruating women obviously need more, however, and should try to eat more iron-rich foods.

Detecting iron deficiency

Severe anemia is immediately obvious because the sufferer becomes very pale. Less severe cases can be detected by blood tests. If there is a low hemoglobin level in the blood, a lack of iron can be confirmed by looking at the red blood cells under a microscope. When iron deficiency anemia is present, the red blood cells become smaller; in other types of anemia they tend to enlarge or remain of normal size. The level of iron in the blood can also be measured to avoid confusion. Treatment is with iron pills, which are taken by the patient until the level of hemoglobin is back to normal. This will be confirmed by a blood test.

Excess iron

Iron overload in the system can occur for a number of reasons, including excessive iron absorption from the intestine, or the genetic disorder hemochromatosis. Excess iron may affect the liver, causing cirrhosis, and it may accumulate in the pancreas, giving rise to diabetes, or in the testes, which may then cease to produce male hormones.

The treatment for iron overload is repeated removal of blood at intervals. This effectively lowers the level of iron in the body. Once cirrhosis of the liver has been established, repeated removal of iron will not cure the condition, but less iron may help to slow down the progress of the disease.

See also: Anemia; Diabetes; Diet; Minerals; Ulcers

Lacerations

Questions and Answers

My husband had his spleen removed after it sustained a laceration in a car crash. Why wasn't it just repaired?

A ruptured spleen is almost impossible to repair because it contains so many blood vessels and bleeds profusely. The only safe thing to do is to tie off the splenic artery and remove the spleen. A person without a spleen is more susceptible to certain infections.

I lacerated my hand and severed a nerve. The surgeons stitched the nerve together, but there is still a numb area. Why is this?

When a nerve is completely severed, only the central portion survives. New fibers will grow out from this living portion, and the severed nerve ends are stitched together to guide these new fibers down the course of the old nerve. This is a slow process, and it may be months before the fibers grow all the way and sensation returns. Nerves can regenerate at a rate of about 0.04 in. (1 mm) per day.

I am expecting my first baby and have heard that an episiotomy is almost routine. Is this procedure absolutely necessary?

An episiotomy is done only when necessary. The object is to prevent vaginal tearing; this may be more extensive and damaging than the controlled incision of an episiotomy.

When I hurt my hand in the garden, my doctor said I must have an antitetanus shot. Why was this?

The organism that causes tetanus, *Clostridium tetani*, is found in soil. It causes disease by producing a toxin that affects the nervous system. *C. tetani* is an anaerobic organism and will flourish only deep in wounds where the supply of oxygen is poor.

Lacerations are wounds where the skin is torn rather than cut. As it takes great force to tear the skin, lacerations are often serious. Internal organs can suffer laceration, too, in which case prompt medical treatment is essential.

Wounds are traditionally divided into five kinds—scratches, abrasions, cuts, lacerations, and puncture wounds. The distinction between cuts and lacerations is often unclear, but in general a cut is a neat incision through the skin, usually caused by a sharp object, such as a knife, whereas a laceration is usually caused by a blunt instrument, leaving a ragged wound with crushing and bruising of the surrounding tissue.

The damage a laceration inflicts depends on the area of the body involved. Lacerations of the hand, for instance, frequently involve damage to the tendons or nerves. On the arms and legs, the impact that causes a laceration may be enough to break a bone. This sort of injury needs immediate medical attention, because if bone is exposed it always becomes infected, making the injury worse. Scalp lacerations bleed profusely because of the rich blood supply to the head, but a rich blood supply also mean that such injuries tend to heal more quickly. Lacerations involving the eyelids or lips need careful treatment so as not to disfigure the person.

Internal damage

The term "laceration" is also applied to damage sustained by internal organs in major injuries, such as lacerations of the spleen and liver. Such lacerations may occur in one of two ways. A violent compression, such as a kick in the abdomen, can cause a ragged tear and profuse internal bleeding. A forceful impact, as in a car collision, could also produce lacerations of major organs.

SKIN LACERATION

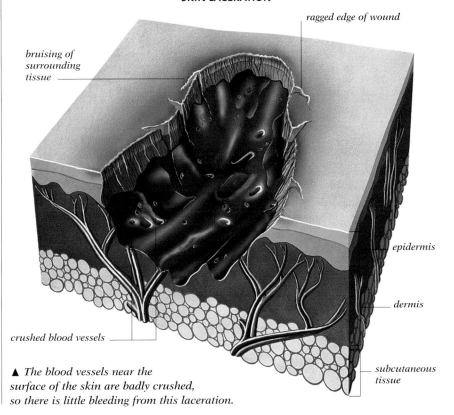

bruising of surrounding tissue

ragged edge of wound

epidermis

dermis

crushed blood vessels

subcutaneous tissue

▲ *The blood vessels near the surface of the skin are badly crushed, so there is little bleeding from this laceration.*

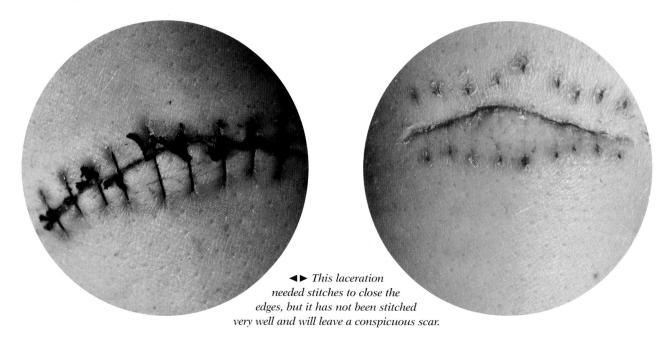

◄► *This laceration needed stitches to close the edges, but it has not been stitched very well and will leave a conspicuous scar.*

Lacerations usually have a ragged edge, and the surrounding skin is bruised. They may bleed only a little, because blood vessels are crushed. Slanting blows may raise a flap of skin; this is particularly likely to happen on the scalp.

Lacerations on the hands are likely to affect nerves or tendons; this effect will be indicated by a loss of some movement, by a loss of feeling, or by a pins and needles sensation. Prompt treatment is essential to avoid disability.

Liver and spleen lacerations are usually indicated by a severe and constant pain in the abdomen; in the case of a laceration to the spleen, there may also be a pain in the shoulder. If the lacerations are severe, there will be internal bleeding, and the patient will be in a state of shock—the skin becoming cold and clammy, and the pulse rapid and weak. An immediate blood transfusion is needed.

Lacerations of the vagina can occur during a difficult birth. If an episiotomy (a surgical cut across the muscle surrounding the opening of the vagina) is not done, the risk of laceration increases. Any laceration of the vagina becomes evident immediately after the delivery, with bright red bleeding from the vagina. Vaginal tears are usually repaired immediately. If the cervix is torn, this usually requires repair only if the bleeding persists.

Treatment

Minor lacerations can usually be treated at home with an antiseptic solution; first, ensure that any dirt is removed. A simple dry dressing is best, because antiseptic ointments left on the wound may make it moist and delay the healing process.

If the laceration is serious, the patient should go to an emergency room. There the wound will be examined to see if any underlying structures have been damaged. If they have not, the wound will be cleaned and foreign material removed. Stitches may be needed.

When important areas have been damaged, the repair will be carried out in an operating room. Sometimes lacerations involve a loss of skin, and a skin graft may be needed at a later date. If internal injuries are suspected, an intravenous infusion may be set up in case a blood transfusion is needed. An abdominal tap may also be performed. A special needle is inserted into the abdominal cavity to take a fluid sample. Liver or spleen lacerations produce a bloody tap.

Most surface lacerations heal within two weeks. Some scar tissue is inevitable, but usually this tissue will become as strong as intact skin. The outlook for an internal laceration depends on its seriousness and how quickly it is treated. Blood transfusion and early surgery to stem bleeding will prevent shock.

What to do
For serious lacerations, call emergency services immediately.
Minor lacerations can be cleaned at home with antiseptic.
Take care not to do more damage. If bleeding is profuse, direct pressure over the wound with a gauze pad or another clean cloth for at least 10 minutes will usually control it.
Laceration of internal organs is usually indicated by a severe pain in the abdomen. If this injury is suspected, call an ambulance immediately. The patient should not have anything to eat or drink, since an anesthetic may be needed.
Foreign bodies, such as metal or broken glass, are best left where they are for a doctor to treat.
If a fracture is suspected, cover the wound and keep the limb still until emergency services arrive.

See also: Abrasions and cuts

Leukemia

Leukemia is a relatively rare disease that affects the blood. Advances in the treatment of leukemia are being made all the time. In some cases it can be cured, and in all cases the patient's life can be prolonged.

Questions and Answers

Can leukemia run in families? My uncle died of leukemia and my father worries that he will die too.

There are a few unusual hereditary diseases that are associated with an increased incidence of leukemia. These are mainly immunodeficiency diseases and those associated with an abnormal fragility of chromosomes. Both of these conditions are rare.

I have heard that X rays can cause leukemia. Is this really the case?

Yes, this is true, but even if you have undergone X rays on many, many occasions it is very unlikely that you will be at an increased risk. People who spend their lives taking X rays have only a slightly increased risk of developing any form of leukemia. In contrast, those who have been heavily exposed to radiation, such as the survivors of the atomic bomb that was dropped on Hiroshima in 1945, have a greatly increased risk.

My friend's brother has developed leukemia. Is this very serious?

Yes, sadly, it is. The outlook for lymphocytic leukemia is better these days, and in some cases a cure can result. However, the outlook for acute myeloid leukemia is not so good. It is always better to have the disease treated in centers where special facilities for treatment are available.

I have been told that leukemia is caused by a virus. Is this true?

One form of leukemia, epidemic in the southeastern United States, the Caribbean, and Japan, has been shown to be caused by a virus called human T-cell leukemia virus type II (HTLV II). Leukemias that occur in animals, such as feline leukemia in cats, have been known for many years to be virus-induced.

Leukemia is a cancer of the blood that usually starts in the bone marrow. Bone marrow is where blood cells are made: these may be red cells, which carry oxygen; white cells, which fight infection; or cell fragments called platelets, which form clots to seal injured blood vessels and prevent bleeding. There are four main types of leukemia, but the common factor in each is the proliferation of abnormal white blood cells. These mutated, often immature white blood cells begin to multiply in the bone marrow (and sometimes in the liver and spleen), before spreading by way of the bloodstream to other parts of the body such as the lymphatic system, the central nervous system, and other organs.

Although leukemia sufferers often have a huge number of white cells in their bodies, these cells are essentially nonfunctioning. Instead they crowd out the red cells and platelets and prevent healthy white cells from forming. As a result, the leukemic patient is unable to fight off serious infections, becomes susceptible to anemia, and has a tendency to bleed easily.

Types of leukemia

Lymphocytic leukemia is a disorder of the lymphoid cells, which would normally mature to form white blood cells called lymphocytes. Myeloid leukemia affects myeloid cells, which mature to form other types of white blood cells called granulocytes and monocytes. Both types of leukemia may appear in acute or chronic forms: the acute form affects very immature cells; the chronic form affects more developed cells. In acute leukemia, the disease develops rapidly and the symptoms are severe and immediately apparent. The white blood cells are very abnormal and their number increases rapidly. Chronic leukemia develops much more slowly. In the early stage of the disease, large numbers of functional cells are still being made, and it is only as the number of abnormal cells increases that the symptoms, which are similar to those of acute leukemia, become apparent. The symptoms may take years to appear and may seem less severe.

The acute leukemias are much easier to treat than the chronic forms and in some instances may be cured completely. The chronic leukemias tend to affect people in middle age and can, if necessary, usually be controlled with interferons or other treatment. However, because of their slow course and the gradual appearance of the symptoms, many people, particularly the aged, tend to die of illnesses that are unrelated to their leukemia.

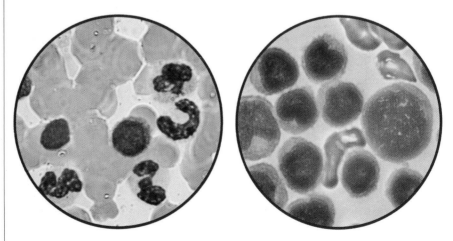

▲ *Through a microscope, normal white blood cells, stained purple, look like this (left). In leukemia, the numbers of white cells, stained purple, are greatly increased (right).*

HOW LEUKEMIA AFFECTS CELLS

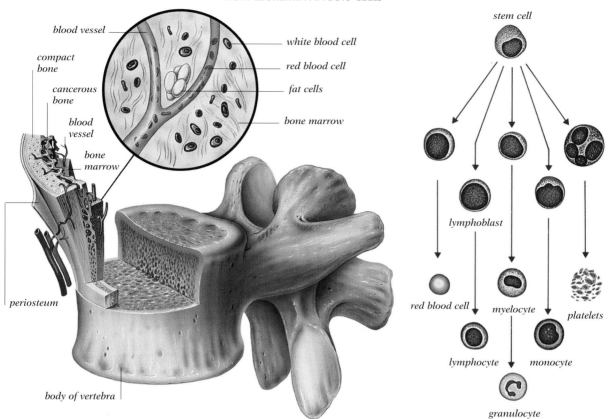

blood vessel

compact bone

cancerous bone

blood vessel

bone marrow

periosteum

body of vertebra

white blood cell

red blood cell

fat cells

bone marrow

stem cell

lymphoblast

red blood cell

myelocyte

platelets

lymphocyte

monocyte

granulocyte

▲ *A cross section of a vertebra (left) with the bone marrow and blood vessels that supply it. The white blood cells are made in the bone marrow, then carried out of the bone in the blood vessels (inset). All the blood cells originate from the same stem cell (right), which is found in the bone marrow. In acute leukemia the white blood cells do not mature properly, the granulocytes never develop beyond the myelocyte stage, and the lymphocytes stop maturing at the lymphoblast stage. Both types of immature white blood cells tend to live longer than normal.*

Incidence

In 2007, approximately 244,000 people in the United States had a history of leukemia—137,000 men and 107,000 women. This statistic includes people who were living with the active disease and those who had been cured. It is estimated that 35,000 new cases of leukemia are diagnosed yearly in the United States. Most cases of leukemia occur in older adults; more than half of all cases occur after age 67. The most common types of leukemias in adults are acute myelogenous leukemia (AML) and chronic lymphocytic leukemia (CLL). The most common form of leukemia in children is acute lymphocytic leukemia (ALL). Leukemia is more common in Americans of European descent than among those of African descent.

What happens in leukemia

In a healthy individual, normal white blood cells cannot reproduce themselves, and after a life cycle of a few days or weeks they are replaced by new cells. With leukemia two things go wrong. First, abnormal white blood cells crowd out normal white blood cells, so

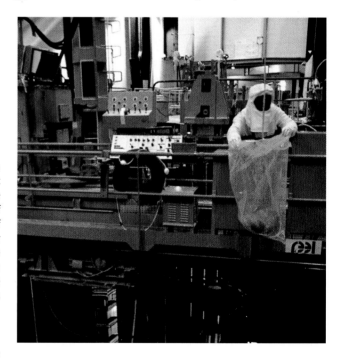

▲ *Excessive doses of radiation can potentially stop the formation of all blood cells. Workers in nuclear energy plants must wear protective clothing.*

that the latter are unable to fight infection. Second, the abnormal cells live longer, and they eventually accumulate and clog up the bone marrow. They then spill into the blood to invade the lymph system, the liver, and the spleen.

Causes

In 97 percent of cases, chronic myeloid leukemia is caused by a chromosomal abnormality known as the Philadelphia chromosome, named for the city where it was discovered. A short section of chromosome 22 is detached and becomes attached to chromosome 9. The Philadelphia chromosome is also found in many cases of acute lymphocytic leukemia. The acute leukemias originate from a single mutation in a white blood cell that alters its genetic structure. There may be several causes for this. It is believed that a virus similar to AIDS may be a cause. Another cause is atomic radiation; there was an enormous increase in cases after atomic bombs were dropped on Japan in 1945. Radiologists, who handle X-ray equipment, also have a slightly higher risk of developing the condition.

Cases of chronic leukemia also increase following exposure to atomic radiation; chronic myeloid leukemia (of the bone marrow) is more common after prolonged exposure to benzene, a constituent of petroleum. Both chronic types occur in 1.5 new cases per 100,000 people each year in the United States; both are fairly uncommon below the age of 20.

Abnormalities of chromosome 21, the cause of Down syndrome, are also linked to a higher incidence of myeloid leukemia.

Symptoms

When the bone marrow teems with the abnormal leukemic cells, it cannot function properly and the patient becomes anemic through lack of red blood cells, is susceptible to infection because of lack of efficient white cells, and bleeds excessively because the blood cannot clot without platelets. Anemia may be one of the earliest signs and sometimes appears before any abnormal blood cells are found. Bleeding in odd places like the gums, easy bruising, and heavy nosebleeds are also warning signs. Infection occurs more commonly, resulting in dental abscesses, sinusitis, or pneumonia. Liver, spleen, and lymph nodes also enlarge; in leukemia the liver and spleen may drop down below the level of the ribs and can be felt on examination.

Diagnosis

Doctors diagnose the disease by examining a blood sample. Because red blood cells are made in the marrow, it is always abnormal to see immature red blood cells circulating. The diagnosis is sometimes made before such abnormal cells appear in the blood by taking a sample of bone marrow. This is done under local anesthetic by inserting a needle usually through the breastbone or hipbone into the marrow cavity (see diagram above).

Treatment

All forms of leukemia can be effectively treated, and most can now be cured. In the case of the chronic leukemias in older people, supportive

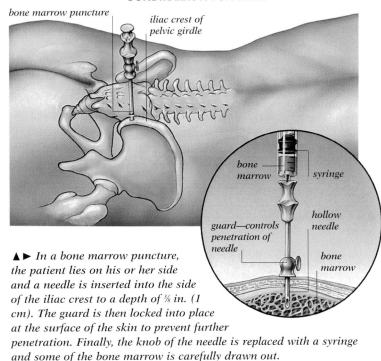

BONE MARROW PUNCTURE

bone marrow puncture

iliac crest of pelvic girdle

bone marrow *syringe*

guard—controls penetration of needle

hollow needle

bone marrow

▲▶ *In a bone marrow puncture, the patient lies on his or her side and a needle is inserted into the side of the iliac crest to a depth of ⅜ in. (1 cm). The guard is then locked into place at the surface of the skin to prevent further penetration. Finally, the knob of the needle is replaced with a syringe and some of the bone marrow is carefully drawn out.*

treatment to sustain the quality of life by treating the effects of the disease may be most appropriate. Alpha-interferons can be effective in normalizing the blood in most cases of chronic myeloid leukemia.

Modern combination chemotherapy can cure up to 80 percent of people under 60 with acute myeloid leukemia. In children with acute lymphocytic leukemia, 70 percent can be cured and 90 percent improved. In adults with this form of leukemia, only about 30 percent can be cured by chemotherapy, and bone marrow transplantation may be necessary.

Chemotherapy involves two broad classes of drugs. The first kills all the white blood cells to get rid of the leukemic cells. When this hospital treatment is finished, the new white blood cells that develop in the bone marrow will be healthy. The second keeps the cancer in remission (slows its progress) and can be taken at home. Alternatively, radiation treatment may suppress the reproduction of cells. A large dose destroys all blood cells, but a small dose affects only abnormal ones.

A more drastic treatment entails killing the patient's marrow and replacing it with a donor's graft. This eradicates any leukemic cells and the remaining normal blood cells that the patient had. The treatment carries the risk that the patient will be attacked immunologically by the donor's cells, however, which perceive the patient's tissues as foreign, and can result in serious complications or even death. Treating the donor's cells to remove these killer lymphocytes before giving them to the patient can prevent this serious complication.

New drugs have greatly improved the quality of life for patients with chronic leukemia, who can sometimes survive for years. As a result of progress in managing leukemia, many patients now expect to be long-term survivors.

See also: Anemia; Cancer

Lice

In the past, because of poverty and poor standards of hygiene, most people were infested with lice. Although far fewer people harbor these parasites, it is still possible for even the most fastidious people to catch lice. Simple and effective remedies are available to treat infestation.

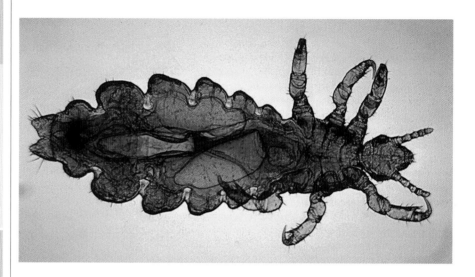

▲ *A female head louse* (Pediculus humanus capitis), *shown vastly magnified.*

Lice are small, wingless, slow-moving, six-legged creatures that seldom exceed ⅛ inch (3 mm) in length. They are unique, for insects, in that they possess seizing claws similar to those of crabs and lobsters. The claws enable lice to grip body hairs or the fibers of clothes. Lice have flattened bodies and are a grayish brown color with darker markings.

Appearance of lice

Head and body lice: The head and body lice, *Pediculus humanus capitis* and *Pediculus humanus corporis*, are similar in appearance, the only difference being that head lice are slightly smaller than body lice.

The features can be easily made out with the aid of a magnifying glass. The head is longer than it is wide with a pair of simple pigmented eyes and a pair of five-segmented antennae. The thorax has fused segments and gives rise to the six legs with gripping claws. The abdomen is long and heavy and has a series of distinct indentations along its edges.

The male is slightly smaller than the female. In the male the rear tip of the abdomen is rounded; in the female it is slightly forked.

Pubic lice: The pubic or crab louse, *Phthirus pubis*, is quite different in shape and, as the name implies, resembles a miniature seashore crab. The head is distinct, but the thorax and abdomen are fused into a single unit so that the whole body appears heart-shaped. The front two pairs of claws are weak and feeble, but the other two pairs are extremely powerful, more so than any of the claws of the head louse or body louse. These hind claws secure the parasite to pubic hairs at a particular site; here the creature remains for long periods, with its mouth parts buried in the skin. These are withdrawn during molting. Pubic lice are seen as small, off-white, yellow, or grayish specks that are attached to the hairs. They live for about one month.

Of the many types of louse, only two main groups—*Pediculus humanus*, which includes the head and body louse; and *Phthirus pubis*, the pubic louse—live by infesting humans and sucking their blood. Fortunately, lice can be dealt with quite easily, but the treatment varies because each type of louse requires different conditions for survival.

My daughter caught head lice at school. Although she was treated successfully—the doctor gave me a special shampoo—I am still worried that the lice have spread. Can someone with head lice get lice elsewhere on the body?

No. There are three types of louse that live on humans—head lice, body lice, and pubic lice. Head and body lice have evolved so that it would be impossible for them to survive in different conditions. The pubic louse may transfer to the hair of the eyelashes, eyebrows, underarms, or chest. Infestation by one kind of louse does not mean that a person will be infested by another type.

I go to garage sales, but my mother keeps telling me that I could get lice from wearing old clothing. Is this true?

Lice will die if they cannot feed regularly and stay at body temperature, so there is unlikely to be any risk of catching lice from clothing bought in a garage sale or secondhand store.

I want to work on a farm but am a little worried about catching lice from the animals. Is this possible?

It is very unlikely that humans would be at risk from the lice that live on animals; these lice would not be able to survive the change of environment. For the same reason, animals are unlikely to catch lice from humans. However, human body lice can live on pigs for a short time.

Should children with head lice be kept out of school?

No, not once treatment has been given. If there is an infestation, school nurses will check each child regularly and ensure that the necessary treatment will be given.

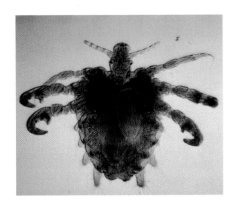

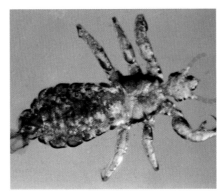

◄ The three types of louse that live off humans—head (opposite), pubic (far left), and body (left)—have evolved in such a way that they require different living conditions for survival.

Effects of louse bites

Disorders caused directly by the bites of head and body lice are called pediculoses. The bites are usually painless but cause itching and may lead to dermatitis (inflammation of the skin). This inflammation is aggravated by scratching, and the result may be secondary infection of the skin with impetigo or boils. Night biting causes loss of sleep in those infested.

In people who remain affected for years, the skin can become markedly altered and heavily bronzed by the deposition of pigment, which is tattooed by scratching. The skin can also become roughened and thickened. These changes are never found in people who acquire only a brief infestation.

Only two major diseases are transmitted by lice: epidemic typhus and relapsing fever. Neither of these conditions is at all likely to occur as a result of a mild infestation.

Head lice

The eggs of the head louse are laid in the hair close to the scalp and are secured to it by a cementlike substance. Each egg is about 0.039 inch (1 mm) long and is visible to the naked eye. After about eight days, the eggs hatch, and the lice begin to feed off the scalp by sucking blood. Over a period of about nine days, the louse molts three times. At the end of this stage, the adult is fully formed and ready to reproduce. Each louse will then live for about two more weeks, during which time the female will lay as many as 10 eggs every night. The effects of head lice vary greatly from person to person. Some people experience only slight itching, while others may be driven to distraction by the itchiness of what may be a swollen and inflamed scalp.

An itching scalp is the most obvious symptom of head lice, but when the head is inspected it is also possible to see the discarded egg casing known as nits, still cemented to the hair, and this will indicate that treatment is necessary.

Treating head lice

The safest way to deal with head lice is to use a special shampoo, preferably containing carbaryl, phenothrin, or malathion, which can be applied directly to the head. It is never necessary to shave the head. The shampoo should be spread onto the palm of the hand and worked well into the hair, avoiding the eyes. This procedure should be repeated until the whole head is moist. It should then be left to dry naturally. A hair dryer should never be used to dry the hair, because heat will weaken malathion and there is also a danger of igniting the lotion. The head should be washed 12 hours later (usually the next morning) and the hair carefully combed out with a fine-tooth nit comb to remove any remaining eggs. Remember that these are usually attached close to the skin. Such a treatment will achieve an almost 100 percent cure rate.

It is now thought possible that some of the lotions that are intended to be left on the head for a longer period (usually for 12 hours) contain chemicals that may be harmful, particularly to children. However, this suspicion has not yet been proved or disproved. As a precaution, it is always best to consult a doctor before using any preparations on the skin, particularly those containing malathion.

Transference of head lice

Head lice transfer easily by head-to-head contact. Young children are more likely to be at risk, since they are often in close physical contact with each other when playing. School medical services are well aware that this is the case and should inform parents if an epidemic of lice occurs.

Brushing or combing children's hair with a fine-tooth comb before they go to bed may provide some protection, because adult

Coping with head lice
DO
Do ensure that your child's hair is brushed and combed thoroughly every night. Injured lice will not survive to lay eggs.
Do inspect your child's scalp regularly, particularly all around the hairline.
Do check the rest of your family if one member is infected.
Do ask your doctor's advice on what special shampoos or lotions you should use if your child is infected.
DON'T
Don't be ashamed if your child catches head lice. Cleanliness provides no defense against these parasites.
Don't keep quiet if your child has head lice. Tell his or her teachers so that the other children can be treated.
Don't try to prevent infection by using special lotions; they will be too harsh on the scalp. Always ask for your doctor's advice if you are worried about lice infestation.

▶ *Because children tend to make close physical contact, they are susceptible to contracting head lice at school. Medicated shampoo provides a complete cure.*

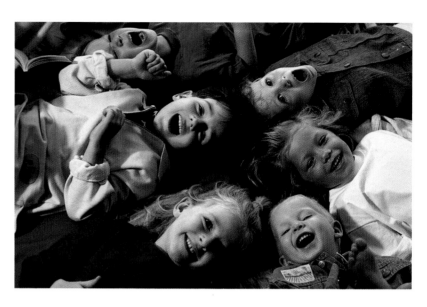

lice that are injured in a comb cannot lay eggs. Keeping children's hair cut short may also provide some protection, but there is little else that can be done to safeguard them from a possible infestation. Since lice are not killed by ordinary shampoo and water, cleanliness will provide no defense; in fact head lice prefer clean hair when they are mating.

Body lice

Body lice occur less frequently than head lice. They need to feed regularly and to live in a constant temperature, so they will thrive under any conditions in which their human host changes clothes infrequently. They have therefore been associated with groups such as troops during wartime and prison populations, where conditions exist in which body lice can develop undisturbed—owing to a lack of soap or washing facilities—and easily transfer from person to person.

The adult female louse lays her eggs in clothing, preferring the safety of the seams where the eggs will be undisturbed. Even when the clothes are removed at night, this may not bring about a change in temperature sufficient to kill the louse and its eggs, so the use of an insecticide is always advised.

Treatment of body lice

Malathion and carbaryl are highly effective. The instructions on the lotion bottle must be carefully followed. Lice will also be killed in extreme temperatures, so washing clothes in hot water (followed by careful ironing of all seams) will ensure that body lice are eliminated.

Diseases caused by body lice

The adult female louse can lay up to 250 eggs. Such a reproductive rate makes it very difficult to prevent the spread of body lice, and their numbers can reach epidemic proportions if the environment is suitable and they are left to reproduce unchecked. Their bites produce itchy inflammations that will alert the infested individual to their presence. Treatment should be sought without delay.

There are a number of louse-borne diseases, the most dangerous of which is typhus. This disease starts with flulike symptoms, followed by a serious fever and rash on the body. It is spread by excretions from the louse. However, this disease is now much rarer than it used to be.

Pubic lice

Sometimes called crab lice or just crabs, pubic lice are usually found living in the pubic hairs. They resemble miniature crabs. They are usually spread by sexual contact, and sex with many partners is one of the risk factors.

There are no measures that can be taken to prevent an infestation with pubic lice. If there is close contact with a person who has crabs—and since they infest the pubic area, this contact is likely to be sexual—lice may well transfer themselves.

Many people are concerned about the possibility of picking up pubic lice in public toilets. The habits of the parasite make this most unlikely. *Phthirus pubis* rarely leaves the body while it is still alive.

Life cycle of pubic lice

Pubic lice thrive in warm conditions, and once a pubic louse has made its way onto the pubic hair, it will lay eggs in a way similar to the head louse. The eggs are cemented onto individual hairs and can be seen by the naked eye. A female pubic louse can lay as many as 50 eggs during her lifetime.

After a month, the pubic lice hatch from their eggs and begin to feed off the human host. The symptoms vary from person to person and are usually at their worst and most irritating during the night. There may be inflammation of the pubic area in addition to an uncomfortable rash.

Pubic lice sometimes spread to the hair of the chest, armpits, eyebrows, and eyelashes, but they are never found on the hair of the head, because these hairs grow too close together.

Other effects of pubic lice

Pubic lice do not carry sexually transmitted diseases but are associated with these diseases, so if pubic lice are present, it is best to have a checkup to make sure no other disease has been contracted. All sexual partners should be checked to see if they need treatment for the infestation by pubic lice.

Treatment of pubic lice

In dealing with pubic lice it is unnecessary to shave the affected area. Sometimes forceps are used to remove adult parasites, but this is often difficult because of their strong attachment to the hair. However, pubic lice can easily be disposed of by applying prescription creams or lotions containing permethrin or lindane, or with a wash such as Elimite or Kwell.

It is important to wash all clothing and linens in hot water to prevent reinfestation.

> *See also:* **Bites and stings; Infection and infectious diseases; Sexually transmitted diseases**

Measles

This common childhood illness is usually mild and harmless. However, the possibility of a severe case and complications means that most parents in Western countries have their children immunized against the disease.

It is neither necessary nor useful. In the past, before immunization and antibiotics, people were put into isolation if they caught measles. However, immunization gives excellent, if not complete, protection (you can have a mild case, even after a vaccination); and modern antibiotics have reduced the dangers of complications.

In any case, in order to have any effect, isolation would have to be much more thorough than is possible in an average home—the disease is extremely contagious. A child with measles should simply be nursed normally at home. There is no reason to keep him or her separated from other children, because American schoolchildren are now given routine immunization.

How do you identify measles for sure when so many illnesses that children get produce a rash?

The only way is to look for what are called Koplik's spots, named after the man who first identified them. These appear in the mouth (on the inner lining of the cheeks) on the third day after the initial symptoms (a fever and runny nose) appear. They look like grains of salt surrounded by a rosy, slightly inflamed area.

I don't know if I had measles as a child. Since I'm hoping to have a baby soon, should I consider being immunized?

Most doctors would not suggest immunization in the case of a woman trying to conceive, especially if there is a chance that she is pregnant—the vaccine could harm the baby. Measles is not nearly as harmful in pregnancy as German measles (rubella).

Before the introduction of measles vaccination, most children caught the measles virus between the ages of one and six. Because a baby has natural immunity inherited from the mother, he or she is protected for several months. However, from the age of about one year, all children are at risk. In older children and adults, the condition is rare. Having measles once provides immunity for life; but, because it is highly infectious, few people who have not been immunized escape it.

Measles in perspective

In most communities of the Western world (where measles has been established for centuries), the condition is mild and hardly ever dangerous. The only worry is its complications.

While the virus has a hold, the body is weak and particularly susceptible to a variety of infections in such sites as the ears, lungs, and eyes. These are bacterial infections, caused by germs that are different in nature from the measles virus. As such they can be controlled with antibiotics. However, if immunization is not given, measles can reach epidemic proportions and put children at risk.

Measles should not be confused with German measles, or rubella. Rubella is a milder infection and less contagious. Adults are likely to be affected as a result of having escaped it as children; in pregnancy it is dangerous and capable of deforming the fetus.

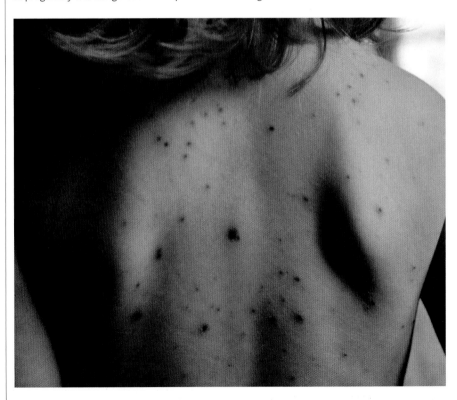

▲ *In severe cases, measles spots can appear all over the body. The most common telltale spots are on the back and arms and inside the mouth (where they are called Koplik's spots). Wherever they are, it is important that the patient does not to scratch them.*

Questions and Answers

I know of a child who was immunized against measles, then caught the disease three years later. How can this occur?

It occurs because the measles vaccine gives only 80 percent protection after the first shot, and 95 percent protection after the second. However, if an immunized child does catch measles, the attack is mild, and there is little or no danger of complications.

Could a new strain of measles appear that would be immune to the usual vaccine that is in use?

This is highly unlikely, mainly because measles has been around for centuries among humans without changing its nature. The measles bug or germ is of a particular type, called a virus. Although some viruses, such as the influenza virus, change their surface coats regularly, making immunization difficult, measles does not.

I've heard that measles is becoming less and less severe. Why should we bother with immunization in this case?

Measles is no less potent a virus than it ever was. The only thing that has changed is the severity of the attacks, and this is on account of widespread immunization.
  Although the measles virus in itself is rarely dangerous, the complications it can cause may be. Long-term lung trouble, deafness, and even blindness may arise if complications are left untreated. Because of this, immunization is a legal requirement for all schoolchildren in the United States.

Is it true that measles can lead to mental illness?

A rare and dangerous complication of measles is encephalitis—inflammation of certain parts of the brain. A tiny proportion of patients who contract encephalitis do, when they recover, suffer from changes of mood and personality.

First signs

The measles virus is passed from person to person, like many other viruses, on the tiny droplets of moisture that people constantly breathe out and in. Following contact with an infected person, there are no symptoms for generally between seven and 12 days, during which time the virus is incubating or multiplying in the cells of the throat and the passages leading to the lungs.

This phase is followed by the two stages of measles itself. The first is called the catarrhal stage, because the virus is confined to the mucous membranes (linings) of the eyes, nose, and mouth. The patient develops what appears to be a heavy cold with a husky cough. The nose is runny, and the eyes are red and watery. There may be a fine, red rash that lasts for a few hours, then disappears.

A parent usually notices that his or her child is sick. Most children have a temperature rising to 100.4°F (38°C). There is a loss of appetite and possible vomiting and diarrhea. Tiny white spots (called Koplik's spots), which are unique to measles, can be seen lining the mouth.

The rash

On the third or fourth day (occasionally the fifth to seventh day), the patient's temperature falls and the rash begins to appear. It is typically a dusky red color, with slightly raised spots that are grouped in patches to give the blotchy appearance that is typical of measles.

The rash starts to form behind the ears, then spreads to the neck and forehead; eventually it will cover the face and trunk and, in severe cases, the limbs. This usually happens over a period of about 24 hours. There is only slight itching and sometimes none at all.

After the rash starts to appear—on the same day—the temperature rises once more. This is usually the time when the patient feels most ill; in severe cases he or she will feel terrible. The cough and inflammation of the eyes are at their worst; light is likely to be irritating to the eyes; any complications, if they are to occur, will begin to develop at this time.

Over the next three days, the rash disappears in the order in which it appeared. A brownish staining of the skin remains, this usually disappears with peeling of the skin. After the rash begins to fade, most patients recover quickly.

The dangers

In a tiny minority of cases the patient has a low resistance to measles; his or her temperature rises uncontrollably, and there is the danger of bleeding, either in the skin affected by the rash or in certain organs. Called "hemorrhagic measles," this condition needs hospital treatment if the patient's life is to be saved. Tiny hemorrhages sometimes occur in the rash of mild measles, but should cause no alarm. However, if bleeding is widespread, a doctor should be called immediately.

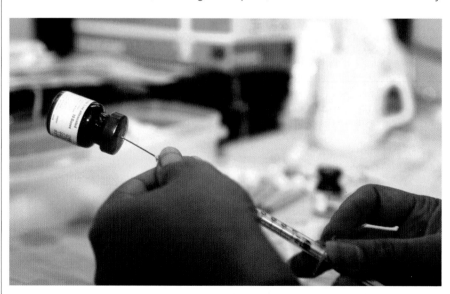

▲ *Vaccination development starts in a laboratory where measles viruses are cultured. The viruses are then made into vaccine doses ready for distribution.*

Home treatment

Mild painkillers—acetaminophen or aspirin for children over 12—can help to bring down the patient's fever.

Use a mouthwash regularly if the mouth is sore from infection.

Give the patient plenty of fluids, especially during feverish periods.

Calamine lotion can be applied to the spots if they itch.

Closing the curtains will soothe irritated eyes.

A simple syrup will help the cough—a pharmacist will advise.

Note: Earache, a congested cough, widespread bleeding of the spots, or unexpected drowsiness must be reported promptly to the doctor.

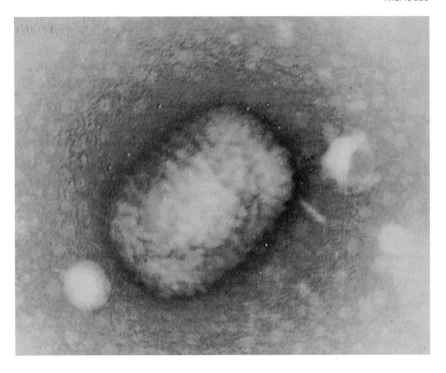

▲ *The virus that causes measles takes 12 days to incubate in the nose, mouth, and eyes after contact with an infected person has been made.*

Ear and lung infection

The measles virus temporarily destroys the lining of the passage leading to the lungs and paves the way for bacterial infection of adjoining or connected areas, such as the ears and lungs. Some patients develop infection of the middle ear (roughly halfway into the ear), with earache and a discharge of pus. When this is observed in a child, parents should report it to a doctor without delay—antibiotics will prevent spread of the infection and will clear it up.

A congested, wheezing cough in a measles patient is a sign of chest infection. Some coughing is normal, but if this produces phlegm and there is wheezing (rather than a dry, hacking, and unproductive cough) antibiotics are essential to prevent lung damage; a doctor should be called without delay.

In severe, untreated cases a chronic (long-term) lung infection called bronchiectasis may develop. Although this can be treated, prevention is worthwhile, as the condition can retard growth.

In young children measles sometimes leads to bacterial infection of the larynx (the voice box), which is situated in the throat. The passage of air is obstructed and a croupy, or hoarse, croaking cough is produced. This is a serious complication; if parents observe such symptoms, they should call a doctor immediately.

Mild conjunctivitis—an irritation that produces a pink hue in the whites of the eyes—is normal in measles. However, if there is a bacterial infection as well, the discharge will be thick and sticky. This can cause scarring of the conjunctiva and blindness if it is left untreated. Again, the doctor should be called if this condition develops.

A further complication that can sometimes develop is measles pneumonia; this is more likely to occur in crowded conditions such as refugee camps. It can also be treated with antibiotics.

Encephalitis

Encephalitis is an inflammation of the brain and central nervous system in response to the presence of the measles virus. It used to be the most dreaded complication of measles. The symptoms are drowsiness, hallucinations, and delirium; these occur about 10 days into the illness. With modern immunization it is rare—developing in one in 1,000 cases—but the condition needs urgent hospital treatment because the consequences can be severe.

Treatment

Mild cases of measles need no treatment other than home nursing. The patient can go to bed when he or she feels too ill to stay up. Some doctors give antibiotics in all cases; others reserve them for severe cases and those with complications. Patients with severe measles need intensive home nursing; however, even these need stay in bed only if they feel too sick to do anything else.

Outlook

One attack of measles gives lifelong immunity, and recovery is usually complete. However, there are rare cases in which a patient has severe complications. In view of this, immunization makes the most sense. It involves two shots (usually given as part of the combined MMR—measles, mumps, and rubella—vaccine), and the possibility of a slight rash and fever 10 days later; these symptoms are not as bad as in normal measles. A booster shot is given a few years later. In measles epidemics patients who are already ill can be protected with a gamma globulin shot.

See also: **Antibiotics; Bacteria; Immunization; Rubella; Vaccinations; Viruses**

Medicines

Constant advances in medical science encourage the creation of new medicines and the improvement of existing ones. Medicines either aid the symptoms of a disease or help its cure.

This depends on what they contain. If a medicine is known to deteriorate or lose its potency with age, it will have an expiration date stamped on its label, and it should not be used after that. To avoid mistakes it is wise to get rid of any medicine that is no longer needed.

My children hate taking medicine. How can I make this less of an ordeal for them and for me?

Try to treat the matter as an ordinary event. If you can, pretend to take some medicine yourself at the same time—colored water will do—and explain to the child that taking it is an important part of getting well. If it tastes unpleasant, don't pretend to the child that it doesn't; give him or her a reward for taking it without fuss.

My medicine has to be taken before meals, but I haven't been eating regular meals since I've been sick. What should I do?

When a medicine is prescribed to be taken before meals, this has nothing to do with what you eat. It simply means that your doctor wants you to take the medicine when your stomach is empty rather than after a meal.

My doctor prescribed tablets for high blood pressure. I feel well again now and my blood pressure is back to normal, so why do I have to go on taking the tablets?

It is the effect of the tablets that has brought down your blood pressure; the underlying tendency to raised blood pressure is still there, and if you stopped taking the medicine, your blood pressure would soon rise again.

Medicines are remedial substances that preserve, improve, or restore health. They are taken by swallowing, by inhalation, by injection, or by application to the skin in the form of a cream or lotion. The first medicines were probably discovered by accident, when prehistoric people found that certain plants relieved pain or helped to heal wounds. Gradually, what was learned by trial and error became an organized body of knowledge; the study and use of medicinal plants. The Chinese practiced an advanced form of herbalism more than 5,000 years ago. However, for the most part illness was seen as either a punishment inflicted by angry gods or the vengeance of enemies; medicines were a defense against evil, and their prescription was often in the form of a spell. In the 15th century, this changed with the birth of the science of physiology, the study of how the human body works; and pathology, the study of disease.

Modern medicines
Some new medicines are still derived from plants and other natural substances, although many more are made in the laboratory from synthetic copies of such natural substances. Pharmaceutical chemists generally prefer to use synthetic ingredients in the creation of new medicines. This is because, unlike their natural equivalents, synthetic chemicals can be measured and their actions predicted to a very high degree of accuracy, making the medicine both safe to use and effective.

Understanding medicines
Using medicine to treat any condition is a matter of cooperation among research chemist, doctor, and patient; its success finally depends on whether the person taking it keeps scrupulously to the right dosage at the right intervals through the day and for the right length of time. Many modern drugs are intended to have a cumulative effect: they are effective only if they are taken in certain regular amounts for a specific period.

It is always unwise, and could be very dangerous, for someone to stop taking a prescribed medicine halfway through its course, just because it seems to have done what was expected of it, or because it is adding to rather than relieving discomfort. In both cases, before stopping the medicine, a person should discuss his or her concerns with a doctor.

How medicines work
Most drugs work by interfering positively with the way in which the body functions. This has always been the case, even when drugs were largely plant substances. The way in which they influence organs in the body depends on what each drug contains and on how it is absorbed.

A medicine may be taken in liquid or solid form and it takes about half an hour to be digested and pass into the bloodstream. Some drugs are destroyed by the digestive process or irritate the lining of the gastrointestinal tract and so are introduced into the body in another way—by injection or inhalation. They then go straight into the body's circulation and start to work immediately.

Medicines that are applied to exterior surfaces of the body take a variety of forms, too. A collodion, for example, is a clear, sticky liquid, which is used to hold the edges of wounds together and to keep dressings in place. Ointments are rubbed onto the skin to reduce soreness and stiffness. Lozenges are held in the mouth and allowed to dissolve in the saliva to soothe any soreness occurring in the mouth or the throat.

The herbal medicines of the past worked gently in or on the body, helping it to heal itself and lessening pain and discomfort. Modern medicines have a great deal more power, enough to rid the body of certain diseases or to correct disorders so that it can work efficiently. In the course of performing these fundamental functions, drugs can cause troublesome side effects.

Medicines in the home

A well-stocked medicine chest is a necessity in the home. Everyone in the family should know where it is; it must be clearly labeled; and, most important of all, it must be kept out of the reach of small children. Any medicines in use should be stored in the chest, so that there is no risk that attractively colored tablets will fall into the hands of small children. Even childproof containers are no match for curious toddlers; self-poisoning is one of the most common causes of accidental death in the very young.

In addition to prescribed medication, a medicine chest might contain simple remedies for coughs, headaches, or diarrhea; first-aid dressings in case of domestic accidents; and a thermometer.

In the unlikely event of an emergency, helpers may not know the name of a victim's doctor, so a list of useful telephone numbers (doctor, hospital, and ambulance services) taped to the inside of the medicine chest and next to the telephone is a sensible measure. Also noted should be the address of the nearest hospital emergency room and that of the local pharmacist.

An envelope containing the medical history of each member of your family could be of great help in an emergency. Mention of their previous illnesses, operations, sensitivities, immunizations, allergies, and any drugs that must be taken regularly could provide vital information in an emergency.

The contents of the medicine chest should be checked regularly. Medicines have a limited life, and any preparations that are no longer needed or have passed their expiration date should be removed and disposed of.

Self-treatment

Many minor illnesses, such as colds or flu, can be dealt with by commonsense over-the-counter treatments at home. There are many over-the-counter remedies that are useful for home treatment. Before any medicine is taken, the label should be read carefully and all instructions should be followed. Many pharmacies provide instructions regarding contraindications, side effects, and possible drug interactions. Instructions will be given about whether or not food can be taken with the treatment.

However, illnesses should not be treated with medicines without medical supervision. If the complaint is minor, if symptoms persist, or if there is any doubt, a doctor should be consulted. For example, only a doctor can tell if a sore throat indicates strep.

Medicine must never be taken if it was intended for someone else or taken from a container without a label. Remedies should never be mixed. Self-treatment should never be continued for too long, and self-diagnosis must not be attempted for persistent symptoms. People who take over-the-counter medicines for weeks to relieve troublesome coughs or digestive problems may have a serious problem that needs medical attention.

The doctor needs to know if a patient has been taking any medicine before the consultation and what the medicine is, since it may have altered the pattern of the illness. Most over-the-counter medicines do not cure diseases; they only relieve the symptoms while nature and time set to work correcting the condition.

Medical necessities

It is best to keep few and simple self-treatment medicines. Pharmacists can advise on suitable remedies to keep at home.

For headaches and fevers: Aspirin (acetylsalicylic acid) or acetaminophen tablets. Nonsteroidal antiinflammatory drugs (NSAIDs), such as Ibuprofen and Naproxen, can also relieve pain. Aspirin tablets must never be given to children under 12; research has suggested that aspirin is connected with Reye's syndrome.

For indigestion: Magnesium trisilicate or calcium citrate tablets, which should be sucked or chewed rather than swallowed. Bismuth in liquid form works more quickly but is less convenient to carry. The tablets can be taken as often as necessary, up to every hour. Two teaspoons (10 ml) of the liquid should be taken about an hour after meals, up to four times a day.

For diarrhea: Kaolin and pectin. The dosage is 4 teaspoons (20 ml) followed by 2 teaspoons (10 ml) every three hours while the diarrhea is severe. The dose should cease once the gastrointestinal tract is back to normal. These medications should never be given to children; a doctor will advise on alternatives. In case of fever, dizziness, bloody stools, or inability to keep down liquids, a doctor should be consulted immediately.

For coughs: Coughing is the body's natural way of clearing the lungs and should be interfered with as little as possible. However, sometimes it is reasonable to use a cough medicine. If a cough persists for more than a week or is accompanied by high fever, shortness of breath, or chest pains upon deep breathing, a doctor should be consulted. If a dry cough interferes with a child's sleep, a pharmacist can suggest a suitable cough syrup.

Other preparations to be kept in a medicine chest include antiseptics such as hydrogen peroxide, iodine, rubbing alcohol, or betadyne to clean wounds; calamine lotion for the skin; cough drops or lozenges for sore throats; menthol and eucalyptus inhalants and rubs; and saline eyedrops. Eye preparations should be used only on medical advice, and the use of laxatives can usually be completely avoided by means of a high-fiber diet.

> *See also:* **Aspirin and analgesics; Fevers; Headache**

Treating young children

Try to deal with your child's taking medicine in a calm, lighthearted way. If you appear anxious, or dramatize the proceedings, your child will take his or her cue from you, and make a fuss about taking the medicine.

Use a dropper to adminster medicine to a child who cannot drink from a cup.

If your child has a bad reaction to a medication, tell your doctor immediately.

Clasp the child's hands in one of yours so that the medicine can't be pushed away or spilled.

Give praise for swallowing—and sometimes give the child a small reward.

Be patient; a child who associates medicine with punishment and anger is bound to resist it.

Mental illness

My teenage daughter has started to have unpredictable mood swings, from elation to depression. Could this be bipolar disorder?

It could be, but at her age it is unlikely. These mood swings are common in teenagers, and the cause is far more likely to be the appearance of a new boyfriend than anything deep-seated. If the moods become considerably more frequent and longer-lasting, you should talk to your doctor.

My husband has always been a little eccentric, and now he's getting worse. When does eccentricity become mental illness?

Strictly speaking, this occurs when those who live with the person are no longer able to cope with his or her behavior. However, passing a verdict of that kind on someone should never be done lightly. In practice it is done jointly by the patient's relatives and his or her psychiatrists.

Experts generally agree that few eccentric people are, in fact, mentally disturbed, because they know what they are doing when they are being eccentric. Quirky behavior is usually a way of gaining freedom of behavior.

My mother has just died, and my father is extremely depressed. Should he see a doctor and get psychiatric counseling?

If you are really worried about your father's depression, go to the doctor yourself and tell him or her about your fears. Older people usually do not approve of trying to cure grief by medical intervention. With gentle coaxing, your father may agree to see a doctor.

You could also try to help him yourself. Talk to him about his sadness, but don't worry if he does not respond at first. Keep encouraging him to find a way of expressing his grief.

The field of mental illness is by no means a clear-cut area of medical knowledge. However, some basic explanations can help in understanding the range of disorders that people may suffer at some time during their lives.

Mental illness is not a tidy subject. Experts may attach names to mental disorders as if there were no doubt that such disorders fall into precise categories; however, often they do this because there is a pressing need to find words for something that defies an easy description.

Most psychiatric experts agree that several mental conditions should not be called illnesses at all, and that categories of psychological problems overlap considerably. However, all the different categories do still exist; if they are approached with caution, they can be useful.

Psychosomatic states
The term "psychosomatic states" is given to physical illnesses that appear as a result of mental pressure. They include headaches, abdominal pain, hyperventilation, skin disorders, and others. In such cases, the patient is not simply saying that there is something wrong in order to gain sympathy: the physical symptoms are real.

Brain damage
There is an array of possible causes of brain damage; for example, head injury, alcoholism, rupturing of a blood vessel in the brain, poisoning, drug abuse, reduction of blood supply, or infection. Senile dementia is a form of brain damage that affects old people; it is brain degeneration that is always caused by a disease.

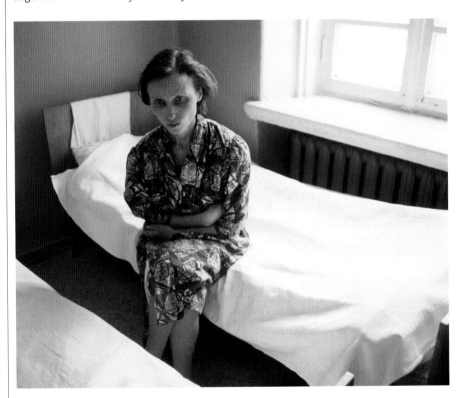

▲ *There are some instances, particularly if a patient is a danger to him- or herself or others, where a stay in hospital may be necessary to treat a mental illness.*

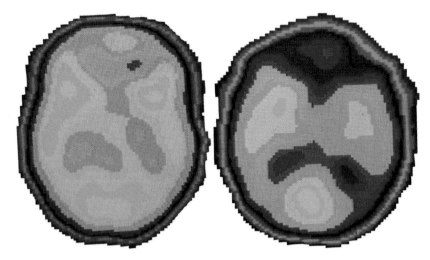

◄ *Variations in brain blood flow are sometimes a feature of certain serious psychiatric conditions; however, diagnosis cannot be made by scanner. These pictures show the difference between a normal person's brain (far left) and that of a person with bipolar disorder (left).*

factor. A question that is commonly asked is whether certain personality types are more prone to mental illness. There is no simple answer to this, because there are so many exceptions to the rule. However, those people who find it most difficult to shrug off life's pressures, whatever their personality type, do tend to be the ones who are most at risk. There is also a significant proportion of highly introverted people who fall into this category.

Psychoses and neuroses

Psychoses are fairly severe disorders and include schizophrenia, some forms of depression, bipolar disorder, and psychopathy. Such conditions often run in families, not only because behavior of parents is copied by children, but also because some of these disorders can be hereditary. A chemical imbalance in the brain is often at the root of such problems. They are characterized by the patient's being unaware that he or she is behaving abnormally.

Neurosis includes problems such as phobias, hysteria, states of anxiety, obsessions, and some sexual difficulties. In such cases the patient is usually aware that he or she is behaving abnormally.

Personality disorders

People with personality disorders usually have problems already mentioned as neuroses, but on a long-term basis and in a more general way. For example, someone with an obsessive personality will show not so much a particular obsession as obsessive beliefs about a number of situations. The beliefs may change from time to time, with a new obsession developing as the old one fades.

The category also includes the hysteric personality; depressed personality; schizoid personality, in which some of the deluded thinking and inappropriate emotions of schizophrenia appear; and psychopathic personality, in which ruthless, selfish actions are carried out for no apparent reason. The psychopath's hallmark is not so much deliberate disregard for others (which implies intent) as a seemingly total lack of awareness of the possibility that he or she should have any regard for others in the first place.

Finally there is the uncommon condition of split or multiple personality. This condition involves radical changes of nature; for example, the sufferer may change from shy to extrovert, from aggressive to submissive, or from childlike to adult.

Those at risk

Mental illness can affect anyone—male or female, young or old, rich or poor—although certain conditions are more prevalent in some groups than they are in others. Depression occurs more in women than men, more in middle-aged people than younger people, and more in the poor than rich people.

Such differences are sometimes caused by external stresses, which act more on some groups than others, but there is also a personality

Symptoms of mental illness

Changes in attitude or behavior, however unexpected, are hardly enough to brand someone as mentally ill. Only if these changes are such that an individual is unable to look after him- or herself, or be accepted by society, is sanity called into question. Even then, it is

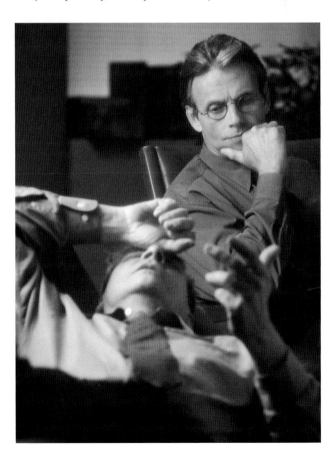

▲ *Psychotherapy and behavior modification therapy are the preferred treatments for less severe forms of mental illness.*

▶ *Four patients attend a group counseling session with a qualified counselor. This type of therapy is useful for resolving shared psychological problems.*

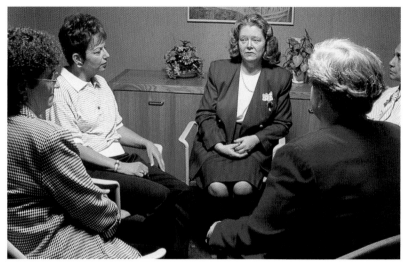

invariably more constructive to use the correct name of the disease rather than the inaccurate and condemnatory terms "mad" and "insane," which are in any case legal, not medical, terms.

The symptoms of a psychosomatic illness, which are those of the illness that is mimicked, are easy to discern.

Similarly, evidence of brain damage is usually easy to recognize. In such a case, the patient shows obvious defects of memory, thinking, coordination, and movement. Sometimes he or she may be subject to bouts of stupor and unconsciousness.

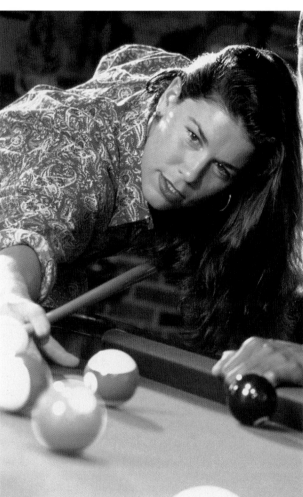

▲ *Patients are encouraged to live as normal a life as possible, and most will benefit from involvement in everyday social activities such as a game of pool.*

Schizophrenia may be more difficult to diagnose. Contrary to a commonly held belief, schizophrenia is not a "split personality." Rather, the condition is characterized by delusional thought, irrational beliefs, and inappropriate emotions, especially a type of foolish giggling for no reason. The patient may also go into a blank stupor in which he or she seems totally divorced from reality.

The symptoms of depression are well known, but it should be remembered that these symptoms may be linked to periods of forced gaiety and excitement (a mark of bipolar disorder), or to periods of apathy and irritability.

The symptoms of neurosis are also clearly evident. For example, in phobias there is an obvious and irrational fear of some object or activity, be it a cat, leaving the house, or sexual encounters.

Compulsions and obsessions show up in a person as an excessive need for him or her to collect things or perform repetitive actions. Hysteria is more difficult to pinpoint: it may involve amnesia (loss of memory), wandering around in a state of confusion, purposeful episodes of arguing or fighting, phantom sensations, and a range of other aberrant patterns of behavior.

Treatment

Nearly all treatment of mental illness starts at a family doctor's office. However, if the doctor cannot handle the case, he or she will refer the patient to a specialist.

Modern treatments of mental illness seldom involve a stay in a hospital; the object is to have the patient live as far as possible in his or her everyday world, attending an outpatient clinic or seeing a psychiatrist for therapy.

Drugs are seldom used in cases of neurosis except to reduce panic. Tranquilizers or sedatives may be used as a first line of treatment to try to relax the patient sufficiently for his or her anxiety to drift away. However, experts are aware that resorting to drugs may be an easy way out because all too often it does not touch the cause of the patient's problems; such drug usage is on the decrease.

In severe disturbances drugs are more helpful, but even here they are likely to do no more than control behavior rather than cure the patient's underlying condition. In some cases this may not matter. For example, if depression or anxiety can be held in check long enough, the patient is often able to gain sufficient respite to fight

Common types of mental illness

CONDITION	MOST COMMON SYMPTOM	TREATMENT
Psychosomatic illness	Mimicry of a real physical illness such as stomach upset, breathing difficulty such as hyperventilation, or headache.	If the problem is sufficiently serious and persistent, psychotherapy is used to discover and remove the underlying cause.
Brain damage	A wide variety of symptoms, including confusion, amnesia, and hallucinations.	Improvement is often not possible; the brain cells do not have the same power to renew themselves as the other cells in the body. The only option may be to teach the patient to make the most of remaining powers or abilities; under expert guidance this can produce good results.
Schizophrenia	Hallucinations; delusions, especially of persecution; and inappropriate emotions.	Drug treatment, psychotherapy, and rehabilitation courses to help the sufferer reintegrate into society.
Depression and bipolar disorder	Anxiety that is deep-seated; extremes of mood, from elation to despair.	Drugs, used with due caution; psychotherapy; or both.
Hysteria	Amnesia; wandering; inability to sense things.	Psychotherapy to discover what caused the condition and to promote recovery.
Phobias	Intense, and apparently irrational, fears of objects or situations.	Behavior modification therapy to reduce anxiety or to teach new constructive patterns of behavior.
Obsessions and compulsions	A need to perform pointless and repetitive actions or to collect things; high anxiety.	Same as for phobias.

back against the condition. A stay in the hospital will always be necessary if a patient's behavior is intolerable for his or her caregivers or others, or if—importantly—it makes the patient a danger to him- or herself or to others.

One radical type of treatment is electroconvulsive therapy (or electric shock treatment), which is not as drastic or crude as it sounds. Controlled electric current is passed through certain parts of the brain while the patient is anesthetized. This can dramatically relieve severe depression and other conditions. However, the depression can return, requiring additional treatment, and the side effect of temporary memory loss is often of concern. ECT is now used much less often than it was in the past.

Living with mental illness
In general, neuroses and the other less severe conditions, such as psychosomatic illness, can be substantially improved or even cured. With the more severe conditions, especially those involving brain damage, there is a mixed outlook. Often the best that can be offered is successful management of the condition.

The trend in modern psychiatry is not only to help patients but also to consider those who live with and care for them. Patients and their caregivers can become frustrated by the fact that many problems can be controlled only temporarily. A caregiver's hopes may be raised, only to be dashed when problems reappear. The resulting disappointment and impatience, however understandable, may be communicated to the patient, and this can have a destructive effect on his or her progress.

An assessment of whether symptoms are likely to reappear is therefore a vital part of a psychiatrist's work. Those who have to live with someone who is mentally ill should also try to cooperate with both doctor and patient: this is in everyone's interest in the long run.

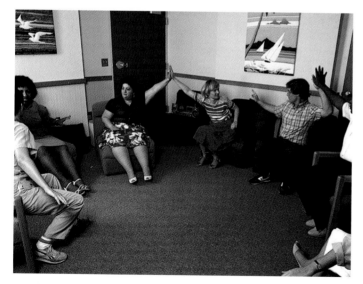

▲ *Treatment for mental illness can take many forms. Here patients in a hospital mental health unit take part in a music therapy session.*

See also: Depression

Minerals

Is it possible to take too large a quantity of minerals?

Yes. Almost all the minerals in the diet can be poisonous in excess, although people rarely suffer from toxicity unless they have taken a deliberate or accidental overdose. An overdose of iron is one of the more common and serious types of poisoning in children, and any iron pills kept at home should be locked up and out of the reach of young, active children. Potassium, given as a medicine, can be dangerous in excess, so the amount prescribed has to be closely monitored.

Do mineral waters contain a higher level of minerals than ordinary tap water?

Ordinary tap water contains plenty of dissolved minerals, and in general the harder the water, the more minerals it contains. Some mineral waters have a higher mineral content, but this depends entirely on what area the water has come from originally.

Are vegetarians and people who eat health foods in danger of a mineral deficiency?

Most vegetarian diets rely heavily on whole foods and grains, which are good sources of essential minerals. The main danger of completely vegetarian diets is a deficiency of iron and vitamin B12.

My 16-year-old son seems to live entirely on candy, potato chips, and cake. Should I give him mineral supplements?

He sounds just like most teenage boys. You will probably find that he does eat a fairly varied diet; it just seems as though it is all junk food. He is unlikely to be short of minerals; his main problem is likely to be a shortage of fiber.

Minerals are an essential part of the diet and perform various functions. A well-balanced diet with plenty of meat, dairy products, and vegetables contains most of the minerals necessary to maintain a fit and healthy body.

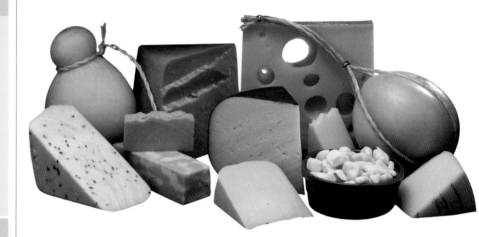

▲ ▶ *All the essential minerals can be found in a varied selection of food and drink.*

Chemists divide all the natural substances in the world into two types of chemicals: organic and inorganic. Organic chemicals, the building blocks of life, contain the three main chemical elements—carbon, oxygen, and hydrogen—and lesser elements such as nitrogen. All the organic chemicals contain carbon. In contrast, the inorganic chemicals do not depend on carbon and can consist of any compound of the remaining 91 naturally occurring elements.

When people speak of minerals in the diet, they are really talking about the few inorganic substances that are necessary for health in addition to the large amounts of organic carbohydrate, protein, and fat that make up most of the diet. The vitamins, which are also essential to a healthy diet, are organic compounds.

What do minerals do?

There are two types of minerals in the body—those that are found throughout the tissues and cells and those that are found only in specific places where they are an essential part of a single key process. In the first category there are three main substances: sodium, potassium, and calcium. These are metals in their purified forms, but in the body they are present in the form of salts. This group of metal salts, with the addition of magnesium, is essential in several processes.

For example, the amount of sodium in the fluid surrounding a cell is much greater than that within the cell membrane; with potassium the opposite is true. This imbalance establishes a tension that makes it possible for living cells to respond to electrical stimulation, such as nerve conduction and muscle contraction (including the heartbeat).

Calcium is the most abundant mineral in the body and is essential for building a healthy bone structure. Exercise is vital to achieve the right balance of calcium, so people who are bedridden are exercised as much as possible to reduce the risk of fractures.

Complex systems control the levels of sodium, potassium, and calcium in the body. About 70 percent of the oxygen breathed in is used to keep sodium and potassium on either side of the cell membranes, and although people tend to think of the kidney as the organ that disposes of waste material, most of the energy that it uses is to regulate the amount of sodium and potassium excreted in the urine.

In contrast, the other types of minerals may be required for only a few specific purposes in the body. Iron, for example, is an essential component of hemoglobin, which carries oxygen

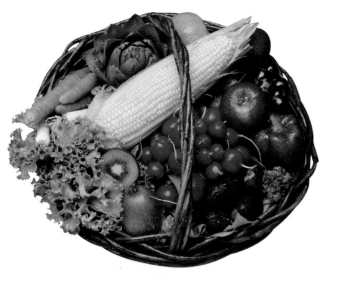

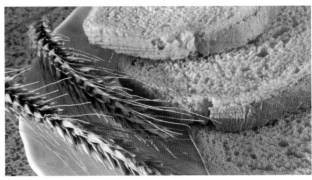

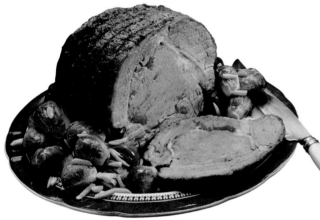

from the lungs to the tissues. Iodine's only role is in the thyroid hormone, which helps control the production and use of energy by the tissues.

What can go wrong?

The essential minerals are found in the soil and are therefore present in vegetables and animal foods. The two minerals that are most likely to be deficient in natural circumstances are iron and iodine. Iron deficiency (anemia) is extremely common in developing countries where the diet is inadequate. Even in developed countries some women are anemic because of the iron they lose each month during their periods. Iodine deficiency can be avoided by using iodized table salt.

Deficiencies of the other minerals are uncommon, although zinc deficiency does occur and extra zinc can improve leg ulcers in old people. It is much more common to encounter poisoning with minerals such as manganese and copper. Copper poisoning, known as Wilson's disease, results from an inherited defect in the way that the body absorbs and stores copper.

See also: Anemia; Calcium; Diet; Iron; Nutrition; Ulcers

Minerals—Their uses in the body

MINERAL	ROLE	SOURCE
Sodium and chloride (together making salt)	Essential components of all organisms. Found in all tissues. The main role of the kidney is to keep them in balance.	All foods, and added in cooking.
Potassium	Tends to act in conjunction with sodium to control all electrical activity in the body.	Fresh fruit and vegetables.
Calcium	Essential for healthy bones, muscles, and nerves, and in mediating hormone effects.	Meat and dairy products.
Phosphorus (phosphate)	In all cells as a basic energy store. Also works with calcium in bones and muscles.	Meat; dairy products; grains; cereals.
Magnesium	Important in many processes in the body, and essential for muscle strength.	Same as for phosphorus; snails.
Iodine	Required for thyroid activity.	Seafood, and added to salt.
Iron	Required to make hemoglobin and prevent anemia.	Meat
Copper	Needed for the cells to handle oxygen.	Seafood and meat.
Manganese	Needed for the control of fats in the body and for the cells to use oxygen.	Same as for phosphorus.
Zinc	Required for many of the body's chemical processes and for healthy skin.	Seafood; whole wheat; grains.
Fluoride (fluorine)	Helps to protect the teeth against decay.	Water and toothpaste.
Chromium	Essential for the handling of sugar.	A balanced diet.

Mumps

As with many common childhood illnesses, children who develop mumps (parotitis) usually have future immunity from the disease. In adults, the infection can be more serious, but symptoms subside after a few days.

Mumps is a common acute viral infection that produces fever and swelling of the salivary glands. The illness is most common in children between five and 14 years old. A small percentage of people contract mumps in adulthood; the symptoms may be severe and complications are more common.

Causes

Mumps is caused by a virus similar to the influenza virus. The virus spreads from person to person by contact with the moisture expelled in coughs, sneezes, and the breath of someone infected. It enters the body through the mouth or respiratory tract and has a two to three-week incubation period. It then affects the glands and, very rarely, the nervous system.

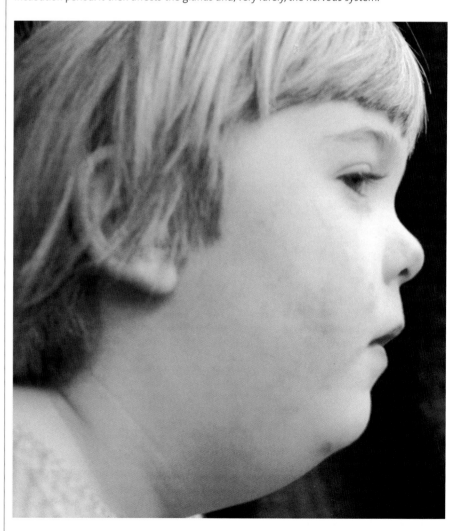

▲ *Mumps usually affects one salivary gland, causing moderate swelling. But if other glands are involved, the swelling spreads.*

Questions and Answers

Is it possible to have my children immunized against mumps virus?

Yes. There is now a safe vaccine that can be given to children after the age of 15 months. Immunization against mumps (as well as against measles and rubella) is required for all children attending school.

I was told mumps had affected only one of my salivary glands. Could I therefore get the illness again?

No. Mumps quite often inflames only one salivary gland and leaves the others unaffected. Because you have had the mumps virus, you now have immunity for life.

My doctor says he is not positive that my sister has had mumps. How can the virus be detected?

Only a blood test will positively identify the mumps virus. However, with a mild case of mumps it often happens that the swelling disappears before the doctor sees it, making a diagnosis more difficult.

My young son has caught mumps. Should I keep his sister away from the school during the infectious period?

Check with your daughter's school, because regulations vary from school to school. However, in general, schools do not now insist on a quarantine period.

My friend's daughter had meningitis as a complication of mumps. Is this common?

Mild meningitis can occur in about 1 percent of cases of mumps. It follows about 10 days after the first symptoms of mumps.
The patient will experience stiffness in the neck, headaches, and sometimes vomiting. These symptoms usually clear up within three or four days, and complete recovery is usual.

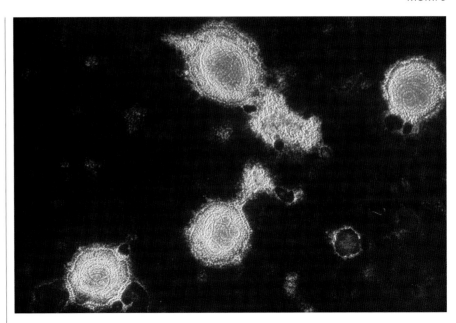

▲ *A colorized transmission electron micrograph of the mumps paramyxovirus. The virus has been magnified 20,000 times.*

Symptoms

The first symptoms are a fever, a sore throat, and shivering, and these can be mistaken for influenza. The gland that is first affected is generally the parotid, the large salivary gland between the upper and lower jaws. This gland becomes tender and swollen, so that it is difficult to open the mouth wide, and eating is extremely painful. The fever increases, and the temperature can rise to 103°F (39.5°C).

It is very rare for mumps to be dangerous, but the virus can cause inflammation in other glands and the nervous system.

Orchitis: Inflammation of one or both testicles occurs in about 20 percent of adult male cases of mumps. A week after the virus has caused swelling of the salivary glands, there is a painful enlargement of the affected testicle. In rare cases this can even occur without a fever or swelling of the salivary glands. Most testicles return to normal size within a week. Even in the most severe cases, when both testicles are involved and they shrink in size following the infection, sterility is rare. Impotence virtually never occurs, even with shrinkage of the testicles.

Oophoritis: Inflammation of the ovaries is uncommon, but it can produce lower abdominal pain and vomiting. The complication subsides within three days and has no long-term effects.

Prostatitis: Inflammation of the prostate gland is a rare complication of mumps. The patient complains of a high fever and of frequent urination a few days after the mumps fever has subsided. No treatment is necessary, and the symptoms soon abate.

Mastitis: The mammary glands rarely become inflamed because of mumps. However, if they are affected, and pain and swelling occur, painkillers and breast support are the treatment.

Encephalitis: This is a rare inflammation of the brain and is the only serious danger from mumps. The patient develops severe headaches, a high fever, and vomiting. In most cases a full recovery occurs. In a small proportion of cases there is permanent disability or even death.

Treatment

There is no curative or specific treatment for mumps. In mild and moderate cases painkillers are the best treatment, and resting in bed is unnecessary. In more severe cases, the patient should stay in bed, keep warm, and drink plenty of fluids when feverish. When swelling of the glands is severe and eating is painful, bland food and adequate fluids are recommended. Painkillers reduce the discomfort, and frequent mouthwashes with a weak saltwater solution will prevent bacterial infection of the gums or salivary glands.

See also: **Infection and infectious diseases; Vaccinations**

Nutrition

The body is like a factory that needs maintenance and fuel, which is supplied by the food we eat. Nutrition is the study of different kinds of foods and the ways that the human body utilizes them.

A list of the body's components will give some idea of the complex chemical structures of which humans are made. For the average person they are: protein (17 percent); fat (13.8 percent); carbohydrate (1.5 percent); water (61.6 percent); minerals (6.1 percent). In fact, the cells of the body are factories that use chemical reactions to convert the components supplied to them in the diet into the products necessary for life and growth of the body.

There are about 48 substances that must be supplied ready-made in the diet, including oxygen and water. All the rest can be manufactured, given these basic essentials. In addition, the body needs a constant reserve of energy to function efficiently. For nutrition to be adequate, it is important not only that adequate nutrients are supplied in the diet but also that the body absorbs them properly.

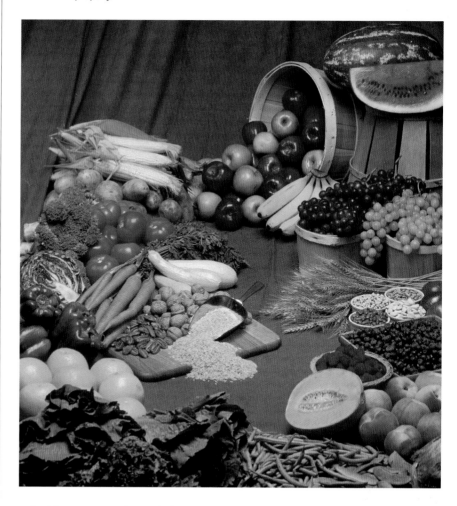

▲ *A healthy vegetarian diet includes vegetables, fruits, nuts, and grains. One standard serving recommendation is three to five servings of vegetables, two to four servings of fruit, two to three servings of nuts, and six to 11 servings of grains each day.*

216

Packed lunches for schoolchildren

A packed lunch can meet children's nutritional needs during the day, but a nourishing meal in the evening to supplement this must be provided. Sandwiches are ideal—bread contains vital nutrients and the fillings can contain a sufficient amount of protein—but lunch ideas need not be restricted to sandwiches alone.

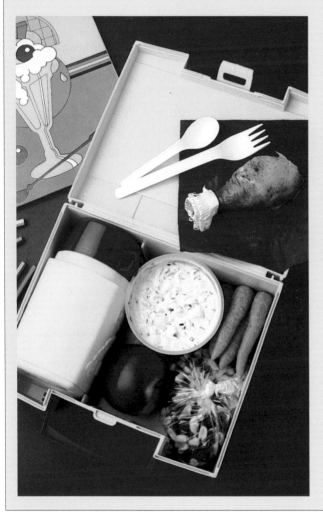

INCLUDE:

• Meat, fish, nuts (containing protein for growth)
• Dairy products (protein and fat for growth and energy)
• Whole wheat bread (carbohydrates, protein, and fiber)
• Fruit and vegetables (vitamins and minerals)

AVOID:

• Candy, jam, cookies, chocolate (all these sweet foods can be replaced with foods that have natural sugars, such as fruit, honey, potatoes, and bread)

A VARIETY OF LUNCHTIME IDEAS:

• Chicken drumsticks
• Cooked meatballs
• Hard-boiled eggs
• Small meat pie
• Slice of quiche
• Tuna salad

FOR COLD DAYS:

• Thermos of hot soup (with chunks of meat and vegetables) plus a fresh buttered roll or bagel

FOR DESSERT:

• Fruit yogurts
• Fruit salad
• Peeled and segmented orange
• Seedless raisins and nuts

PACKING:

• Use plastic boxes or save yogurt, margarine, or cottage cheese containers.
• Wrap carrots or celery in wax paper. Use aluminum foil for sandwiches.
• Remember to pack a fork, a spoon, and some napkins or tissues for wiping hands.

Fuels for the tissues

The body's basic fuels are fats and carbohydrates, and the energy they produce is measured in calories. People take in these fuels from animal and plant products, and the body converts them into assimilated forms for uptake into the cells.

Fats are converted into fatty acids and triglycerides, which are carried in the blood as complex lipoproteins. These are then taken to the adipose (fatty) tissues for storage; or, if they are needed, they can be "burned" chemically to provide energy.

Carbohydrates are mainly converted into sugars, especially glucose. This is the body's principal fuel. It is easy to transport, and the cells can use it conveniently. Glucose can also be made in the liver and other tissues by breaking down protein. Some cells, especially in the brain, require glucose as an energy source. This is stored in the form of glycogen and can be readily converted to glucose when needed. A minimum level of glucose is essential for the brain cells to function.

Proteins are broken into their basic components, amino acids. From amino acids the cells make their own proteins. They are not usually used as fuel, but when other sources of energy are lacking, they can be metabolized for this purpose. In cases of starvation the muscles waste away as the body burns up their protein components in an effort to maintain the glucose level of the blood at an appropriate level.

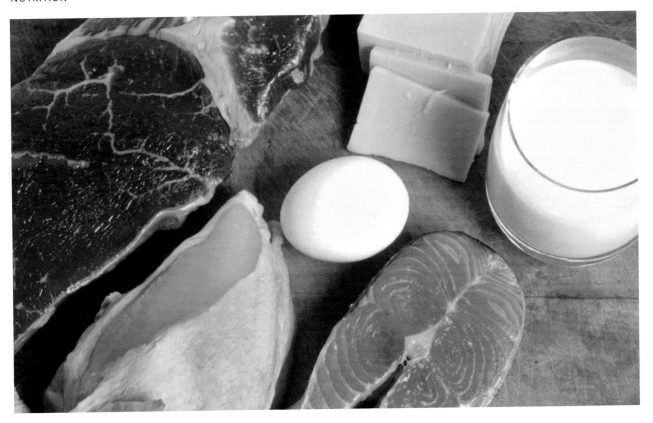

▲ Meat and fish are a good source of proteins and amino acids. Dairy products such as milk, cheese, and eggs provide vitamin D and calcium, which helps the bones to grow.

Essential nutrients

The body also requires some chemicals that it cannot make for itself. However, these can usually be stored, so a person may be able to survive for months, or even years, without them before the effect of any deficiency in the diet is felt. Oxygen is necessary at all times, and a lack of water will be felt in a day or two, since this cannot be stored in any quantity. The nutrients that people need include vitamins, essential elements and minerals (including those that are required in only minute amounts), fatty acids, and some amino acids.

Vitamins are essential in small amounts to help the body function. Different vitamins work in different ways. For example, once it is in the body, vitamin D acts like a hormone, coordinating the distribution of calcium and bone growth. Vitamin K helps control the clotting of blood. Vitamins are soluble in either water or fat. This is important, because if the absorption of fat is abnormal, owing to some disease in the intestines, then the fat-soluble vitamins will not be absorbed into the system. The fat-soluble vitamins are A, D, E, and K. Other vitamins are water-soluble.

Some constituents of the diet may interfere with the absorption or use of vitamins. It has been suggested that nicotinic acid, present in cereals, may be chemically bound to some of the other constituents; this binding would make it unavailable for use.

Food preparation may also affect some water-soluble vitamins. Folic acid is often destroyed through prolonged cooking or canning. (Nicotinic acid and folic acid are included in the vitamin B group.)

Mineral elements that are needed for adequate nutrition include carbon and hydrogen, which are so abundant that deficiency is practically impossible.

Sodium and chloride, the constituents of common salt, are essential to human biochemistry. Salt is widely distributed in foods, and deficiencies are found only when the body's requirements are greatly increased through abnormal losses. For example, when people who live in hot climates sweat excessively, the ensuing salt loss may be sufficient to require extra dietary supplements.

Calcium is an important constituent of bones and other tissues. The body's calcium usage is carefully regulated by a hormone system that includes vitamin D.

Iron is essential for the manufacture of hemoglobin, the vital oxygen-carrying substance in red blood cells. Some iron is also essential in the makeup of some of the enzyme systems in cells that provide energy to be used by the cells.

Minute quantities of other elements (trace elements) are also needed. Iodine, for example, is essential to the manufacture of thyroid hormone.

Fluorine, contained in fluoride, is necessary to prevent tooth decay; and in areas of low fluorine level, this is sometimes added to water supplies. Other trace elements such as copper, cobalt, and manganese are needed for various enzyme systems.

Amino acids are nitrogen-containing compounds that are the basic building blocks of the much larger protein molecules. The cells can manufacture many amino acids, but nine amino acids must be supplied ready-made in the diet. Different foods have different proportions of these essential substances; a mixture of food proteins must be eaten to ensure an adequate diet.

Linoleic acid and alpha-linoleic acid are fatty acids that are essential for the body to function properly. They are components of cell membranes and are needed for oxygen use and energy production, control of substances flowing in and out of cells, and hormone regulation. Deficiencies of fatty acids are rare.

Principles of good nutrition

It is important to eat the right kinds of food in the right quantities. The maintenance of good health depends on much more than simply getting enough calories and the basic vitamins and minerals.

The first requirement is that a person should not exceed the amounts necessary to maintain an optimum weight. By far the most common form of malnutrition in the United States is caused by excessive overeating, leading to obesity and all its attendant physical and psychological problems. The Centers for Disease Control and Prevention report that 34 percent of American adults aged 20 years and older are overweight, another 34 percent are obese, and another 6 percent are extremely obese. A similar increase has occurred in children. Regardless of the type of food that is eaten, obesity occurs when a person's calorie intake consistently exceeds his or her energy expenditure. Obesity is more common in lower-income groups than in high-income groups, and it is twice as common in African-American women as it is in Caucasian women. The difference between African-American and Caucasian men is less marked. Obesity is associated with a reduced life expectancy and a number of serious diseases such as diabetes, atherosclerosis, high blood pressure, and arthritis, in addition to various social disadvantages.

There is no easy answer to obesity nor any miraculous drug that can control food intake. The only effective cure is to establish new eating habits that involve strictly limited amounts of the appropriate foods. Obesity is encouraged by diets that are high in fat. This is because, weight for weight, fats provide nearly three times the calories of carbohydrates or proteins.

The second requirement is to avoid foods that are known to cause diseases. The principal disease of concern is atherosclerosis, which is a disease of arteries that results in a diminished capacity to carry blood. It is the cause of conditions such as heart attacks, strokes, limb gangrene, serious kidney diseases, dementia, and other severe disorders. Atherosclerosis has a number of causes, but among the most important is the excessive intake of saturated fats. Most of these are of dairy origin. It is not the amount of cholesterol in the diet that is of primary concern, but the total intake of saturated fats that a person consumes.

The third requirement is to ensure an adequate intake of dietary elements that prevent diseases. For example, people who eat a diet high in soluble, but nonabsorbable, fiber—such as that found in oats and wheat germ—have a much lower incidence of intestinal diseases such as colitis, diverticulitis, and colon and rectal cancer. Colorectal cancers are one of the three most common causes of deaths from cancer. Fiber also has the advantage that it can bind some of the cholesterol entering the intestine from the liver as a constituent of bile into an insoluble form. Cholesterol that is bound in this way is lost from the body in the feces.

Antioxidants

Another class of dietary elements that can prevent disease are the antioxidant vitamins and the flavonoids. Vitamins A, C, and E are antioxidant vitamins; to be effective as antioxidants, they must be

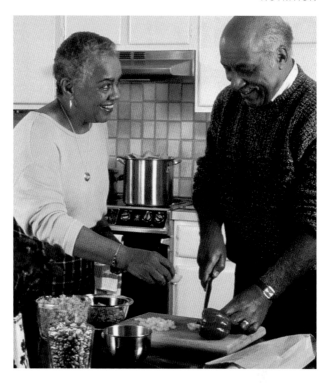

▲ *The key to proper nutrition is an adequate daily intake of protein, carbohydrates, fats, vitamins, and minerals, which should be maintained throughout a person's life.*

taken in much larger quantities than are necessary to prevent a vitamin deficiency. Less than about 0.05 ounce (1 g) of vitamin C and less than 0.01 ounce (0.3 g) of vitamin E taken daily are unlikely to be of much value as antioxidants. Flavonoids are compounds that are found in many fruits and vegetables and in red wine.

Antioxidants are important because many disease processes that damage the body do so by the production of powerful chemical elements called free radicals. These can start destructive chain reactions in the cells and tissues. Antioxidants mop up free radicals before they can cause harm.

The use of antioxidants may decrease the incidence of heart disease and cancer, and it may also remove lipids and cholesterol from the blood vessels, but this is not proved. Excessive intake of vitamins, especially fat-soluble A and D vitamins, is always dangerous because the excess is not excreted as it would be with water-soluble vitamins.

A good balance

A healthy balanced diet is one that is high in fruit and leafy green vegetables, to provide slow-release carbohydrates, fiber, and flavonoids. It should be low in fats of all kinds, especially dairy fats and their products, and moderate in protein, such as that found in cheese and red meat, because too much protein is associated with fat; and the diet may be supplemented by antioxidant vitamins.

> See also: **Antioxidants; Calcium; Diet; Fats; Glucose; Iron; Minerals; Obesity; Protein; Salt; Vitamin A; Weight**

Obesity

People are called "obese" if more than one-third of their body weight is fat. Obesity can happen to anyone, and not only is the excess weight unattractive, but, more important, it is a serious health hazard.

According to some estimates, in countries like the United States up to half the population carry too much fat and many are obese. Obesity can be prevented by calorie management, although once obesity occurs, it is often difficult for people to achieve their ideal weight.

Causes

Obesity is caused by eating too much, that is, more food than the body uses, so that the surplus is stored as fat. When overeating occurs for many years and the surplus fat is not burned up, weight will be gained. For example, if a person eats one slice of bread more than he or she needs every day, after 10 years the stored food will weigh about 40 pounds (about 18 kg), and the person will weigh 40 pounds more than his or her ideal weight.

To a certain extent, obesity runs in families. The cause may be genetic inheritance—some people are more likely to become obese than others, given the same food intake and energy expended—but often obesity occurs from learning bad eating habits from the family.

Emotional factors can play an important part in causing obesity. When people are depressed, they often turn to food for comfort—and over time, weight gain is the result. Their large size may then be a cause of depression, and they will eat more and get even fatter—making obesity a self-perpetuating condition.

My friend eats the same amount as I do, is about the same height as I am, but is of average weight, whereas I am fat. Why is this?

The way in which people's bodies use food varies widely. People who use their food fuel economically become obese more easily than those who use it extravagantly, because they burn off less energy for the same amount of work. You may also find that you are getting less exercise than your friend, so that you are expending less energy. Finally, you may have acquired an excess of fat as a child, so that even if you eat the same as your friend, you are still not losing your excess stored fat.

My son is seven and is very fat. Will he lose weight as he gets older, or will he be an obese adult?

Unless your son loses weight now, he is likely to be overweight as an adult. Some fat children do lose weight in adolescence, but you can't count on this. Assume that your son is likely to remain fat and help him change his eating habits to prevent this.

Is it true that gland trouble can cause obesity?

People are rarely overweight because of an underactive thyroid gland or overactive adrenal glands, and in these cases there are other symptoms.

Is it true that obese people feel the cold less than thinner people?

Fat tissue is an efficient insulator—in fact this is one of its functions. People who have more fat should not feel the cold as much, since they have insulation under their skin. The exception is people who are overweight as a result of thyroid hormone deficiency: they feel the cold far more than others.

FEMALE HEIGHT	SMALL FRAME	MEDIUM FRAME	LARGE FRAME	MALE HEIGHT	SMALL FRAME	MEDIUM FRAME	LARGE FRAME
4' 8"	88–94	92–103	100–115	4' 8"	101–109	107–111	115–130
4' 9"	90–97	94–106	102–118	4' 9"	104–112	110–121	118–133
4' 10"	92–100	97–109	105–121	4' 10"	107–115	113–125	121–136
4' 11"	95–103	100–112	109–124	4' 11"	110–118	116–128	124–140
5' 0"	98–106	103–115	111–127	5' 0"	113–121	119–131	127–144
5' 1"	101–109	106–118	114–130	5' 1"	116–125	122–135	130–148
5' 2"	104–112	109–122	117–134	5' 2"	120–129	126–139	134–153
5' 3"	107–115	112–126	121–138	5' 3"	124–133	130–144	139–158
5' 4"	110–119	116–131	125–142	5' 4"	128–137	134–148	143–162
5' 5"	114–123	120–135	129–146	5' 5"	132–142	138–152	147–166
5' 6"	118–127	124–139	133–150	5' 6"	136–146	142–157	151–171
5' 7"	122–131	128–143	137–154	5' 7"	140–150	146–162	156–176
5' 8"	126–136	132–147	141–157	5' 8"	144–154	150–167	160–181
5' 9"	130–140	136–151	145–164	5' 9"	148–158	154–172	165–186
5' 10"	134–144	140–155	149–169	5' 10"	152–162	159–177	170–191
5' 11"	138–148	144–159	153–174	5' 11"	156–167	164–182	174–196
6' 0"	142–152	149–163	157–179	6' 0"	160–171	169–187	178–201

Recommended weight for females and males

This table shows ideal weights (in pounds) for males and females. Bone structure influences ideal weight; if a person has a large frame, he or she will weigh more than a person with a small frame, even if they are both the same height. If a person is too heavy or too light and finds it difficult to reduce or gain weight, he or she may have a problem that requires medical attention.

Questions and Answers

I recently stopped smoking and have put on 20 lb. (9 kg). Is this more dangerous to me than if I had continued to smoke?

No. Many people who give up smoking put on weight, usually because they replace addictive smoking with a greater appetite for eating. However, studies have shown that the increase in weight under these circumstances is less dangerous than continued smoking, although clearly it is better to give up smoking without becoming obese.

I am a woman in her forties with three grown children. I don't really overeat, and I seem to be as active as I always was, but I'm obese. How could this have happened?

It happened gradually. If you have been eating only a small amount above your daily calorie requirement, then it will take many years for this excess to accumulate into obesity.

Another possible factor is that women usually acquire weight in pregnancy and may not lose it afterward; therefore, several pregnancies could have left you with a considerable excess, which you will not lose unless you eat less than you require.

Finally, women use up lots of energy caring for young children. If your food intake stays the same, you will put on weight when your children leave home and you have less to do—and as you age and your metabolism slows.

I know that my teenage daughter binges on huge quantities of food at least twice a week, yet she is not obese. Why is this?

Your daughter may be burning up all the calories that she consumes, in which case she should eat smaller amounts of food at regular intervals. Alternatively, she could be suffering from bulimia—binge eating followed by self-induced vomiting. If she seems preoccupied with her weight and you suspect she has bulimia, take her to see your doctor, who may recommend psychotherapy.

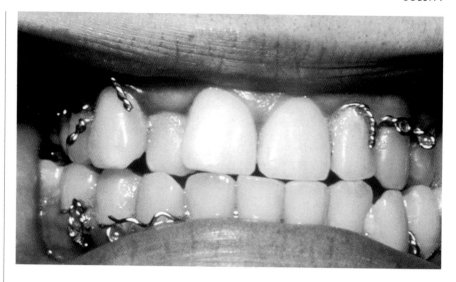

▲ *Wiring together a person's teeth is an extreme measure that can be taken to cure obesity. It is used only as a last resort when all other methods have failed.*

Medical findings

In rare cases a medical problem causes obesity. An underactive thyroid gland or overactive adrenal glands can result in weight gain, as can rare medical causes such as congenital syndromes involving hormonal abnormalities, and birth defects that affect appetite regulation.

Research has also identified a group of proteins called leptins that are involved in the regulation of metabolism and appetite. Deficiencies of leptins or of their receptors lead to obesity and sometimes cause diabetes in mice. The role of leptins in human obesity is still under investigation.

Development of obesity

When a person consumes more food than the body needs, the liver converts the surplus into fatty acids. These fatty acids are carried in the bloodstream to the fatty (adipose) tissues located around the body, where they are converted into storage fats and kept inside the cells.

When fat is laid down in excess, it appears where the body tissue is most abundant— initially this is usually in the buttocks and the abdomen, followed by the thighs and arms. People may develop fat deposits in slightly different places and at different rates, but most people follow this pattern.

Health risks

Most people dislike being overweight because they feel that it makes them unattractive, but there are also some serious medical dangers that are associated with obesity. Being slightly above the ideal recommended weight for an individual's height, build, and age—by 5 percent or so—is probably not a great risk to health. However, if a person's weight is much over this amount, he or she will be prone to many other complications in addition to the emotional and social problems that obesity can cause.

One problem is that the extra weight an obese person carries is distributed mainly in the central parts of the body, where it puts extra strain on the joints, particularly the knees. This leads to the early development of osteoarthritis (wear and tear of the joints), which is likely to become a painful problem in early middle age.

In addition to this, obese people who consume large amounts of certain foods and neglect others may suffer from malnourishment due to a lack of protein or essential vitamins and minerals.

Obesity can also cause mild diabetes, which in turn may cause serious complications in the small blood vessels of the eyes and kidneys. Since there is an increase in available fats, especially cholesterol, in the circulation, the obese person also tends to develop gallstones and, to a lesser extent, gout.

Fatty infiltration

More serious problems arise when fatty infiltration impairs the efficiency of the abdominal muscles. This impairment inhibits movement of the diaphragm and makes breathing inefficient, possibly leading to lung disorders and shortness of breath. For similar reasons, obese people have a high incidence of lung complications when they have a general anesthetic before an operation.

Atherosclerosis

Obese people tend to have high levels of fat in their blood, and for this reason they have an increased risk of developing atherosclerosis—thickening and hardening of the arteries that impairs blood circulation.

As a result, there is likely to be an increased chance of thrombosis of the arteries that supply vital organs such as the brain and heart. This can cause strokes and heart attacks. If the blood supply to the kidneys is threatened, the blood pressure will rise and kidney failure may result.

Life expectancy

Because of these complications, obese men and women have a reduced chance of living to a healthy old age. Indeed, some insurance companies have calculated that if a man is 25 pounds (11 kg) overweight, his life expectancy will be reduced by one-fourth.

▼ *In recent decades, a dramatic increase in cases of type II diabetes in U.S. children seems to be closely linked to obesity.*

Dieting

The main treatment for obesity is gradual dieting. That is, the gradual overeating that has caused the condition must be reversed so that less food is eaten than is required for the energy expended by the person in his or her daily activities. In addition, the output of energy should be increased through exercise and movement.

Ineffective shortcuts

Dieting is never easy, since it requires extreme willpower to change the eating habits that have been acquired over a lifetime, and for this reason, many obese people try various shortcuts—none of which are an effective alternative to sensible dieting.

The first of these is the crash diet. It is possible for a person to lose a large amount of weight very quickly, but studies have shown that crash dieters almost always gain back the weight and return to their previous size within a year or two of dieting.

Another method is to take amphetaminelike pills. These help reduce a person's appetite, but at the expense of dangerous side effects to the heart and brain. Such pills are also addictive.

Other, much safer, drugs have been developed, including non-absorbable bulking agents, statin drugs such as orlistat that block the action of digestive fat-splitting enzymes, and serotonin reuptake inhibitor anorectic agents such as sibutramine. Although these modern antiobesity drugs can help to control appetite, however, most of them are at least mildly addictive, none actually "burn up" fat, and weight is rapidly regained once the pills are stopped.

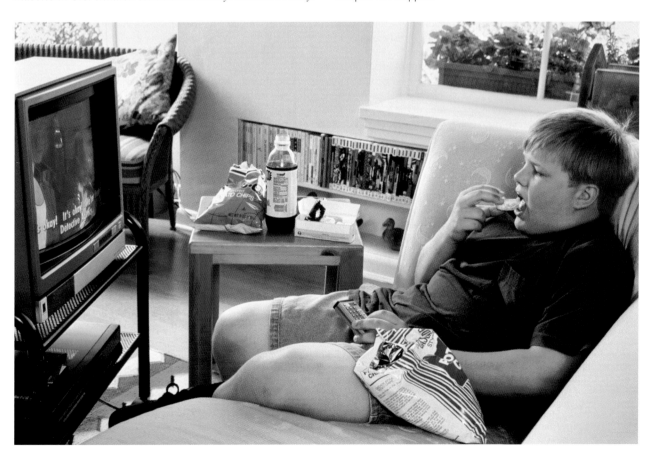

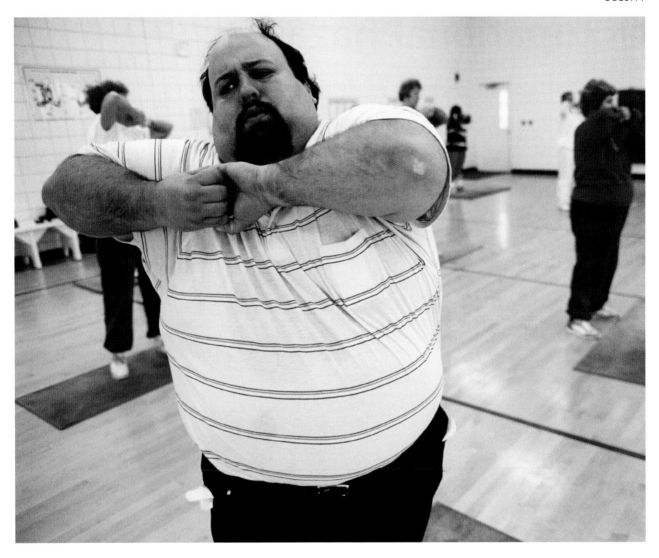

▲ *To achieve long-term weight loss, obese people must consistently eat less and expend more energy through exercise.*

Extreme measures

When obesity becomes life-threatening, people may resort to jaw-wiring, which is the temporary wiring together of the jaws to prevent the person from taking in solid food—resulting in a great loss of weight. However, the weight is usually rapidly regained when the wires are removed.

Various operations have also been tried to help very obese people lose weight when everything else has failed. Sometimes the stomach walls are stapled together to reduce the volume of the stomach so that the person feels full more quickly and stops eating sooner. However, the stomach may still be stretched by overeating, and if the staples break, major surgery may be required. Another method involves removing or reversing segments of the small intestine, or bypassing it, so that less food is absorbed. However, these procedures can cause serious malnutritional problems, and patients risk complications such as leakage of the intestinal fluid, internal bleeding, blockages, infection, and even death.

Lifestyle changes

Obese people who genuinely want to lose weight and to remain slim must completely alter their previous lifestyles and eating patterns. In particular, they must change any bad habits, such as eating only junk food. They may also find it helpful to seek medical advice as to the most suitable diet for weight reduction and for fostering and maintaining sensible and healthy eating habits.

Diet clubs and organizations such as Weight Watchers may help obese people to lose weight and learn about nutrition, which is important, because they need to develop and maintain healthy eating habits after they reach their ideal weight. The clubs also offer the encouragement and support of other members who have a similar problem.

In addition to reorganizing their eating habits, obese people need to increase the amount of exercise that they get—particularly if they lead a mainly sedentary life.

> *See also:* **Anorexia and bulimia; Birth defects; Cholesterol; Depression; Diabetes; Diet; Dieting; Exercise; Fats; Heart attack; Heredity; Stroke; Weight**

Occupational hazards

Every year, occupational hazards result in disease, injury, and sometimes even death. People encounter a variety of potential problems in the workplace, and many of these can be prevented.

Questions and Answers

I read that inhaling some kinds of dusts found at work can be dangerous. Why is this?

Although it is not desirable to have any foreign particles enter the lungs, some dusts are more harmful than others. A stonecutter who works only with marble and inhales its dust has practically no chance of getting lung disease. Yet if he were working on sandstone, the risk of lung disease and death caused by the dust would be high. The reason for these differences is not fully understood. Many dusts, such as asbestos, are a special danger and can cause cancer of the lung and the pleura (lining of the lung), as well as the disabling disease asbestosis.

I have heard mixed reports about whether computer screens are safe to use. What are the health risks?

Reports on the risks to health from radiation as a result of using computers are very mixed, but prolonged use of terminals may cause physical problems such as eyestrain; headaches; pain in the back, neck, arms, and fingers (carpal tunnel syndrome); and more general stress. Some of these ailments can be avoided if the terminal is set in a properly designed workstation. Regular breaks should be taken away from the computer screen, with at least 10 minutes' rest every hour.

We have a representative in our office whose sole concern is health and safety. Why do we need one?

Every year thousands of office staffers are injured at work. Half of the injuries are caused by falls, such as tripping over carelessly placed wires or objects. These accidents can be easily prevented, and a safety representative is very helpful in assessing the potential dangers to the staff and advising the management accordingly.

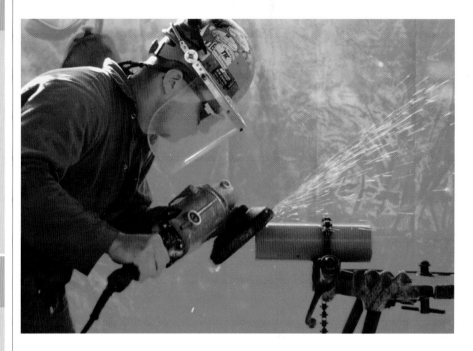

▲ *This industrial worker wears a special helmet with a visor to protect his face from the dangerously sharp bits of metal that are flying off the metal tube he is grinding.*

Health hazards associated with work have existed for centuries. In the last few hundred years, with the development of industrialization, very specific occupational hazards have been recognized. While industry was slow to acknowledge and deal with the problems, safety measures are now regarded as a high priority by many employers and labor unions.

Apart from the personal toll that such occupational disease and injury can bring, there is a heavy economic price to pay. Millions of working days are lost each year in the United States through work-related health problems.

Many of the most serious occupational hazards have been brought under control by legislation. However, the risks can never be eliminated completely as new products and working methods are devised and tried. There is also the reality that accidents with machinery can never be totally eliminated, because of human error. However, these accidents can be minimized. Employers should ensure that safety standards are maintained, and staff members should always adhere to safety regulations.

Hazardous materials

Occupational hazards may arise with the use of gases, liquids, or solids. Substances can enter the body through the lungs.

One dangerous metal is lead, a toxic substance that has been used in the manufacture of batteries, rubber, paint, roofing, and soldering material. It can enter the body through the inhalation of small dust particles and fumes or by ingestion. The earliest symptoms may include fatigue, headache, loss of appetite, constipation, and mild abdominal pain. Acute poisoning can result in severe abdominal pain, muscle weakness, kidney damage, convulsions, coma, and death.

Questions and Answers

I often have to work night shifts. Will this affect my health?

About 20 percent of people enjoy working nights; another 20 percent dislike it intensely and have to quit. No studies have shown any difference in causes of death between day and night workers, but if you have been working during the day and then are put onto a night shift, it can take time for your body to adapt. Research shows that there is a slightly higher incidence of cancer in people who are not exposed to normal diurnal and nocturnal light and dark cycles.

I work near a hot furnace. Will the high temperatures harm me?

The body can usually adapt to raised temperatures, but if physical labor is involved, and if the salt and water lost during sweating are not replaced, you may suffer from heatstroke or heat syncope, leading to unconsciousness. Treatment involves cooling the body and rest. If you become used to high temperatures, heat tolerance is likely to be greater and the chance of problems reduced.

I am a smoker. Can smoking increase the risk of my getting a work-related disease?

Yes. Smoking is likely to increase your risk of developing a number of health problems. One problem is that smoking damages the airways, undermining the natural defense of the lungs and allowing harmful substances easier access into your body.

Why are substances thought to cause cancer still used in industry?

It is not possible to eliminate these substances entirely from many industrial processes. However, the Occupational Health and Safety Administration constantly studies these substances to establish safe levels and safeguards to protect workers. Companies that do not follow these guidelines risk legal action.

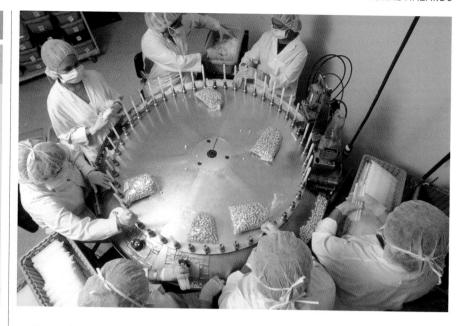

▲ *These pharmaceutical workers packaging pills are wearing sterilized gowns, masks, and gloves to prevent any diseases or infections from reaching the consumer.*

Mercury, a silver-colored liquid that has been used in some thermometers, is another hazardous metal. It has been used in the electrical industry to manufacture fluorescent lamps and precision instruments, as well as in dentistry.

Mercury poisoning causes jerky movements starting in the fingers, irritability, and drowsiness. In the final stage, the person becomes mentally disturbed. Other symptoms include sore throat and gums, vomiting, and diarrhea. Compounds from mercury can also be dangerous when they occur in the form of industrial effluents. The effluents are absorbed by fish, which are then eaten by people. The poisoning results in blindness, mental deterioration, lack of coordination, birth defects, and even death.

Cadmium, a soft metal that is used for increasing the hardness of copper, and as a protective plating for other metals, is particularly dangerous. Once a person has inhaled or ingested a certain amount, there is no known cure. Poisoning can be gradual because the amount of metal in the body builds up slowly. However, at a critical point the lungs and the kidneys will cease to function properly, causing death.

Chromium, a silver-white, hard, brittle metal, is used to make various types of steel, including stainless steel, and high-speed tools. Its compounds are used in chrome plating as well as the production of pigments in paints and inks. It is also used in leather tanning, in timber preservation, and in photography and dyestuffs. The major danger of chromium is that even slight contact with dilute solutions can cause skin ulcers.

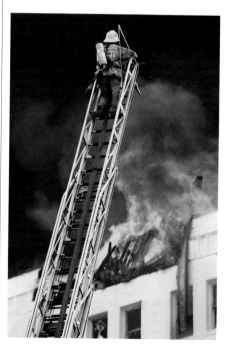

◄ *Firefighters face many occupational hazards that can result in injury or death from falls, burns, and smoke inhalation.*

The inhalation of fine droplets or mist containing chromium salts can cause ulcers inside the nose. Although lung cancer has not been associated with chrome plating, it has been linked with the manufacture of chromates. Asthmatic symptoms can occur, as can sensitivity to chrome—a strong reaction to chrome following symptoms of exposure.

Many liquids are classed as solvents, and employees in nearly all occupations are exposed to them. Solvents evaporate very quickly, and the vapors can enter the body by inhalation through the lungs, the skin, and, more rarely, the digestive system. Once they enter the body, they can attack the liver, the heart, the lungs, and the nervous system.

Solvents are found in inks, varnishes, glues, cleaners, dry-cleaning fluids, and many other substances. Some of the most dangerous ones may be pleasant to smell, while others that are foul-smelling can be quite harmless.

Trichlorethylene smells good, but it can cause loss of consciousness and death. Benzene is another pleasant-smelling solvent, used in the manufacture of artificial leather, some detergents, pesticides, and paint removers. It can cause dizziness and coma. When poisoning is chronic, leukemia may result.

Because of the dissolving properties of solvents, they can attack the skin and cause skin inflammation (dermatitis). Contact with solvents should be strictly limited.

All isocyanates are dangerous. They are used in the manufacture of a variety of polyurethanes that are used to make foams, adhesives, lacquers, and paints. Overexposure to isocyanates that are in the air can lead to painful skin inflammation, eye irritation,

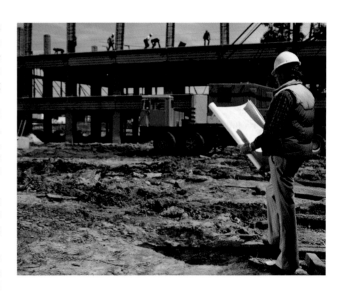

▲ *Thousands of construction workers are injured or killed in accidents on construction sites each year, most commonly from falls, but also from electric shocks, collapsing structures, fires, explosions, welding, and machinery.*

and breathing difficulties, including severe asthma. Some people can also develop sensitivity to isocyanate.

Dust is the biggest killer in industry. Some dusts are relatively harmless, but others are deadly. There are four basic categories. The

Emergency first aid

To give first aid in an emergency, first see if the patient is breathing. If breathing has stopped, either start mouth-to-mouth resuscitation, or if the patient's mouth is burned with chemicals, start cardiac compression. Next, check for serious bleeding. Control bleeding by pressing at the site of the wound with a sterilized pad or with your fingers. Raise the injured limb, if possible, to help slow the blood flow. If the patient is unconscious, make sure that he or she can breathe and the throat is not obstructed. Place the person in the recovery position; get expert help immediately.

OTHER INJURIES	TREATMENT
Burns and scalds	Cool the area by flushing with plenty of clean, cool water. Then cover with a sterile dressing or clean material. Do not apply any ointment, or burst any blisters, or remove any clothing sticking to burns.
Chemical burns	Remove contaminated clothing, taking care that you do not contaminate yourself, and dilute the chemical by flushing with plenty of water. Then apply a dry dressing.
Chemical in the eye	Quickly flush the open eye with clean, cool water and continue for at least 10 minutes.
Foreign body in the eye	If the object cannot be removed easily with the corner of a clean piece of material or by flushing with water, send the patient to the hospital.
Broken bones	Unless there is a danger of further injury, do not move the patient until expert help arrives.
Electric shock	Do not touch the patient until the current has been switched off. If breathing has stopped, give mouth-to-mouth resuscitation or cardiac compression and call for expert help.
Gas inhalation	Move the patient into fresh air, but wear suitable breathing equipment so that you do not become a victim yourself. If breathing has stopped, give mouth-to-mouth resuscitation or cardiac compression.
Amputation of finger	Keep pressure over the stump to prevent arterial bleeding. Wrap the finger in an ice pack. Rush the patient and the protected dismembered finger to the hospital.

I've heard that if a man works with dangerous substances his wife can be affected. Is this true?

Yes. This can happen if proper precautions and hygiene are not followed. Cases of lead poisoning have been seen among families of lead workers who went home without changing their work clothes. Employees can also carry contaminating fibers home on their clothing. However, strict regulations are ensuring that such risks are a thing of the past.

I work in industry and am planning to have a baby. Are there any health risks that could affect my pregnancy?

There are laws to protect women from most dangerous hazards, such as lead. Other risks can include waste anesthetic gases to which operating room staff members can be exposed; these gases can cause miscarriages and birth defects. Radiation is a danger, and a fetus is 10 times as vulnerable as an adult. Mercury and its compounds, which can produce mental abnormalities in children, are a potential problem. It should be remembered that the fetus is at risk from all toxic substances that are transferred via the mother. Therefore, smoking and drinking alcohol in pregnancy are not recommended.

I use a pneumatic drill whose noise level is controlled. Could the vibrations affect my body?

The major hazard for people using vibration tools is vibration white finger; the blood supply to the fingers is impeded and the fingers appear pale and can tingle and feel numb. At a certain stage, the tissue damage becomes permanent. People with poor circulation should not do this sort of job. Others should wear warm clothing and padded gloves when using the tools. Where possible, employees should be in a warm environment to ensure good circulation in the extremities. Hours for this type of work should be strictly limited.

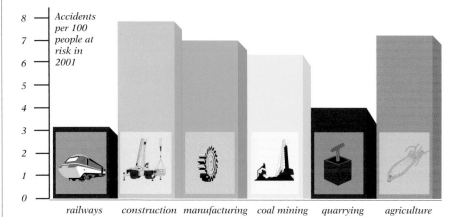

INCIDENCE OF ACCIDENTS AT WORK IN THE UNITED STATES

Accidents per 100 people at risk in 2001

railways · construction · manufacturing · coal mining · quarrying · agriculture

▲ *The graph shows hazardous occupations, as measured by the number of accidents recorded at work. Many other jobs also involve health hazards for workers.*

first category is nuisance or inert dust such as plaster of paris, starch, and portland cement. Such dusts can accumulate in the body without producing a serious reaction. Second, toxic dusts include lead and chromium compounds. They can have serious effects on specific organs in the body such as the kidneys and the nervous system. Third, dusts that produce allergic reactions, such as some wood dusts and fungus spores from grain, can cause eczema and asthma. Fourth, there are some dusts, like asbestos and coal dust, that alter the lung tissue, making the lungs inefficient. These cause death and serious disability in hundreds of people.

The danger of dusts depends not only on the type of dust but on the amount and the time over which it is breathed in. It is often more dangerous to inhale small quantities of dust repeatedly over a long period than to inhale a large amount of dust in a short period.

Healthy lungs can cope with a certain amount of some dust and fumes without any ill effects. However, the body's defense mechanisms may be unable to cope with the onslaught of dangerous or excessive dusts. This is why elimination of dust in the working atmosphere is so important, and why protective clothing and respiratory equipment must be used.

In many industries, working with deafening noise used to be accepted as part of the job. However, it is now a hazard for which there are controls and preventive measures.

Basic preventive measures are to deaden the noise of machinery, and instruct workers to wear earmuffs or plugs that reduce sound levels.

Occupational injuries

Every year, some people employed in manufacturing jobs die as a result of an occupational accident or disease. Some jobs have a notoriously high risk of death, such as lumberjacking or working on oil rigs. Other jobs are not dangerous in themselves, but they involve machinery that can give rise to accidents if misused.

A number of accidents occur through the use of unguarded machinery. Laws declare that all machinery must be safeguarded, but some employers try to cut corners and do not always ensure that these safeguards are taken. Moreover, some employees believe that

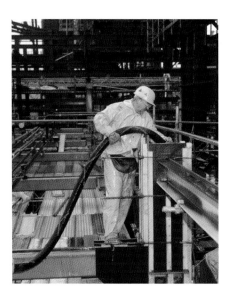

► *Factory workers at oil refineries risk injury or death from accidents involving gas leakages or explosions.*

Occupational hazards

HAZARD	INDUSTRY	ENTRY MODE	SYMPTOMS	TREATMENT	PREVENTION
AIDS	Doctors, dentists	Needle-stick injuries	Fever, fatigue, attacks of shingles or herpes	Anti-HIV drugs but no cure	Care with needles, proper disposal of blood-associated equipment
Asbestos	Many, including shipbuilding, pipe and boiler lagging, building	Inhalation	Breathlessness, dry cough, cancer of the lung or pleura (lining of thorax and lungs)	Remove from further exposure to inhalation and relieve symptoms	Enclosing dust-producing process, wearing masks and gloves, using substitute materials
Cadmium	Plating on metals; production of alloys, paints, enamel, and pigments	Inhalation or ingestion	Irritation of eyes and nose, breathlessness, coughing, vomiting, headache, diarrhea, colic, kidney damage	Symptomatic only	Enclosing process, wearing masks and gloves, monitoring of the environment
Chromium	Auto industry, steel, pigments, leather tanning, photography	Inhalation	Ulcers on skin, especially nasal membranes; asthmatic symptoms	Ointment and local treatment of ulcers	Enclosing process, environmental monitoring, wearing masks and gloves
Hepatitis	Laboratory and hospital workers	Contact with infected blood or excreta	Weakness, loss of appetite, malaise, jaundice	No specific treatment; hepatitis A often self-limiting	Safety clothing and protocols to avoid contamination
Isocyanates	Manufacture of foams, adhesives, synthetic rubbers, paints, polyurethane	Vapor inhalation or skin contact	Dermatitis, coughing, eye irritation, asthma, and breathlessness	Removal from contact, symptomatic treatment	Exhaust ventilation, wearing masks and gloves
Lead	Batteries, rubber, paint, roofing, and soldering	Ingestion, inhalation	Headache, convulsions, constipation, coma, abdominal pain, muscle weakness, kidney damage	Removal from exposure, chelation to remove lead and change properties, oral penicillamine	Exhaust ventilation, personal hygiene, regular analysis of blood and urine, environmental monitoring
Mercury	Electrical industry, fluorescent lamps, dentistry	Inhalation, ingestion, absorption through skin	Jerky movements, irritability, drowsiness, bleeding gums	Removal from source of contact	Enclosing process, exhaust ventilation, wearing masks and gloves
Noise	Boilermaking, drop-forging, shipbuilding	Ears	Deafness	Remove from further exposure	Reducing machinery noise, wearing earplugs
Radiation	Medicine, luminous dials, atomic energy and weapons, welding checks	Irradiation, ingestion of contaminated particles	Burns, scaling of skin, loss of hair, cancer, cataracts, dermatitis, genetic damage	Symptomatic; immediate removal from contamination	Screening from source; monitoring; wearing masks, gloves, and protective clothing
Silicosis	Pottery, mining, quarrying, sandblasting	Inhalation	Dry cough, bronchitis, breathlessness, severe respiratory disablement	Remove from further exposure, treat symptoms	Wearing masks and gloves, damping dust, enclosing process
Solvents	Inks, glues, varnishes, paints, degreasing and dry-cleaning agents	Inhalation, skin contact, ingestion	Many, due to damage to nervous system, liver, heart, lungs; dermatitis	Various; remove from exposure	Exhaust ventilation, monitoring environment, wearing masks and gloves
Vibration	Building, welding, forestry	Contact with tool	Pale, numb fingers	Removal from contact	Warm environment, wearing masks and padded gloves
Wood dust	Lumberyards, wood polishers, furniture	Inhalation and skin contact	Dermatitis, respiratory irritation, nasal cancer	Symptomatic	Dust extraction, wearing masks and gloves

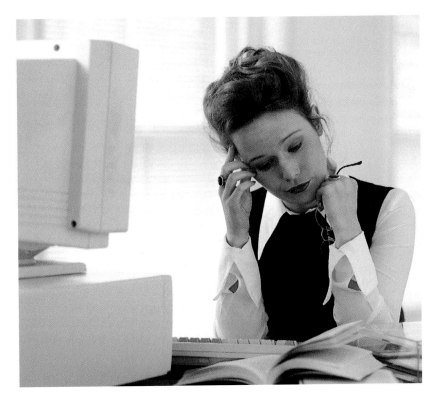

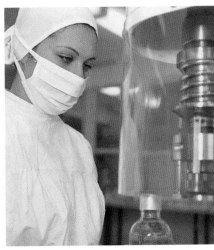

▲ *Laboratory accidents that may lead to contamination can be avoided by following safety procedures.*

◄ *It is important for computer workers to ensure that they are sitting correctly when they are working at a computer screen, and take regular breaks to rest their eyes.*

certain safeguards are slowing their output and costing them pay. Such people may deliberately remove the safeguards and so risk losing a limb.

Machinery maintenance is especially hazardous because safeguards often have to be removed for access. Unfortunate mistakes, such as failing to switch off the power supply, can be the cause of other serious injuries. Many injuries in factories are caused through the misuse of hand tools. Eye injuries from fragments of metal flying off drills, or chips of stone or metal split off in hammering, are common. Employees do not always like wearing eye protection, but such a basic precaution prevents minor eye injuries.

Certain types of hand tools such as chain saws can cause a condition that is known as "vibration white finger." The symptoms are pale or blue tingling fingers. This can progress to pain, or loss of sensation. There is no known cure for white finger. Because the injury causes a cold-sensitive spasm of the arteries, employees who must use vibration tools should wear padded gloves and keep their hands as warm as possible.

Falls in factories account for another high proportion of occupational injuries. Many of these falls occur on a level floor and are a result of clutter from boxes and various other items left lying around. Spilled liquids and general untidiness can also cause falls. Trailing wires, filing cabinet drawers left open, and poorly lit stairs are other avoidable traps that can cause accidents.

An increase in the use of computers has brought about a new set of work-related injuries, which can be divided into three basic groups: repetitive strain injury (RSI), back and neck problems, and eyestrain.

RSI is a disorder that results from performing repetitive tasks over a prolonged period of time. Although RSI disorders such as "writer's cramp" were reported among clerks as an epidemic in London in the 19th century, the term "repetitive stress injury" originated in the 1970s when video display units (VDUs) were introduced in the workplace. The most common forms of RSI are carpal tunnel syndrome (caused by irritation and compression of the median nerve at the wrist, which results in numbness, pins and needles, pain, and lack of mobility in the wrist) and tendon injuries (caused by inflammation of the tendons, as in tendonitis, or the tendon sheaths, as in tenosynovitis, both of which result in pain in the hands and fingers).

The most common types of computer-related disorders are back and neck problems, with the accompanying pain. Such disorders often develop when workers remain in a sedentary position for long periods. Eyestrain also affects people who sit for long hours in front of a computer screen; it can lead to headaches and migraines.

Preventing injury

Many occupational injuries can be prevented by following safety regulations. Employers should actively enforce these regulations, and employees should make sure that they wear any safety equipment their employer provides for them. Employees also have a responsibility to encourage better office and factory maintenance. To help prevent computer-related disorders, workers should correctly position their chairs and screens in their work stations, check their posture, try not to remain in the same position for too long, and take breaks. Although occupational hazards will always exist, simple precautions can reduce the various risks that people encounter as part of their job.

See also: **Birth defects; Burns; Hepatitis; Leukemia; Ulcers**

Osteoporosis

Questions and Answers

This condition of unusually light and fragile bones causes 238,000 hip fractures in the United States each year. Women are four times more likely than men to suffer from the disease. However, osteoporosis is preventable.

My grandmother has a humpback. It seems to have occurred gradually since her 70th birthday. She calls it her dowager's hump and says that it's not worth worrying about because it doesn't hurt. Is she right? What caused it?

A dowager's hump is the result of osteoporosis, in which the bones become smaller, lighter, and less robust than normal. Over the years, some of the bones in your grandmother's spine have become squashed and others have collapsed into a wedge shape, so that the spine has bent into a hump. Your grandmother is right not to worry about it; it is not life-threatening, it often causes no pain, and severe cases are rare.

Can I avoid osteoporosis if I drink plenty of milk?

Some of the constituents of milk are essential for bone growth, but milk cannot prevent osteoporosis, which is a condition of old age and its accompanying changes in the balance of the body's hormones or chemical messengers. By all means drink plenty of milk, but don't expect it to work wonders.

Is it true that women on hormone replacement therapy (HRT) do not develop osteoporosis?

Hormone replacement therapy (HRT) may be given to women who suffer from severe problems associated with menopause. One of these problems is the failure of the ovaries to produce the hormone estrogen, and it is thought that a lack of estrogen is a cause of osteoporosis. HRT usually consists of estrogen and progesterone. Evidence suggests that HRT does seem to prevent or reverse osteoporosis to some extent, but HRT is now known to pose some serious health risks, which must be weighed against its few and relatively slight benefits.

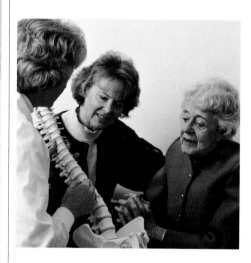

▲ *Elderly people are prone to osteoporosis. The weakened bones can cause minor deformities, falls, and fractures.*

The bones in the body are not dead, as some people imagine. They are living material that is constantly changing. When such changes involve a loss of bone, the condition is called osteoporosis.

Causes

The most common cause of osteoporosis is aging. From middle age onward everyone's bones become lighter. This change is generally more marked in women after they have been through the menopause. However, it is only when an excessive amount of bone is lost that the symptoms of osteoporosis arise.

There are other, more complicated causes of osteoporosis, most of which are rare. In such cases the loss of bone is usually a result of drastic changes in the body that have been brought about by another illness. In these instances, the osteoporosis is described as secondary, since it is an effect of the initial (primary) illness and will disappear if the primary illness is cured. Many cases of secondary osteoporosis are diseases of the hormonal system.

There is one relatively common secondary cause that is generally described as immobilization—a term meaning simply that the patient must stay in bed for some reason. Therefore, osteoporosis is often seen in the bones of a single limb, which cannot be moved because of pain, paralysis, or a broken (fractured) bone.

Symptoms

Osteoporosis may cause no symptoms at all, or it may give rise to bone pain and backache. In advanced cases there may be deformities such as loss of height or a bent spine. The bones tend to break easily from even minor accidents or trivial strains.

The most commonly caused fracture is the collapse of one of the spinal vertebrae (small bones). This may not hurt, or it may cause severe pain over that bone, which tends to improve without treatment over two or three months. In the long run, several of these fractures may occur and cause the spine to shorten and bend.

The other common fracture site is the hip, which is particularly vulnerable in older people, whose poor balance and general stiffness make them likely to fall. If an elderly patient has osteoporosis, a relatively minor trauma will often be enough to break the hipbone.

Diagnosis

The diagnosis of osteoporosis is confirmed with X rays and bone densitometry nuclear scans, which can measure bone density and estimate the risk of future osteoporotic fractures. Women generally have these tests done when they reach menopause.

Blood tests may be used in order to rule out another disease that has similar symptoms or to see whether there is a disease, such as an overactive thyroid, that may be causing secondary osteoporosis.

HOW OSTEOPOROSIS AFFECTS THE SPINE

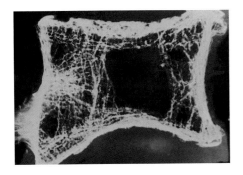

▲ *This X ray of a normal vertebra shows bone with both a normal calcium content and a regular structure.*

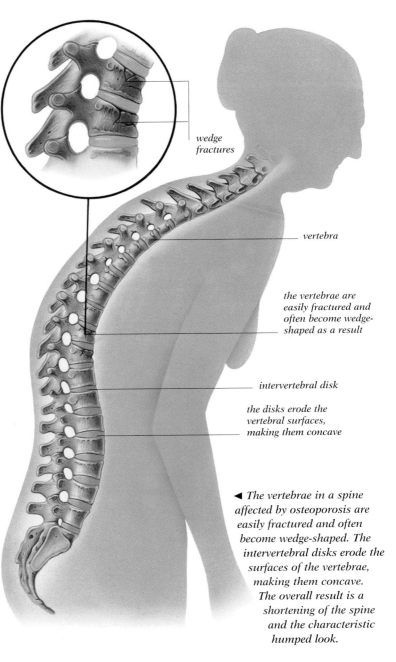

▲ *Osteoporosis in this vertebra shows up clearly. The affected areas look blacker than normal bone would.*

wedge fractures

vertebra

the vertebrae are easily fractured and often become wedge-shaped as a result

intervertebral disk

the disks erode the vertebral surfaces, making them concave

◄ *The vertebrae in a spine affected by osteoporosis are easily fractured and often become wedge-shaped. The intervertebral disks erode the surfaces of the vertebrae, making them concave. The overall result is a shortening of the spine and the characteristic humped look.*

Dangers

Left untreated, osteoporosis can seriously restrict mobility and cause disability. Repeated fractures may confine a sufferer to a wheelchair. Hip and other types of fractures that cause immobilization are associated with a high death rate in elderly patients.

The associated back troubles may also affect the nerves leading from the spine to the limbs, causing considerable pain and weakness. In the most advanced cases, the back can become bent almost double, and breathing may become very difficult.

Treatment

The patient should make efforts to become as mobile as possible. Regular exercise promotes strong bones and also prevents their deterioration. Following a fracture, the patient is encouraged to start moving at the earliest possible opportunity. To give the bones the best possible conditions for growth, a calcium-rich diet is advised. For women, hormone replacement treatment (HRT) may help retard further bone loss, but this must be considered against the increased risk of heart disease, breast cancer, and stroke. Alendronate is a drug that can build bone and prevent fractures, although its optimal use has not yet been discovered.

Outlook

Although aging, lack of exercise, and a calcium-poor diet can all aggravate osteoporosis, the disease can be prevented with calcium supplements, regular exercise, and, if the disease is really severe, HRT. There are drugs that can prevent or slow the rate of osteoporosis, so no one should needlessly have to suffer this debilitating disease without any alleviation.

See also: **Calcium; Diet; Exercise; Fractures**

Oxygen

People cannot live for more than a few minutes if their oxygen supply is cut off. Oxygen is the single most important substance on which human life depends; therefore, breathing and the transportation of oxygen throughout the body are crucial functions for human existence.

Oxygen is an odorless, tasteless, and colorless gas. Its main source on Earth is from living green plants. Oxygen also makes up about one-fifth of the air that people breathe, and the function of the lungs, the heart, and the blood vessels is primarily to carry oxygen from the air to the body's cells, where it is needed to produce the energy that the tissues need to stay alive.

What oxygen does

Oxygen is essential for the production of energy in the body. An automobile burns gasoline with oxygen, and a log fire uses both wood and the oxygen in a room to produce heat; the body's cells use oxygen in exactly the same way: they burn up their fuel—usually in the form of sugar—with oxygen to produce energy. This chemical reaction produces the same waste products in automobiles, log fires, and the body's cells—carbon dioxide and water. Although some of the body's cells are able to function for a short while without oxygen, the brain cannot manage without it.

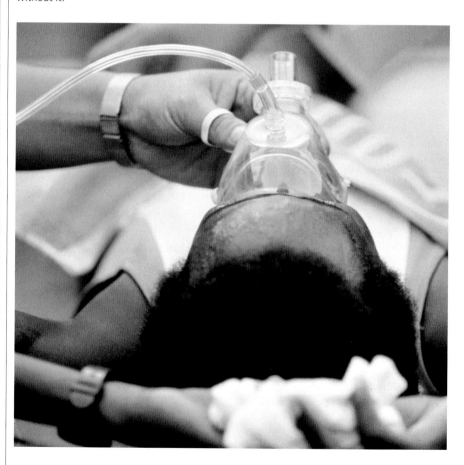

▲ *Oxygen-enriched air is being given to this athlete through a face mask after he was injured while running a marathon.*

THE PATH OXYGEN TAKES THROUGH THE BODY

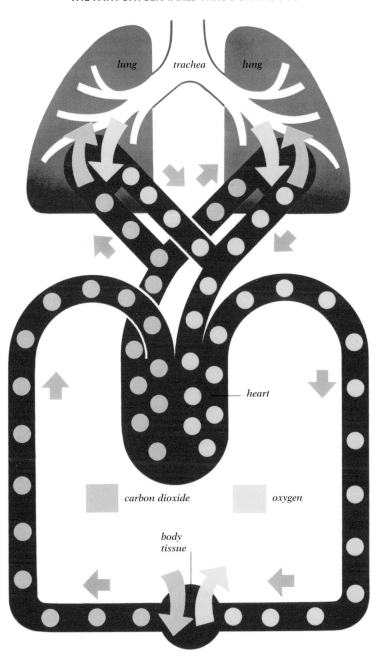

lung   *trachea*   *lung*

heart

carbon dioxide   *oxygen*

body tissue

◄ Oxygen from the lungs is transported around the body in the blood. The cells exchange oxygen for carbon dioxide, which is returned to the lungs and then exhaled.

embolus or blood clot, or pneumonia) and those with heart complaints that keep the lungs short of blood (for example, congestive heart failure). A lack of oxygen shows up as blueness around the lips and tongue, a condition that is called cyanosis.

Hemoglobin is the red pigment in blood that takes up oxygen in the lungs and carries it to the tissues where it is released. Saturated hemoglobin is hemoglobin that is full of oxygen; it is red. Hemoglobin with insufficient oxygen looks purple. Therefore, an excess of low-oxygen hemoglobin leads to the blue look of cyanosis.

Associated conditions

Almost any type of lung condition can lead to the patient's developing a low level of oxygen in the bloodstream. Chronic bronchitis is perhaps the most common of these complaints, and it is often combined with emphysema. Emphysema is a disease in which the lung tissue is destroyed to such a great extent that fewer air sacs than normal are available for the exchange of oxygen between the blood and the tissues.

A lack of oxygen is also associated with acute attacks of asthma. The condition is prevalent during severe spasms among asthmatics, which may also lead to chronic bronchitis.

Pneumonia may also lead to cyanosis, and it may be necessary to give oxygen to people who have suffered from a heart attack, because the flow of blood—and therefore the delivery of oxygen to the body's tissues—will have been drastically reduced by the attack.

Giving extra oxygen

An oxygen mask is the most common way for oxygen to be administered to a patient. The type of mask that is used in hospitals allows doctors to regulate the percentage of oxygen in the air that the patient breathes. The aim is to raise the amount of oxygen in the bloodstream until it reaches normal levels. The level of oxygen in the blood can be monitored by taking samples of arterial blood.

Oxygen from the air is inhaled, then absorbed by the lungs and carried in the blood to all the body tissues. When the amount of oxygen needed for a particular physical task is greater than that available at the time, the difference is known as an oxygen debt. A person makes up the shortfall in oxygen supply by panting and breathing in deeply, so as to take in as much oxygen as possible—for example, immediately after a period of strenuous physical exertion.

Oxygen deficiency

There are two main groups of people likely to suffer from a shortage of oxygen in the blood: those with a lung disease (such as pulmonary

Some people find wearing an oxygen mask over the face very uncomfortable, so they may be given oxygen through nasal cannulas instead. These are simply tubes which run under the nostrils, and through which the extra oxygen can be inhaled by the patient as needed. A tube can also be inserted directly into the windpipe—a medical process known as transtracheal oxygen.

Babies and small children can be put inside an oxygen tent. If the baby has been born prematurely, the oxygen can be fed directly into the incubator. Great care is needed in giving oxygen to premature babies, because too much can lead to a disease that causes blindness.

The oxygen cycle

Green plants are the main source of oxygen for all animals, including humans. In plants a chemical reaction called photosynthesis is initiated by sunlight. Carbon dioxide and water absorbed by the plant form starch in the leaves and release oxygen. Oxygen is breathed in by animals, and carbon dioxide is exhaled and used by plants, forming a continuous cycle of interdependence. Animals, including humans, eat plants, and the starch is broken down into sugars that release energy when they react with oxygen.

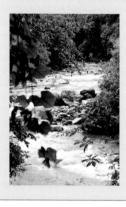

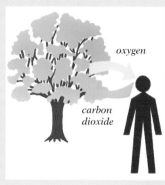

oxygen

carbon
dioxide

Oxygen chambers

Low levels of oxygen in the body's tissues may be treated by putting the patient into a small chamber with oxygen which is more concentrated than usual, and which is also supplied at a higher than normal pressure. This is called hyperbaric (high-pressure) oxygen. The treatment has a small but valuable place in modern medicine. It is used to treat carbon monoxide poisoning, or when people are distressed from inhaling acrid smoke, or in cases of gas gangrene.

High concentration

If a person on a ventilator (artificial respirator) breathes a high concentration of oxygen—more than 60 percent—for a prolonged period of time, he or she can develop a lung injury.

Another potential problem with oxygen therapy is its effect on patients with a chronic obstructive pulmonary disorder (COPD) such as emphysema, or chronic bronchitis. For some reason, when a patient with chronic obstructive pulmonary disease is given oxygen, his or her breathing can slow or stop.

Because of such problems, the level of oxygen that is administered to a patient in a hospital is always carefully controlled and monitored.

See also: **Body structure; Heart attack; Pneumonia; Sugars**

▼ *Sea air is thought by some to be especially invigorating because it has a higher proportion of ozone, a form of oxygen.*

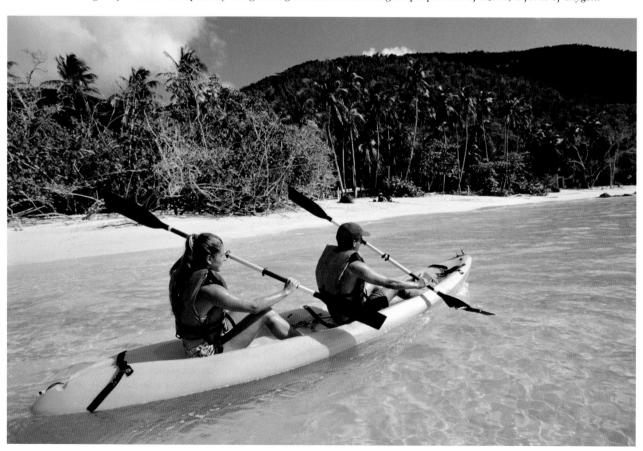

Pain

Questions and Answers

Pain is the body's protective warning system, signaling injury and disease. It tells people to avoid harm and to seek medical attention for painful illnesses or injuries.

Why can pain cause a person to faint?

The parts of the brain that receive and analyze painful stimuli have close connections with the parts that have overall control of blood circulation, the heartbeat, and the condition of the peripheral blood vessels. Even a small degree of pain causes some change in a person's pulse rate, blood pressure, or both. If pain is severe, the circulation can be swamped by these influences: the blood vessels dilate and the blood pressure drops so low that unconsciousness results. This process is the same for any severe unpleasant stimulus, though people vary as to what degree of pain causes fainting.

Does acupuncture work only psychologically to relieve pain?

Psychological factors are very important in any method of pain relief, because of the considerable psychological component in our appreciation of pain. However, it is likely that there is a genuine physiological mechanism at work in some methods of acupuncture.

Is it true that some people feel pain more easily than others?

Yes. The threshold above which a person interprets a stimulus as being painful varies hugely for both psychological and physical reasons. Hence, different people require different amounts of painkillers or local anesthetics for pain caused by identical stimuli.

Can chronic pain cause a person to become emotionally disturbed?

Severe depression can result from prolonged suffering. Often the personality seems to be changed as the pain takes over the person's whole life. However, such severe pain is not very common.

Pain can come in many forms. Individual sufferers may describe it as sharp, dull, aching, gripping, or throbbing. Minor degrees of pain are normal functions of the body and also part of its repertoire of sensory contact with the outside world. Through the experience of pain, people learn to avoid unpleasant elements in the world; the prospect of pain warns a person against repeating an action that has caused him or her pain in the past.

In disease, more severe and distressing pain arises generally from the persistent presence of some harmful stimulus in a particular part of the body. Occasionally, pain may be caused by a malfunction, due to some kind of damage, of the nerve fibers that carry and analyze painful stimuli within the nervous system.

A large section of the nervous system participates in the sensations of pain, from the peripheral nerves to the most sophisticated thinking areas of the cerebral cortex in the brain. There are many different types of pain. Each depends on various stimuli that cause it, and the way in which those stimuli are analyzed by the nervous networks in the spinal cord and brain. Cultural and social factors also play an enormous role in determining the mind's response to the perception of pain.

The purpose of pain

The ability to feel pain is vital to the well-being of humans. This can be seen from situations in which the whole or parts of a person's body lose their ability to discern pain. In leprosy, for example, the nerves to the hands and feet become so damaged that pain is no longer felt in these areas; as a result, sufferers damage their hands and feet continually and sometimes unknowingly without feeling any pain.

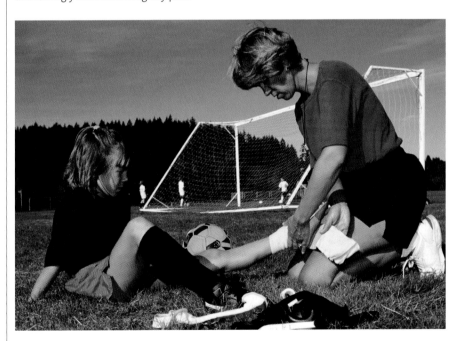

▲ *Pain acts as a warning to a person that part of the body has been injured. He or she should then seek medical attention if further damage is to be avoided.*

PATHWAYS OF PAIN

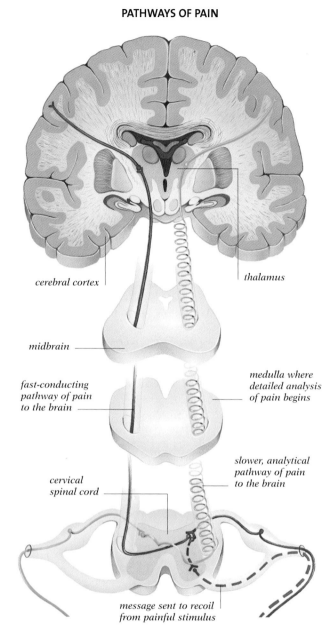

cerebral cortex

thalamus

midbrain

fast-conducting
pathway of pain
to the brain

medulla where
detailed analysis
of pain begins

slower, analytical
pathway of pain
to the brain

cervical
spinal cord

message sent to recoil
from painful stimulus

▲ *A representation of nerve pathways to the brain. (In reality,
the fiber pathways are straight, not coiled as shown).*

A few people are from birth in the dangerous state of being unable to feel any pain; they must be protected from injuring themselves. Such injuries would cause severe physical damage to anyone who did not heed the warning messages conveyed by the pain system. People do not touch boiling saucepans, for example, because the very few times they have done so, the pain has reminded them of the tissue damage that can occur.

Pain from the internal organs warns a person in the same way of the presence of a disease. For example, indigestion may warn a person to eat less rich, spicy food during his or her next meal. The paradox is that while the most distressing aspect of a disease may

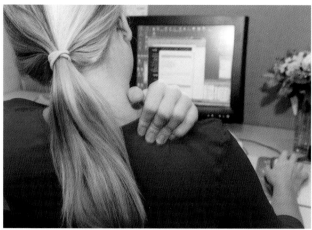

▲ *A stiff, painful shoulder is one of the first signs of
repetitive strain injury (RSI).*

be pain, it is pain—its character and its position—that enables a doctor to detect the cause of the complaint and prescribe treatment. When a person has abdominal pain, it is dangerous for him or her to cover it up with painkillers, since this may mask the development of painful symptoms that could herald the presence of a serious disorder. However, once a doctor is sure of a diagnosis, any painful symptoms can be treated as necessary.

How pain occurs

Painful stimuli inside or outside a person's body excite otherwise unspecialized nerve endings in the skin and elsewhere. The nerve endings are attached to nerves of two different types: one is fast-conducting and conveys its information to the spinal cord rapidly; the other also takes its information to the spinal cord, but more slowly. This helps the brain to distinguish between two types of pain—pricking pain that is felt immediately, and can therefore be reacted to, or pain that is dull and aching.

Peripheral nerve endings make many contacts with the network of fibers in the spinal cord. The fibers are responsible for the initial analysis of all sensations, but pain in particular. A second nerve fiber then takes this more organized information upward to the brain. Again this happens by two different pathways—one leads to the thalamus (the main sensory relay station deep in the brain) fairly directly; the other takes a more branching course, making many connections with centers in the brain stem before it also arrives at the thalamus. This enables the cortex—the part of the brain where pain is actually perceived—to obtain fast reports of the painful situation, and also more slowly arriving but more heavily analyzed information coming by the slow pathway.

The thalamus, which analyzes information for presentation to the cerebral cortex, has rich connections with the areas of the brain that are concerned with the maintenance of emotional tone and the areas concerned with arousal. As a result, before the perceiving brain receives information, especially of painful stimuli, it is already aware of a person's emotional state and is affected by his or her levels of arousal.

The final arbiter as to whether pain is perceived is the cerebral cortex. It seems that large areas of this part of the brain participate

Can a man really feel the physical pain of his partner's childbirth?

Probably not. However, if a man is very close to his wife or partner, his brain may synthesize some of the distress (if any) of childbirth, although this is unusual. Of course, not actually feeling the pain does not mean that the man is not affected in other ways.

When someone loses the sensation of pain in a leg—owing to a disorder of the nerve, for example—isn't this a good thing?

No. In such a situation the warning value of pain is lost and the person will not notice minor injuries. Such injuries may then progress to ulcers that can cause serious damage to the limb. Pain is a helpful sign that gives a person warning signals of actual or potential damage to tissues.

Is there any truth in the theory that twins, although they may be separated by many miles, can feel the pain of each other's injuries?

No. There is no real evidence that this happens and no theoretical way in which it could happen.

I have seen TV programs showing religious initiates walking over red-hot coals with no shoes on. Do these people feel any pain?

At the time, probably not. The situation is similar to that of a soldier who may feel no pain from even a severe injury received in battle. If the mind is sufficiently diverted, either by the induction of a religious trance or by the fear and excitement of a battle, the brain does not pay sufficient attention for the painful sensations to reach the person's consciousness.

Another factor is that there is considerable cultural pressure on religious initiates to hide their pain from others. Even if the pain penetrates their personal threshold, their minds may be able to erect a barrier.

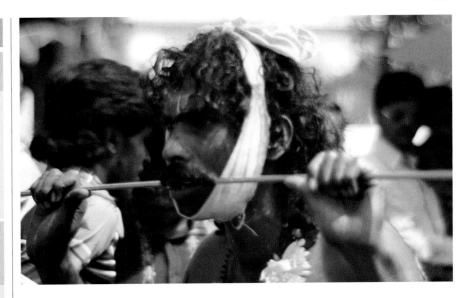

▲ *Some cultures make a virtue of pain and of the idea of "mind over matter." In this Thai Pusau ceremony, a celebrant has both cheeks pierced by a metal rod.*

in this complex form of perception. The frontal lobes, especially those parts concerned with the analysis of emotions—that is, the parts of the frontal lobes that connect with the limbic system—seem to be important for the perception of painful stimuli as unpleasant. People who have lost the use of this part of the brain report that although they can feel pain, they are not upset by it. The parietal lobes of the brain seem to be important in the localization of the painful stimulus, but they also participate in the perception of the sensations associated with pain.

Types of pain

Skin pain: This is usually localized. It is a sensation of either pricking or burning or a combination of both, according to whether the fast- or slow-conducting nerve fibers or both are stimulated.

Internal pain: This is more variable—it has different qualities, such as sharp or dull pain—and tends to be poorly localized. It is perceived as deeper and often of a duller quality than skin pain. The stimulation of combinations of different sensory fibers may produce a variety of stabbing, pressing, or constricting pains, and these may be felt coming from the internal organs.

Referred pain: Pain from any internal organ may seem to come from areas of the body some distance from the position of that organ. This is because the nerves from the organs are received, and their messages analyzed, by parts of the spinal cord that also deal with those areas to which the pain seems to be referred. Thus, pain coming from the heart may be felt in the center of the chest and also in the left arm and in the jaw. This is because the pain messages spill over from their spinal analyzing centers into neighboring zones. By careful questioning of a person in pain, doctors can usually get a clear idea of the organ involved. Not all organs refer their pains to distant sites; however, those that do always do so in characteristic distributions.

Pain from the nervous system: Damage to the peripheral nerves rather than the

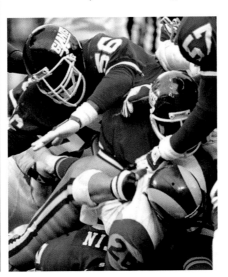

◄ *The threat of injury, and the pain that is associated with it, is common in a contact sport such as football.*

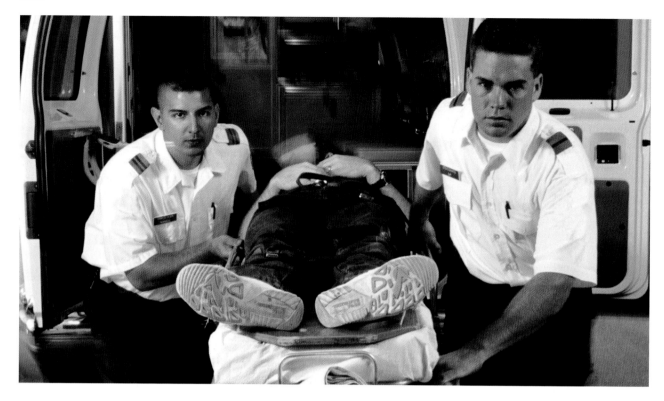

stimulation of these nerves by harmful stimuli may be the cause of pain. For example, pressure on the median nerve in the wrist may cause pain and tingling in the hand. The sensation may spread up the arm to other parts of the body, again because of the connections in the spinal cord.

"Slipped" disks in the spine can cause pressure on the sensory nerves as they enter the spinal cord; since the nerve being pressed carries impulses from the back of the leg, the pain is felt by the sufferer as traveling down the back of the leg.

Damage to the spinal cord itself, from pressure that is due to tumors or inflammations such as multiple sclerosis, also causes pain. This pain may be sent to the part of the body whose sensations are analyzed by the segment of the cord that has been affected.

Damage to other parts of the central nervous system may also cause pain. In particular, damage to the thalamus due to minor strokes may cause very unpleasant sensations and pain, since the nerves that organize the incoming stimuli become disorganized and interpret ordinary sensations as painful.

Phantom pains: When a limb has been amputated, the nerves remain in the stump. If they are stimulated by the swelling or scarring of the remainder of the limb, the brain actually registers the pain as if it were coming from the lost leg or arm. After a while the brain usually reorganizes its perceptions so that any pain is actually felt in the stump alone; however, initially the site of the pain is perceived according to where the nerves originated.

Psychological aspects of pain

The state of a person's mind is an important factor in his or her perception of pain, because large areas of the nervous system participate in feelings and responses to painful stimuli. This state of mind is strongly influenced by the situation in which

▲ *One person might faint from the pain of an injury that another person perceives as merely uncomfortable.*

a particular painful sensation occurs, and the cultural and social background against which people's attitudes to pain have developed.

In the heat of a battle, soldiers may feel no pain even though they have suffered substantial injuries, partly because the mind is being distracted by the battle itself. Also, in a highly stressful situation such as this, the brain produces morphine-like substances called endorphins that can, for a time, abolish pain totally. Later, however, when a soldier has calmed down, the pain may become unbearable, although the injury itself is no more severe.

During yoga or meditation, the mind may be diverted away from painful stimuli by the deep contemplation of other things, so that what seem to be feats of endurance—such as lying on beds of nails and walking over hot coals—can be achieved. It is likely that people undergoing such an ordeal are not actually feeling the pain in the same way that they normally would. They have managed to distract the mind from the unpleasant significance of the stimuli that are still undoubtedly reaching the brain.

The psychological effect of prolonged pain may be pronounced. Severe pain can begin a cycle in which the mental ability of the sufferer to cope with pain is eroded gradually, and causes a change in the person's personality. The person begins to concentrate unduly on the pain and begins to perceive the pain as more severe than it really is. People who suffer constant and prolonged pain often become depressed. Pain management that is swift and effective is vital once the cause of the pain is known.

See also: **Slipped disk; Stroke**

Paralysis

Questions and Answers

My cousin's legs have been paralyzed for some time. Is there any hope of recovery for him?

It depends on the cause. If his paralysis followed an injury, there is less hope than if he was suffering from a disease that caused paralysis. However, even if the motor nerves have been badly damaged, there is often some degree of recovery, which may even allow him to walk again and lead an almost normal life.

My father's stroke paralyzed his right side. Has the stroke damaged that side of his brain?

It's the brain damage that causes the stroke. Since the nerves to the muscles cross over at the bottom of the brain stem, damage to one side of the brain causes paralysis of the other side of the body. Your father has suffered damage to the left half of his brain, opposite his right paralyzed side.

Does a stroke victim always recover from the paralysis?

If the patient survives the acute stage, there will be some recovery after a stroke. Recovery depends on the extent of the brain damage and on whether or not any other body functions have been affected. Most people show considerable powers of recovery.

Why do paralyzed people tend to develop bedsores?

When we are asleep, we move around so no part of the body rests in the same place for too long, because the skin cannot cope with the pressure of body weight for long. Paralyzed people cannot relieve this pressure and need to be turned regularly to prevent bedsores. That is why badly paralyzed people are difficult to take care of at home.

There are many different types of paralysis, ranging from a weakness in one muscle to an inability to move at all. However, it is possible that the cause of the paralysis can be corrected and the outlook can be optimistic.

One of the most important functions that enables people to exist independently is the ability to move about and manipulate objects using different parts of the body. In addition to the muscles that are needed for these obvious external movements, other muscles are needed to breathe, eat, and speak. Paralysis causes the temporary or permanent loss of some or all of these muscular activities. A complex motor system controls movements, and it can be attacked on many levels by different diseases and injuries.

What is paralysis?

Paralysis is the loss of normal functioning of the muscles to a part of the body. When this happens a person feels a weakness when he or she tries to use that part of the body. When

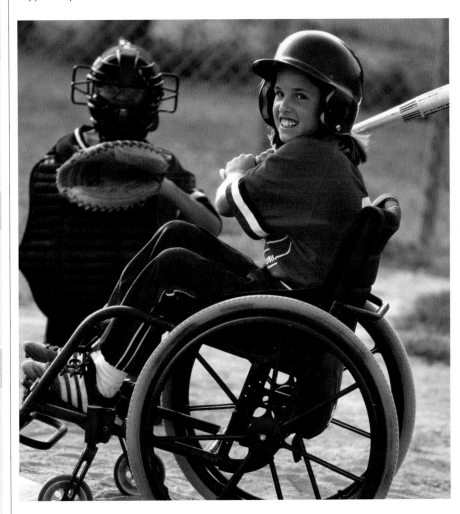

▲ *Children with muscular dystrophy meet to take part in outdoor activities. Specially adapted wheelchairs give body support and mobility—keeping them as active as possible.*

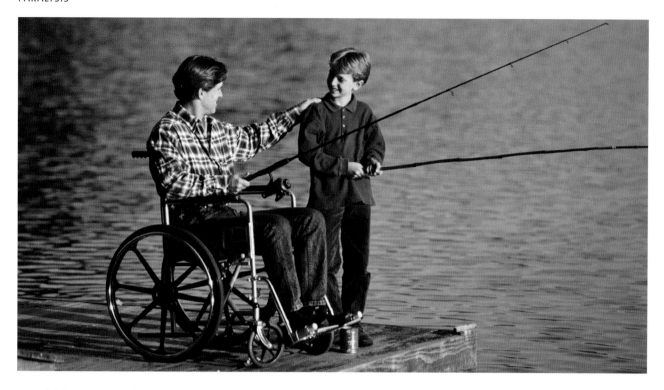

▲ *Indulging a passion for sports is one way of adjusting to and overcoming a disability.*

paralysis affects the arm or leg muscles, walking will be difficult or the grip will lose its strength. If the muscles affected are those related to speech, paralysis may cause slurred or incoherent speech. If the eye muscles are affected, double vision may be experienced. The common factor in all these symptoms is that some or all of the muscles are not working properly. The term "paralysis" is also sometimes applied to loss of other functions, especially sensation.

How does paralysis occur?
The muscles are made up of tiny fibers that are grouped together in bundles, which are each connected to the fiber of a single motor nerve cell or motor neuron in the spinal cord. Motor neurons are closely connected with many other nerve networks in the spinal cord, and also with fibers of the nerves that descend from the brain. Paralysis can happen as a result of damage to, or malfunction of, any part of the neural network. The area that is damaged will dictate the type of weakness experienced.

The muscles
When paralysis is caused by a disease of the muscles, the effect is usually felt on both sides of the body, and it generally affects the shoulder and hip muscles most strongly. Diseases such as muscular dystrophy that affect the muscles and cause paralysis may be present from birth, or the cells of the muscles may become inflamed, a condition called myositis. When these diseases strike, in addition to being weak the muscles often waste away, making the affected part of the body look thin. Walking may be difficult because the hip muscles are involved, and if the disease is severe enough, the leg muscles may become totally paralyzed. Paralysis of the shoulder

muscles will make shaving and hair-brushing more difficult, even if the hands retain their ability to grip things. The diseases of the muscles that cause a degree of paralysis vary enormously in their severity; often the paralysis is only partial. In myositis, there may be pain as well as weakness, since the inflammation causes the muscles to swell.

The muscle-nerve junction
The connection between the surface of the muscle fibers and the nerve fibers is not direct; there is a very short gap across which tiny quantities of chemical transmitters jump when the nerve is activated. In a disease called myasthenia gravis, the receptors on the muscle fibers, to which the transmitter jumps, are reduced in numbers as a result of autoimmune damage, and weakness ensues. This paralysis is progressive; the muscle gets weaker the more it is used but recovers with rest. The first muscles to be affected are usually those that keep the eyelids from drooping, but the shoulder and hip muscles, and muscles affecting the voice, swallowing, and breathing may be involved. Breathing, for example, may become so difficult that artificial help is needed. When the throat muscles are affected, a drink may be regurgitated or go down the wrong way into the lungs and cause the patient to choke.

Damage to the motor nerves
Weakness and paralysis of some groups of muscles can occur as a result of damage to the nerves that serve those muscles. For example, the ulnar nerve, which passes down the arm, is rather exposed at the back of the elbow and may be damaged if the elbow is jarred continually. This jarring will lead to paralysis in the muscles of the hand. The grip will become weaker, because the thumb cannot be brought across to meet the fingers when a person is trying to grasp something in the hand. Individual motor nerves may be damaged by a prolapsed disk in the spine. As the nerves emerge

SPECIFIC CAUSES AND AREAS OF PARALYSIS

Questions and Answers

Can a boy who is paralyzed in both legs have sex later in life?

This depends on the cause of the paralysis and its severity. Many men whose legs are paralyzed have an active sex life and produce children. If the spinal cord has been seriously damaged, however, impotence can result. An enjoyable sex life need not include penile penetration.

Why are some paralyzed limbs stiff while others are limp?

When nerve tracts are damaged as in a stroke, a small sensory stimulus such as a passive muscle stretch may be enough to produce tight reflex contraction and hence severe stiffness. This is called an upper motor neuron lesion. Conversely, a lower motor neuron lesion cuts the spinal motor reflex circuit so that the fibers of the brain can't act, and flaccid paralysis results.

If my legs become paralyzed, will I lose all sensation in them?

Not necessarily. In some kinds of paralysis, it is possible for just the nerves to the muscles to be affected, leaving nerves to the sense organs intact. Then, although you may not be able to move your legs, you may still feel sensation in them. Sometimes, both sets of nerves are affected; then sensation will be affected too, and feeling in the legs will be lost.

Can hysterical paralysis be long-term or permanent?

Hysterical paralysis is rare. If the psychological process causing the hysteria continues, paralysis may last some time; but hysterical paralysis is easy to recognize, and treatment of the psychological condition can reverse it. Simply telling the person that he or she is not really paralyzed may bring on other symptoms, so it is important to get to the root of the psychological condition.

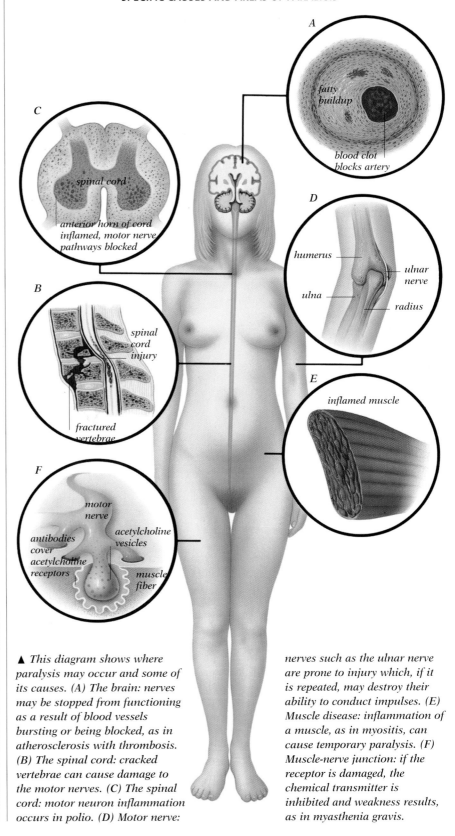

▲ This diagram shows where paralysis may occur and some of its causes. (A) The brain: nerves may be stopped from functioning as a result of blood vessels bursting or being blocked, as in atherosclerosis with thrombosis. (B) The spinal cord: cracked vertebrae can cause damage to the motor nerves. (C) The spinal cord: motor neuron inflammation occurs in polio. (D) Motor nerve: nerves such as the ulnar nerve are prone to injury which, if it is repeated, may destroy their ability to conduct impulses. (E) Muscle disease: inflammation of a muscle, as in myositis, can cause temporary paralysis. (F) Muscle-nerve junction: if the receptor is damaged, the chemical transmitter is inhibited and weakness results, as in myasthenia gravis.

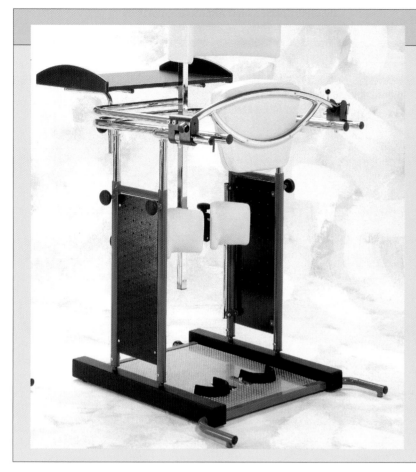

from the spinal cord, the prolapsed disk may put pressure on the nerve or nerves. The paralysis affects only part of the leg or arm, and unless the damage is severe or prolonged, relief of the pressure on the motor nerve will remove the paralysis.

The spinal cord

Damage to the spinal cord usually involves damage to the nerve fibers that carry instructions from the brain down both sides of the body. The area of the spinal cord that has been damaged will determine which parts of the body are paralyzed. Both legs may be paralyzed (paraplegia) or all four limbs may be affected if the damage is in the neck (quadriplegia). The spinal cord may be damaged in an accident in which the backbone or neck is broken or displaced; there may be blood vessel damage due to clots or hemorrhage; or there may be inflammation caused by multiple sclerosis. If the cause of the paralysis can be removed, there may be almost immediate relief. Another cause can be simply a depressed fragment of bone that presses on the spinal cord.

Diseases of the spinal cord can cause paralysis. For example, polio, which used to be a common disease, is a viral infection of the spinal cord. Polio starts with paralysis of an arm or a leg and may progress to involve the entire body.

The nerve fibers that run from the brain to the spinal cord carry instructions to the muscles. The fibers cross over from one side to the other at the bottom of the brain stem as it meets the spinal cord.

Damage to the nerves above this crossover point will cause weakness in the opposite side of the body. A common cause of this type of paralysis is a stroke, which is caused by damage to the brain, usually by a hemorrhage or blocked vessel. If the part of the brain that is supplied by a blocked or burst blood vessel includes the motor nerves, then the opposite side of the body becomes paralyzed. Strokes usually cause paralysis suddenly, and the brain often recovers well. Paralysis caused by a brain tumor develops slowly.

The outlook following paralysis

The cause of the paralysis will determine the recovery time. Some diseases that cause paralysis will resolve without treatment. Similarly, most people who are admitted to the hospital totally paralyzed on one side because of a stroke can later walk out of the hospital, albeit with a limp. Multiple sclerosis can wax and wane, or be progressive. However, treatment is always necessary to maintain the health of the affected limbs. Physical therapy and careful nursing are vital.

During convalescence, occupational therapists will help the paralyzed person to make the most of any remaining abilities so that some independence can be retained. Recent research suggests that the spinal cord might be able to regenerate somewhat after injury.

See also: **Slipped disk; Stroke**

Parasites

Some kinds of viruses, bacteria, fungi, protozoa, worms, flukes, ticks, lice, bugs, flies, and leeches are the cause of hundreds of human diseases. Hygienic practices and better sanitation can help to prevent such diseases.

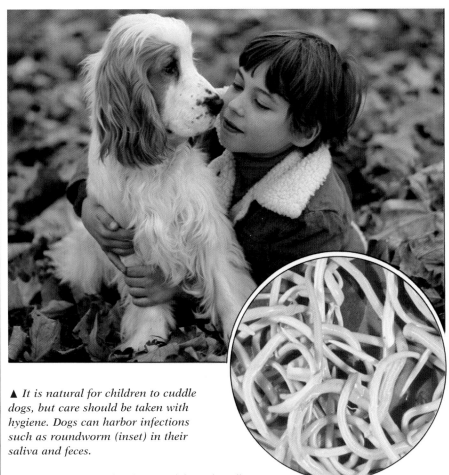

▲ *It is natural for children to cuddle dogs, but care should be taken with hygiene. Dogs can harbor infections such as roundworm (inset) in their saliva and feces.*

Parasites live in or on their hosts and depend totally upon the host for survival. People and animals are troubled by numerous types of parasites, which can be as small as one cell (like the malarial parasite) or up to 65 feet (20 m) long, like a fish tapeworm.

Parasites can damage hosts in different ways. Some feed directly upon tissues; for example, the liver fluke feeds on liver cells. There is also the hookworm, which lives on its host's blood.

Many parasites are more common in poorer, tropical countries. The better the sanitation and living conditions in richer countries, along with easier access to medical care and a cooler climate, the less likely it is for parasitic diseases to be transmitted.

Threadworms are perhaps the most common disease-causing parasites in countries like the United States. They inhabit the large intestine and lay eggs around the anal skin during the night. The eggs cause intense itching. Disadvantaged children in families where hygienic practices are lacking are most commonly affected by threadworms.

Fleas, head and body lice, and mites are also relatively common. They differ from parasites that infest the liver or the intestines because they live outside the body and feed exclusively on their hosts' blood.

The parasitic lifestyle

Parasites have adapted and modified their way of life to the lifestyles of their hosts. They can overcome immune defenses, so the body can do very little to fight the parasite.

Parasites have voracious appetites. For example, each tiny hookworm consumes 8,000 times its own weight in human blood each day. Parasites produce eggs or larvae at such a colossal rate to ensure that reproduction takes place and that their new hosts are infected. Ascaris is a common type of parasitic worm, infesting at least one billion people around the world. Transmission takes place when the host eats food that has been contaminated with infected feces. Once it is established in the body, the parasite lives in the small intestine. Parasites living in tissues or in the bloodstream depend on mosquitoes or other biting insects (called vectors) for transmission. Their larvae or reproductive cells are microscopic. They have to be produced in massive quantities to ensure that an insect becomes infected each time it bites the host.

How parasites are spread

The eggs, cysts, or larvae of many parasites are found in the feces of human or animal hosts. In some countries, human feces are still an

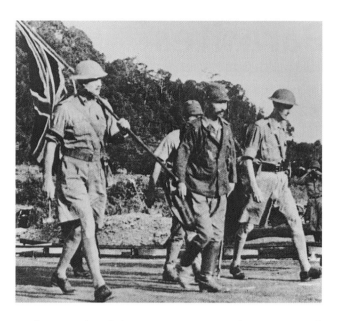

▲ *The surrender of Singapore to Japan in February 1942 and other conflicts resulted in years of captivity for some Allied servicemen. Many of those who survived Japanese prisoner of war camps returned with serious parasitic diseases.*

important source of fertilizer and are spread over the land. In poorer countries, generally, the facilities for disposal of sewage are not always adequate.

Flies and cockroaches spread eggs directly from the feces of one host to the food of another. Transmission can also take place when dirty hands touch food. Water from wells and rivers is easily contaminated by unhygienic disposal of feces and sewage.

Soil that has been contaminated with feces often harbors larvae that are able to penetrate the bare feet of the next host. Hookworm is transmitted in this way. Feces may also contain eggs or cysts that infect secondary hosts like cows or pigs (in cases of tapeworm) and freshwater snails (in cases of bilharzia). In this way, parasites multiply and are spread farther afield.

Obviously, better sanitation and more careful disposal of feces would interrupt the life cycles of all these parasites, helping to bring the diseases that they cause under control. Better hygiene and more care when handling food are also essential to prevent parasitic diseases.

Meat infestation can be a serious problem, for developed countries as well as developing nations. For example, pork can contain one million larvae of the parasite *Trichinella* in a small fraction of an ounce (a single gram). Eating even a very small quantity of such infected meat can be potentially dangerous. Careful, thorough cooking is necessary to make all meats safe.

Another transmission route for parasites is by insect vectors. A vector becomes infected when it bites the host. The parasite multiplies within it, and the infected vector is soon able to pass the disease on to new hosts with each bite. In this way, flies can spread amebic dysentery, and anopheles mosquitoes can spread malaria. One way of controlling such diseases is by attacking the insect vector. Breeding grounds can be destroyed by draining mosquito-ridden swamps and spraying them with insecticides.

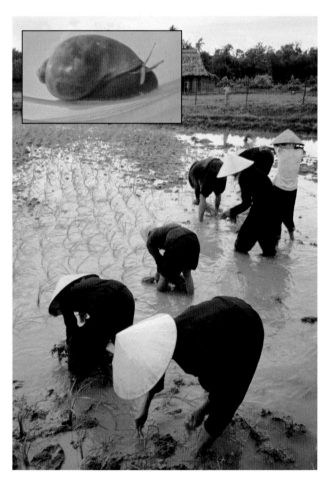

▲ *Workers who plant rice in watery fields in Asia are likely to become infested by schistosomiasis, which is carried by larvae of the freshwater snail (inset).*

Questions and Answers

Can a parasite live in a human without revealing its presence?

Yes. Many intestinal worms cause no symptoms at all in well-nourished people. The parasite will not cause too much harm, for if the host dies, so does the parasite. A check on the health of ex-soldiers who had been prisoners in Asia during World War II showed that many still had parasitic infestations. Some of these had been present without symptoms for decades.

I have been losing weight since returning from Pakistan. Could the weight loss be the result of a parasitic disease?

Parasitic diseases may cause weight loss, as can many other illnesses. You should consult your doctor, who can carry out tests to discover the cause.

Is it true that dogs carry parasites that can be transmitted to humans?

Dogs can harbor around 40 different infections harmful to humans, including several types of parasite. The most dangerous parasite is a small tapeworm, which lives in the dog's intestines. Eggs are discharged with the feces. Contamination of food leads to a severe infestation of larval cysts that can develop in the liver and lungs. This condition is called hydatid disease.

Toxocariasis is another common and serious infestation that can cause blindness in young children. It is caused by a small worm that wanders around the human body. Fecal contamination of food is the source of infestation.

Can parasites be spread to humans through blood transfusions?

Malaria may be spread by transfusion if medical facilities are poor. Donated blood is usually checked thoroughly for diseases before it is given in a transfusion.

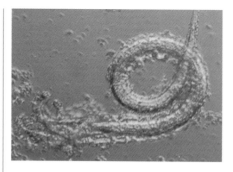

▲ An ancylostoma larva, which causes hookworm infestation in the intestines.

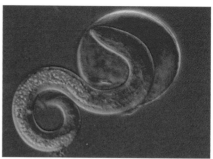

▲ The hatching of the ascaris larva, which infects the intestines and stomach.

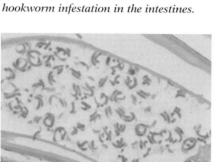

▲ Onchocerca parasites, which cause river blindness, live in the skin nodules.

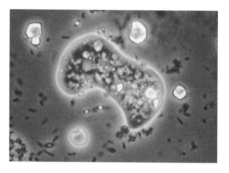

▲ Entamebae in contaminated food and water cause amebic dysentery.

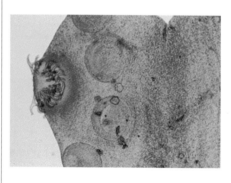

▲ A tapeworm (taenia) attaches itself with its hooks and suckers to the intestine.

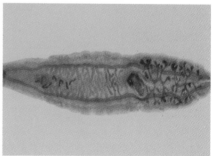

▲ The liver fluke (clonorchis) infects the liver and bile duct.

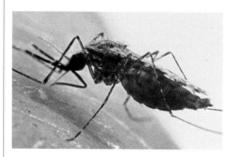

▲ The anopheles mosquito is an insect that transmits malaria through a bite.

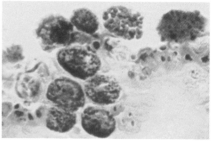

▲ Malaria parasites (plasmodium) line a mosquito's stomach.

The most common parasitic diseases

INFESTATION	PROPER NAME	WHERE PARASITE LIVES IN BODY	HOW TRANSMITTED	HARMFUL EFFECTS	PEOPLE AFFECTED	PLACES WHERE MOST COMMON
Malaria	*Plasmodium vivax, P. falciparum, P. ovale, P. malariae*	Bloodstream; liver	Mosquito bite	Recurrent fever; anemia; ill health; miscarriages; often causes death	Over 300 million each year	Africa; Latin and South America; India; Southeast Asia; Asia
Amebic dysentery	*Entameba histolytica*	Large intestine	Flies spread cysts from feces; these contaminate food and water	Diarrhea; dysentery; liver abscesses	About 500 million at any time	All parts of the world, but Africa, Latin America, Asia especially
Hookworm	*Ancylostoma duodenale* and *Necator americanus*	Intestines	Eggs passed in the feces hatch in the soil; larvae burrow into bare feet	Weight loss; anemia; malnutrition	About 1 billion	Africa; Asia; Latin America and South America
Bilharzia	*Schistosoma mansoni*	Veins around intestines and bladder	Larvae live in fresh water and burrow through human skin; they develop into snails	Damage to the liver and bladder; often fatal	About 200 million	Africa (Egypt especially); China; Latin and South America; Asia
Filariasis	*Wuchereria bancrofti; Brugia timori*	Lymph vessels	Mosquito bites	Elephantiasis	Over 120 million	Asia; Africa; parts of Latin and South America
Ascariasis	*Ascaris lumbricoides*	Intestines and stomach	Eggs from feces spread by flies; found in contaminated food and water	Heavy infestation causes malnutrition with obstruction of the intestine	Over 1 billion	All parts of the world; especially Africa, Asia, and Latin America
River blindness	*Onchocerca volvulus*	Adults live in nodules beneath the skin; larvae live in the tissues and eyes	Bites from blackflies (*Simulium damnosum*), which live only in rapid-flowing rivers	Blindness; skin damage	About 18 million	Africa; parts of South America
Guinea worm	*Dracunculus medinensis*	Beneath the skin of feet and legs	Larvae live in water fleas, which contaminate drinking water	Increased risk of foot and leg ulcers	About 80,000	Africa; Asia
Tapeworms	*Taenia solium* and *T. saginata* (beef and pork tapeworms); *Diphyllobothrium lata* (fish tapeworm)	Intestines	Cysts and larvae infest meat and fish; these mature into adult tapeworms if meat is not properly cooked; smoked and cured meats are common sources	Malnutrition and anemia; the pork tapeworm can kill if cysts form in the brain; tapeworms may not produce symptoms	Over 100 million	Many parts of the world, especially Africa, South America, Asia, Scandinavia (fish tapeworm)
Liver fluke	*Clonorchis sinensis*	Liver and bile duct	Cysts are present in raw fish	Liver damage and obstruction	Over 20 million	Asia
Threadworms (pinworms)	*Enterobius vermicularis*	Large intestine and anus	Contamination of bedding; clothing; dirty hands; fingernails	Itching; can cause secondary infection through irritation	Over 400 million	Worldwide

Prevention of a parasitic disease

If you live in or visit a country where parasitic diseases are a problem, these rules will help you to stay healthy.

Check that drinking water is safe to use. If you are in doubt, drink only boiled water or use purifying tablets that contain chlorine.

Never eat food that has been left in the open or exposed to flies. Eat food that has been cooked recently and thoroughly. Wash hands and maintain hygiene when handling food.

Wash all fruit and vegetables in clean water before eating. If possible, use detergent.

Avoid exposure to insects. Wear sensible clothing and use insect repellent sprays and gels containing DEET. Use mosquito nets, or burn pyrethrum mosquito coils at night.

In malarial regions, take antimalarial pills and use mosquito nets. Seek your doctor's advice before going on your trip.

Do not swim in canals or rivers.

Do not walk around with bare feet.

Detection of a parasitic disease

Your doctor will perform the following tests if you report feeling unwell after returning from an area where parasitic diseases are common.

Blood tests: Blood is first examined under the microscope for signs of any of the nonspecific changes found in parasitic infestations—for example, disordered white blood cell counts and anemia. Blood is then checked carefully. Malarial parasites, trypanosomes (which cause sleeping sickness), and the larvae of some filarial worms can all be seen under a microscope.

Stool tests: A fresh stool sample is examined under the microscope for the eggs, cysts, and larvae of parasites. Almost all of the parasites produce eggs with a characteristic size and shape. Finding and recognizing them requires skill. Several stool samples may be necessary if the infestation is not a heavy one.

Urine tests: In diseases such as bilharzia the urine may contain eggs. These eggs may be detected by using a technique of centrifugation or filtration. The resulting sediment is then examined under a microscope.

Effects of parasites

Parasites can cause considerable harm, but the damage to the host may not appear for a long time. Infestation with ascaris or tapeworms, which live in the intestines and feed on partly digested food, may not be noticed by a healthy host. In developing countries, where many people do not have the food they need for good health, such parasites contribute to the widespread problem of malnutrition. Sometimes the damage done to the host is so severe that whole populations have chosen to move away from villages rather than remain exposed to a debilitating disease.

Treatment

Drugs are available to treat most parasitic diseases, and treatment is usually simple. However, when the host suffers damage over a period of many years, treatment to kill the parasite may come too late. Drugs cannot undo the liver damage that occurs in schistosomiasis or the deformity caused by elephantiasis. Drug treatment is not always practical for dealing with large communities. Some drugs are too toxic for use on a large scale and have to be carefully supervised. Whatever the treatment, it is vital to focus on prevention, too, so that reinfection becomes less likely.

Outlook

Many parasitic diseases have proved difficult to eradicate completely, and preventive programs can be costly. Poorer countries that have the worst problems with parasites often have inadequate resources to deal with the problems. There have, however, been advances in recent decades. As basic hygiene, sanitation, and health improve throughout much of the world, the parasitic diseases of poverty are becoming less inevitable.

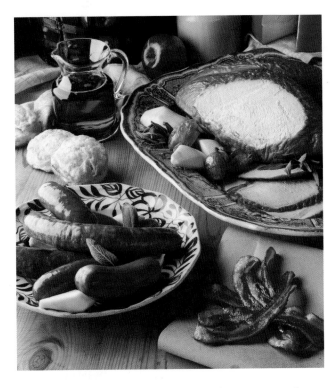

▲ *Cooking pork thoroughly —for example, sausages and bacon—helps ensure that any parasitic larvae contained in the meat are completely destroyed.*

See also: **Hygiene; Lice**

Personality

Personality is what makes someone an individual, different from everyone else. What each person inherits and what he or she experiences in life are factors that influence the development of the personality.

Yes. A baby not only is absorbing information all the time but is more sensitive to his or her environment during this time than at any other time in the future. A child who has been overprotected in the first five years, for example, will tend to be hesitant about making contact with other people later in life; or if a child was not given enough affection in the first two years, his or her emotional responsiveness is likely to be stunted.

Studies have revealed patterns of behavior (which often repeat themselves over generations) that illustrate this. For example, girls who were cared for in a sensitive and intelligent way find it easier to give this sort of mothering to their children, who will, in turn, develop the same sensitivity.

Parents who physically damage their children also tend to pass on similar patterns of behavior: their children may become the same sort of parents. It seems that such parents have a lower sense of their own worth and find it hard to make their own children feel valued.

There is a school of thought that maintains that certain personality traits are more prevalent among criminals of both sexes than among noncriminals. The criminal type tends to be antisocial and impulsive, and cares little for the feelings of other people. This type of person also tends to be highly extroverted and emotional. These qualities may add up to a criminal personality, if such a term can be defined. However, in personality there really are no hard and fast rules.

Personality is often defined as the more or less constant pattern of behavior and way of thinking and feeling that characterizes an individual. Generally, an individual's personality remains much the same throughout his or her life. This means that a happy-go-lucky child will usually develop into an optimistic adult. Similarly, timid young people will generally maintain their nervousness and reserve as they get older, unless powerful influences combine to alter their apprehensions. This is not to say that individuals cannot modify their personality type if they really want to, but the process can take considerable effort over a long period of time.

Traits of personality

Perhaps the most easily noticed parts of personality are character traits, which are qualities that a person exhibits in certain situations. Honesty, meanness, perseverance, laziness, kindness, stubbornness, patience, courage, and modesty are all examples of character traits. Although a person may be said to possess a given trait, he or she will not, and is not expected to, display that trait in all circumstances. For example, a man may be scrupulously honest in all his business deals yet may take office stationery home without a second thought. A woman may be generous to her neighbors and friends yet could be thrifty to the point of meanness with her own family.

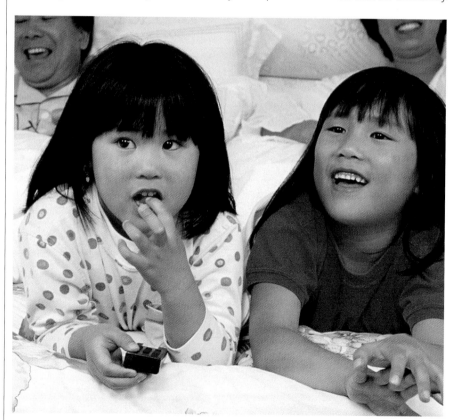

▲ *In any family it is normal for the children to have different personalities: the boisterous and outgoing child is quite normal, and so is her quiet, reflective sister.*

A child may be highly willful and aggressive at school, yet meek and mild at home. In spite of such variability, however, character traits are usually regarded as being part of the permanent personality if they occur regularly in a person.

Roles

The roles that people play in life are not attributes of personality in themselves, but they very much affect when and where people display various traits of their personality. For instance, in order to be successful, a man may find that, in his role of sales manager at work, he has to be aggressive, dominating, and quick to make firm decisions without consultation. At home, on the other hand, these qualities might be almost absent. His sales team would regard him as dominant in personality, whereas his wife may even think of him as quite submissive. The different roles he plays all appear to be very real parts of his personality.

Society encourages people to play roles by supporting them when they fit the stereotype for a particular role. Similarly, society tends to reject those people who do not fit a particular stereotype. A politician who admitted in public that he believed the opposing party had made a good decision or had a good policy on something would soon lose his job, whatever the facts of the matter. A mother who confessed that she felt no affection for her newborn child would probably be branded as cruel and inhuman.

Counselors not infrequently have to deal with clients whose personality lies more in the role that society has given them than in traits that they possess themselves.

Personality types

Since the display of a wide range of different traits is a matter of occasion and circumstances, many scientists have looked for broader classifications that describe a person better and more consistently. Perhaps the simplest classification is that developed by the English psychologist Hans Eysenck, who has reduced the variables to three: extroversion (as opposed to introversion), emotionality (versus stability), and tough-mindedness (as against tender-mindedness).

Everyone has these qualities to some extent, but the usefulness of Eysenck's system is that, instead of saying a person is or is not an introvert, for example, the three qualities can be estimated on a rating scale, giving an idea of just how extroverted, emotional, or tough-minded a person actually is.

It is also possible to show that these qualities are related to a person's speed of learning and various other phenomena that, on the surface, seem to have little to do with personality itself. The evidence implies that these three personality factors are real in themselves, rather than something observed by one person in one situation, as can happen with traits such as courage and honesty. Therefore, the three qualities could be built-in, and can be likened to continuous pressures that move a person to act in a certain way. Even when there may be circumstances in which, say, an emotional person finds it better to go against his or her natural inclination, the pressure to act emotionally will still be there.

Inherited or acquired?

Anyone who has brought up more than one child will be aware that children from the same family can show very different personalities almost from the moment they are born. This implies that some

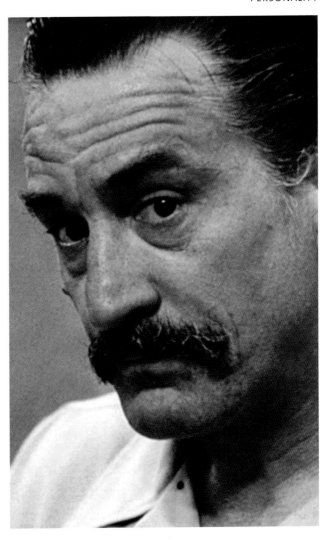

▲ *Some actors and actresses can submerge themselves totally in the parts they play to project a different personality in every film. Robert De Niro has this ability. TV stars, such as Oprah Winfrey, project a particular personality on screen, which may be very different from their off-screen personality.*

aspects of personality are probably innate and may be determined genetically. However, since parents can, unknowingly, bring up successive children in very different ways, researchers have studied to what extent identical twins—who develop from a single egg and therefore have an identical genetic program—raised together have similar personalities. Results from the research show that identical twins are much more similar than fraternal twins—who develop from separate eggs and so have a different genetic makeup—or nontwin siblings (also different genetically) in their measures of emotionality, sociability, and tough-mindedness.

This suggests that in some respects personality is a matter of inheritance, but inheritance should not be thought of as the only factor, or even the most important factor, determining an individual's personality. Rather, many facets of the personality are influenced heavily by a person's experiences in life. For example,

I have often heard the term "split personality." Is there such a thing?

Yes, but it is rare. People with this condition behave in radically different ways at different times, almost as if more than one person inhabited the same body. Strictly speaking, the condition is known as "multiple personality."

Although it may be confused with schizophrenia—which means "split mind"—split personality has nothing to do with that condition. In schizophrenia, the patient's speech and thought processes are often split up and confused, whereas in multiple personality each personality within the same body is lucid and coherent.

Why do some people become so violent when they are drunk? My boyfriend seems to turn into a different person when he's had a lot to drink, and I become very afraid of him.

Aggression is a powerful element in every personality. It shows itself more in some people than in others, and most people succeed in keeping it in check. However, alcohol seems to release, or relax, the control mechanisms, and latent aggression may emerge.

Alcohol in large quantities also clouds judgment and acts as a depressant, which may put the drinker in a bad mood. These three effects combine to produce a cocktail, which can—as you say—make your boyfriend seem to be a different person.

Are twins likely to have the same personality or similar personalities?

Identical twins develop from the same egg, are of the same sex, and resemble each other closely, suggesting an identical genetic program. Fraternal twins develop from two separate eggs, are not necessarily of the same sex, and may not resemble each other physically. It does seem that identical twins are far more similar in personality than fraternal twins, who may have completely different personalities.

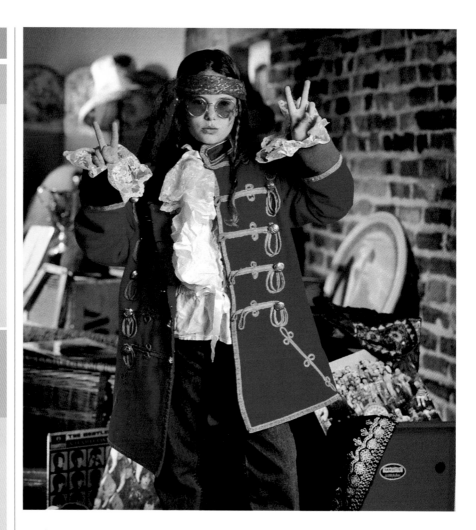

▲ *The games children play often reflect their personalities. When dressing up, an extroverted child will usually choose flamboyant clothes that attract attention.*

similarities in personality between fraternal twins, who generally have much the same upbringing but different genetic influences, show clearly the powerful influence of a person's upbringing. At the same time, the different ways in which an individual can behave in various circumstances—a timid, introverted person finding the courage to address a meeting on an issue about which he or she feels strongly, for instance—shows that people can change certain aspects of their personalities if they have to.

Abnormal personalities

One of the most significant consequences of measuring individuals' degrees of extroversion, emotionality, and tough-mindedness is the discovery that many of the mental illnesses and conditions dealt with by psychiatrists are associated with extremes of one or more of the personality characteristics described by Eysenck's tests.

Neurotic conditions, such as phobias, obsessions, and compulsive behavior, are generally associated with extreme emotionality. In addition, people who tend to become severely depressed often show the same high emotionality; however, in such cases this is combined with very low extroversion—that is, depressed personality types tend to be highly introverted. Hysterical people, on the other hand, show high emotionality combined with very high levels of extroversion.

Psychotic individuals, such as psychopaths and schizophrenics, differ from neurotic, depressive, and hysterical individuals in that they are often unexceptional in their degree of

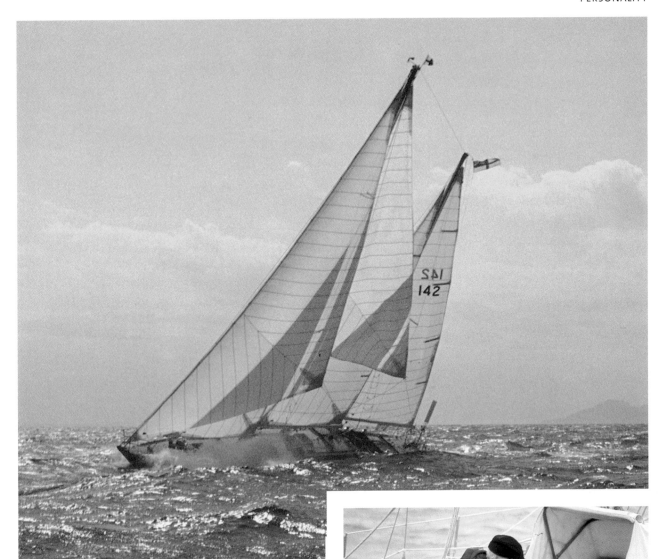

▲ *Those hardy individuals who sail single-handed around the world must have an unusual degree of self-reliance to endure the stark loneliness of months at sea on their own.*

▶ *Francis Chichester on his yacht Gypsy Moth IV, on his famous solo circumnavigation.*

emotionality and extroversion. However, they are rated as extreme for tough-mindedness—so much so that the scale for tough-mindedness is actually called the "psychoticism scale."

Many criminals have been found to rate extremely high on all three of Eysenck's variables.

Changing personality

To some extent, all forms of psychotherapy are concerned with modifying how a person acts, thinks, and feels. This, by definition, is changing that individual's personality. A marital problem or some other relationship problem may, at least in part, be caused by a so-called clash of personalities, and its solution may involve getting the partners to change the way they behave, think, and feel.

Phobias and similar problems are often treated by reducing the anxiety of the person in question—through behavior therapy, for instance. If this is achieved, the patient will, on a personality questionnaire, seem to be less emotional—that is, this aspect of his or her personality will have been changed.

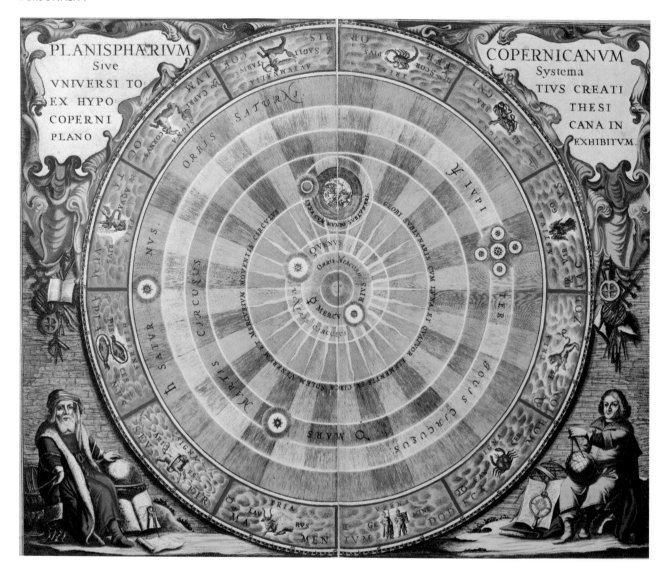

▲ *It is sometimes suggested that personality is predetermined by the astrological sign of the zodiac (a cyclical chart of the 12 signs, or constellations, as shown above) under which a person is born. Astrologers believe that certain personality traits are common to people who share the same birth sign.*

One fact has arisen from therapists' attempts to facilitate such personality changes in their patients. The neurosis of a shy, reserved introvert is much easier to cure than a similar condition in a brash, outgoing extrovert. Similarly, it is generally easier for a therapist to change an introvert into something of an extrovert than to quiet an extrovert and give that patient the reflectiveness of an introvert.

Influences on personality

It has already been mentioned that personality is modified as a person matures; however, other influences can also have effects of varying magnitude. Long periods of stress will increase a person's emotionality and aggressiveness and may also make that individual more reserved.

Patterns of upbringing will also have some effect on a child's personality, although it is not easy to predict what the effect might be. For example, a child may follow the pattern set by one or both parents, or may rebel against both. Certainly parental influence is a very important factor, particularly in the first five years of a child's life. Studies have shown that some patterns of behavior are repeated in succeeding generations.

There is also no doubt that personality in its widest sense can be affected by the long-term effects of alcohol or drug abuse, by traumatic shock, and by brain injury.

What is less obvious, however, is just how constant the broad outlines of the personality of an individual remain, even when he or she is faced with powerful outside influences. The personality does not change under duress; rather, people change the way they display their personalities.

See also: **Depression; Drug abuse; Genetics; Stress**

Physical fitness

How quickly will my body adapt itself to my new fitness regimen? At the moment I ache all over.

You may be doing too much too soon; slow down a bit. As you get fitter, you will be able to do more without feeling such ill effects. Your body has probably been under-used for a long time; don't expect it to be in prime condition after only a few days or weeks. There shouldn't be too much suffering involved in getting fit; more discomfort should be felt during exercise than afterward.

Does the ability to remain fit lessen as you get older?

Yes, it is more difficult to get fit and stay fit as you age, so you should exercise regularly as the years go by. You don't need to do this to excess, but anyone over 70, for example, should make a habit of walking a few miles every day.

Are children naturally physically fit or do they have to work at fitness?

The younger children are, the less they have to work at their physical fitness. As they grow older, though, the situation changes; there will be a noticeable difference between the performance of teenage athletes and their untrained friends. People from their twenties onward definitely need regular exercise for real fitness.

I used to jog a lot before I became pregnant. Is it OK to continue?

If you have not had any problems during pregnancy or any bad pregnancies previously, there is no reason why you should stop. If you have had trouble, you should cut down or stop for the first trimester. During the second trimester you will probably feel fine; by the final trimester you may feel a bit large for too much exercise.

All age groups are much more concerned with physical fitness now than ever before. However, people should ensure that if they embark on a fitness program, they choose one to suit their age and capability.

There is no doubt that to see someone like Michael Johnson sprinting his way to a world record in his prime was to witness one of the fittest people who ever lived. However, it is equally obvious that people do not all need to be so fit to lead a happy and contented life. How much exercise does a person need to keep the body fit enough to deal with the demands of everyday life, and what is the best way of getting that exercise?

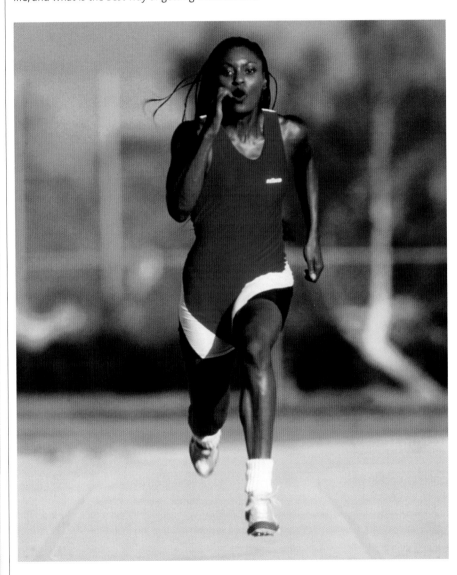

▲ *Few people are at the peak of their physical fitness throughout life. However, only top athletes need to be supremely fit. For other people, gentle, regular exercise is all they need to feel and look healthy.*

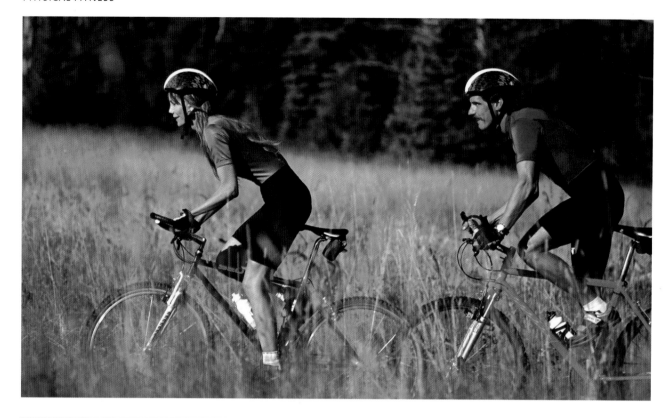

Getting fit

DO

Do warm up properly. Injuries occur when you start a heavy workout without an adequate warm-up period. Runners should do a few stretching exercises to keep supple and repeat these during the cooling-off period.

Do use proper equipment. This is particularly important in relation to training or running shoes. Always buy the best shoes for your feet.

Do eat sensibly. If you are overweight you must not combine a crash diet with a sudden fitness program; in fact, your appetite may increase if you exercise more than usual.

DON'T

Don't rush into your fitness program; you could injure yourself. The older you are, the more slowly you must start; if you are over 35 and are concentrating on jogging, for example, you should start with a week of brisk walking.

Don't exercise if you have a cold or flu, or if you feel an infection coming on.

Don't get cold. Injuries can be prevented by wearing warm clothes in cold weather.

▲ *Regular exercise doesn't have to be boring. Thousands of people take up physical activities for recreation, either through clubs or with friends.*

Generally, it is true to say that most of the people would feel a lot fitter, and maybe live longer, if they exercised regularly and took more care of their bodies.

Keeping fit is very much concerned with the way that a person chooses to lead his or her life. An office employee whose only exercise is walking between the subway station and home will not be as physically fit as a bicycle courier who rides many miles in a day.

Fitness has two roles to play in each person's attitude toward positive health. First, a person must keep up a minimum level of fitness to keep the body looking good and feeling well so that he or she can enjoy life to the fullest. Second, a person must be physically fit enough to be able to manage the physical loads that his or her daily activities and leisure pursuits demand.

Why bother to keep fit?

There are two important reasons why people should always try to remain physically fit. By far the more important is that they will simply feel better; the ordinary tasks of everyday living seem so much easier to cope with when the body is in good shape. The main reason why so many joggers have taken to the parks and sidewalks is that they have discovered this simple fact.

The second important part of keeping fit is the effect it is thought to have on life expectancy. If physical fitness does prolong life, that result is almost certainly due to the benefit fitness gives to the heart, lungs, and blood vessels, which are all involved with delivering oxygen to the tissues.

Ideal pulse rates during exercise

AGE	MINIMUM	IDEAL
Women		
20–30	130	155
30–40	125	150
40–50	115	140
50–60	110	130
60–70	100	129
70+	95	115
Men		
20–30	135	165
30–40	130	160
40–50	125	150
50–60	115	140
60–70	105	130
70+	100	125

This panel shows the pulse rate you should be aiming for if you are trying to do your heart any good.

Any exercise that increases the heart rate is useful, even brisk walking. The easiest way to take your own pulse is to stop exercising and time your pulse over the next six seconds, multiplying by 10 to get the heart rate in beats per minute. The minimum column shows the lowest effort that will improve your heart; the figures in the ideal column are about three-quarters of the maximum possible rate, and this level does the most good.

GETTING THE MOST FROM EXERCISE

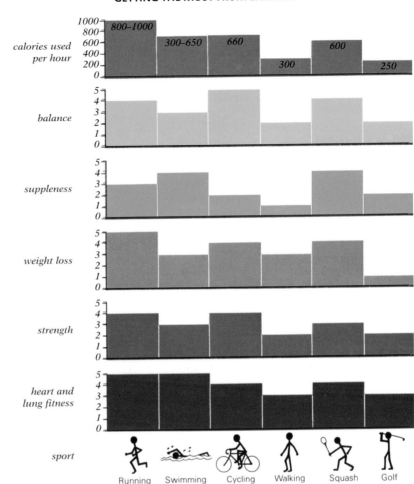

▲ Each area of fitness is graduated from one to five, with five as the most effective.

It is a simple fact that people who live in the West are most likely to die of a disease affecting the heart or the blood vessels caused by the twin evils of high blood pressure and atherosclerosis. If exercise does have a helpful effect on life expectancy, it acts by preventing or delaying the effects of these disease processes. However, physical fitness certainly has no known effect on the chances of suffering from other fatal diseases, such as cancer.

Scientific studies

Scientists (epidemiologists) who study the effects of disease on the population as a whole have for some years been looking at the possible beneficial effect of physical fitness on the heart and blood vessels. There are many different studies that indicate a reduction in the number of heart attacks in people who are physically active compared with those who are less active, or sedentary. One study showed that people who were on the move and ran up and down stairs several times a day were less likely to develop heart trouble than people who were simply sitting down all day. And while it is too early to say that exercising definitely reduces the chances of having a heart attack, there is a definite correlation between fitness and avoiding heart trouble.

How can people tell if they are fit?

When people talk about physical fitness, they usually have some specific objective in mind. Sports people will get fit in time for the baseball or football season, for example, and the level of fitness that they accept as adequate will depend on what they want to do and on how well (and at what level) they want to perform. Perhaps a better question is: how can a person tell if he or she is unfit?

The main signs of unfitness are breathlessness and sweating on relatively minor exertion. If a person cannot climb up three flights of stairs without breaking into a sweat, then he or she is unfit; also, if a person gets so breathless when walking up the same three flights that he or she cannot carry on a normal conversation, he or she is also unfit.

Apart from the ability to exert a lot of energy in a short time, when a person climbs stairs, for example, he or she should also have a reasonable amount of endurance. Nobody under the age of 70 (who is not disabled) should feel unable to manage a level four-mile walk at a reasonable pace. For more active sports, a person would have to be much fitter.

Finally, there is the question of actual physical strength. In these days of relatively mechanized living, there are few tasks that need an enormous amount of physical strength. Many people have felt the worse for wear as a result of moving some heavy piece of furniture at some time, and this is fairly normal.

When people's bodies are not up to the physical tasks that they attempt, it is of course reasonable to say that they are unfit. However, there is no reason to suppose that people are improving their life expectancy by building up muscular strength; it is the fitness of the heart and lungs that probably matters more from this point of view, although there are actually few forms of exercise that do not increase muscle strength to some degree.

How do you get fit?

The capacity of the heart and lungs to carry oxygen to the tissues of the body seems to be the key to the sort of fitness that leads to physical well-being and possibly a longer life. Scientists can measure this by looking at the amount of oxygen the body can consume during the course of one minute while someone is exercising hard. In a healthy 20-year-old man this may be around 1½ fluid ounces (45 ml) of oxygen consumed per 2.2 pounds (1 kg) of body weight during the course of 1 minute; the figure for women is about 0.3 fluid ounce (10 ml) per minute less. Oxygen consumption falls in everyone after the age of 20. In a highly trained endurance athlete, such as a top-class marathon runner, the figure may be as high as 2½ fluid ounces (80 ml) per 2.2 pounds (1 kg) per minute. Very unfit people can sink to a figure of around 0.85 fluid ounce (25 ml).

The type of exercise that improves the degree of oxygen uptake and the overall efficiency of the heart and lungs is called aerobic exercise. In simple terms, this means the sort of exercise that makes a person breathless while he or she is doing it. Endurance exercises—such as running, swimming, and walking, as well as the many ball games and team games that involve a lot of running—are all good forms of exercise that improve oxygen uptake and therefore the level of fitness of the heart and lungs. The most efficient, convenient, and inexpensive form of exercise for most people is probably running. However, the most important thing about choosing a basic form of exercise in a fitness program is that it should be an exercise that the person enjoys and is prepared to go on doing for years.

Nevertheless, improvement of the function of the heart and blood vessels is not the only thing that matters when overall fitness is considered. It is also important to develop the body so that it is well balanced and supple, as well as being reasonably strong. Running or jogging does all of these things, except developing suppleness; therefore, some stretching exercises must be done for overall fitness. Swimming, on the other hand, is a particularly good all-around approach to achieving fitness; and for those who are motivated best by some direct form of competition, all the common racket games like squash, tennis, and badminton have excellent effects on fitness. Finally, for those who find fitness easiest to achieve when some form of travel is involved, hiking and cycling are the obvious activities.

Whatever form of exercise a person chooses, it has been shown that any reasonably intensive training program will improve oxygen consumption of the body by as much as 30 percent in the course of a few weeks. In middle-aged men who were given a very gradual increase in the amount of exercise that they were doing, it was found that increases of up to 20 percent could easily be obtained.

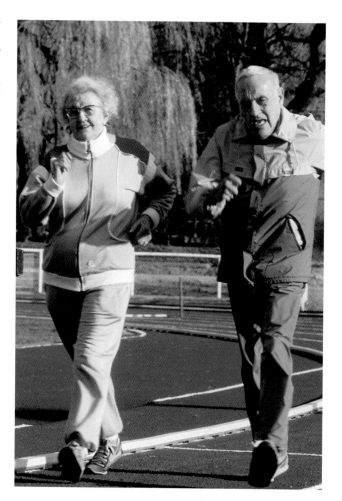

▲ *There are hundreds of activities that promote physical fitness. The keynote is activity, whether in the workplace or at play. Getting any sensible regular exercise is going to be good for people, so they should choose the type that best suits their age, lifestyle, and preference. Physical fitness will improve a person's health and outlook and may even prolong life— whether a person is 25 or 75.*

The main thing to remember about starting to get fit is not to expect too much too soon. However, with perseverance it should be possible for a person to produce a noticeable change in his or her feeling of well-being in the course of only a few weeks by a simple program that involves walking and running.

One noticeable change that has taken place in Western society in recent years has been in the number of people who are prepared to take hard exercise to keep themselves physically fit. Although they may have no thought of going out and winning world-class athletic events, these people are motivated by the thought that, through being fit, they can function better in business and socially; and, of course, in the process they realize that they might well be prolonging their lives.

> *See also:* Exercise; Oxygen; Heart attack; Sports medicine

Physical therapy

Questions and Answers

Is it true that electrotherapy treatments can be dangerous?

In unskilled hands, electrotherapy could be dangerous. However, physical therapists are trained in the use of this equipment and will ensure that the patient is protected.

After nine holes of golf my hip begins to ache and sometimes gets quite painful. I try to keep playing and work the pain away. Is this sensible?

Pain is usually a danger signal that something is wrong. It would be advisable to see your doctor and not to try to work through the pain, since this may make the problem worse. Your doctor may think that physical therapy will help with this problem.

I recently had a gallbladder operation and have been told to do breathing exercises. Why?

Pain in the abdomen will make you breathe more shallowly. This can cause some of the small air spaces in your lungs to collapse and can lead to pneumonia. Deep breathing helps prevent this.

My child suffers from cerebral palsy and has regular physical therapy. Will she ever be able to manage without it?

A child with cerebral palsy has to learn to sit up, walk, and control bodily movements until he or she gains independence. This requires an intensive course of treatment in the early years. As the child is more able to fend for him- or herself, the physical therapist will teach the parents how to encourage the child further, and gradually there will be no need for continuous treatment. However, you can always ask a physical therapist for advice.

Physical therapy has to do with mobility. It uses physical methods, including manipulation and massage, plus a range of other techniques, to give relief from pain and restore movement after an injury or disease.

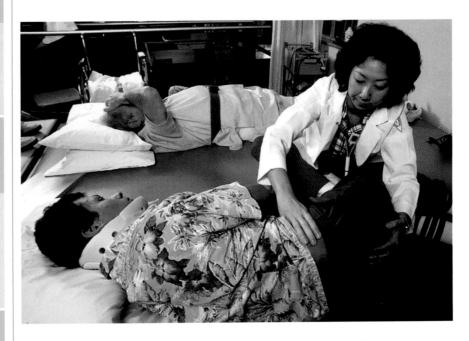

▲ *A physical therapist works to mobilize a patient's lower spine. Back pain can be highly disabling, but manipulation may resolve the problem and bring welcome relief.*

For many people, the words "physical therapy" conjure up an image of an arthritic limb being massaged, but in fact such therapy covers a broad range of treatments. The term "physical therapy" is derived from two Greek words: *phusis*, meaning nature; and *therapeutike*, meaning healing.

Physical therapy is a necessary adjunct to many treatments of disease, disability, and injury. In addition to its traditional role of treating rheumatic aches and stiff joints, physical therapy can help restore limbs to their normal function after an injury, help pregnant women to prepare for childbirth, and teach children with physical disabilities to control their limbs. Physical therapy also helps many postoperative and bedridden patients to breathe, trains those who have suffered brain or spinal damage to relearn mobility, and teaches paralyzed patients to use other muscles so that they can have more independence and control over their lives.

Physical therapists are highly trained health care personnel. They study anatomy (the structure of bones, muscles, blood vessels, and nerves), physiology (how the body works, including breathing, digestion, and circulation), pathology (how disease affects the body), and psychology, as well as therapeutic exercises and techniques of healing. In addition to their wide variety of manipulative skills, they have machines and aids at their disposal. They use treatments that range from simple to highly complex and include various techniques to strengthen muscles; mobilize joints; relieve aches, pains, and stiffness; and teach coordination and walking.

Methods

Physical therapists' work involves manipulation, mobilization, and massage, to get the patient and his or her temporarily immobile limbs moving. Manipulation is a method used to make joints and tissues more flexible. Finger and hand movements are used to apply pressure, for example, in cases where joints, although not dislocated, have moved slightly out of alignment and have become stiff or fixed. Many back complaints benefit from this treatment. Forceful, finely isolated pressure can relieve pain when a nerve has become inflamed or pinched. Skill is needed to know precisely where and how to apply pressure to obtain a satisfactory result. Unskilled manipulation can be dangerous. Similar skills are used to mobilize joints and relieve pain. Often, less force and more gentle pressure are needed than in manipulation, and the benefit comes not from one or two treatments by the physical therapist, but from repeated movements in which the patient has to work with the therapist. Exercises are used to restore strength to weakened muscles. Hands are used to massage and manipulate soft tissues around the joints to improve blood flow and assist limb movement. Some modern massage techniques are based on Swedish methods.

Techniques

In addition to their manipulative skills, physical therapists use a range of techniques that require specialized equipment. The most recently introduced technique is electrotherapy or electroshock therapy, in which low- or high-frequency electricity is used for its healing effect on the skin, muscles, and other tissues.

Electrotherapy comes in a variety of forms. Shortwave diathermy is a high-frequency current that penetrates deep into the tissues and is used to relieve deep-seated pain in joints such as the hip. Pulse magnetic field therapy, in which pulses of magnetic energy are passed through the limb, is used to heal fractures. A combination of high- and low-frequency currents that penetrate deep into the tissues is used in inferential therapy to increase circulation and reduce pain. Low-frequency currents initiate muscle contractions in limbs that have been affected by disease or injury.

Pain can also be reduced by transcutaneous nerve stimulation, in which a low electric current is passed through the tissues, thereby stimulating nerves near the surface of the skin.

Ultrasound is used on soft tissue, muscles, and ligaments; high-frequency sound waves cause vibration and a warming effect to relieve pain, decrease inflammation, improve circulation, and restore movement in the fluid components of the tissues. For pain relief and improved circulation, infrared irradiation from a lamp, or a hot pack, can be used. There is also a wide range of traditional treatments. Cold therapy is applied in the form of ice wrapped in towels or crushed ice in water, and it is used to suppress pain and relieve swelling. By reducing blood flow, cold therapy can reduce inflammation, and it is a convenient method of treating hand, foot, and knee injuries.

Hydrotherapy involves exercising in warm water in special pools. The heat helps muscles to relax and relieves pain. Exercises aim to restore muscle power and make movement easier. Hydrotherapy is widely used for paralysis and rheumatic disorders.

Paraffin wax can be used to treat painful joints in the hands. Hot wax is molded around the fingers, and since it prevents heat loss, the heat is retained for a long time. Finally, there are techniques that can be used to facilitate movement. Facilitatory techniques are used when there is abnormal movement or no movement of a limb; the aim is to make the limb more efficient by working through nerve reflexes and nerve stimulation.

A combination of all these techniques may be used. The choice will depend upon the physical therapist's assessment of the patient's condition and his or her knowledge of which techniques produce beneficial results. Weakened and damaged muscles and

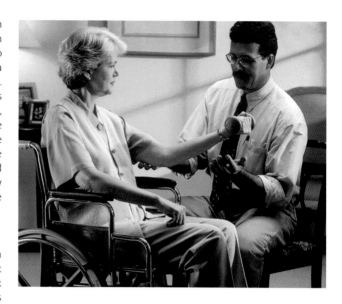

▲ *A wheelchair-bound woman keeps in shape with physical therapy. A range of equipment and techniques are used to strengthen joints and muscles and restore normal movement.*

tissues cannot be strengthened by the physical therapist alone; effort has to come from the patient too. The physical therapist will teach, assist, encourage, and demonstrate, but the patient must follow the treatment consistently and make an attempt to fight his or her way back to health.

Uses of physical therapy

Physical therapy is used in a wide range of problems that may arise because of disease, disability, or injury.

Neurology: Neurological conditions occur in the central nervous system, when the nerves in the brain or spinal cord are damaged by disease or injury, or when there are disorders of the peripheral nerves. Central nervous system disorders can have such diverse causes as traffic accidents, strokes, and congenital or birth disorders such as cerebral palsy. Muscles cannot move unless messages are transmitted to them along the spinal cord. Muscles will also not be able to move if nerves are damaged. If a nerve in a finger is cut, it will cause a loss of sensation and a loss of movement in the finger. Much more serious paralysis results if the spinal cord is cut or if certain areas of the brain that control movement are affected. If the spinal cord is cut below armpit level, paraplegia is the result. Injuries higher up produce tetraplegia or quadriplegia. Damage to the brain from a stroke or severe head injury can produce hemiplegia.

Paralysis can result from congenital conditions such as spina bifida, or diseases such as multiple sclerosis, in which the myelin sheath that allows the nerve to conduct its electrical message becomes damaged and prevents proper functioning of the nerve.

A patient with hemiplegia may suffer from visual disorientation, in which he or she sees only half of each visual field. This is distressing, and the patient will have to be trained to adjust to the environment. In all cases, the therapist will try to stimulate the nerves, inhibit abnormal movements, correct imbalance, or improve the strength of normal muscles to take over extra work from those that are permanently damaged. For instance, the arm muscles of a

Questions and Answers

I always thought that an osteopath was the same as a physical therapist, but a friend said this was wrong. Who is right?

Your friend is correct. Osteopaths are physicians who have been through medical school; physical therapists have not.
Physical therapists cover a wide sphere of practice, specializing in manipulation and often working as part of a health care team. Osteopaths treat skeletal disorders.

My father recently had a stroke and has lost movement and feeling in his right arm. How can physical therapy help him when he cannot feel anything?

Physical therapists are trained to treat not only loss of movement but also loss of sensation. They will be able to help your father by retraining the nerve pathways that have been affected by the stroke to adapt to new patterns of movement.

I am paralyzed from the waist down and am confined to a wheelchair. Is there any point to physical therapy when I'll never walk again?

Many patients who are confined to wheelchairs live full, active lives. Some travel, play sports, go to work, and raise children. To help such people achieve independence, a physical therapist teaches them the basic activities that will produce the strength and stamina to maneuver their wheelchairs, so they will be able to engage in activities as fully as possible.

I woke up the other morning with a stiff and painful shoulder. Could a physical therapist treat this?

Yes. It would be best to see your doctor first, and if he or she thought it warranted further treatment, he would refer you to a physical therapist who would find the source of the pain and treat it.

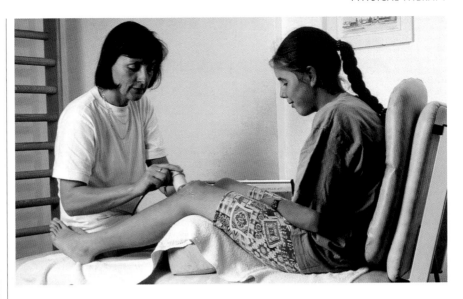

▲ *Ultrasound is an addition to the physical therapist's armory for treating damaged tissues—particularly in arthritis. Very-high-frequency sound waves are passed into the body, decreasing inflammation, improving circulation, and relieving pain.*

patient whose legs are paralyzed can be strengthened to enable him or her to propel a wheelchair, and to transfer to a toilet, bath, or bed.

Obstetrics and gynecology: Some therapists work chiefly with pregnant women. At prenatal classes they give information about relaxation, breathing, how to push and use muscles correctly during labor, and what actually happens during birth. Therapists can give advice about correct posture, so that the extra weight of the baby in the womb will not lead to backache. Postnatal sessions not only improve general physique but also teach the importance of exercise to restore the normal strength of the pelvic floor muscles, which support the abdominal organs, including the bladder. Weakness following childbirth can lead to urine leaking from the bladder, a condition called stress incontinence. Guidance can also be given on the correct way to lift and carry, so that lifting the baby will not lead to aches and pains.

Orthopedics: This branch of medicine deals with deformity of the bones because of accident, disease, or congenital complications. These deformities, which include fractures, sprains, and amputations, can be treated surgically or by mechanical means. Broken bones generally require support from a plaster cast, and the limb may be immobilized from three weeks to two months or more. When the cast is removed the limb is stiff, and treatment is needed to strengthen and restore it to normal mobility. Different techniques of manipulation, mobilization, and massage will be needed depending on whether or not the affected limb is weight-bearing (as a leg is, for instance). Less severe than broken bones, but more common, are injuries to ligaments and muscles. It is important that these are treated quickly, especially for injured athletes, so that the full function of the limb can be restored.

When a patient has lost a limb, the physical therapist will be involved in choosing an appropriate artificial limb. The patient is taught to move the limb correctly so that bad habits do not develop in the early stages of rehabilitation. With the right prosthesis and physical therapy many patients are able to resume normal activity and live full and active lives.

Pediatrics: Pediatrics covers diseases and injuries to children. Many techniques used for adults also apply to children, but there may be complications because the child is still growing. Physical therapists work very closely with other members of the health team, such as play therapists, occupational therapists, and speech therapists, so that a full relationship with the child is developed and he or she suffers as little as possible during treatment.

Respiratory care: Physical therapy is necessary when respiration is impeded, because in such cases, chest diseases, such as asthma, bronchitis, and pneumonia, can occur.

Following surgery, the effects of an anesthetic can produce secretions that need to be removed from the lungs. In all of these cases, the physical therapist will teach the patient postural drainage

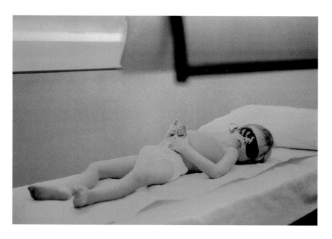

▲ *In liver disease, bilirubin causes yellow staining in the skin (jaundice) and itching. Blue light therapy converts the bilirubin to a form that can be excreted in the urine.*

techniques to remove the secretions. In conditions such as cystic fibrosis, it may be necessary to percuss the chest (a form of beating) to dislodge the mucus from the bronchi.

Intensive care: Patients who are seriously ill are cared for in an intensive care unit, where a physical therapist is an important member of the extended team. He or she works with patients who have been involved in serious accidents, when there may be severe head injury, and on patients who have had chest, heart, or abdominal surgery. Physical therapists keep the limbs of unconscious patients mobile and monitor any chest condition. Patients in intensive care units are often on respirators, and a physical therapist must work to keep the airways clear and the chest free of secretions, both by agitating the chest with hand massage and by using suction methods.

Rheumatology: This encompasses a group of diseases including rheumatoid arthritis and osteoarthritis. Rheumatoid arthritis (inflammation of the tissues around the joints) attacks several joints at once, such as the fingers and toes, whereas osteoarthritis usually attacks a single joint that has previously been damaged through injury or wear and tear. The term "rheumatism" is often used to cover symptoms that arise from these conditions, such as lumbago. If a patient has a painful joint in the hand, wrist, elbow, or foot, a physical therapist can support the joint with a splint.

Burns: Physical therapy is important in the treatment of burns. When the burn covers a joint, the scar tissues contract as they form across the joint, and this will restrict movement. During the healing process, the soft area underlying the skin has to be mobile. Massage is needed to keep the tissue stretched, and exercises are used to keep the joint moving. When a patient has extensive burns, the exercises may be done under water in warm saline baths, after the dressings have been removed. The warmth of the water relieves pain and aids movement. Ultrasound is also often used to soften scar tissues by agitating the cells of the tissues to decrease inflammation and improve local circulation.

Intellectual impairment: The various degrees of intellectual impairment are usually classified into two main groups: the severely impaired, who require constant care and attention because serious brain damage prevents them from responding to treatment, and

those who are intellectually impaired but can still learn to wash, dress, and feed themselves with a minimum of help.

If a child is intellectually impaired, treatment starts very early. The child will be encouraged to learn the simple, everyday movements of sitting, standing, walking, and climbing. Treatment is aimed at giving the child maximum independence as early as possible so that he or she will be able to carry out simple activities such as going for walks, taking a bus, or going to the store.

Frequently, mental impairment is combined with motor disability. In this condition the skilled techniques of the physical therapist can help correct imbalance and achieve normal movement patterns.

Cancer: Many forms of cancer can now be cured, but the disease can result in paralysis, pain, muscular weakness, and fractures. Even when a patient has a terminal illness, the physical therapist will use massage, mobilization, and exercise to retain full movement of the limbs for as long as possible.

Geriatrics: Geriatric medicine is the care of elderly people. During the aging process elasticity in tissues lessens, and the result can be stiffness and pain. The physical therapist will treat these symptoms with massage, mobilization, or other techniques, such as one of the forms of electrotherapy.

Lack of mobility in older people, however, can lead to other symptoms. For example, a broken leg considerably limits movement, and this limitation in turn can lead to circulation problems and result in congestion of the lungs. In this instance, patients will also need to have respiratory care. Age can cause problems with balance, and patients may need to be retrained to control their balance by following a specific exercise program, usually done in front of a mirror.

One neurological disease that sometimes affects older people is Parkinson's disease, which produces a tremor in the limbs. A number of facilitatory techniques, which have been developed through many years of research, are used to teach patients how to easily change their walking pattern.

Cardiac surgery: In the cardiac unit the work of the physical therapist begins two or three days before surgery. Physical therapists will get to know the patient and teach him or her certain movements and exercises. These will help the patient as soon as he or she regains consciousness following surgery. The patient will need to know how to handle a machine that will assist his or her breathing, how to carry out exercises that will help him or her to breathe properly, and how to cough. It is very painful to cough following major heart surgery, but coughing is necessary to remove secretions from the lungs. When the patient is able to get out of bed, he or she will be given a program of graduated exercises to help improve stamina and regain normal patterns of movement.

Physical therapists work closely with their colleagues in the health care team, including occupational therapists and, when the patient has had a stroke, speech therapists. All of these therapists could be involved in assessing the patient's needs in preparation for his or her discharge from the hospital.

Aside from specialized functions of physical therapy, simply getting a patient out of bed regularly is very important. Pneumonia, deep vein thrombosis in the legs, and bedsores are just a few of the problems that can be avoided in this way.

See also: Fractures; Pain; Paralysis; Pneumonia; Sprains

Pneumonia

Questions and Answers

Is double pneumonia worse than the ordinary type of pneumonia?

In the past, one of the most common forms of pneumonia was lobar pneumonia, in which one complete lobe of one of the lungs became infected, usually with the pneumococcus bacterium. (There are three lobes on the right lung, two on the left.) In double pneumonia, more than one lung was infected; this was obviously a more serious condition than involvement of only a single lung. Pneumonias involving more than one lung have a higher mortality than those that are confined to a single lung.

When my father had pneumonia he received treatment from a physical therapist that involved hitting him on the chest. What good could this have done him?

The physical therapist is vital in the treatment of pneumonia to ensure that all the infected secretions of the inflamed mucous membranes are brought up from the depths of the lungs and coughed up. Thumping the chest wall is one technique that a physical therapist will use to loosen the secretions, and some patients find that it brings relief from breathlessness. However, it does not affect the rate of recovery from the pneumonia.

Does pneumonia tend to be worse in people who suffer from asthma?

The main problem in people who suffer from asthma is that their bronchial tubes tend to become constricted (narrowed) easily. Any infection in the chest will increase this problem; there doesn't have to be full-blown pneumonia for someone to get a bad asthmatic attack. However, when an asthmatic does have pneumonia, it will definitely tend to constrict the bronchial tubes, and this will make the condition worse.

Pneumonia—acute inflammation of the lungs—used to be one of the great killers, attacking the young and fit almost as readily as the aged and infirm. Treatment with antibiotics has now made it possible to save countless lives.

Pneumonia usually occurs as a result of a bacterial infection, but it may also arise from a viral or fungal infection or from inhaling foreign matter into the lungs. Owing to treatment with antibiotics, fewer people now die of pneumonia. However, the aged, people with chronic lung disorders, and those already weakened by other diseases remain at risk.

Causes

To understand how pneumonia affects the lungs, it is important to look at their structure. The breathing tube that supplies air to the lungs is the windpipe (trachea). This splits into two branches (the bronchi), which in turn divide into three main branches on the right and two main branches on the left. Each of these branches supplies one lobe of one of the lungs: there are three lobes on the right and two on the left, separated from each other by thin membranes of fibrous tissue. Each

LOBAR PNEUMONIA

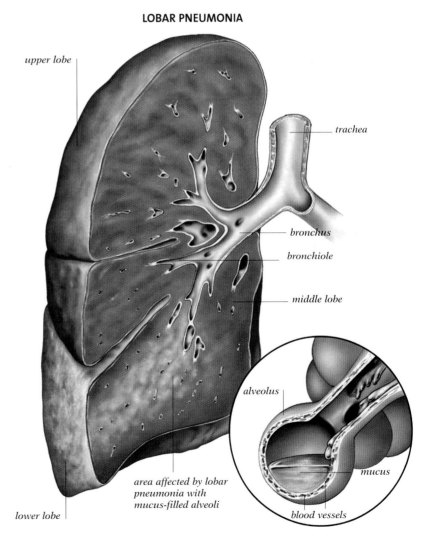

upper lobe

trachea

bronchus

bronchiole

middle lobe

alveolus

mucus

area affected by lobar pneumonia with mucus-filled alveoli

lower lobe

blood vessels

261

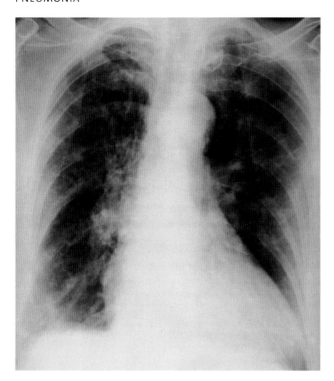

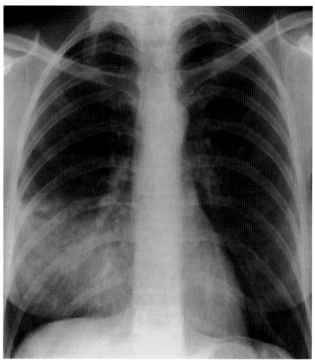

of the main bronchi then splits down into finer branches that supply all of the tiny air sacs (alveoli) where oxygen finally crosses from the air inside the lungs into the blood.

When the chest is infected, the lung tissue becomes inflamed. If the inflammation is confined to the bronchi it is called bronchitis, and it results in a thickening of the membrane that lines the bronchi and the production of large amounts of secretions from the glands in the bronchi.

In pneumonia, the infection occurs in the smaller bronchi (the bronchioli) and the alveoli, which become solid with secretions, rather than filled with air. This process is called consolidation. On a chest X ray the affected area shows up as a white patch, rather than as the black area that would be seen in healthy lung tissue. The congestion of the lungs may severely affect breathing.

There are two main types of pneumonia. Lobar pneumonia was, in the past, the more common of the two. It is nearly always caused by the pneumococcus bacterium. Only one lobe of the lung tends to be involved, and this lobe becomes consolidated while the rest of the lung remains relatively normal.

Bronchopneumonia can be caused by many different sorts of organisms, but usually one of several bacteria is responsible, the most common of which is the *Haemophilus influenzae* bacterium. Other kinds of bacteria that can cause bronchopneumonia include the pneumococcus and the staphylococcus. Staphylococcus is the

▲ *A chest X ray reveals the type of pneumonia. Bronchopneumonia (above left) is distinguished by white patches on all or part of a lung; note those on the right lung (left-hand side of image). Lobar pneumonia (above right), involves the whole lobe.*

▼ *Bronchopneumonia caused by the pneumococcus bacterium.*

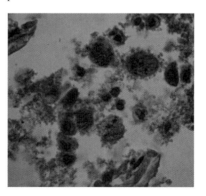

more serious. This kind of bronchopneumonia tends to appear after an attack of flu, and may cause death even in people who were previously healthy.

Bronchopneumonia is characterized by small patches of consolidation that appear all over the lungs. These patches may be concentrated in one lung, or even in one part of one lung, but a whole lobe is not involved. Bronchopneumonia can occur at the same time as bronchitis, and it often results when bronchitis spreads to involve the rest of the lung tissue. This frequently happens to people who have chronic (long-term) chest problems, but it is also common for people to get acute bronchopneumonia in addition to chronic bronchitis.

Viruses can cause pneumonia, but more often a primary viral infection in the upper part of the respiratory tract (the throat and nose) is followed by a secondary bacterial infection in the lungs.

Other microscopic organisms, such as chlamydia (which causes psittacosis, a disease caught from caged birds), rickettsia (which causes typhus and Q fever), and mycoplasma (a funguslike organism), can also cause pneumonia. People with AIDS are particularly likely to develop a severe pneumonia caused by the organism *Pneumocystis carinii*.

Pneumonia may also arise as a result of a blockage of one of the main bronchial tubes, for instance from cancer of the bronchus. Similarly, chronic disorders of the bronchus, such as bronchiectasis (in which the bronchi continually produce pus as a result of a chronic

Questions and Answers

Can people's lungs be permanently damaged by pneumonia?

Yes. Some of the bacteria that cause pneumonia, such as the staphylococcus, can lead to the formation of abscesses that remain as a scar even after treatment. However, most cases of pneumonia can now be treated with antibiotics and recovery of the lungs is complete.

I've heard that a simple cold that spreads to the chest can cause pneumonia. Is this true?

Yes, infections in the upper part of the respiratory tract—the nose and throat—can be a cause of pneumonia. The original infection is usually due to a virus, but as a result of this a bacterium can become established lower down in the chest, causing pneumonia.

Are inhalations with steam good for people who have pneumonia?

Inhalations with steam, or with a substance called tincture of benzoin, were used much more in the past than they are today. However, they may very well make people cough up infected phlegm and feel better. A more modern form of inhalation is with drugs that widen the bronchial tubes. These are given as a vapor through an oxygen mask.

Why are elderly people more prone to pneumonia?

Anyone who is weak, either through age or through illness, will be prone to pneumonia, and for this reason it is often what finally leads to the death of people who are already ill with some other disease. The resistance of the body to infection is reduced, and once pneumonia has become established, an elderly patient may be too weak to cough up all the infected secretions, so that the infection becomes worse. This leads to a further weakening of the patient, who then has even less ability to clear the sputum.

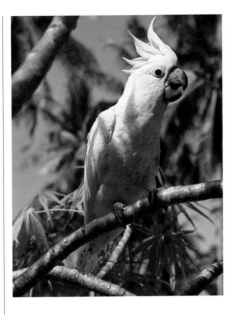

▲ *Though beautiful to look at, the cockatoo may transmit the chlamydia virus, which causes psittacosis—a type of pneumonia. However, it is fairly uncommon.*

How to prevent pneumonia

Stop smoking, especially if you have long-standing chest trouble.

If pneumonia is prevalent in your area and you are at high risk, ask your doctor to immunize you against influenza.

If you have lung disease, ask your doctor to immunize you against pneumococcus.

Don't wait for a chest ailment to get better on its own; seek medical attention immediately.

Avoid crowds during the flu season.

Keep up a high level of nutrition and health—all types of pneumonia pose the worst threat to the weak, the elderly, and people who are debilitated.

infection that also destroys the normal bronchial wall), can produce pneumonia by blocking the tubes and allowing pus to be sucked back into normal lung tissue.

Finally, pneumonia can result from inhaling foreign objects, such as loose teeth or peanuts, into the lungs. This is called aspiration pneumonia. However, the main kind of aspiration pneumonia occurs as a result of unconsciousness, because when a person is unconscious the coughing mechanism that normally prevents food and other foreign substances from going down the wrong way is absent. Therefore, it is important for unconscious patients to be watched carefully so that no such inhalations occur, for example, when general anesthesia is given, or when emergency resuscitation is needed.

Symptoms

The main symptom of pneumonia is a cough, which varies according to the type of condition. In bronchopneumonia with added acute bronchitis, infected (yellow or green) sputum may be produced; in a viral pneumonia there could be a dry cough with no sputum at all.

In bronchopneumonia there is usually a cough, although it is not the main symptom. Lobar pneumonia is characterized by fever, and unless the patient is treated with antibiotics, he or she will have a very high temperature. Since the whole lobe is involved, the inflammation may spread to the lining of the pleura, causing pleurisy, which will result in the additional symptom of pain on coughing or on taking a deep breath.

In bronchopneumonia caused by bacteria, the symptoms tend to vary according to how much extra bronchitis there is. However, there is nearly always more sputum produced in bronchopneumonia than in lobar pneumonia, and pleurisy is a less common occurrence. The patient usually has a raised temperature, but it is not as high as in lobar pneumonia.

Bronchopneumonia is more likely to affect older people and those who are sick or infirm. Often there are fewer symptoms in older

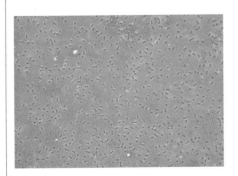

▲ *In lobar pneumonia, a sputum sample examined under a microscope will reveal the presence of pneumococcal bacteria.*

Causes and treatment of pneumonia

TYPE	CAUSE	SYMPTOMS	TREATMENT
PNEUMONIAS CAUSED BY A BACTERIUM			
Lobar pneumonia	Pneumococcus bacterium	Cough, pain on breathing, fever. Rust-colored sputum.	Antibiotics
Bronchopneumonia	Various organisms, particularly *Haemophilus influenzae*	Cough is the main symptom, but there may also be fever. Green or yellow sputum.	Antibiotics appropriate to the organism concerned
Pneumonia leading to abscess formation	Staphylococcus and klebsiella bacteria; anaerobic bacteria	A severe feverish illness with a cough	Antibiotics
Aspiration pneumonia	Various organisms. As a result of inhalation, usually while patient is unconscious.	Fever and cough. Often causes lung abscess.	Antibiotics
PNEUMONIAS NOT CAUSED BY A BACTERIUM			
Viral pneumonia	Chicken pox, influenza	Cough and fever without much sputum being produced	Antibiotics if the lungs then become infected by a bacterium. Ventilation on a respirator may be required.
	Respiratory syncytial virus	Occurs in newborn babies. Causes breathlessness.	
Pneumocystis carinii pneumonia	Immune deficiency allowing infection with *P. carinii*	Slight fever, weakness, breathlessness, and cyanosis	The drug pentamidine isethionate
Q fever	Rickettsia virus	Cough and fever, not much sputum	Tetracycline or erythromycin
Mycoplasma	Very small bacterial organisms, but with no thick cell wall	Cough and fever, not much sputum	Tetracycline or macrolides

people than in people who are young and fit, even though when the disease occurs in older people, it may cause death after a long illness.

In the rare forms of pneumonia caused by organisms other than bacteria, the symptoms vary, but by and large, fever is common. Changes in the lungs are obvious in X rays; the cough and sputum production are less than in bacterial pneumonia.

Dangers and complications

One of the most common complications of all kinds of pneumonia is pleurisy. This may lead to a pleural effusion (a collection of fluid within the pleural cavity). If this fluid then becomes infected, it leads to pus formation in the pleural cavity, causing emphysema.

Pockets of pus can also form within the lung, causing a lung abscess. This is especially likely to develop in staphylococcal pneumonia and in a rare form of lobar pneumonia called klebsiella, as well as with pneumonia caused by anaerobic bacteria (bacteria that do not need oxygen to survive). Lung abscesses are a serious problem and occur only as a result of severe lung infection.

In general, though, rather than giving rise to other complications, pneumonia is a complication of other diseases. It is for this reason that pneumonia, usually severe bronchopneumonia, may be fatal, because it is so often the final event in the life of someone who is already very weak, sick, or aged.

Treatment

In fit people, treatment with antibiotics is generally all that is necessary. However, in older people, or people who already have a chronic chest disease or another illness, it is important to make sure that the secretions in the lung produced by pneumonia are coughed up and not allowed to remain in the chest, where they can cause further problems. The physical therapist has a vital role to play in helping people with pneumonia to clear these secretions. Drugs that are inhaled as a vapor through an oxygen mask may help to widen the bronchi, which tend to narrow in pneumonia.

Outlook

The outlook in pneumonia depends on the age and state of health of the patient. A young, fit person who gets lobar pneumonia should make a total and rapid recovery, whereas an aged person with chronic bronchitis who has probably already had a number of attacks of bronchopneumonia is at some risk of dying if he or she has a further attack. Pneumonia in someone who is very weak as a result of disease can be fatal, even with antibiotic treatment.

See also: AIDS; Antibiotics; Bacteria; Cancer; Physical therapy; Staphylococcus; Viruses; X rays

Poisoning

Do all poisons cause deep unconsciousness in the victim?

No. Tranquilizers and sleeping tablets will lead to coma when taken in an overdose, but others such as acetaminophen and aspirin can leave the patient wide awake for as long as 48 hours or more after being taken. Corrosives that burn the esophagus also leave the patient awake, so the state of consciousness is not a good guide to the severity of poisoning.

What is alcohol poisoning?

Alcohol can slowly poison the liver and cause cirrhosis, a disease that can be fatal. Large, unaccustomed amounts of alcohol taken in a short time can cause a coma or death. Alcohol can make the body susceptible to acetaminophen (Tylenol) poisoning; for this reason, most painkillers cannot be given to alcoholics. In children, alcohol, even in small amounts, can result in unconsciousness. It can also increase the effects of medicines such as tranquilizers, sleeping tablets, and pills for hay fever or motion sickness, and lead to drowsiness and unsteadiness.

What can I do to reduce my family's risk of poisoning by medicines?

If you buy medicines such as painkillers or cold remedies, ask for as few as possible. Don't get twice the amount you need "so that they'll be there for next time"; 25 tablets should be the maximum. When buying medicines for a child, tell the pharmacist this, and give the child's age. Adults' medicines should never be given to children. Prescription tablets should always be kept in childproof bottles and put away out of reach of children. Return any unused medicines to your pharmacist if a medication is changed or a course of treatment is finished.

A large number of everyday household substances contain poisons, and because they are so common, it is easy to overlook their potential dangers. Beware of carelessness, which can all too easily lead to tragedy.

Doctors consider poisoning a modern epidemic. Millions of people are accidentally poisoned every year and there are around 5,000 deaths each year from foodborne diseases alone.

Accidental cases of poisoning, either in the home or at work, are often the result of carelessness or industrial incidents. Other cases can be a result of deliberate self-poisoning; the number of such cases has increased dramatically in recent years. Whatever the cause, many of these cases can be avoided. By examining the problem and the areas of greatest risk, everyone can play a part in preventing some of these tragic events. It is vital, for instance, to be aware of the potential danger of many commonplace substances used daily in the home.

ORGANS AT RISK

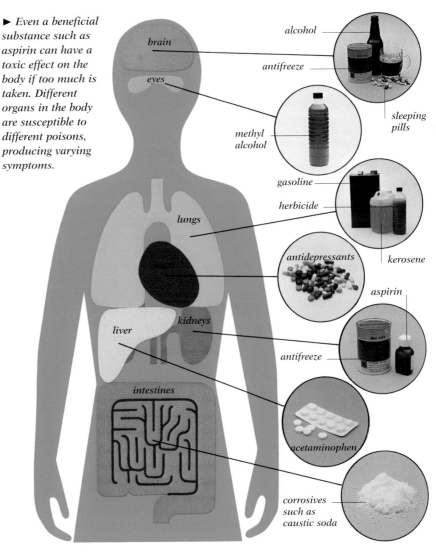

▶ *Even a beneficial substance such as aspirin can have a toxic effect on the body if too much is taken. Different organs in the body are susceptible to different poisons, producing varying symptoms.*

brain

eyes

alcohol

antifreeze

sleeping pills

methyl alcohol

gasoline

herbicide

kerosene

lungs

antidepressants

aspirin

heart

kidneys

liver

antifreeze

intestines

acetaminophen

corrosives such as caustic soda

Are there any aerosol sprays that are poisonous?

Most aerosols, including bug sprays, are not poisonous, or are not potentially very dangerous. An exception is oven cleaner, which contains a caustic substance that could burn the skin. With any aerosol it is important to read the manufacturer's instructions carefully to see what precautions should be taken and what the hazards are. If an aerosol is accidentally sprayed into the eye, keep the eyelid open to allow as much of the substance to evaporate as possible and wash for several minutes under a running faucet. Some aerosols can be dangerous if directly inhaled.

Can poisoning occur in people in the form of epidemics?

Yes. An epidemic of poisoning is said to occur when a single agent is responsible for poisoning a large number of people. This can occur through contaminated food or water supplies. The relevant authorities take great care to prevent this. However, in 1981, in Spain, a large epidemic of poisoning was caused by contaminated cooking oil; outbreaks on a smaller scale also occur from time to time.

Can exhaust fumes from vehicles cause poisoning?

Yes. Exhaust fumes from any type of vehicle contain the highly poisonous gas carbon monoxide, so a vehicle engine should never be left running in an unventilated space. Care should also be taken to ensure that the exhaust pipe does not leak, because, even in small amounts, the gas might build up on a long drive and cause sickness, headaches, or even death. Until recently, gasoline also contained lead compounds, which were given off in exhaust fumes. Lead can cause brain damage in high concentrations, especially in children. Leaded fuels have now been banned in many countries, including the United States.

DANGERS IN THE KITCHEN

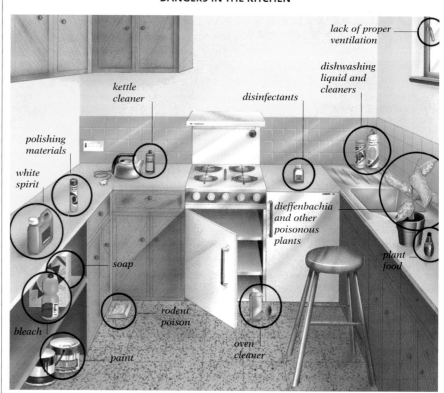

lack of proper ventilation

dishwashing liquid and cleaners

kettle cleaner

disinfectants

polishing materials

white spirit

dieffenbachia and other poisonous plants

plant food

soap

rodent poison

bleach

oven cleaner

paint

▲ *Kitchens are dangerous places for children. Many products and plants are poisonous and should be kept high up or in locked cupboards. All gas appliances need ventilation.*

Those at risk

The possibility of accidental poisoning is present throughout a person's life. However, there are certain ages when people may be particularly at risk of accidental or intentional poisoning.

When young children start to explore their surroundings, it is natural for them to put objects or liquids into their mouths, particularly if the objects are small or brightly colored. Children aged two to five years are especially at risk of poisoning by materials they find within their reach.

Teenagers often suffer emotional conflicts. Some of them seek to resolve these conflicts by taking an overdose of painkillers, sleeping tablets, or medicines that have been prescribed for their parents. Their intention is very rarely to take their life. More often it is to attract attention and indirectly to seek help, or to avoid a difficult situation. Doctors and psychologists use the term "suicidal gesture" to describe this kind of behavior. However, some teenagers accidentally die because they underestimate the effects of the poisonous substances that they take.

Both suicidal gestures and genuine attempts can occur in adults who are severely depressed. In the elderly especially, suicidal intentions can be provoked by factors such as chronic illness or pain, loneliness, and depression, and poisoning is more often fatal in this age group than in any other.

What is a poison?

It is difficult to say precisely which substances are poisonous. Even water or oxygen, when present

▶ *A scan of a brain affected by carbon monoxide, which is very poisonous, shows reduced activity in the dark blue areas.*

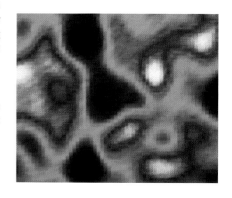

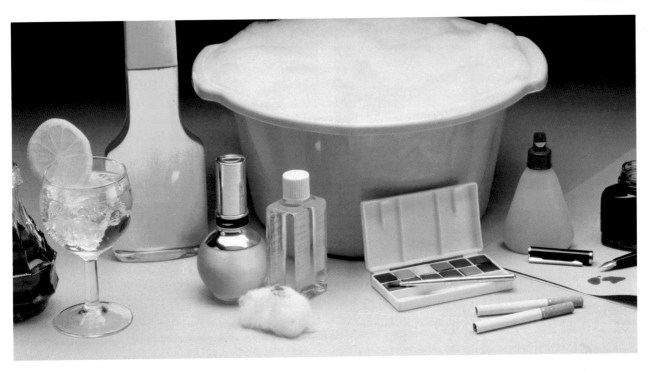

▲ *Many people do not realize the potential danger of common products. Vinegar, detergents, cigarettes, alcohol, perfume, cosmetics, ink, gum, and paints can all be lethal.*

in excess, can damage the body. Also, many lifesaving medicines can be fatal when taken in large doses. A poison is best defined as any substance consumed in sufficient quantity to damage the normal working of the body.

Poisons include a vast range of substances that can enter the body through the skin, mouth, or lungs. They include stings by insects such as bees and wasps, and venom from poisonous fish, spiders, or snakes. Gases, fumes from industrial works, vehicle exhausts, and fires can also be poisonous. Fires kill people as often by poisoning as by direct burning or lack of oxygen, since fabrics and plastics burning in enclosed spaces can rapidly produce large amounts of highly toxic fumes.

Food—particularly meat and dairy products—can cause poisoning when it has not been properly prepared or refrigerated. Food poisoning usually causes vomiting and diarrhea, which clear up in a few days but can occasionally be more serious.

Some common plants, such as deadly nightshade, yew, and laburnum, contain poisonous substances. In remote parts of the world, indigenous peoples use these natural poisons in hunting.

Many tablets, medicines, and domestic products that are commonly found in most homes can also be dangerous. As most of them will not have a warning of "poison" written on them, it is worth knowing which ones are more likely to be toxic.

How a poison acts

Poisonous substances do their damage in a variety of ways. Sleeping pills, tranquilizers, excessive alcohol, and a number of other substances can depress the working of the brain to the extent that it no longer maintains respiration; death results because oxygen is not taken in through the lungs. Some poisons act by blocking the action of vital enzymes necessary for cell function. Cyanide, for instance, inhibits certain enzymes and prevents the cells from using oxygen.

Other poisons will act directly on one or more of the body's organs. For example, antidepressants can cause serious abnormal rhythms of the heart. If any type of petroleum compound is swallowed, it may pass through the system and out of the body, but if any amount reaches the lungs it can cause a type of pneumonia that is very difficult to treat. This is why a person who has swallowed gasoline, or similar oily products, should not be made to vomit: some of the vomit may be taken into the lungs.

Corrosive substances burn the body tissues and if swallowed may burn the mouth and the esophagus. More rarely, they may actually burn through the esophagus, causing a perforation requiring surgical treatment. Milk can help dilute and neutralize corrosives, especially if given at an early stage. Vomiting is not likely to be helpful in this case and may cause further damage.

The ethylene glycol in antifreeze is converted by the body to oxalic acid, a substance that can damage the brain and kidneys. Some antifreezes also contain methyl alcohol, which the body converts into substances that damage the optic nerves and cause blindness. Other products, such as model aircraft fuel and rubbing alcohol, also contain methyl alcohol.

Acetaminophen, when taken in an overdose, leads to liver damage. At first there are no symptoms, but damage can be done to the cells in the liver because a small amount of the drug is converted into a poisonous substance. There are antidotes that can be very effective in preventing liver damage, provided they are given within 24 hours. Aspirin can also be poisonous, but it has no known antidote. Of the many other poisons, each has its own toxic effect on the body, so that a doctor can often suspect a certain poison has been taken simply because of the signs or symptoms.

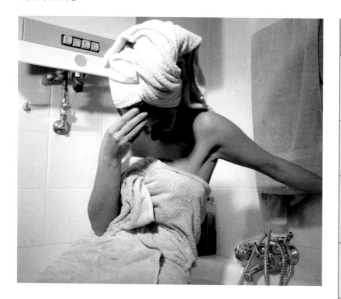

▲ *Dizziness and headaches due to carbon dioxide poisoning can result from gas leakage in a defective boiler heating system.*

Symptoms

Vomiting is one of the most important symptoms of poisoning; it is usually due to irritation or burning of the stomach but sometimes occurs because the poison has reached the part of the brain that controls the vomiting reflex. Convulsion is a symptom that can occur with some types of drugs for depression. Other symptoms of poisoning include drowsiness, coma, and pain. Vomiting, drowsiness, and coma should always be taken seriously and help should be sought immediately. Some painkillers may cause no symptoms, but with most other poisons symptoms appear early if large doses are taken.

Treatment

In all cases of poisoning or suspected poisoning, the victim should be taken immediately to his or her local doctor or the emergency room of a hospital. This is also necessary when the victim has taken an overdose of tablets but there are no symptoms, since some medicines can have delayed effects. If possible, the patient should be accompanied and any tablets or household products that may have been taken should be brought along, with their containers.

It is sometimes possible and advisable to give immediate first-aid treatment in the home. If a child has swallowed some pills and is conscious, it is sensible to attempt to induce vomiting by putting a finger down his or her throat. If this is not successful, do not persist; seek help at once. If the child has swallowed something believed to be corrosive, vomiting should not be induced, since this may cause further damage as the substance is regurgitated. Instead, the local emergency service should be called immediately.

Hospital treatment for any type of poisoning depends on the kind of poison and the amount that has been taken. Sometimes a drug called ipecac may be given to produce vomiting, or the stomach may be washed out with warm water passed through a tube. All these measures prevent the poison from being absorbed further and reaching the bloodstream. Special techniques include giving lots of fluids so the poison is flushed out through the

Preventing accidental poisoning

Bottles of cleaning fluids and bleach must never be left on the floor or stored at floor level in unlocked closets. The danger areas are: kitchen, bathroom, under the stairs, garage, and garden shed.

Closets containing dangerous substances must be locked or kept out of a child's reach. Medicines must always be kept in a locked closet and never left lying about in a room.

Never transfer any substance—whether it is poisonous or not—into an unlabeled container, particularly one such as a soft drink bottle or beer bottle. All household maintenance items, hobby items, and medicines should be clearly labeled.

Wash your hands immediately after handling any poisonous substance. Wash out used containers such as cans and buckets. Never leave them in the kitchen or near food.

Never keep unused drugs or medicines from an old prescription. Return them to your pharmacist, or if there are only a few tablets or drops of medicine left, flush them down the toilet.

Some medicines are packaged in the form of a pleasant-tasting syrup and many tablets also come in attractive colors and flavors. Never encourage children to take their tablets or medicines by pretending that you or they are taking sweets.

If you think someone has swallowed a poisonous substance, do not panic. By keeping a cool head and taking the right steps, you can still prevent serious damage. If in doubt, always consult your doctor or get to the hospital as soon as possible.

kidneys; in very severe cases, the patient may be put on a dialysis (artificial kidney) machine. This treatment is normally used for aspirin poisoning. Dialysis machines are also able to remove certain drugs from the bloodstream.

In a few cases, such as poisoning that is caused by taking iron tablets or certain types of painkilling drugs, antidotes can be given that bind with the poison or counteract its effects. However, in most cases, only skilled nursing care and medical supervision are needed while the body overcomes the poison in its own way.

Outlook

Following treatment for poisoning, the patient usually does not suffer any aftereffects. Delayed reactions are rare, but if corrosives have been swallowed a doctor will examine the patient after a certain interval to see if the substance has had any side effect on the swallowing mechanism. A person who has taken poison when disturbed might attempt to do so again. Such people should be treated with great care and sympathy.

See also: Alcoholism; Aspirin and analgesics; Bites and stings; Depression; Environmental hazards; Food poisoning; Iron; Medicines; Occupational hazards; Oxygen; Pneumonia

Preventive medicine

"An apple a day keeps the doctor away" is obviously an oversimplification, but the principle holds true: health care and preventive medicine, both public and personal, will certainly reduce the chances of disease.

I'm fed up with all this talk about health care and preventive medicine. Surely, if you give up all the things doctors want you to, life won't be worth living.

The old saying "an ounce of prevention is worth a pound of cure" has a lot of truth in it, and never more so than today, when it seems likely that the most dramatic advances in saving lives lie in preventing diseases rather than in curing them.

The only thing that most doctors suggest you give up altogether is smoking. Most of the other preventive measures that may be advised amount to adjustments or changes in routines, like getting additional exercise, rather than giving things up. Far from cramping their style or limiting their pleasures, most people find that adopting a simple, sensible program for taking care of the only life they have actually increases their zest for living.

There are two broad categories of preventive medicine: public health or community medicine, and personal health. Public health medicine is generally concerned with such things as ensuring that water is pure, food is safe, and waste and garbage are properly disposed of.

Personal health or personal preventive medicine depends on the efforts of each individual, and is mainly concerned with making sure that a wide range of preventable disorders are avoided by having immunizations, taking safety precautions both at home and away, getting adequate sleep and exercise, and changing habits, such as smoking, that are likely to lead to disease. There is a strong link between public health and personal preventive medicine.

Public health

The great improvements in public health—and the associated huge leap forward in life expectancy—that took place in the first part of the last century were due not so much to advances in medical care as to the effect of considerably improved living standards. They were also due to the control and prevention of diseases such as cholera, diphtheria, and tuberculosis by mass public health programs.

Are regular medical health checkups really worthwhile?

Yes, there is growing evidence that they are. Many potentially serious conditions can be detected by examinations and tests before they give rise to any symptoms, and if treatment is given at this time the chances of either curing the condition or preventing it from developing are much higher.

What can I do during my pregnancy to help ensure that my baby is healthy?

Don't put on too much weight—eating enough for two is a myth and will spoil your figure afterward. Get enough exercise, probably more than you would normally, and get plenty of rest and sleep, particularly during the final three months. Make sure that you have your prenatal checkups and try to attend the classes. Avoid smoking altogether because it can seriously harm the baby. Alcohol should be avoided as well. However, there is no need to give up intercourse during pregnancy; not only does it not harm the baby, but it gives you and you partner some scope for inventiveness.

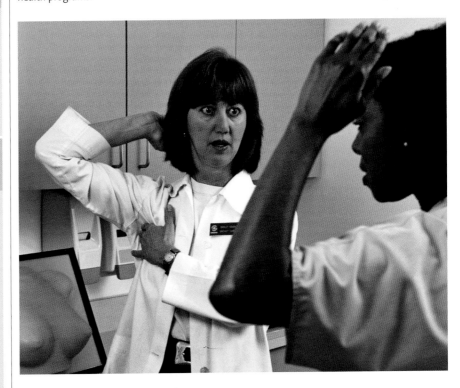

▲ *Breast cancer is one of the leading killers of women. However, a doctor can show a woman how to check her breasts for any lumps that could be malignant and thereby catch the cancer before it develops beyond the stage where it is treatable.*

269

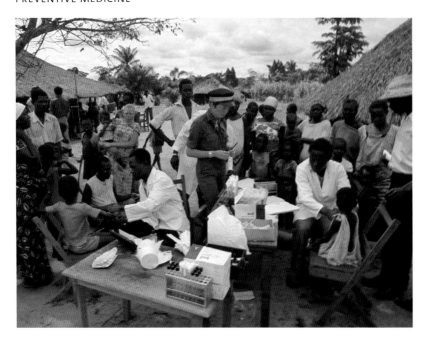

▲ *People living in some developing countries have benefited enormously from medical care and public health measures that prevent unnecessary death.*

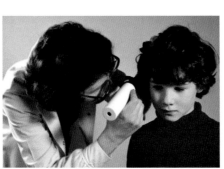

▲ *Worldwide campaigns have made the public aware that good dental care will prevent tooth decay and gum disease.*

Of course, the continued maintenance of high standards of public health remains vital to people's safety and health. No one needs to be reminded of the vicious and devastating nature of the epidemics that do still occur from time to time when the vigilance of the public health authorities slackens.

The second big leap forward in public health took place in the middle part of the 20th century and was based on the discovery of powerful new lifesaving drugs, particularly antibiotics. The development of radically new surgical techniques and substantial improvements in prenatal and infant welfare were also important. However, there is still room for further advances to be made in all these fields.

Personal preventive medicine

The real potential growth area in lifesaving lies in a different direction. For although the field of preventive medicine at the public level has been mined extensively, people have hardly begun to understand the possibilities in the field of personal health, let alone to exploit them.

Personal health is currently the most potent weapon people have in the crusade against unnecessary death and disability, and holds promise of saving more lives than any other area of medical advance.

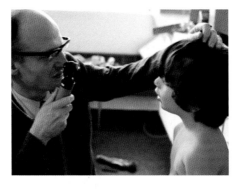

▲ *Routine eye tests are imperative to detect problems with vision which, because their onset is so gradual, are likely to be ignored.*

▼ *The ear is one of our most complex and sensitive organs, and it is prone to problems. Regular examination is very important.*

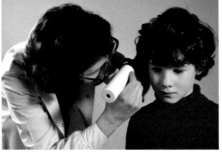

What is more, it is not a field in which humankind is waiting for some crucial new discovery or some major breakthrough in technique; it is simply a question of applying what is already known.

Early diagnosis

Early diagnosis is an area of preventive medicine that holds enormous lifesaving potential. Many people die unnecessarily, not because they have a disease for which there is no cure, but because they do not go to their doctor for investigation and treatment soon enough.

One hundred years ago most deaths occurred because no effective treatment was available for most serious illnesses, and, in these circumstances, failure to diagnose disease early made little difference to the outcome. Today, with the rapid advances in medical treatment, early diagnosis is vital in preventing unnecessary deaths, because many of the modern treatments are curative only if they are applied in the first stages of the condition. Therefore, many deaths, permanent disabilities, and cases of chronic ill health are due not to the inability of doctors to effect a cure, but to delay on the patient's part in seeking medical attention early enough to benefit fully from current techniques.

Questions and Answers

Is it good preventive medicine to stop eating fatty foods?

It is certainly good preventive medicine to take care about what you eat, but there is no reason to avoid fatty foods altogether. Many doctors believe that eating foods rich in saturated (animal) fats or in cholesterol increases the risk of developing heart and circulatory diseases, although most of the cholesterol in the blood is produced by the body itself. What is important in healthy eating is to have a nourishing diet in which the five essential ingredients—carbohydrates, fats, proteins, vitamins, and minerals—are all present in well-balanced quantities, and to remember that all foods taken in excess of what your body can utilize will turn into fat.

Does an apple a day really keep the doctor away?

Not exactly, but taking sensible care of your health certainly does. What is most likely to keep you out of the doctor's office is staying away as far as possible from smoking, underexercising, overeating, and stress. Daily fruit and vegetables certainly help.

Is it a good idea to have inoculations before going abroad?

Many parts of the world, particularly countries outside North America and Europe, do have health hazards, such as yellow fever or typhoid. It is good sense to have inoculations if you are traveling to countries where certain diseases are endemic.

If I take care of myself, will I live longer?

Life expectancy is determined by heredity, environment, and how long you have already lived. By taking precautions you will remain healthier longer, and with luck you will reach your maximum life span. The single most important thing you can do to live longer is to avoid smoking.

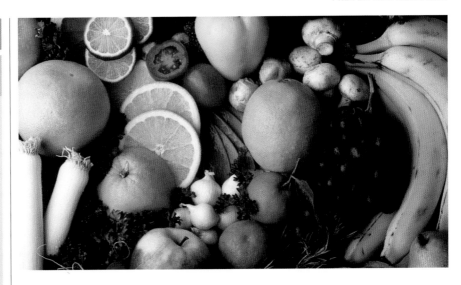

▲ *A balanced, healthy diet may not prevent illness by itself, but it can help keep the body fit and ready to fight off any problems that might occur.*

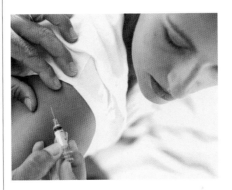

▲ *Throughout their early years and until they leave school, children are given immunizations to prevent them from catching certain diseases.*

▼ *Blood pressure problems affect many people and are a major cause of ill health. Advances in equipment now allow patients to monitor their own blood pressure.*

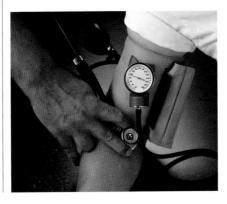

Health education

It is clear that the limiting factor in many cases of illness today lies not in what the doctor can do, but in whether the patient comes to him or her in time. A surefire method of helping to persuade people to seek medical help early is therefore likely to be even more effective in saving lives than some new medical discoveries. The prime aim of health education is to make people more aware of what they can do for themselves by increasing their knowledge of what makes them tick, and by telling them about how they themselves can affect their own health.

Many schools offer a comprehensive program in health education. Both boys and girls are taught about diet, exercise, and personal hygiene. They are also taught about safety in the home, keeping the environment clean, and ecology. The program may involve sex education, including family planning and how to avoid the spread of sexually transmitted diseases. Reproduction and contraception may also be explained so that unwanted teenage pregnancies can be avoided. Emotional health and social relationships are also discussed in the program, as well as the importance of seeking therapy for family-related problems such as parents' alcoholism, drug addiction, and child abuse

Early health education can teach children about the dangers of bad habits, but, more important, it can point the way toward a more positive attitude to healthy living. If children are to benefit from adults' examples, and if

PREVENTIVE MEDICINE

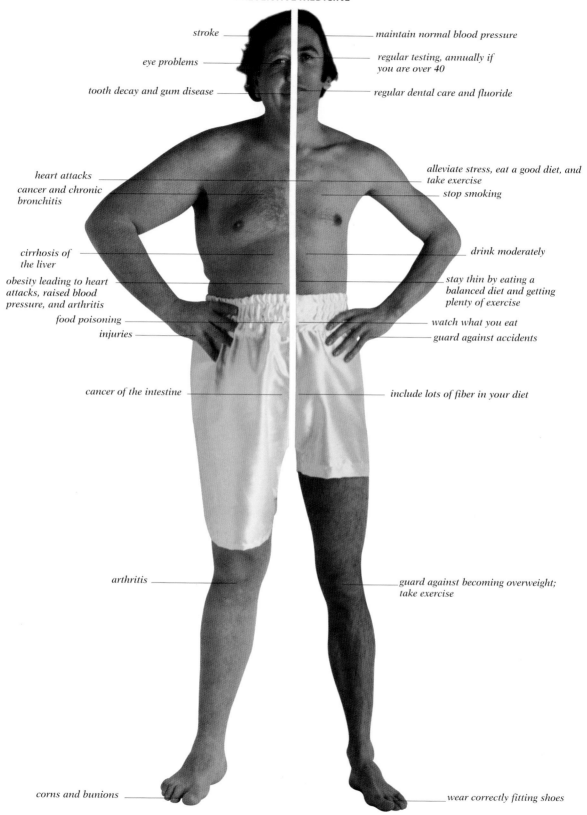

stroke — maintain normal blood pressure

eye problems — regular testing, annually if you are over 40

tooth decay and gum disease — regular dental care and fluoride

heart attacks — alleviate stress, eat a good diet, and take exercise

cancer and chronic bronchitis — stop smoking

cirrhosis of the liver — drink moderately

obesity leading to heart attacks, raised blood pressure, and arthritis — stay thin by eating a balanced diet and getting plenty of exercise

food poisoning — watch what you eat

injuries — guard against accidents

cancer of the intestine — include lots of fiber in your diet

arthritis — guard against becoming overweight; take exercise

corns and bunions — wear correctly fitting shoes

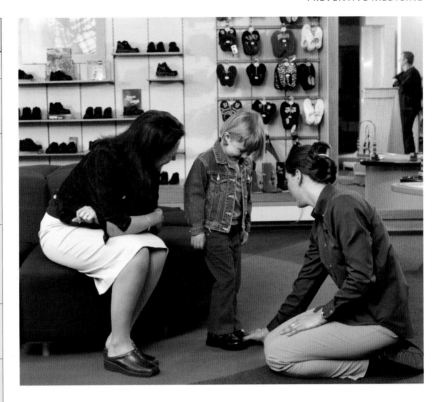

▲ *Foot problems in adults are very often the result of wearing ill-fitting shoes from childhood onward; this is why taking proper measurements is so important.*

what they learn at school about health education is to be reinforced at home, adults must educate themselves. They need to know about how the body works, basic nutrition, preventive health care, dental hygiene, and the importance of exercise.

Preventive medicine for all

Achievements in the control and prevention of infectious diseases tell a remarkable success story. The development and implementation of immunization techniques are partly responsible, as is the important part played by measures designed to prevent the organisms that cause disease from ever reaching the body, particularly the public health measures that are implemented to ensure the safety of food and water, and the efficient disposal of sewage. However, outbreaks of preventable diseases—especially gastrointestinal infections—will still occur unless adequate personal and domestic hygiene is maintained.

Checkups

Many people wonder whether regular medical checkups are a worthwhile preventive measure. It is true that people can drop dead on their way home from a health checkup at which nothing was found wrong with them, because some serious conditions cannot be detected by any form of screening. It is also true that not all doctors agree about the validity of checkups; some feel that abnormalities found, for example, in blood tests do not necessarily indicate that the person will develop a disease if nothing is done about them.

On the other hand, there is no doubt that regular checkups do pick up unsuspected conditions that may require treatment, and

conceivably save lives. This fact alone makes regular checkups well worth doing. The areas in which regular checks are most important are the eyes, ears, teeth, weight, heart and circulation, lungs, urine, and blood, plus breasts and a gynecological examination for women. The ideal person to carry out a health check is the family doctor, since he or she is probably the only person who knows enough about the patient to be able to put the findings into the right perspective.

Health checks are not always covered by health insurance plans. Nevertheless, many doctors are prepared to do them, much as they will carry out medical examinations for either insurance or employment purposes, and for a similar fee.

Health checks are carried out routinely on children throughout their school years, and the suggested frequency in adult life, when they are done on a voluntary basis, is every five years until the age of 45, and every one or two years after that.

Maintaining health

An apple a day doesn't necessarily keep the doctor away, but the golden rule in personal preventive medicine is for people to take the best possible care of their health, which should include eating a well-balanced diet with plenty of fruit and vegetables—this is the thread that should run throughout life.

See also: Antibiotics; Diet; Exercise; Food poisoning; Hygiene; Immunization; Infection and infectious diseases; Smoking; Tuberculosis

Protein

Questions and Answers

What happens if you don't eat any protein?

Protein is an essential part of the diet. If people are starving, they usually do not have enough protein or energy-producing food, so the body breaks down its own protein to act as a fuel, losing much muscle bulk. Lack of protein in a normal-calorie diet leads to a condition called kwashiorkor, which mainly occurs in young children.

Is too much protein bad for you?

Normally, the body metabolizes excess protein to produce energy. Protein imbalances in the body can be a sign of disease. Some tumors produce antibodies, increasing the globulin level in the blood. In conditions such as meningitis, protein levels around the brain and spinal cord are raised. Kidney failure can allow albumin from the bloodstream to leak away.

My father has kidney failure and the doctors have put him on a low-protein diet. Why?

One of the tasks of the kidneys is to remove waste products, many of which result from the body's use of protein. The main waste product is urea, which is formed as a result of protein breakdown. If the protein level is kept low in the diet of someone with failing kidneys, less urea is produced, so that there is less work for the kidneys to do.

Is protein the best sort of food to eat if you want to put on weight and build yourself up?

If you actually want to build up your body's muscle content and strength, the way to do it is by exercise that encourages the muscles to grow. Just eating more protein without any exercise, however, would simply be an expensive way of putting on fat.

Most people think of protein simply as an important part of the diet. In fact, everything from the color of the hair to inherited talents is determined by the way people's bodies are genetically programmed to make proteins.

The three main classes of food are proteins, fats, and carbohydrates. Fats and carbohydrates supply our energy needs, while proteins are the actual building blocks from which the body is made. A minimum intake is needed to maintain the body's reconstruction and repair processes so that it remains healthy, especially in growing children.

What is protein?

Protein molecules are twisted chains of smaller compounds called amino acids, which are vital to the body's survival. Proteins are the only major food group to contain nitrogen. Twenty amino acids make up all the proteins found in food; eight are essential to the diet, since the body cannot make them itself. The other 12 can be made in the body, although its ability to do this sometimes fails. Acids and enzymes in the digestive system break down food protein into its constituent amino acids. These can then be absorbed by the intestine, passed on to the liver, and enter the bloodstream.

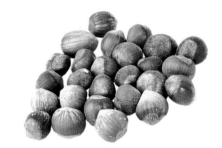

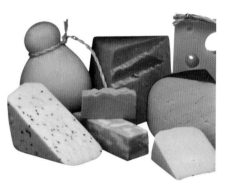

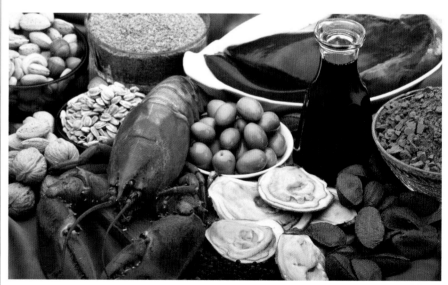

▲ *These foods contain relatively high amounts of protein. Cheese contains about 0.88 oz. (25 g) of protein in every 3.5 oz. (100 g) of weight. Prime beef contains 0.75 oz. (21 g). Proteins in nuts range from almonds at 0.65 oz. (18.6 g) to hazelnuts (top photo) at 0.44 oz. (12.6 g). Oysters, although still high in protein, contain only 0.29 oz. (8.2 g).*

STRUCTURE OF PROTEIN

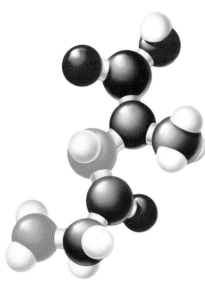

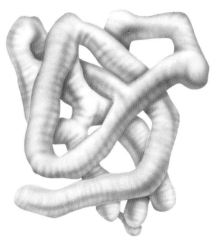

▼ *Protein chains are linked to parallel chains or are coiled around themselves to give the more complex secondary structure. The regularly wound coils of a helix (a spiral staircase shape) shown below are held in place by bonds (dotted lines) linking the oxygen and hydrogen atoms in different amino acids. Each amino acid also has a side chain called R (purple); the constituents of the R chain vary according to the individual amino acid.*

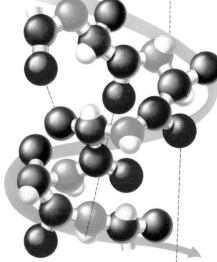

▲ *Proteins are composed of chains of amino acid molecules, each of which is made up of atoms of carbon (black), hydrogen (white), oxygen (red), and nitrogen (blue). There are 20 different amino acids generally found in proteins. The number of amino acids, and the order in which they are arranged in a particular protein chain, make up the primary structure of proteins. Shown above are two amino acids linked in a protein chain.*

▲ *The third structure of a protein concerns its overall three-dimensional shape. Some proteins, including the enzymes, are curled around themselves into entwined knots to give a globular shape. However, there is a great variety and range of proteins according to their composition, size, and shape—those which have a purely structural function (the building blocks) are less convoluted than the enzyme above.*

Although tissues such as the liver can store some amino acids taken into the body after a protein meal, the body has no major store of protein or amino acids. Fat and carbohydrate, in contrast, can both be stored in large quantities.

What does protein do?

The most important role of protein within the body is as a building block. People's tissues are made with protein, and the central substance of connective tissues holding the various organs and tissues together is a protein molecule called collagen.

Enzymes are also protein molecules. They act as catalysts for the chemical reactions the body depends upon. Proteins also circulate in the blood. The small molecules of albumin help keep fluid in the bloodstream; the larger group of globulin proteins includes the immunoglobulins or antibodies, the body's main defense against infection.

Some hormones are proteins, and they are also vital to the overall functioning of the body. Insulin is an example

of a protein hormone; it is made of two protein chains linked together. The body's entire protein structure is renewed about once every 60 days. Food and recycled body proteins replenish the blood, liver, and other tissues, and cells drain this supply to make new proteins.

Protein and genetics

Heredity is based on a code passed from one generation to the next, telling the cells how to make proteins. Information in the chromosomes specifies the amino acid sequence in each body protein. Every inherited characteristic, from eye color to musical talent, originates in coded instructions passed on by the parents. As far as scientists know, these coded instructions concern only the way in which cells are told to make proteins.

See also: **Diet; Fats; Genetics; Heredity; Nutrition**

Pulled muscles

Questions and Answers

A pulled muscle is an unavoidable hazard, particularly for people who regularly participate in sports. However, the inconvenience caused is usually minimal, treatment is simple, and recovery is rapid.

If I pull a muscle during a game of basketball, should I stop playing, or is it safe to finish the game?

This depends on the severity of the injury. If it is serious you should stop taking part in all sports until the damage has healed completely. For minor injuries, you can continue if the muscle is supported with adhesive strapping or a firm bandage.

A pulled, strained, or overstretched muscle is one of the least severe of all the injuries that can occur to any part of the bodily structure. More severe types of injury include sprains and tears of the body's muscles and ligaments, and various fractures of the bones and joints.

Causes

A pulled muscle can happen in an accident or during exercise. The type of injury varies. For example, people may drop their share of a load they are helping to carry, causing a sudden sharp movement or moment of acute tension on a particular muscle. Attempting to lift something that is too heavy, or lifting awkwardly or incorrectly, can have similar results.

A powerful movement that twists a part of the body into an unnatural position, as often happens in baseball or basketball, may also stretch muscles beyond their natural limit.

This kind of strain is less likely to occur in children, young people, and those who have trained themselves to make the necessary movements or sustain the loads on the muscles involved. Some movements, however, are likely to result in a pulled muscle no matter who makes them. Occupations and activities such as heavy manual work and strenuous athletics therefore entail a high frequency of muscular injury.

Should a pulled muscle always be rested or should it be exercised?

Both. Initially, the muscle needs rest, but as the injury improves it should be exercised more often. Each person can usually gauge how much to do, but should put the strained muscle through its normal range of movements as soon as possible. Pain will be felt beyond a certain point, but exercise should continue to just short of this point. Repeat each exercise up to 12 times, holding the position for 10 seconds each time. Gradually increase the range of movements and the amount of weight on the injured muscle.

Symptoms and sites

Pulled muscles can occur in virtually any part of the body. Stress from lifting is likely to be felt in the muscles of the lower back or abdomen. Sudden head movements or whiplash accidents, in

Does massage help pulled muscles?

Yes. Unless the pull is extremely painful, massage will help relieve the discomfort and can also benefit the muscle itself. Use a steady kneading movement—with oil to make the massage more effective—for 10 to 15 minutes, placing consistent pressure on the affected area with the balls of the thumbs.

My boyfriend pulled a thigh muscle playing baseball and had something sprayed on it to remove the pain. What was it?

It was probably ethyl chloride, which will freeze the injury so that no pain is felt and the muscle does not go into spasm. It has very little real value.

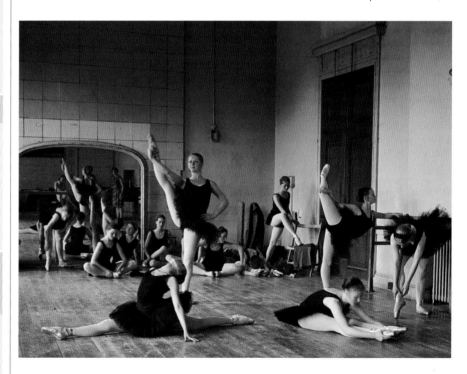

▲ *Professional dancers take care to avoid pulling a muscle by doing warm-up exercises before their demanding performances.*

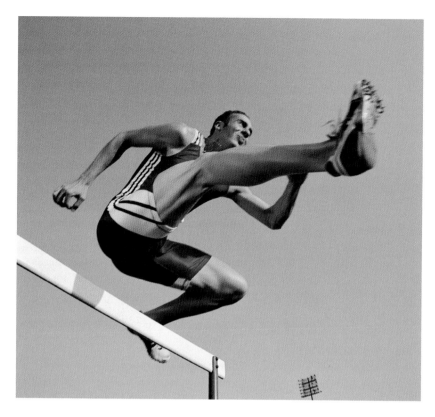

▲ *Athletes such as hurdle jumpers can often suffer from pulled muscles due to the great strain that is put on the muscles of the back, hips, thighs, calves, and feet.*

Home treatment for a pulled muscle

Apply a cold compress immediately to the affected area.

Soak a cloth in cold, not iced, water and wring it out.

Loosely bandage it over the injury and leave until it begins to dry or becomes warm.

Remove the dressing, resoak it, and repeat the procedure.

After 24 hours, apply heat treatment for 15 minutes every day until the muscle can be freely moved without pain.

If you do not have a heat lamp, use a heating pad or a hot water bottle covered in a cloth.

Apply the pad or hot water bottle with the affected part unclothed.

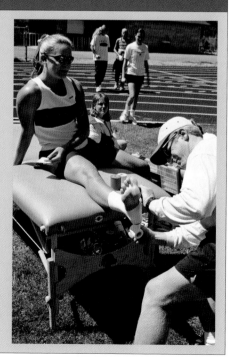

which the head is jerked sharply backward or forward, will give rise to pulled muscles in the neck. The shoulders, arms, and hands are at risk in boxing and weight lifting. Ball games, sprinting, and gymnastics place a particular strain on the muscles of the hips, thighs, calves, and feet.

The principal symptom of a pulled muscle is pain, and, if the pull is severe, the muscle may also become weak and unable to support any weight. It is usually the fibrous meat of the muscle that is affected. Tendons are damaged only by injuries severe enough to tear them from the bone.

The actual damage done can vary—the muscle fibers may simply be overstretched or they may be torn. In severe cases, the pain will be immediate and acute enough to stop the injured person from using the muscle until it has had time to heal. In slight pulls, the pain may not be felt until the next day and then subsides quickly, without much inconvenience or interruption of normal activities.

Treatment

Distinguishing between a simple pulled muscle and more serious damage, such as an underlying fracture, is obviously vital but may be difficult in some instances. In all cases of musculoskeletal injury there may be pain, tenderness, and loss of use of the injured part. Sometimes it will be clear that the injury is only a strain, or a definite fracture. Extreme caution is needed until a doctor has examined the injury and taken an X ray. Until this has been done it is safer to treat the injury as though it is a fracture.

Most pulled muscles can be treated by simple measures at home. A cold compress is helpful in limiting the amount of swelling and bruising that develops. After 24 hours, heat is also useful in increasing the blood supply to the damaged area and in making it less painful and easier to move.

A pulled muscle should initially be rested and then gradually used again as it recovers. A doctor should always be consulted if there is any doubt about the exact course to follow.

Outlook

With care and common sense a pulled muscle should heal with no difficulty, and normal use should be quickly restored.

See also: Fractures; Occupational hazards; Sports medicine; Whiplash injury

Rabies

Is it possible to survive rabies?

Without early vaccination, the disease is almost invariably fatal. However, there are several well-documented cases of survival. One of these was a young boy in the United States who was bitten by a rabid bat. He was given both serum and vaccine right away. He survived even though he developed signs of the disease. In another case, a laboratory worker inhaled droplets of the virus and he too was given the vaccine.

Can you catch rabies from infected humans or is it always caught from animals?

Rabies is nearly always caught from animals, though there were two reported cases of human-to-human spread. These occurred when the eyes of two people who had died were used for corneal grafts. Both the donors had died of rabies and both the recipients subsequently caught the disease and died. These are the only two proven cases of transfer.

Do I need the rabies vaccine if I go on vacation to India?

No; the vaccine is not given as a preventive measure. The risks are low unless you are in contact with animals, but you should always avoid stray dogs, and do not stroke any dog that you meet: rabies can enter the body through minor cuts and scratches.

Can you really get rabies months after being bitten?

Yes. The incubation period varies from days to years, although the disease usually appears within 20 to 90 days of being bitten. The period is shortest in children who have been bitten on the face, and longer if the site of the bite is far from the brain.

Rabies is a potentially fatal disease of the nervous system, caused by a bite from an infected animal. It is rare in the developed world; cases in the United States are usually from bats, or dogs that have been bitten by wild animals.

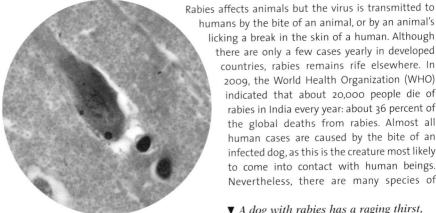

▲ *The virus that causes rabies.*

Rabies affects animals but the virus is transmitted to humans by the bite of an animal, or by an animal's licking a break in the skin of a human. Although there are only a few cases yearly in developed countries, rabies remains rife elsewhere. In 2009, the World Health Organization (WHO) indicated that about 20,000 people die of rabies in India every year: about 36 percent of the global deaths from rabies. Almost all human cases are caused by the bite of an infected dog, as this is the creature most likely to come into contact with human beings. Nevertheless, there are many species of

▼ *A dog with rabies has a raging thirst, yet terror and spasms occur at the sight of water. This is known as hydrophobia.*

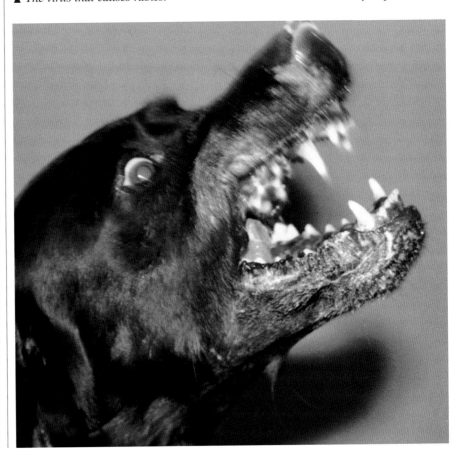

animal that can have rabies, and in northern Europe, for example, the fox is the most common carrier of the disease, while in South America it is the vampire bat. In the United States, the raccoon is one of the most common carriers of the disease. Ninety percent of human cases arise from domestic dogs, many of which have been infected by wild animals.

Causes

Rabies is caused by a virus. Although there is only one type of virus that causes the disease, there are about five other similar viruses that have been found in various parts of Africa. Two of these viruses are reported to cause a similar infection in the human brain.

Rabies is found almost everywhere in the world, although in most places it is confined to the wild animal population, and only very rarely does it actually spread to human beings. Transmission of the disease occurs when an

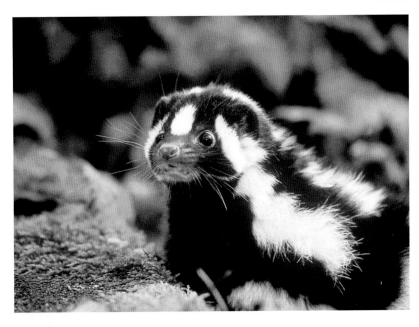

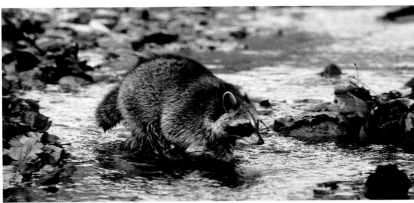

◄ ▲ *Although only a few cases of rabies are reported each year in the United States, certain wild animals, such as the skunk and the raccoon, are common carriers of the virus. The reason humans rarely catch the disease is that they do not often come into contact with wild creatures. It is important to remember not to go near any animal that appears to be sick or is acting strangely. The virus is highly potent and can be passed through saliva, or in moisture droplets in air.*

infected animal bites another animal or a human. The rabid animal will eventually die of the disease, so biting another animal ensures the survival of the rabies virus.

The virus attacks the nervous system and alters the behavior of some animals once they are infected, so that they become uncharacteristically aggressive and attack whatever comes near them—humans or other animals alike. This characteristic is important to the survival of the virus, and is brought about in part by hydrophobia, the major symptom of rabies, which is a thirst for water accompanied by terror and spasms at the sight of water. By keeping the pool of affected animals small and isolated, the disease can be made self-limiting.

Once the infecting virus has made its way through the skin, it may act immediately or it may lie dormant for some time. The incubation period has been known in some

ANIMALS THAT CARRY RABIES

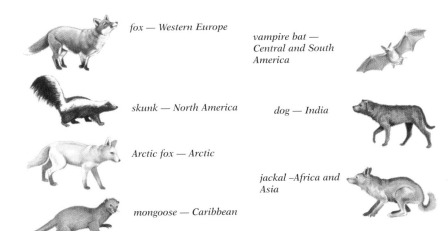

fox — Western Europe

vampire bat — Central and South America

skunk — North America

dog — India

Arctic fox — Arctic

jackal –Africa and Asia

mongoose — Caribbean

cases to extend to years before symptoms appear. Generally, though, the incubation period ranges from 20 to 90 days. After the initial infection through the skin, the virus enters the nerves of its victim and works its way up the nerves through the nerve cells until it reaches the brain. Once it has become established in the brain the symptoms of the disease break out.

That the virus has to make this journey through the nerves explains why the incubation period seems to be longer in those people who are bitten on the foot compared with those who are bitten on the hand or the face: the farther the virus has to go from the site of entry to reach the brain, the longer it takes for the symptoms of rabies to appear.

Other methods of transmission

A bite is not the only way that the disease can be transmitted. It is possible for the virus to enter the body through a cut or scratch in the skin, so even a lick from an infected animal can transmit the disease. There is even a documented case of someone's becoming infected with the virus by inhaling droplets of virus-carrying liquid. This has happened in laboratory accidents, and in even more bizarre circumstances, for instance as a result of breathing in a cave atmosphere contaminated with the urine of infected bats.

Symptoms

Rabies is a form of encephalitis; that is, the symptoms are due to an infection of the tissues of the brain. The best-known symptom of rabies is hydrophobia. This symptom is unique to rabies and follows a set pattern when it occurs. A patient may feel very thirsty, but as the water is given, he or she will recoil at the sight of it and have spasms of the throat. This may progress to real terror at the sight of water or even just the mention of it. The fear will be accompanied by generalized convulsions, and back-arching spasms similar to those shown by patients suffering from tetanus.

The symptoms of hydrophobia do not appear until the rabies is quite well developed. The disease usually starts with a few days of ill health, fever, sore throat, and muscular aches. Although they are typical symptoms of a viral infection, with rabies there is also restlessness and insomnia accompanying the early nonspecific symptoms. Another, more specific symptom in the early stages is that there is pain and tingling at the site of the bite.

Progress of the disease

After the hydrophobia has begun, the disease progresses to a more generalized involvement of the nervous system. Physical spasms become more frequent and violent and any one of the spasms can end in death. The patient may have episodes of wild, confused excitement alternating with lucid periods. There is often an exaggeration of such automatic functions as salivation and sweating; the equivalent of the frothing at the mouth of a typical rabid dog. Eventually the victim lapses into a coma and dies. This particular form of the disease is known as furious rabies and it is the

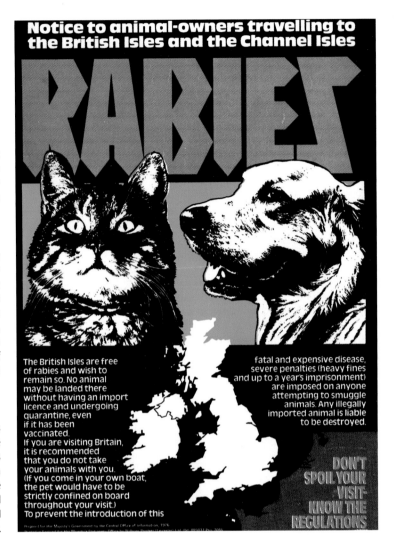

▲ *Great Britain is rabies-free, and there are strict controls that allow pets into the country only after a period of quarantine.*

pattern that most patients follow. The progress of the disease is different in about one-fifth of patients, with paralysis being the major feature. The paralysis begins at the legs and ascends the body in a symmetrical pattern. Hydrophobia may then occur, but it tends to happen later in the disease. Oddly enough, this type of rabies seems to be common in people who have been bitten by rabid vampire bats.

Diagnosis

One of the problems that a doctor will face is in proving the diagnosis with a laboratory test. Samples of blood and other body fluids from an infected patient must be considered highly infectious, and there are limitations about which type of laboratory can handle such specimens. In this respect the disease is classed in the same way as dangerous viral diseases such as Lassa fever.

A blood test is not always helpful, since the level of antibodies to the disease (which give the diagnosis) does not begin to rise until some time after the symptoms have started to develop.

Sometimes, a small sample of skin is taken, preferably from around the hairline area, which, when it is treated in a special way, will reveal the rabies virus in the tiny nerves.

Finally, there is another method of making a diagnosis of rabies, which would be used only if other methods were impossible. It involves making a tiny hole in the patient's skull and taking some brain tissue for examination under the microscope in the laboratory. This will show conclusive signs of the disease.

It is very important that the diagnosis of rabies should be confirmed immediately. In a developed country such as the United States, rabies is so rare that there are only a few cases each year, and it is very unlikely that a case of rabies will come to the attention of a doctor who is familiar with the disease. Extensive public health programs may have to be undertaken as the result of a single case, so it is very useful to have confirmation. Doctors in the United States can get assistance with a diagnosis from the Centers for Disease Control.

Treatment

There is no cure once rabies has become established in a patient, and it seems almost inevitable that people with the disease are going to die. However, most cases of rabies occur in developing countries where the advanced facilities needed to treat the disease are almost nonexistent. Ironically, rabies is extremely rare in technologically advanced countries, such as the United States— countries that are able to provide the intensive care that may help patients with rabies survive.

Treatment of rabies consists of putting affected patients on a respirator (breathing machine) and maintaining support of vital functions, such as their heartbeat and the urine output of their kidneys, in the hope that they may recover. There have been three such recoveries recorded; all the patients who recovered had been vaccinated very shortly after their exposure to the disease.

There is some hope that the antiviral substance interferon will be of some value in treating the disease. However, the prognosis for someone with an established case of rabies is not optimistic.

Prevention

Although there is treatment for rabies, it needs to be administered immediately to have a chance of being effective. Often, particularly in developing countries, this does not happen, or people simply do not realize that they have been put at risk—particularly if the affected animal does not display any obvious symptoms. Because of this, the potentially long incubation period of the virus, the only really effective way of dealing with the disease is by prevention.

Vaccination

The basis of rabies control throughout the world, then, must be prevention, since cure of the disease seems unlikely. People who are at risk are given vaccinations, and people who may have suffered a bite from an infected animal not only are given a course of vaccinations but may also be given protection in the form of immunoglobulins (antibodies) that are prepared from the blood of someone who is immunized against the disease. In countries that cannot afford to prescribe human immunoglobulin, it is standard procedure to use antibodies that have been raised in horses, although this carries a risk of reaction to the horse serum itself.

In the past, the common vaccine that was used against rabies contained viral matter raised on nervous tissue. This required large amounts of vaccine to be given, with a risk of a reaction to the nervous tissue, which could in a very few cases be fatal. The vaccine is still the most widely used worldwide, but there is a newer vaccine that is raised on tissue in a cell culture. This type of vaccine is safer, and fewer injections are needed.

See also: **Bites and stings; Immunization; Infection and infectious diseases; Paralysis; Tetanus; Vaccinations; Viruses**

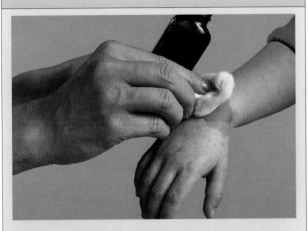

Immediate first aid

Steps to take if you are or your child is bitten by an animal that has the remotest chance of having rabies.

Scrub the wound under a running tap with soap or detergent and water for at least five minutes.

Remove any dirt or foreign material from the wound.

Rinse with plain water.

If possible, rinse the wound with a virus-killing fluid like iodine tincture or, failing this, any strong form of alcohol.

Seek medical help urgently. Don't leave it till you get home, particularly if you are on vacation.

Leave the wound open, if possible.

Afterward, at the doctor's office or at the hospital, the following steps may be taken.

The doctor will thoroughly cleanse the wound, and he or she will trim the edges of the wound if necessary.

He or she will decide whether to give the patient either a rabies antiserum or immunoglobulin, or a course of rabies vaccine.

Rashes

A rash is any redness of the skin or outbreaks of spots. In medical terms it can indicate a condition that is affecting the whole body, or it may be a localized inflammation of the skin.

My friend has a rash on her hands and arms. She says it's dermatitis but isn't catching. Is this true?

Yes, probably. "Dermatitis" means inflammation of the skin. A few types like impetigo, ringworm, and scabies can be spread by direct contact, but usually the condition is due to the skin's sensitivity to a substance or to an emotional or nervous disorder, and is not contagious.

Why should chicken pox spots not be scratched?

It is simply to avoid getting scars. If chicken pox spots are not scratched there is a good chance that they will heal without leaving scars. Scratching may infect the spots, and make them larger and deeper so they are more likely to leave permanent marks.

What is the best thing to put on a measles rash?

Nothing at all. The eruption is dry, does not form sores or ulcers, and will follow the natural course of the condition. Since nothing will make any difference, either to the illness or to the rash itself, it is best to leave the rash alone.

What's the difference between a rash due to an infectious disease and one due to an allergy?

The rashes of common infectious diseases differ from each other in appearance, and rarely form welts or irritate so acutely. Also, a person with an infectious disease will probably have a fever and feel ill, while someone with an allergy usually feels no other effects. There is nothing specific about an allergy rash except when it consists of raised areas or welts with white centers surrounded by a red area. These usually irritate considerably.

A rash may be an outward sign of a condition affecting the body as a whole. Infectious fevers, emotional disorders, and allergies may all have accompanying rashes.

However, rashes are equally likely to be an indication of a localized disorder in the skin, the kind of inflammation that is commonly called dermatitis. Included in this type of local inflammation are diaper rash, prickly heat, eczema, and fungal infections.

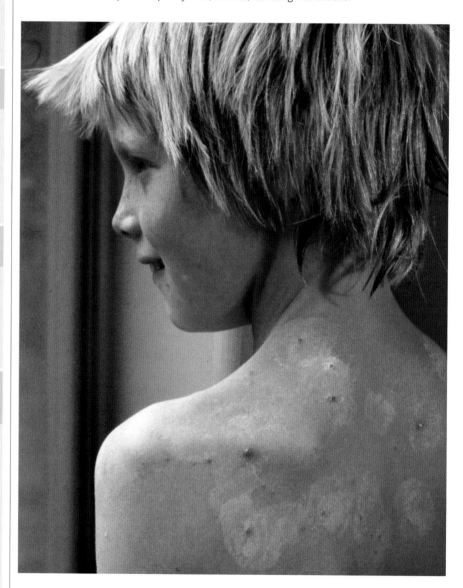

▲ *A chicken pox rash causes itching, but remedies such as calamine lotion, oatmeal baths, oral antihistamine, and diphenhydramine cream can soothe the irritation.*

Types of rashes

Rashes take many different forms. A rash that is present at the start of an illness is called a primary rash. The rash may subsequently change in character and appearance during the course of the causative disease, owing to complications or in response to the treatment used. New rashes or changes in the original rash are called secondary eruptions, and each has its own set of characteristics.

Primary rashes

The most common of the primary rashes shows as areas of redness known as macules. Any abnormal change in the color of the skin over a limited area qualifies as a macular rash; the redness itself is known as erythema.

Sometimes, in the early stages of measles, the rash consists of hundreds of tiny red spots, each spot discrete or separate from the others.

In other cases the spots enlarge until they run into each other to form blotchy patches. This is called a confluent rash. Usually, if a thumb is pressed on a part of the rash the area will not fade, but a white area may remain temporarily. This is an important diagnostic feature and is characteristic of many conditions; it is especially noticeable in typhoid fever.

The second common type of rash consists of spots which are not necessarily red but project above the surface of the skin. They can be felt as small raised pimples if a fingertip is run over the skin, in contrast to a macular rash which is not raised. The pimples are

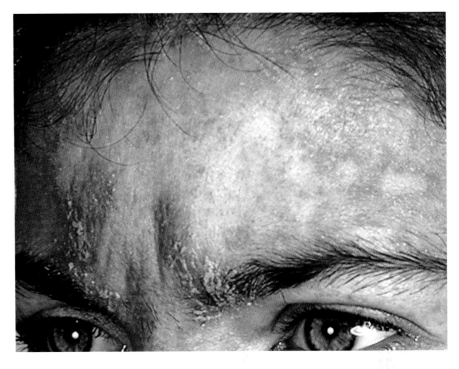

▲ *Seborrheic dermatitis is a skin rash that, in adults, commonly occurs on the face. It is characterized by patches of scaly red and itchy skin, which eventually flakes.*

known as papules, and the rash is called a papular rash. A maculopapular rash has both macules and papules.

When the rash is made up of pimples containing a clear or milky fluid doctors refer to it as vesicular, and each pimple is a vesicle. Chicken pox and herpes simplex are typical vesicular rashes.

A rash may also consist of raised areas of skin much larger than papules. These are known as welts, and they are usually white at the center and pink or red at the outer edge. This type of skin eruption, called urticaria or hives, is usually highly irritant and indicates an allergic reaction that releases histamine into the skin, causing inflammation.

Secondary rashes

In some cases a primary rash, whatever its type, simply fades away or resolves as the condition improves, without going through any secondary stage and without leaving scars or any other aftereffects. Secondary eruptions are quite common, however, and may manifest themseves in a variety of ways.

Often the area of skin covered by the rash peels away. This normally occurs if the original rash was a dry macular or papular one or, as in some cases, a mixture of the two. The type of rash usually seen in the later stages of chicken pox, by contrast, is pustular: that is, the spots have become infected pustules, containing pus. This type of moist lesion will dry out to form a crust or small scab. New skin will grow under the scabs, which will eventually separate and drop off. If the deeper layers of skin have been affected, as when chicken pox spots are scratched, there may be scarring in the form of pockmarks, or tiny pits in the skin.

Other types of secondary rash include a thickening of the area of the skin concerned, giving it a leathery look and a texture that is

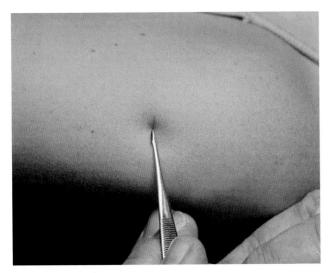

▲ *During an allergy scratch test, the arm is scratched to expose the dermis layer; then a foreign substance is applied. If a reaction occurs, the substance is confirmed as an allergen.*

The doctor gave my husband a very effective ointment for a rash he had last year. I now have a similar rash. Would it be a good idea for me to use some of this ointment that was left over?

No, it wouldn't. It is possible that you are right and that your rash has the same cause as your husband's. Still, using the remaining ointment could be dangerous for at least two reasons. First, using a medicine of any sort—other than those you can buy over the counter—that has not been prescribed for you personally is very risky. People can, and do, injure themselves in this way. Second, the skin can develop sensitivity to any medication. Never put anything stronger than calamine lotion on your skin without first consulting your doctor. Remember that the skin, although tough in some ways, can be very individual and temperamental in its reactions. This is why great care is taken in the diagnosis and treatment of skin conditions.

Every few months I develop an irritating rash on my hands. My doctor says it isn't anything serious, but what could be wrong with me?

Since your rash occurs intermittently and your doctor has ruled out a serious disorder, it may be due to a condition, like nervous tension, that comes and goes. It could possibly result from periodic exposure to something which triggers an allergic reaction in you. Since the rash develops on your hands, this is likely to be a substance you touch or handle. Try to remember if you had any particular worries at the times the rash has occurred, or if it coincided with doing a job that involved handling something unusual, perhaps while gardening or using household chemicals. To pinpoint the precipitating factor you may need to keep a detailed diary of everything you do, including items you touch. The only real cure is to track down the cause so that you can try to avoid it in the future.

Rashes associated with infectious diseases

Chicken pox	Small flat spots that turn into small blisters. These become pustules which burst to form scabs. The rash starts on the trunk, itches, and lasts about a week.
German measles	Tiny red spots, often very faint, appearing first on the face and spreading down to the trunk.
Herpes	Painful small blisters forming in groups.
Measles	Tiny red spots first on the forehead and behind the ears, spreading down to the chest and abdomen. The rash is preceded by small white spots inside the mouth, takes two days to develop fully, and starts to fade after about a week.
Scarlet fever	Flat red spots, most marked at the armpits, and elbow and groin creases, leaving a clear area around the mouth.
Syphilis	A faint copper-colored rash in the secondary stage of the disease, most often on the trunk, palms of the hands, soles of the feet, and the forehead. A blood test can confirm the diagnosis.
Typhoid and paratyphoid	Crops of a dozen or so rose-spots, about ¼ in. (0.6 cm) across, on the chest and abdomen, for two to three days.

characteristic of long-term inflammation or chronic inflammation. Similarly, permanent discoloration or pigmentation of the skin may develop in the area of the rash.

Finally, entire areas of skin may break down, exposing the underlying or subcutaneous tissue. Without this protective covering of skin, ulcers can form which are very likely to become infected by bacteria from the atmosphere, especially in moist, heavily contaminated environments. This sometimes happens with diaper rash, cold sores, or rashes from shingles.

Treatment

Rashes as such do not require or benefit from any particular treatment, except that needed to treat the underlying condition.

If itching is a problem, calamine cream is as effective as any other nonprescription preparation that is available, and has the advantage of cheapness. If this is not adequate to control the irritation, a doctor may prescribe a short course of antihistamine pills or syrup. Antihistamine cream should never be used to treat rashes that are irritating or itchy. It is now clear that this can give rise to an allergy to the antihistamine itself, making it dangerous to use on a future occasion which might be a real emergency.

If the papules or pustules of a rash burst, or if there are ulcers present, a mild antiseptic cream or lotion can be useful in preventing any infection.

▲ *Rashes are commonly caused as a side effect of drug treatment such as antibiotics. A drug-induced photosensitivity caused this patient's rash.*

See also: Allergies; Chicken pox; Measles

Rheumatic fever

Rheumatic fever is one of the most dangerous childhood diseases, since it may lead to long-term problems with the heart valves. Although relatively rare in developed countries, it is still a big problem in less developed countries.

Rheumatic fever is caused by an infection with a streptococcus bacterium and usually follows a sore throat. Rheumatic fever affects different systems of the body, with the result that it has different effects on those who have suffered from the disease.

Although rheumatic fever occurs mainly in children and adolescents, the damage it causes to the heart may persist, leading to long-term heart trouble. In fact, cardiac surgeons are still performing operations to repair heart valves damaged years ago by the disease.

Rheumatic fever used to be a common disease in the United States—in 1950, about 15,000 Americans died as a result of rheumatic fever. However, the development of antibiotics in the late 1940s, offering an effective treatment for streptococcal infections, led to a consistent decline in the incidence of the disease. By 1980, the number of rheumatic fever cases had dropped so low that doctors were no longer required to report it. However, in 1985 there was a resurgence of rheumatic fever—perhaps due to the emergence of more virulent strains—and it has continued to take its toll.

Questions and Answers

I had rheumatic fever when I was a child. The doctor has told me that I'll have to take penicillin before I go to the dentist. Why is this?

Your original attack of rheumatic fever was caused by an infection with a streptococcus, a kind of bacterium. The reason why you are given antibiotics before dental treatment is that anyone who has heart abnormalities as a result of rheumatic fever is at risk of developing an infection in the heart valves, particularly after dental surgery. Small amounts of bacteria are released from the mouth and may enter the bloodstream where they can infect abnormal heart valves. This can be prevented by using the antibiotic.

Do you always get heart trouble after a bout of rheumatic fever?

No. It is very possible to have the disease without developing any heart trouble. Generally, severe long-term heart trouble occurs only after repeated or very prolonged attacks of rheumatic fever; it is much less likely to result from a single attack.

Is it possible to get rheumatic fever when you are an adult?

Rheumatic fever is a disease of childhood and adolescence. It rarely occurs after the age of 18.

I used to hear about rheumatic fever a lot, but not so much nowadays. Is it now rare?

It is still prevalent in some less developed countries, but it is less common in the United States and other developed countries due to the more widespread use of antibiotics to treat streptococcal infections. It was almost eradicated in the United States in the early 1980s, but resurged in 1985 and incidences have continued to occur.

RHEUMATIC MITRAL VALVE

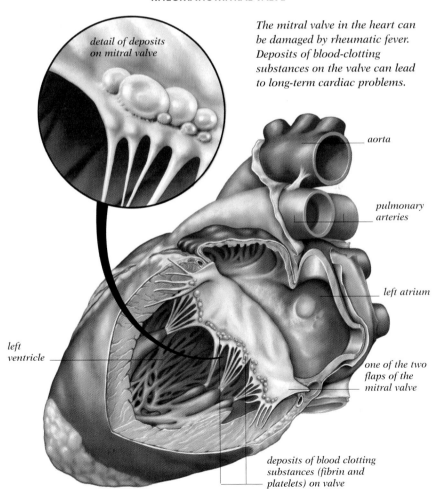

detail of deposits on mitral valve

The mitral valve in the heart can be damaged by rheumatic fever. Deposits of blood-clotting substances on the valve can lead to long-term cardiac problems.

aorta

pulmonary arteries

left atrium

left ventricle

one of the two flaps of the mitral valve

deposits of blood clotting substances (fibrin and platelets) on valve

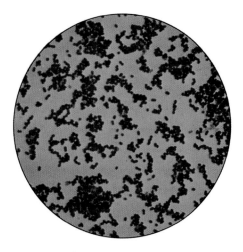

▲ *Rheumatic fever is caused by strains of the streptococcus bacterium, shown above stained and magnified more than 300 times.*

More than 3,000 Americans die each year from rheumatic fever or heart disease caused by it.

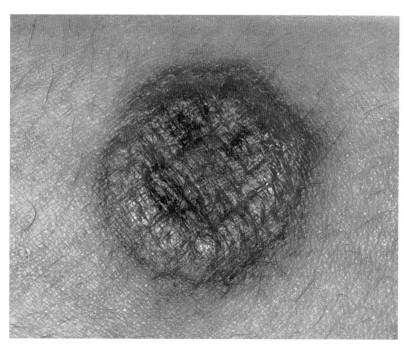

▲ *This type of rash, known as erythema marginatum, is a typical symptom of rheumatic fever and can appear on various parts of the body.*

Causes

Rheumatic fever is caused by a streptococcus bacterium belonging to a strain known as Lancefield group A. Only a tiny proportion of the population are at risk of getting the disease even if they develop a sore throat from this bacterium, but there is no way of knowing who is susceptible.

A streptococcal sore throat results in the formation, by the immune system, of large numbers of specific antibodies to antigens (chemical groups) on the surfaces of the streptococci. Both the lining membranes of joints and the lining of the heart carry chemical groups that closely resemble those on the streptococci. The result is that the antibodies attack both the joints and the heart. This is called an autoimmune process. The effect on the joints is transitory and seldom of long-term importance, but the effect on the heart valves is permanent and may be serious. Heart complications tend to be more severe and develop more quickly where there are poor living conditions, overcrowding, and little access to health care.

Symptoms

Rheumatic fever produces a variety of symptoms. It is characterized by a generalized feeling of illness, with fever and tiredness, pallor, loss of appetite, and loss of weight.

Rheumatic fever causes an inflammation of the joints (that is, rheumatism—thus the name). The disease affects mainly the larger joints of the hips and knees and has a curious tendency to move from one joint to another, so-called flitting arthritis.

The disease also affects the skin, producing a typical rash that consists of a red line enclosing pale areas (erythema marginatum). Additionally, gristly nodules can be felt under the skin over bony protrusions such as the wrists, knees, elbows, and ankles.

Most important, and more worrying, rheumatic fever affects the heart. There is inflammation of the fibrous lining of the heart and the heart muscle, which may lead to heart failure. The inner lining of the heart, or endocardium, may be affected: this is potentially serious because it can lead to abnormalities of the heart valves.

Finally, the disease can affect the nervous system, causing chorea or Saint Vitus' dance. This is characterized by writhing movements of the trunk and the limbs, and facial grimacing. The movements are made worse by excitement and disappear when the child is asleep. This seldom lasts for more than a few weeks but may recur.

Dangers

The main danger is that the child will have repeated attacks of the disease, which can lead to the development of problems with the heart valves. In the past, it was this that led to people's becoming cardiac cripples, often at a very young age. Although disease due to atherosclerosis (hardening of the arteries) is now the most common heart problem, this was not always so: rheumatic heart disease once had this distinction. There are many people still alive with long-term heart troubles from rheumatic fever.

Treatment and outlook

Once the diagnosis has been made, the mainstay of the treatment consists of rest, and regular large doses of aspirin. When heart failure has occurred, children are often given steroid drugs instead of aspirin to cut down the inflammation of the heart. It usually takes about six weeks to recover.

Once the child is well, it is important to prevent further attacks, since every bout can cause additional injury to the heart. For this reason, an antibiotic, usually penicillin, is given until age 18.

See also: Bacteria; Heart disease; Sore throat; Streptococcus

Ringworm

Ringworm is a contagious fungal infection that affects the feet, nails, scalp, armpits, or groin. However, even severe cases of this common skin disease usually respond well to treatment.

Questions and Answers

When I was young, children often had to be kept in isolation for months and had to have their heads shaved because of ringworm. Why does this never seem to happen nowadays?

This type of suffering, which was once commonplace, has now been prevented because of antibiotics taken by mouth that are effective in curing stubborn ringworm of the scalp which resists local treatment with creams. Despite this, however, children should be kept away from school while they have ringworm to avoid spreading the infection.

I have had recurring athlete's foot for years, but now I notice with alarm that one of my toenails has become very gnarled and odd-looking. Is there any connection, and, if so, what can I do about it?

The ringworm fungus that causes athlete's foot can also lodge itself and grow underneath the toenail, eventually leading to the condition you describe. You should seek prompt medical attention for this problem before it spreads further, or you may lose the nail entirely.

Why was it that when I had a ringworm infection my doctor told me I should lose weight?

Overweight people have more folds in their skin, and it is in these folds that ringworm fungi can thrive. Losing weight is good for your health regardless.

Why is it that wearing nylon underwear in summer gives me an itchy infection in the vaginal area and in my groin?

The combination of a warm, enclosed atmosphere and the retention of perspiration that has no chance to evaporate creates ideal conditions for the growth of the fungi that cause ringworm.

The name "ringworm" is a somewhat misleading term for this condition. The disease has nothing to do with worms and does not always manifest itself in the shape of a ring. It is caused by a contagious infection of the body with one of a variety of fungi. The specific areas of the body most likely to be affected are the feet, nails, scalp, armpits, genital areas, and groin.

Wherever they become established, ringworm fungi work in the same way. Feeding first on the dead tissues of the epidermis, the outermost layer of the skin, they then eat their way into the living tissues beneath, producing a raised red ring or, alternatively, an extensive sloughing off of the skin which leads to a graying, scaly appearance. The exact symptoms of ringworm vary with the area of the body infected, but itching, which may be very intense, is a symptom common to all types.

Areas of infection

Ringworm of the scalp is the condition that helped give the disease its name. This is

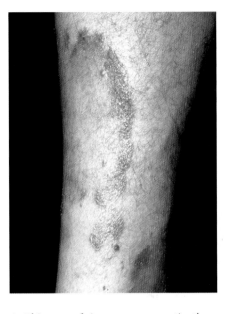

▲ *This case of ringworm on a patient's lower leg shows the raised red rings and scaly appearance caused by the fungal activity of this infectious disease.*

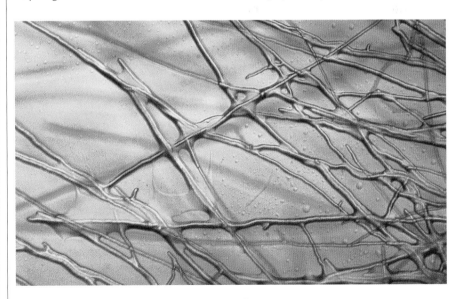

▲ *A micrograph of the* Trichophyton mentagrophytes *fungus shows one of the types of fungus that causes the unpleasant and itchy affects of ringworm.*

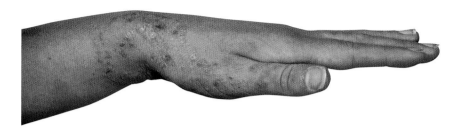

▲ *The ringworm fungus eats its way into the skin, often causing scaling or the outbreak of red, itchy blisters.*

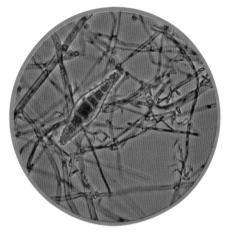

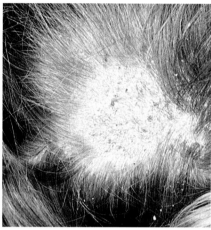

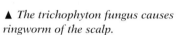

▲ *The trichophyton fungus causes ringworm of the scalp.*

▲ *Ringworm grows outward and gives the scalp a patchy appearance.*

epidermophyton fungus or by means of the closely related fungus called trichophyton. The symptoms are similar to athlete's foot, but both toenails and fingernails may also become affected. In severe cases, the area of skin around the deformed nail may also be red and itchy.

The epidermophyton fungus also causes ringworm of the genital or groin areas, called dhobie itch. Like the other ringworm fungi, this one thrives in damp, warm conditions; for this reason, infection is most common in people who wear tight-fitting underwear and trousers. It is also a problem for the obese and is especially prevalent in men and women of all ages in hot weather, when sweat becomes trapped in the groin area.

Treatment and prevention

The exact treatment of ringworm depends on the site of the infection and the infecting fungus. For athlete's foot, antifungal powders, creams, and sprays are excellent. For these to be effective, however, their application must be combined with rigorous attention to foot hygiene and thorough drying of the feet, particularly between the toes. Similar chemical remedies can be effective in treating ringworm of the

because the fungus usually grows outward in a ring, and as the inner area begins to heal up, the red, itchy area spreads in a circle of ever-increasing diameter. As this spread takes place, the hairs in the center snap off and leave a stubble overlying the scaly skin. As the skin heals in the center of the ring, new hairs begin to grow, giving the scalp an even more mottled appearance. Ringworm of the scalp is usually due to an infection by the trichophyton fungus. It is particularly common in childhood and spreads rapidly through schools.

The fungus that usually infects the feet is called epidermophyton and causes the common condition known as athlete's foot. The infection usually begins between the toes, starting as small blisters and spreading out to form large red areas. Sometimes the soles of the feet may be infected too, leading to scaly gray areas and flaking off of dead skin. Athlete's foot, which spreads rapidly through direct contact via the floors of bathrooms and changing rooms, can be irritatingly itchy and painful. There is also a risk that infective bacteria may enter the skin and cause secondary infection if the skin surface becomes broken and living cells are exposed to the air.

Sometimes athlete's foot may spread to the toenails, causing them to become abnormally thickened and ridged. The fungus can also set up a reaction in other parts of the body. In a typical case, watery, itchy blisters appear on the fingers of a person suffering from athlete's foot.

As well as being involved in athlete's foot infections, the nails are also prone to ringworm on their own account, either by the

nails, but in severe cases, an antibiotic will be prescribed.

Ringworm of the scalp is also treated with antibiotics, although mild cases may respond effectively to antifungal creams. As with athlete's foot, ringworm of the scalp demands close attention to hygiene. The scalp must be washed and dried regularly, and all brushes, combs, and the towels that are used must be sterilized. With dhobie itch, in addition to antifungal preparations, cleanliness, thorough drying after washing, and wearing sensible clothes are essential.

Most ringworm infections are now treated with imidazole, triazole, or allylamine antifungal drugs, which are available in oral preparations or creams. Although many of the antifungal ointments, powders, and sprays for the local treatment of mild ringworm are available over the counter from drugstores without a prescription, it is always wise to get medical advice if these prove ineffective. The doctor will be able to prescribe stronger treatments, including antibiotics if necessary, and give useful advice on how to clear the problem up and prevent it from recurring. To prevent ringworm from spreading, it is a wise precaution to ensure that anyone suffering from a ringworm infection does not share towels, combs, or similar items with other members of the family.

> *See also:* **Antibiotics; Athlete's foot; Blisters; Hygiene; Infection and infectious diseases; Obesity**

Rubella

Rubella, or German measles, is a common virus infection that is mild in children but damaging to a developing baby if a pregnant woman catches it. Immunization is now available that gives women lifelong protection.

Questions and Answers

I missed my rubella immunization when I was in school. I am now married and my doctor recently told me I needed immunization. He said I must not get pregnant for a while. Why did he advise a delay?

The vaccine used for immunization is not as harmful as the rubella virus itself because it is a strain that has been changed by laboratory conditions. If you were to become pregnant after being immunized, however, you would be subjecting the baby to some risk. It is best to avoid pregnancy for at least two months, by which time the live vaccine will have disappeared.

I am six weeks pregnant and my son has rubella. What should I do?

See your doctor, who will be able to tell from your medical records if you have been immunized. If you are immune, you have nothing to worry about. If not, you may need treatment to prevent you from getting the infection, and tests to check that your baby is normal.

My sister is six months pregnant and has rubella. Is the baby at risk?

By six months your sister's baby will have developed all the essential organs and systems, so the baby is unlikely to be affected. However, your sister should see her doctor as soon as possible for reassurance.

When I was young we used to hold rubella parties so all the children could catch the illness and become immune. Why not do this today?

Years ago if a child had rubella, all the neighborhood children would be invited over to catch it. The only trouble was that it did not protect all children. Today, there is a vaccine that gives 100 percent protection. The vaccine may be less fun, but it is a lot safer.

Rubella is a common, mild virus infection that occurs mostly in children. Infection appears to be most likely in the spring or summer months and it seems to run in four- to six-year cycles of minor epidemics. Rubella very rarely causes serious illness in an adult or child, and once diagnosed the illness can usually be ignored.

However, rubella can be very damaging to a fetus in the early stages of development in the mother's uterus, causing serious abnormalities if the mother catches rubella in the early months of pregnancy. It is thus important to ensure that pregnant women do not catch rubella.

Cause and symptoms

Rubella is caused by a virus found in the nose and throat of the patient. Like most viruses living along the respiratory tract, it is passed from person to person by tiny droplets in the air that is breathed out. Rubella is transmitted from a mother to her developing baby through the bloodstream via the placenta. The virus has an incubation period of two to three weeks, during which time it becomes established. However, the patient shows no symptoms.

The illness is also called German measles, taking its name from measles proper. This is because, in some cases, the initial symptoms are similar: a runny nose and mild conjunctivitis followed by a rash. Measles can be a serious illness, but rubella is often so mild that it passes unnoticed. In most cases, there are only two symptoms. A rash appears on the face and neck, spreading to the trunk and limbs, and some of the lymph nodes swell and become tender. The rash appears as tiny pink dots under the skin on the first or third day of the illness and disappears within four to five days with no staining or peeling of the skin. The doctor will usually look at the rash and feel for enlarged nodes at the back of the neck to confirm the diagnosis. In older people, nodes may also

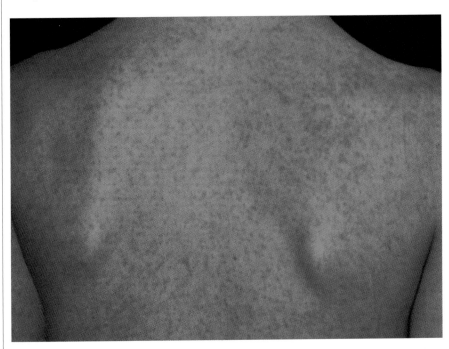

▲ *A common symptom of rubella is a rash of fine pink dots under the skin.*

swell in the armpit or groin. The nodes swell because they are producing antibodies to destroy the virus.

Some patients develop a low fever, but this rarely rises above 100°F (38°C). A joint may become inflamed and develop mild arthritis, but this disappears after a period of rest. Very rarely, nerves become affected by the virus, with accompanying weakness or numbness.

Cases are often difficult to diagnose because the symptoms are so mild. Similar symptoms can be produced by other viruses, but the rubella virus is the only one known to damage developing babies.

Risks

The earlier in pregnancy the virus infects the fetus, the greater the risk of damage. If it is caught between conception and four weeks, 50 percent of babies are affected, if between five and eight weeks, 35 percent are affected, and if between nine and 17 weeks, 12 percent are affected. Older fetuses are well enough developed for the virus not to harm them.

The defects rubella can cause include heart defects, eye defects, bone defects, encephalitis (inflammation of the brain), retarded growth, deafness, enlarged spleen and liver, and nerve defects (which can cause mental disability). Often two or more defects occur together.

The reason developing babies are so susceptible is that while they are forming they have no defense against such viruses and the replicating virus disrupts the developing cells. The mother's antibodies cannot help because they do not all cross the placenta to the fetus's bloodstream.

Immunization and tests

Immunization now gives lifelong protection against rubella. A single dose is needed and is given between the age of one and 13 years. Its only side effect can be transient arthritis.

Routine immunization of adolescent girls is not advised because of the dangers of inadvertent administration during unsuspected pregnancy. Testing for immunity should be done and each case handled separately. People on steroid drugs or those with a serious illness should not be immunized.

Women who did not catch rubella as a child, or are unsure about their status, or are likely to get pregnant in the future should have a blood test to see if they have natural immunity; if not, they should then be immunized.

Treatment and outlook

There is no treatment to cure rubella; only the body's own defenses, or antibodies, will kill off the infection. Most patients hardly know they are ill (apart from the rash), but some may get a sore throat. Aspirin

Protection for women

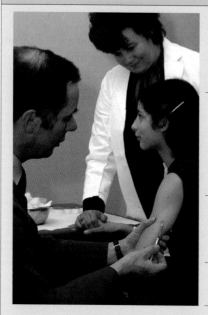

If you have or your child has rubella, you should inform your child's school or your own place of work. This is important, particularly if you are or your child is likely to come into contact with women who are pregnant.

Be sure to avoid your doctor's office or any prenatal clinics if you have rubella. If you have been in contact with someone who has rubella but are unsure whether you are immune, you should check with your doctor first before making your appointment.

There is no need for strict isolation, but it is best to stay at home for four or five days and mention that you have rubella to all contacts, especially females.

All children from one year to puberty should be immunized.

Women who are not pregnant, but might be in the future, should check whether they need immunization. This will involve having a blood test.

If a pregnant woman develops rubella in the first three months of pregnancy, the obstetrician will confirm the diagnosis by taking one or more blood tests. The risk of abnormalities in the baby will be explained to her and she may be offered amniocentesis, a test in which a sample of developing cells from the uterus is tested for abnormality. There is no guarantee that abnormalities will show up on the test, and the mother may decide to take the risk. If the tests show abnormalities, she may wish to consider terminating the pregnancy.

A pregnant woman who is in contact with rubella need not worry if she has been immunized or knows she is immune. A blood test can confirm this.

A shot of antirubella antibody can be given to a woman who has not been immunized and is in the first three months of pregnancy. However, not all doctors will recommend this route.

In general, just contact with rubella is not medical grounds for abortion. It is necessary to prove that infection has taken place. If an abnormal baby seems likely, consult your obstetrician who will be able to advise you on your options.

gargles will help, as will painkilling drugs. Usually, doctors offer no treatment other than rest if the patient feels unwell. Many adults will be able to continue work and most children will be able to attend school, depending on the school rules, throughout the illness. Pregnant women should keep away from anyone who has rubella, or who may have been in contact with others who have it.

The rash disappears after a few days, but the swollen glands may last for up to a week. Recovery may take as long as a month if complications occur.

See also: Arthritis; Fevers; Immunization; Measles; Rashes; Vaccinations; Viruses

Salt

Salt has many vital functions in the body and, with water, is one of the body's most basic constituents. By regulating fluid levels, salt controls many of the body's vital mechanisms.

The exact cause of high blood pressure is not known, but it is likely to be due to a few factors, including heredity. However, there is some evidence to suggest that salt may be an important factor. For example, the disease is more common in countries where there is a high salt intake. There is little doubt that the body's salt-retaining mechanisms are involved in setting the level of blood pressure higher than normal. Very low-salt diets can also be successful in lowering blood pressure, so it would seem that salt plays an important part in the disease, even if it is not the sole cause. You may be able to reduce your risk of getting high blood pressure by using less salt.

Salt is found in the earth and in seawater and is isolated by evaporation and crystallization from sea water and other water impregnated with particles of salt. Salt is a very simple chemical compound composed of two elements, sodium and chlorine, which give it its chemical name, sodium chloride. In the body, salt is dissolved in water, and in this medium the sodium and chlorine parts separate and move independently as sodium and chlorine ions, or electrically charged particles similar to atoms.

Both sodium and chloride ions are important for normal body functioning. In practice, when doctors refer to salt retention and loss, they mean sodium retention and sodium loss, with the assumption that chlorine always coexists with sodium.

Where is salt found?

Salt is found in all the body's fluids, but much more is present in the blood and the extracellular fluid, where it is needed for efficient functioning, than in the fluid contained in the cells.

A balance is maintained between the extracellular fluid containing sodium and the similar solution inside the cells, which contains the complementary element potassium. All cells have a mechanism for pumping sodium outward while keeping potassium inside. This is called the sodium pump and most of the body's energy is taken up in the ceaseless activity of such tiny

The tendency to retain salt, which happens in heart failure, can be helped by reducing salt in the diet. This will in turn reduce the volume of blood, since it depends chiefly on the amount of salt in the body. If the volume of blood in the circulation is reduced, the condition will improve. Diuretic drugs, which are used to treat heart failure, act on the kidneys to increase the volume of urine excreted and reduce reabsorption of water and salts into the blood. It thus seems reasonable to cut down salt intake while increasing the amount going out.

Probably not. Severe salt loss can bring about cramps, but this is unlikely in a temperate climate. Night cramps are common and can be alleviated by taking quinine pills before going to bed.

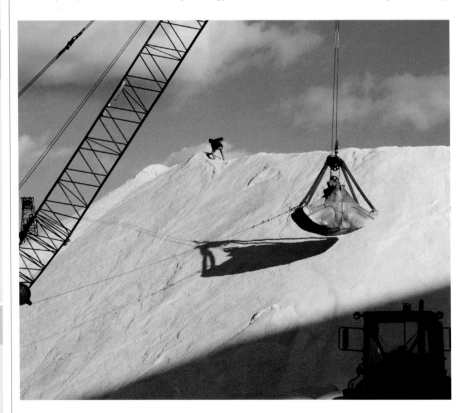

▲ *Industrial cranes at a salt mine excavate salt, which is then processed and cleaned before ending up as free-flowing table salt or rock salt.*

HOW SALT LEVELS ARE CONTROLLED

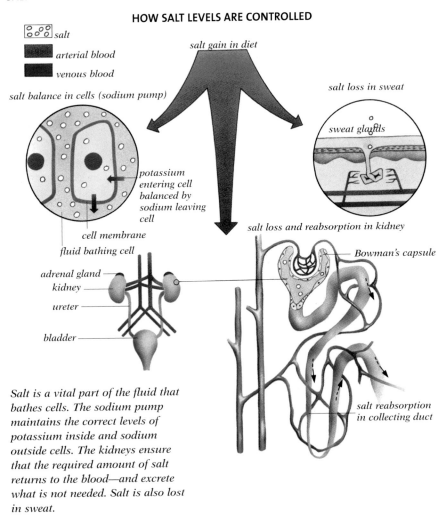

salt

arterial blood

venous blood

salt balance in cells (sodium pump)

salt gain in diet

salt loss in sweat

sweat glands

potassium entering cell balanced by sodium leaving cell

cell membrane

fluid bathing cell

salt loss and reabsorption in kidney

adrenal gland

kidney

ureter

bladder

Bowman's capsule

salt reabsorption in collecting duct

Salt is a vital part of the fluid that bathes cells. The sodium pump maintains the correct levels of potassium inside and sodium outside cells. The kidneys ensure that the required amount of salt returns to the blood—and excrete what is not needed. Salt is also lost in sweat.

the body tends to follow by osmosis (the process whereby a substance, such as water, passes across membranes from a weaker solution to a stronger one) and is retained. Water will therefore leave the kidney tubules when they have lost salt, and pass into the blood, which has a higher salt content than the kidneys.

The kidneys have an important function in regulating the salinity (salt level), acidity levels, and volume of the urine, but the delicate balance can be disturbed, particularly when chemicals act directly on the kidneys. For example, the steroid hormone aldosterone encourages the kidneys to retain more salt than usual, and other steroid hormones, such as cortisone, have a similar but less marked effect.

Since the volume of blood is controlled chiefly by the level of salt, any decline in the amount of blood reaching the kidneys will send a signal that the salt level is too low. The kidneys will respond by tending to retain salt in an effort to restore the blood to its normal level. The kidneys function in this way when there are heart problems. The salt levels then increase, giving rise to greater amounts of fluid in the circulation. Eventually, there is too much blood for the heart to cope with and heart failure sets in. This is the reason why diuretic pills, known as water pills, are used to control heart failure: their function is to make the kidneys lose sodium in the urine. Salt loss through sweating is less easy for the body to control, so when someone is in a hot climate, for example, he or she should use more salt than usual; otherwise, serious illness can result.

pumps. The cells therefore act in a way similar to single-celled animals in the ocean, which keep their salt levels low compared with the water surrounding them.

Function and sources of salt

Salt has the important function of maintaining the body's fluids at an optimum level. This occurs because the volume of a fluid depends directly on the amount of salt dissolved in it. Thus, since the amount of salt in the body is itself rigidly controlled, the volume of blood and other fluids is thereby regulated.

We use salt in its pure form but it is also present in meat and vegetables, and in large quantities in some processed foods like French fries and peanuts and in smaller quantities in other foods such as breakfast cereals.

How salt level is controlled

The body loses salt in excretion of urine and sweat. The kidneys regulate the amount of water in the body and maintain body fluids at a constant concentration by filtering blood and excreting waste products and excess water. Salt and other substances are reabsorbed from the tubular fluid in the kidneys, and the water also needed by

Salt loss

When there is a loss of salt, the body attempts to keep enough fluid in the circulation for the heart to work effectively. Eventually, it is unable to meet the body's requirements and the person collapses.

Dehydration through sweating, vomiting, and diarrhea can all cause a lack of salt, particularly in babies and small children whose salt level is normally low, so they can afford to lose much less. The treatment is to give large doses of water with salt (saline), usually by intravenous infusion. Salt loss and water loss almost always are observed together and so are treated accordingly. Salt loss also occurs when the body fails to produce steroid hormones, although this condition involves less water loss. Low blood pressure and a tendency to collapse are among the symptoms of such failure, which is a known characteristic of Addison's disease.

See also: **Cramp; Diet**

Scarlet fever

Questions and Answers

Once one of the most dreaded diseases of childhood, scarlet fever is now far less prevalent and its symptoms are less severe. Prompt treatment with penicillin minimizes any complications and leads to a complete cure.

In my grandfather's time, scarlet fever used to be a common cause of death among children, but now you rarely hear about it. Is this because of modern antibiotics?

Partly. Treatment of streptococcal infections, particularly sore throats, with antibiotics may make scarlet fever less likely to develop. Also, streptococcus, the organism that causes the disease, is a lot less virulent now: that is, it causes less serious symptoms. This change in the pattern of behavior of the streptococcus began at the end of the 19th century, before antibiotics were invented; nobody knows why.

Is scarlatina the same as scarlet fever?

Yes. Some doctors used the word "scarlatina" to describe mild cases of the disease because it helped to allay the fear that many people had of the illness.

My grandmother said that you could tell that a person had scarlet fever because there was a white line around the mouth. Is this true?

There is often a pale area around the mouth in an otherwise red face: doctors call this circumoral pallor. However, this sign is not specific to the disease; it is also a sign of measles, for example.

Are people who have scarlet fever isolated?

No. In the past, they were rushed off to a fever hospital, but now 24 hours of penicillin usually stops the disease from spreading.

Is there a scarlet fever vaccination?

No. There are many different strains of streptococcus, so a vaccine wouldn't necessarily protect you against the disease.

Scarlet fever is an infectious disease that is caused by a bacterium. It is characterized by a sore throat and a red, if not actually scarlet, rash. Treatment with penicillin will prevent complications and effect a complete cure.

Causes

Scarlet fever is caused by a bacterium called *Streptococcus pyogenes*. To differentiate one type of bacterium from another, medical researchers grow them separately on bacteriological plates that contain blood.

◀ Streptococcus pyogenes, *the bacterium that causes scarlet fever, is betahemolytic: it breaks down blood to leave a clear halo around its colonies.*

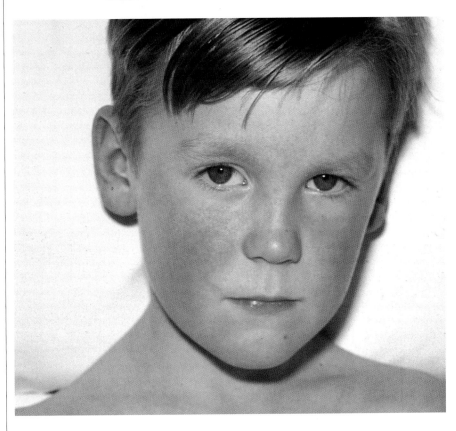

▲ *The bacterium* Streptococcus pyogenes *infects the throat, but its toxins produce symptoms throughout the body, causing rashes on the face and elsewhere on the body.*

Some types of bacterium break down the blood to leave a clear ring around the little colonies of bacteria. This phenomena is called hemolysis (blood breaking). *Streptococcus pyogenes* is a betahemolytic bacterium: that is, it breaks down blood completely, leaving a clear halo around each colony.

This halo indicates that the streptococcus must be producing and excreting a toxic substance, since the bacterium is having an effect beyond the bounds of the colony itself. In fact, it is the organism's ability to produce toxins that leads to scarlet fever, since the organism itself infects only the throat. The toxins' effects, particularly the rash, show up all over the body.

Symptoms

Scarlet fever usually starts within two to four days of incubation, although the incubation period can last between one and seven days.

One of the most characteristic aspects of the disease is that it starts in a dramatic manner, with a sudden temperature accompanied by vomiting and a sore throat. At this stage, the tonsils are infected and have a whitish crust, or exudate, on them. Less serious infections do not cause vomiting, and nowadays the disease can be so mild that children do not even have a sore throat.

The day after the disease starts, the rash that gives it its name breaks out. This is a diffuse reddening of the skin caused by all the little blood vessels opening up. If someone presses down over an area of affected skin, the skin will whiten with the pressure. The rash starts on the face and then spreads down to affect the rest of the body. The farther away from the face it gets, the likelier it is to form actual spots rather than a uniform redness: these spots tend to be found on the legs and to a lesser extent on the hands. The rash usually lasts for about two or three days.

While the rash is appearing and then fading away, there are a series of changes that affect the tongue. First, there is a creamy white exudate all over it, with the tongue's little papillae pointing up through it. This is known as white strawberry tongue. As the exudate peels off, the tongue is left rather red and raw, with its papillae still showing prominently to make it look like a strawberry. This is called red strawberry tongue.

One of the most typical and striking effects of the disease then occurs as the rash begins to fade. The skin starts to peel off and, in more serious cases, it may peel off in great sheets (desquamation). In

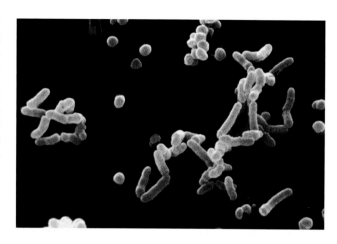

▲ *This scanning electron microscope image shows streptococci bacteria, which cause scarlet fever as well as infections such as meningitis, toxic shock syndrome, and tonsillitis.*

the past it was not uncommon to see an entire cast of a hand in the form of dead skin; nowadays such occurrences are extremely rare.

Although the disease is nearly always caught from a sore throat, there are other ways it can be communicated. It may enter the skin through a wound of some sort, and in the past it was not uncommon for infection to enter through the womb or the vagina during childbirth.

Dangers

Infection can spread to the ears, causing otitis media and also to the lymph glands where it may produce a serious abscess-forming illness. Infection may also lodge in the nose: this is a trivial complication with few or no symptoms, but it can lead to the spread of the disease as a result of droplet infection when one of the carriers sneezes.

Other problems result when the body's immune (defense) system produces antibodies to the streptococci that attack the body's own tissue (autoimmune disease). The first is nephritis, in which the kidneys become inflamed; the second is acute rheumatic fever, in which a rash, joint pains, and even heart damage may occur as a result of the body's sensitivity to the streptococcal toxins.

Treatment and outlook

Scarlet fever is treated with penicillin: this drug kills the bacteria in the throat and stops them from producing the toxin that gives rise to the disease. Even minor cases are treated this way, because after 24 hours of treatment with penicillin, the organism is no longer infectious.

See also: **Bacteria; Infection and infectious diseases; Rashes; Rheumatic fever; Sore throat; Streptococcus**

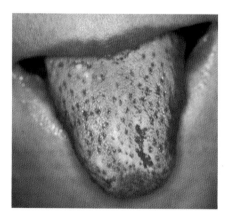

▲ *White strawberry tongue is one of the early symptoms; later the tongue turns red.*

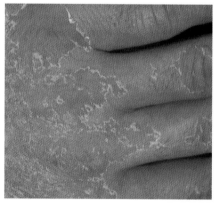

▲ *Once the rash fades, the skin on the hands will begin to peel off.*

Scoliosis

Early recognition and careful treatment can reduce the potentially crippling effects of scoliosis—a condition characterized by curvature of the spine that can cause deformity in children and is more common in girls than in boys.

Scoliosis is the name given to a side-to-side curvature of the spine. There are two basic types. In the first, the curve is mobile (that is, it can be straightened by stretching or leaning); in the second, the curve is fixed and permanent. Scoliosis occurring in a mobile spine is called postural scoliosis. When the trouble is centered in the spine itself, the condition is called structural scoliosis, and this condition can produce serious secondary effects.

Scoliosis is described by indicating the region and direction of the convexity of the deformity. Cervical scoliosis, which may be right or left, is rare, but right or left thoracic scoliosis is very common. The lumbar region is too short to accommodate scoliosis on its own.

Postural scoliosis

The most common cause of mobile scoliosis is having one leg shorter than the other. The patient leans toward the side with the longer leg in order to keep upright, curving the spine. The scoliosis produced can be eliminated by wearing a shoe rise, or insert, on the side where the leg is shorter.

Another cause is a tilt of the pelvis, usually due to excessive tightness and shortening (contracture) of the hip muscles. Because the spine is attached to the center of the pelvis, the lower part of the spine must bend sideways when the pelvis is tilted. Therefore, the upper part must twist in the opposite direction.

Another form of postural scoliosis is caused by unbalanced spasms of some of the large muscles that lie to the sides and back of the vertebrae. This can sometimes result from the condition commonly called a slipped disk, in which material squeezed out of the pulpy center of a disk puts pressure on the nerve roots emerging from the spinal cord. This spasm is a protective response by the muscles and does not cause permanent scoliosis. It may, however, last for a considerable time if the underlying condition is not treated.

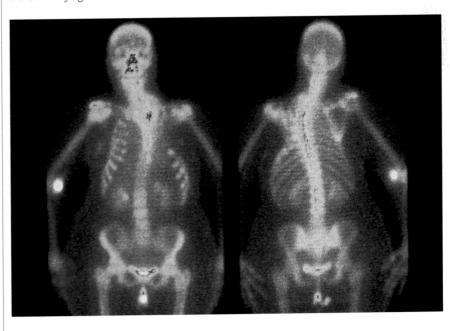

▲ *Colored whole-body scan of a patient showing scoliosis (curvature) of the upper spine. The patient is shown from the front (left) and from behind (right).*

Curvature of the spine

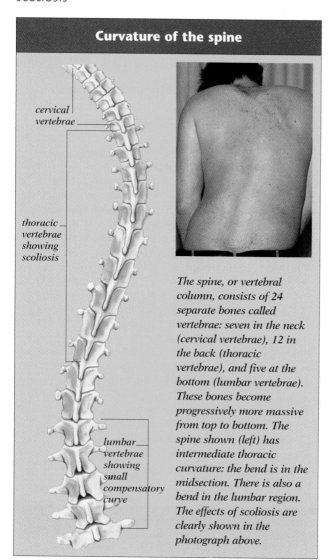

The spine, or vertebral column, consists of 24 separate bones called vertebrae: seven in the neck (cervical vertebrae), 12 in the back (thoracic vertebrae), and five at the bottom (lumbar vertebrae). These bones become progressively more massive from top to bottom. The spine shown (left) has intermediate thoracic curvature: the bend is in the midsection. There is also a bend in the lumbar region. The effects of scoliosis are clearly shown in the photograph above.

which the structural protein collagen is weaker than normal; and a form of scoliosis that starts in early infancy and may either recover spontaneously or progress to severe deformity. Such cases of structural scoliosis are always associated with actual abnormality in the bones and some rotation of the vertebrae. The deformity does not alter with changes in posture. The secondary curves that necessarily form as a result of the primary deformity will often, in time, also become fixed.

By far the most common cause of structural scoliosis is not actual disease or abnormality of the bones or of the surrounding muscles but a condition known as idiopathic adolescent scoliosis. The word "idiopathic" simply means "of unknown origin." Some experts, however, believe that the condition is the result of unbalanced muscular development. This form of the disorder usually becomes apparent before puberty, between the ages of eight and 10, and, unless treated, continues to progress until the growth of the skeleton is complete in the early twenties. Scoliosis appearing before or during adolescence should not, however, be assumed to be of this type. All children found to have scoliosis should be checked to ensure that none of the above-mentioned conditions is present.

Idiopathic adolescent scoliosis is five times more common in girls than in boys and tends to run in families. It is best detected by inspecting the spine from behind while the person bends forward 90 degrees with the hands clasped in the midline. The two sides of the body are then compared. If scoliosis is present, there will be an asymmetry of the ribs and the back muscles, which will appear to bulge on one side or the other. If the angle of the sideways curve to the long axis of the spine is less than 30 degrees, the outlook is excellent: about 70 percent resolve spontaneously. If it is more than 30 degrees, the outlook is less certain. In most cases, the only actual symptom is the deformity itself and even severe scoliosis is not usually painful. However, later in life arthritis can develop, giving rise to backache.

Most seriously, however, secondary curvature of the upper spine can compress the lung on one side and prevent it from expanding. This can lead to diminished lung function and poor respiratory performance. In addition, the blood vessels in the compressed lung offer increased resistance to blood flow so that the heart has to work harder to maintain the circulation through the lungs. The result may be a dangerous condition known as corpulmonale.

Treatment and outlook

Mild curves can be prevented from deteriorating by wearing a special brace, which must be worn continuously for months or even years. More severe cases require correction by special traction exercises or by wearing plaster jackets. However, most severe cases require an operation aimed at straightening out the curve and joining the bones of the spine together with a bone graft. Operations of this type result in considerable improvement in the appearance of the back and prevent the curve from getting worse again.

The principal danger of scoliosis is that it will progress to a more severe curve during the years of growth. This will cause more deformity, which not only is unattractive but may cause difficulties in walking and sitting. Thanks to modern methods of early recognition and careful treatment, severe deformity can usually be prevented. Once the child has stopped growing, the curve will not become any worse.

These forms of scoliosis, which are caused by factors external to the spine itself, can easily be distinguished from the structural form of scoliosis by a simple test. When the person concerned sits down squarely, the pelvis automatically becomes level and the sideways curvature in the spine disappears (best viewed from behind the patient). When the scoliosis is due to structural changes in the spine itself, sitting does not change the visible curvature.

Structural scoliosis

Structural, or fixed, scoliosis arises in childhood and can have a variety of causes. There may be abnormalities in the shape of one or more bones of the spine at birth, or there may be a curvature caused by certain paralytic conditions such as poliomyelitis (polio), in which an imbalance of the strength of the muscles around the spine can cause it to become curved in compensation.

Other causes include: cerebral palsy; rare failures of muscular development (dystrophies); a genetic disorder called neurofibromatosis (von Recklinghausen's disease), in which there are multiple benign tumors of small nerves; the genetic condition Marfan's syndrome, in

See also: **Protein; Slipped disk**

Sexual abuse

Questions and Answers

I am a teacher. What should I do if I think one of my pupils is being sexually abused at home?

You must approach someone who is professionally trained to handle this type of situation; your school probably has guidelines and your principal will know about them. Perhaps there is a therapist or counselor already attached to the school. Ignoring a situation where sexual abuse is taking place can have serious consequences; however, false accusations can be extremely damaging to the alleged assailant. The type of case you describe must be handled by experienced individuals with extreme care and sensitively.

Can a person suffer sexual abuse that is not physical? I think my sister might be being abused by her boyfriend in this way.

Many therapists agree that if a person is continually subject to verbal abuse and comments that make him or her feel threatened or degraded sexually—for example, if your sister's partner makes demeaning and critical sexual remarks, using sexual names or making her feel she has to engage in unwanted sexual acts—then this is a type of sexual abuse. Your sister should seek help; it could be that she needs to get out of this relationship.

I was sexually abused by my stepfather from the age of 11 until I left home at 16. I never told anyone. I am now 23, and have never had a boyfriend; I find it difficult to trust people and to form friendships. What can I do?

You need professional help so that you can accept what has happened, recover fully, and move on. If there is a doctor you know and trust, visit him or her for advice and a referral to a good therapist or counselor.

Sexual assault is usually defined as any sexual contact or attempt at sexual contact that takes place without the victim's consent or that occurs in circumstances where a person is unable to give such consent. Any sexual assault is an instance of sexual abuse; however, sexual abuse is commonly sustained over a period of years.

Many people associate the term "sexual abuse" with sexual relations that take place between family members, such as between parents and children, or brothers and sisters; however, sexual abuse can take place outside a family as well.

Abuse is a misuse of power; sexual abuse might involve marital rape, nonconsensual incest, sexual verbal or physical harassment, child molestation, sexual touching—any kind of sexual relations that involve coercion, force, or intimidation, or when the victim is not in a position to give consent (for example, if he or she is a minor, has been drugged, or is too drunk or intoxicated to know what is happening). However, because abuse, as opposed to assault, usually takes place over a period of time, it almost invariably involves attack by someone the victim knows, such as a family member, partner, friend, colleague, or friend of the family.

Sexual abuse is common, but the figures sometimes quoted—such as that more than one in four girls and one in six boys in the United States have suffered such abuse by the time they are 18 years old—might call into question exactly what is meant in many of these cases by "sexual abuse." An exact definition is key in this respect.

Causes

By definition, victims of sexual abuse do not cause or invite the abuse to take place. Only the person initiating the sexual contact or harassment is responsible.

A perpetrator of certain forms of sexual abuse—for example, rape—is thought to abuse primarily out of anger, out of a need to feel powerful. Because he (or, very occasionally, she) wishes to control or dominate the victim, control and domination may be the sole motive.

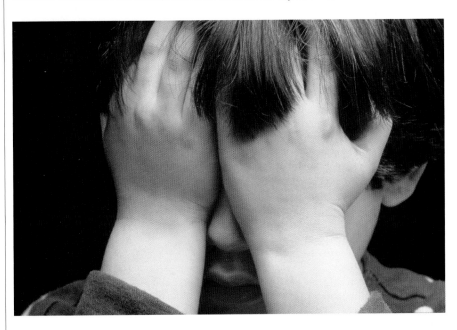

▲ *A child who has been sexually abused will be unhappy, lack confidence, and feel general depression and despair.*

Figures suggest that about a third of sex offenders have been abused themselves—in terms of sexual abuse, physical abuse, or emotional neglect—by one or both parents, by primary caregivers, or by some kind of authority figure before the age of 16 years. The abuser was often someone other than their parents. About 60 percent of those abused had been separated from their biological parents as children. Many sex offenders have a history of drug and alcohol abuse.

Symptoms of abuse; stages of recovery

A victim of a serious sexual assault, such as rape, initially experiences shock; this might be emotional as well as physical, and could be expressed in a controlled or withdrawn manner, or it might be extremely expressive, including crying, screaming, or shaking.

He or she will probably have trouble communicating to others what has happened. Estimates suggest that only about a third of victims of a sexual assault actually report it to the authorities, either at the time of the attack or later on.

A victim of rape or of some other form of serious sexual abuse is then likely to go through a stage of denial. He or she may try to carry on life normally, in an attempt to forget about what has happened or—when the abuse is sustained over time—what is continuing to happen. This is an attempt to deal with the confusion and turmoil he or she is feeling. Victims of sexual abuse may also attempt to convince themselves that the assault did not really take place; or if it did, that it is unlikely to happen again.

At a later stage the victim often reexperiences his or her initial feelings of shock; such feelings are usually triggered by memories of the assault itself. Feelings of depression, anxiety, and shame often become worse around this time. Later still, the victim of a serious assault often comes to experience intense feelings of anger, often toward him- or herself, his or her friends or family, a partner, society, the legal system, or all men or women.

Other symptoms that may occur after any form of sexual abuse include sleeplessness, nightmares, flashbacks, a sense of vulnerability and loss of self-confidence, mistrust of others, fear of being alone, overeating or loss of appetite, feelings of grief and despair, and stress-related illnesses and complaints.

Treatment and outlook

Clearly the first step in a person's recovery from sexual abuse involves removal of the source of that abuse. Often such a situation must be handled with extreme sensitivity, particularly when the abuser is a family member. In some circumstances, it is the victim who must leave or be removed from the situation where he or she is being abused. Apart from treatment for physical symptoms, anyone

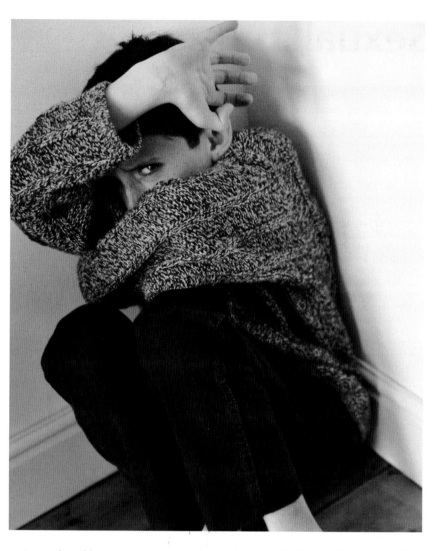

▲ *In a vulnerable young person, systematic abuse instills fear and a distrust of people. These feelings can be overcome with therapy.*

who has suffered serious sexual abuse over a prolonged period will almost certainly require professional counseling and therapy.

The emotions and physical symptoms that the victim experiences are seen by many therapists as part of the natural process of coming to terms with what has happened and moving toward recovery. With skillful support and therapy, a victim of abuse can eventually overcome feelings of despair and vulnerability, and can learn to direct feelings of anger and blame toward the assailant.

The final stage in the recovery from the assault is what is termed "integration," or "closure." As the victim integrates the thoughts and feelings stemming from the abuse into his or her life experience, he or she begins to be able to cope.

With support, education, and time, the victim should eventually feel able to carry on with his or her life.

See also: **Child abuse; Depression; Drug abuse; Sexually transmitted diseases**

Sexually transmitted diseases

Questions and Answers

Is it possible to have a sexually transmitted disease without knowing it?

Yes. People can carry the germs causing these diseases and are unaware that they are infected. For example, about 80 percent of women who turn out to have gonorrhea have no idea that anything is wrong with them. Anyone who has casual sex or sleeps with a number of partners should be checked at a clinic or by a doctor at regular intervals.

Is it possible to catch an STD from a dirty toilet seat?

This virtually never occurs, except in the case of trichomoniasis. Sexually transmitted diseases are caught by having sexual intercourse with somebody who already has the disease, even if he or she is not aware of it.

Is it possible to get vaccinated against an STD?

Not at present, although a vaccine for genital herpes has been developed in a British research unit and vaccination against gonorrhea may become possible. Because these diseases do not produce any protective antibodies, it is possible to be infected with them several times. Although one attack of measles produces lifelong immunity, it is possible to be infected with gonorrhea several times because no protective immunity results.

Is there any way of knowing if somebody has an STD?

Only by doing medical tests. If a person changes partners often, he or she is likely to get infected at some time. Use a condom with a new partner until you know the person well enough to be sure of him or her.

Sexually transmitted diseases (STDs) are infections that are contracted during sexual activity. Early diagnosis and prompt treatment with appropriate drugs are essential to avoid side effects such as infertility.

Sexually transmitted disease is in fact not a single disease but a collection of several different conditions that are grouped together because they are all acquired as a result of sexual intercourse with a person who has the infection. AIDS is a condition caused by the complex HIV virus that is, among other ways, sexually transmitted. Research into HIV and AIDS is extensive, and while some progress has been made, there is still no cure for what is usually a fatal condition. Syphilis, gonorrhea, genital warts, chlamydial infection, and genital herpes are prone to complications, some of which can be very serious; less serious sexually transmitted diseases include trichomoniasis, monilia, and pubic lice.

HIV and AIDS

Acquired immunodeficiency syndrome (AIDS) is the most serious of the sexually transmitted diseases. Since the first official AIDS cases were reported in 1981, more than 30 million people have died of the disease worldwide.

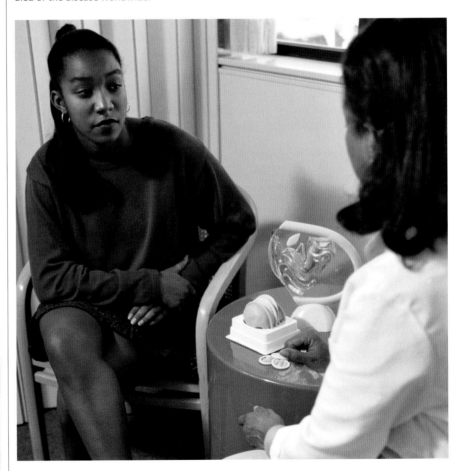

▲ *Young people are particularly at risk when it comes to sexually transmitted diseases because of greater sexual freedom at an increasingly earlier age.*

AIDS is caused by the human immunodeficiency virus (HIV), which is usually acquired during sexual contact through the blood, vaginal fluid, or semen. It can also be transmitted through infected needles or blood transfusions, or from an infected mother to her child through the blood or breast milk. When a person is infected with HIV, the body makes special antibodies to try to fight the virus off. A person is diagnosed as having HIV when a blood test finds these antibodies in the blood; the person is then said to be HIV-positive. In 2009, more than 33 million people around the world were HIV-positive.

HIV slowly wears down the immune system, reducing the number of helper T lymphocyte cells, also called T4 cells, that help fight off infections. When an HIV-positive person has less than 200 T4 cells, he or she has developed AIDS (the average healthy person has 500 to 1,500 T4 cells in 1 ml of blood). About 1.8 million people around the world died from AIDS in 2009.

The development from HIV to AIDS may happen quickly or take 10 or more years. Symptoms of HIV include fevers, night sweats, diarrhea, and swollen lymph nodes. AIDS-related symptoms include severe weight loss and brain tumors. Once AIDS has developed, opportunistic infections occur—most commonly, pneumocystis pneumonia; a skin cancer called Kaposi's sarcoma; cytomegalovirus, which affects the eyes; and candida—until one or a combination of such infections proves fatal.

There is no cure for HIV or AIDS. Drug treatment with highly active antiretroviral therapy (HAART) given to people who are HIV-positive has decreased the death rate from AIDS. However, HAART has to be taken for the rest of the patient's life to be effective and some patients have such severe side effects that they are unable to take it.

Syphilis

Syphilis is considered one of the more serious sexually transmitted infections because it is likely to result, if untreated, in permanent disability or even death. The bacteria are spread from one person to another during intercourse. They can also be passed from an infected mother to her child during pregnancy; therefore the baby may be born with congenital syphilis. Routine blood testing of all expectant mothers and the treatment of those found to be infected have made congenital syphilis a rare condition.

The incubation period of syphilis varies widely, as do the symptoms of the first or primary stage of the disease. This makes for enormous difficulty in the early recognition of the disease, which is essential for a total and permanent cure to be achieved.

An indication of syphilis is a single painless ulcer (chancre) appearing where the germ has entered the body; in or around the genitals, anus, or mouth. The ulcer heals by itself, and because of this, many people fail to consult a doctor. An added complication is that sometimes a chancre does not appear at all. For this reason, it is essential for anyone who thinks that he or she may have been in contact with a sexually transmitted disease to seek advice from a doctor or treatment center, because a cure can be guaranteed only if treatment is given in the early stages of the disease.

Gonorrhea

Gonorrhea is another bacterial disease that is very common. It is contracted by sexual intercourse with an infected person. About 80 percent of infected women have no symptoms and are generally unaware that they have it. Some have pain passing urine (dysuria) or cystitis and some develop lower abdominal pain from infection of the fallopian tubes, which can lead to pelvic inflammatory disease and subsequent sterility. Diagnosis is not easy; it is best carried out by a doctor or treatment center. It consists of finding the bacteria in specimens obtained during a vaginal examination. In men inflammation of the testes can occur. In less than a week after being infected, pain on passing urine develops, followed by a profuse discharge of pus from the opening at the end of the penis, the urinary meatus. The diagnosis of gonorrhea is confirmed by discovering bacteria in the discharge.

Treatment in both sexes is usually by a single dose of penicillin, given either as an injection or as capsules; abstention from

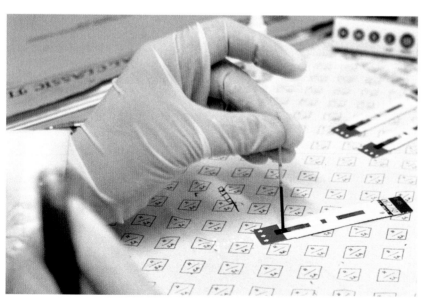

▲ *Blood samples of pregnant women are tested for HIV in a clinic in Soweto, South Africa. Sexually transmitted diseases are particularly dangerous for pregnant women, since they can pass the diseases to their babies, which can, in some cases, endanger the babies' lives.*

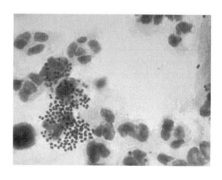

▲ *Diagnosis of gonorrhea is made by microscopic examination, which reveals the presence of the bacteria* Neisseria gonorrhoeae *in the specimen. This is taken from the vagina or, in men, from urinary discharge.*

Questions and Answers

Can an STD make it more difficult to get pregnant?

Yes. STDs are more likely to cause permanent damage in women than in men. One of the most serious ways they can affect women is to make them sterile because the tube down which the monthly egg or ovum passes becomes blocked due to disease.

Does either urinating or taking a shower after sexual intercourse have any effect in reducing the risk of getting an STD?

Washing the sexual parts thoroughly with soap and water and passing urine after sex can reduce the risk of catching a sexually transmitted disease, especially in men, but they do not eliminate the risk. Using a condom offers a much greater degree of protection.

Can one become immune to STDs?

Unlike diseases such as measles, an attack of one of the sexually transmitted diseases does not protect against future attacks. Sexually transmitted diseases can be caught many times, and people do not generally become immune to them.

Can STD affect an unborn baby in the womb?

Yes. Syphilis may cause stillbirth, miscarriage, deformities, or even death of the baby after birth. Therefore all expectant mothers have blood tests for syphilis during pregnancy; if they test positive, treatment can be given to protect the baby. Genital herpes can also be fatal if passed by a woman to her baby during childbirth; if there are open vesicles at the time of birth, the baby will be delivered by cesarean section. Gonorrhea and chlamydia can affect a baby's eyes if the bacteria are active when the baby is born. AIDS can be transmitted before birth from an infected mother to her baby.

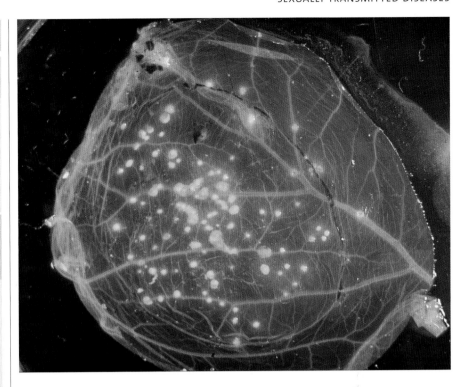

▲ *A microscopic view of the genital herpes virus, which causes painful blisters. There is no cure, and genital herpes has reached epidemic proportions in the United States.*

alcohol and sexual intercourse for several weeks is also important. The relief of symptoms after treatment is dramatic, but supervision must be maintained to ensure that the cure is permanent and complete. An attack of gonorrhea confers no immunity for the future. Patients should ensure that all those with whom they have recently had sexual contact are made aware of the facts and go for examination. The use of a condom during intercourse gives considerable protection to both partners. Gonorrhea is not hereditary, but a gonococcal infection can be passed on to babies and young girls, either during birth or by close contact with an infected mother.

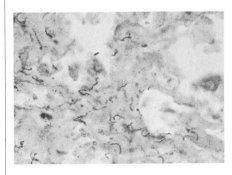

▲ *Syphilis is an infection caused by the bacterium* Treponema pallidum. *The characteristic threadlike spiral cells of the bacteria are visible.*

▶ *Syphilis sufferers may also develop a papular rash, characterized by small, solid elevations of the skin, that appears on the palms of the hands and the soles of the feet.*

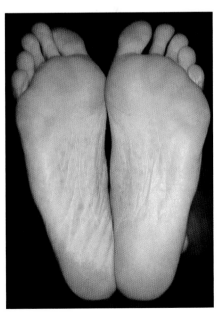

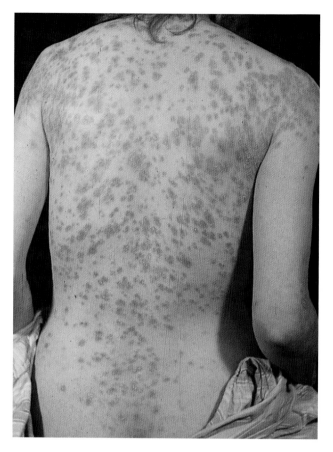

both. PID is a serious condition that may cause severe and persistent pelvic pain and commonly leads to female infertility.

NSU

What was once called nonspecific urethritis (NSU) is now known to be caused by germs called *Chlamydia trachomatis*. The number of cases continues to increase at a rapid rate, making chlamydial infection more common than all the other sexually transmitted diseases together. Chlamydial germs are very much smaller than most bacteria and can survive only inside cells. It is for this reason that the cause of what was called nonspecific urethritis took so long to be established. Some cases get better quickly and present no problem, but in other cases recurrences are common. Chlamydial STD in males is urethritis or inflammation of the urethra that is now clearly distinguished from the other main cause of urethritis, which is gonorrhea. Since the treatment, management, and implications of gonorrhea and chlamydial infection are quite different, when a specialist suspects chlamydial infection, he or she will make sure, by means of microscopic examination and laboratory tests of the discharge, that it is not in fact a mild case of gonorrhea. The main symptom is a discharge from the tip of the penis. The discharge is usually clear white to gray in color, not the creamy yellow matter that is characteristic of gonorrhea, and it is similar to semen in appearance. The quantity varies a great deal but is usually a small amount, sometimes no more than a moistness at the tip of the penis. The second common symptom is pain on passing urine, the severity of which is extremely variable. Often there is no pain at all or there is just irritation.

Chlamydial infection in women may, like gonorrhea, initially be symptomless, but almost all cases of chronic pelvic inflammatory disease (PID) are caused by chlamydial infection or gonorrhea or

Genital herpes

Genital herpes is a sexually transmitted disease that has reached epidemic proportions in the United States. The main problem is that, being a virus, herpes cannot be cured and so each new sufferer adds to the pool of carriers. There are two types of herpes simplex virus, both of which cause painful blisters (vesicles), localized swelling, and sometimes fever. HSV 1 was at one time mainly found around the mouth (cold sores), but possibly as a result of widespread oral sexual practices, HSV 1 is now the most common cause of genital herpes. HSV 2 is spread by sexual contact and the blisters can be found in and around the genitals, around the anus, and on the bladder, buttocks, thighs, and legs of both sexes. This condition exists in two states: latent and active. After the first attack, the virus travels up a local sensory nerve and then lies dormant in the body. It waits until an attack is triggered, then emerges again, usually in the same spot time and time again, as a painful blister. During latent periods when no blisters are open, sexual partners will not catch herpes from the carrier, but the carrier is extremely contagious when blisters are open. It is possible that the carrier will be unaware of their existence if the vesicles are inside the vagina, on the cervix, or in the urethra. Attacks appear to be linked to physical and emotional low points, such as during times of depression or stress, illness, just before a period, or during bad weather, or to local stimulation of the affected areas.

Genital herpes is painful and depressing to an adult, and it is often fatal if it is passed by a pregnant sufferer to her baby as the baby passes down the birth canal. A pregnant woman who has suffered genital herpes, even if she has not had an attack for some time, should always tell the medical team about her condition. They will monitor her during the pregnancy and, if there are open vesicles at the time of birth, the baby can be saved if delivered by cesarean section.

Because a virus is entwined with the cells of the host, and anything that harms the virus invariably harms the host, genital herpes cannot yet be cured, but there are ways of speeding up the recovery time from attacks and making them less unpleasant. Keeping the affected areas clean and dry will stop secondary infection. Salt baths and cold compresses will ease pain. Staying free of stress and healthy will help the body erect defenses against attacks. In most cases attacks will come most months for the first year and gradually tail off, becoming less frequent as the years go by.

Although there is no cure for herpes, the severity and frequency of relapses of the disease can be markedly reduced by means of the drug aciclovir (Zovirax) taken by mouth. Since genital herpes has been linked to cancer of the cervix, women sufferers should have regular Pap smears at least once a year.

Genital warts

It has been known for some time that sexually promiscuous women are much more likely than those in single relationships to develop

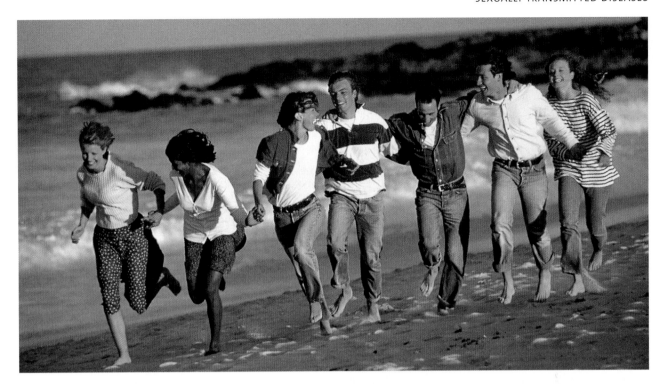

▲ *Young adults under the age of 25 are at the highest risk of being infected with STDs.*

cancer of the cervix. The link is now known not to be genital herpes but genital warts, which are commonly transmitted sexually. The virus that causes genital warts is the human papillomavirus (HPV) and it is this virus that contributes to the causation of cervical cancer. A vaccine against strains that cause about 70 percent of cervical cancer and 90 percent of genital warts was approved for use in the United States in 2006.

Identifying discharges

Women often worry that vaginal discharge or a change in what is normal for them may mean that they have caught an STD. However, although a vaginal discharge should not be dismissed as trivial, and tests and treatment may be required, many discharges are in fact normal, and only a few are caused by a serious condition. The quantity of the discharge, which is often what gives rise to alarm, can vary widely from one woman to another and is particularly likely to increase in certain situations. What is important, in relation to the possibility of infection or other disease, is not the quantity but the quality or type of discharge.

Clear mucous discharges are unlikely to be caused by disease, but a discharge that is discolored, causes soreness or irritation of the vagina or vulva, or has an unpleasant odor is much more likely to be related to infection of the female genital organs. A thin, yellow discharge is suggestive of trichomonas infection; a thick, white discharge is characteristic of thrush (monilia); and brown discharges are decomposed blood, which is an indication of internal bleeding. This is most likely to be due to erosion or ulceration of the neck of the womb or cervix, but it can be caused by cancer of the womb and must therefore always be investigated.

If an unpleasant discharge continues for more than a week, a doctor should be consulted or a woman should attend a special clinic without delay, especially if it is accompanied by fever or abdominal pain, if there is a possibility of STD, if the discharge is bloodstained or brown and a menstrual period is not due, if it is accompanied by pain on passing urine, if there is soreness and irritation with discharge, or if it has an unpleasant odor. A doctor will ask about the type of discharge and recent sexual relationships. He or she will probably examine the vagina with a gloved hand and with a plastic or metal instrument, using a light to see inside. He or she may take specimens from the vagina and neck of the womb and possibly also from the urethra and rectum for laboratory analysis.

STDs and young adults

Half of all young Americans will get a sexually transmitted disease by the age of 25. Genital warts, chlamydia, and trichomoniasis account for the majority of all the new cases of STDs. Teenagers 15 years and older who have had sex have the highest STD rates of any age group in the country. The reason for this large number of cases may be attributed to the development of new contraceptives since the 1960s, which has led to an alteration in attitudes and habits in sexual behavior and, consequently, greater sexual freedom at an earlier age. However, a more open approach to sex demands a need for more awareness and thoughtfulness toward one's partner, rather than less. Young people can suffer from ignorance or embarrassment about asking about methods of protecting themselves from sexually transmitted diseases.

Prevention

Several precautions can be taken to reduce the chances of getting a sexually transmitted disease. Abstinence and avoiding sex with more than one person can reduce the risk. Condoms and a

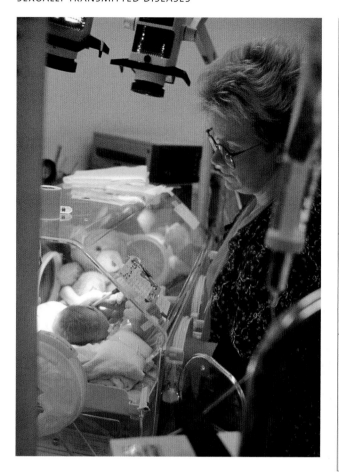

Pregnancy and STDs

The effects of an STD can be serious and even life threatening for a pregnant woman and her baby, with complications that can include early onset of labor, premature rupture of the membranes surrounding the baby in the uterus, and infection of the uterus after the baby is delivered. Infants of women with sexually transmitted infections may suffer from severe health consequences if an STD is transmitted to the developing fetus in utero (inside the uterus) or during delivery. For example, syphilis infection in the mother can cross the placenta and infect the baby in the uterus, leading to congenital syphilis. HIV can also cross the placenta and infect the baby. Chlamydia, gonorrhea, hepatitis B virus, and herpes simplex can infect the infant during the birthing process as the newborn travels through the birth canal.

Some of the health effects from STDs include stillbirth (baby is born dead); low birth weight (less than five pounds); eye infections from chlamydia or gonorrhea; pneumonia; sepsis (severe infection in the baby's blood); blindness; neurological damage; deafness; acute hepatitis; meningitis (infection of the membranes surrounding the brain); and liver disease.

To identify and treat STDs and reduce health risks for the mother and baby, it is recommended that at the first prenatal visit, a pregnant woman and her sex partners are counseled on the health dangers associated with STDs. The pregnant woman should be offered a voluntary HIV test, a blood test for syphilis, a blood test for hepatitis B infection, and tests for chlamydia and gonorrhea. If a woman is at risk, she should also have a blood test for hepatitis C infection. She should also have a Pap smear if one has not been done within the preceding year.

▲ *Sexually transmitted diseases can have tragic consequences for a baby born to an infected mother. The baby may suffer from jaundice, anemia, a swollen liver and spleen, fever, and skin rashes and sores. Even worse, some babies with syphilis are stillborn, or die soon after birth.*

spermicide should be used for sexual intercourse of any kind. Using a condom will give both partners a considerable degree of protection against all forms of STD. Water-based lubricants should be used rather than oil-based lubricants, which damage rubber. For both the man and the woman a thorough cleansing of the genital area with soap and water before and after intercourse will kill a large proportion of the bacteria with which they may have been contaminated. For men, if they pass urine this has the additional benefit that it is likely to flush out of the urethra any microbes that may have entered during intercourse. Urinating will have the same effect in women, but they have the disadvantage that sexually transmitted diseases usually develop in the vagina and in the neck of the womb rather than in the urethra.

Women often debate the value and advisability of douching, either to prevent or to treat discharges. Douching is a misguided practice. There is nothing positive in its favor and there is a risk that any infected material could be flushed upward into the uterus rather than be washed out, which is undesirable. The most useful thing that women can do is to soak in a hot bath, allowing the water to flow freely into the vagina. Unless someone is advised to do so by a

doctor, antiseptic lotions or ointments should never be applied either inside or outside the genitals, and strong antiseptic should never be used in the urethra or vagina; it could lead to serious, permanent internal damage.

Where to go for help

If someone thinks that there is even a remote chance that he or she might have some form of STD, the best procedure is to go to a doctor or treatment center immediately to find out. Some hospitals have a separate department of genitourinary medicine where tests can be carried out and advice can be given. Alternatively, anyone worried could telephone the STD National Hotline: 800-227-8922. The AIDS National Hotline is 800-342-2437.

Any information that is obtained at the treatment center is strictly confidential, and patients will usually be referred to by a number so that their anonymity is completely preserved. No information will be given about a patient in response to queries from a spouse or partner, friends, parents, school, employer, or anybody else. Patients' notes are kept separately from any medical records that may exist elsewhere so that there is no possibility of any cross-reference being made between them. The staffs who work at such centers are there to help, not to judge, and the atmosphere is usually very friendly and helpful.

See also: AIDS; Bacteria; Contraception; Viruses

Shock

A person who is pale, cold, and clammy after an accident is almost certainly suffering from shock. Speedy treatment by blood transfusion can often be a lifesaver to the shock victim.

There is a big difference between the way that most people use the word "shock" and the way that doctors use it. In an everyday sense, people talk about a sudden event giving rise to an unpleasant surprise, or shock. On the other hand, to the doctor, "shock" is a medical condition in which the failure of the circulatory system, for one reason or another, is a central feature. Sometimes the different uses of the word cause confusion.

Psychological shocks

It would be wrong to ignore totally the effects of sudden unpleasant psychological shocks: they can often cause considerable distress and can even precipitate serious psychological illness. However, this is likely only in people already at risk of some sort of psychological illness.

Sudden psychological shocks can cause collapse on their own: people may faint at the sight of a gruesome automobile accident, and it is not uncommon for people to faint when they are given bad news. Also, an unpleasant or horrifying experience can lead to the development of serious symptoms of anxiety that may last for some time: this is particularly likely in the case of victims of violent crime.

One of the psychological shocks that most people have to experience at some time is the death of a close friend or relative. If the death occurs unexpectedly, the initial horror of the event may leave someone numbed, and the deep sadness may take some time to sink in. Even if the death is expected, the finality of bereavement is still an event that will change a person's life and outlook.

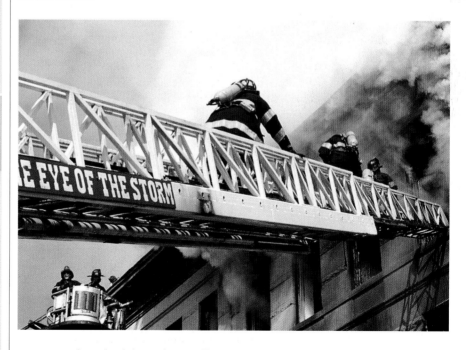

▲ *In second- or third-degree burns affecting more than 10 percent of the body surface, the victim will usually be in a state of shock. This condition is provoked by the loss of large quantities of fluid (and its constituent proteins) from the burned area. Shock can be fatal if not rapidly treated by intravenous fluid replacement.*

Just after the death of his wife, my friend of mine seemed quite calm, but a few weeks later he became really miserable. Was he suffering from delayed shock?

People often talk about "delayed shock," though to the doctor this term does not have any special meaning. It is most often used to describe the way in which the full sadness of bereavement may take days or even weeks to sink in. The period immediately after loss can seem unreal, and the bereaved person can be in a daze.

My father died after going into shock after a heart attack. Could he have been saved by surgery?

No, it is very unlikely. The sort of shock that happens after a heart attack is called cardiogenic shock, and the problem is caused because the damaged heart lacks the strength to pump adequate blood around the body. It is very hard to treat because the only way to get the blood around the body is by making the already damaged heart work harder.

My best friend was killed in an automobile crash, and I felt weak and wobbly for days. Was I suffering from shock?

The shock of losing your best friend was undoubtedly responsible for the unusual symptoms you experienced. However, doctors are much more likely to use the word "shock" to describe the sort of collapse that follows from the loss of blood after an accident, rather than the psychological shock that you experienced.

Can a person die of shock?

If you are talking about the medical use of the word (meaning collapse of the heart and circulation), then certainly a shock can be fatal. However, psychological shock alone is unlikely to cause death in a fit person, although it might be fatal in someone already suffering from a heart condition.

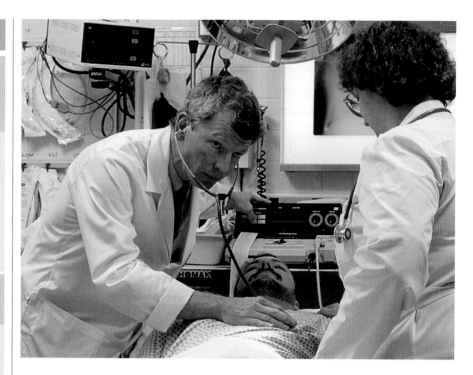

▲ *A male patient receives emergency coronary care from a hospital trauma team. A heart attack is one of the most common causes of shock. Careful and constant monitoring of the patient's heart rate is required to help restore stability.*

These different shocks are the bumps and bruises that people usually have to experience during their lives. If the shocks are severe enough and a person is vulnerable, then they may take their toll and leave some psychological scar. However, these events are not what shock means in the medical sense; it is something much more immediate and easy to recognize. The failure of the circulation is the basic problem, and treatment is the province of the hospital physician or surgeon rather than the counselor or psychiatrist.

What is shock?

Shock develops because of the way the heart and circulation work together. If for some reason the heart fails to pump properly or there is not enough blood for it to pump, then insufficient blood will be circulating to sustain the vital functions. This can be brought on by a variety of factors, ranging from loss of large amounts of blood to failure of the heart itself.

For the heart to pump in the correct manner, it has to be primed with blood, and there must be some blood in the system for the heart to get up enough pressure to push the blood around. Normally, blood leaves the heart and travels throughout the body in arteries. Larger arteries give way to smaller ones, called arterioles, which have thick muscular walls. If blood pressure goes down, these arterioles can constrict so that there is less space for the blood to flow through. This causes the pressure to rise again because the blood is being squeezed into a smaller space than before.

This system of constriction of the arterioles, called vasoconstriction, is one of the body's ways of maintaining the correct blood pressure when things go wrong. If the pressure falls too low, blood cannot flow around all the tissues. In fact, when the system fails—after excessive bleeding, for example—shock occurs.

Hypovolemic shock

There are several types of shock. One of the most common results from the massive loss of fluid (blood or water) that can follow from critical injury or illness. This is termed "hypovolemic shock." Second- and third-degree burns can provoke shock because of the extensive fluid loss that occurs in the burned area.

MEASURING CENTRAL VENOUS PRESSURE

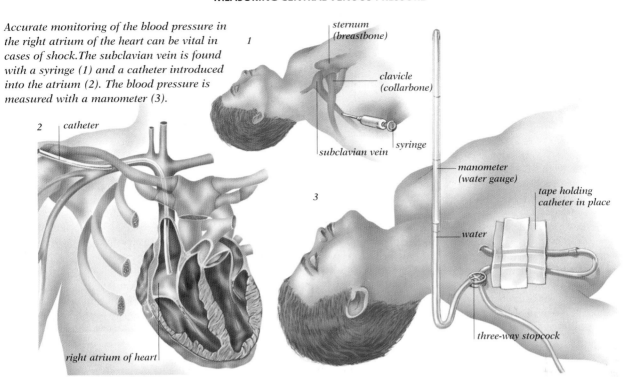

Accurate monitoring of the blood pressure in the right atrium of the heart can be vital in cases of shock. The subclavian vein is found with a syringe (1) and a catheter introduced into the atrium (2). The blood pressure is measured with a manometer (3).

1

sternum (breastbone)

clavicle (collarbone)

subclavian vein

syringe

2 catheter

manometer (water gauge)

tape holding catheter in place

3

water

right atrium of heart

three-way stopcock

Fluid loss does not result only from accidents. It is not uncommon for there to be serious bleeding from ulcers in the stomach. In these cases, large amounts of blood are either vomited or passed through the rectum. Patients suffering from this sort of gastrointestinal bleeding can arrive in the emergency room in a state of extreme shock.

Large blood loss can also occur during childbirth (intrapartum hemorrhage), though with blood transfusions shock under these circumstances has become increasingly rare. Similarly, diarrhea, particularly in young children, can cause severe dehydration, which in turn can provoke shock.

Septic shock

Some infections can cause shock, though in this case the mechanism underlying the shock is different. Infection in the blood may lead to the production of toxins. These toxins seem to have a direct effect on the blood vessels in the tissues, causing the venules (very small veins) to become widened and very leaky. Blood becomes pooled in the venules, and insufficient amounts return to the heart and therefore the blood pressure falls. This is known as endotoxic or septic shock.

Cardiogenic shock

Another major cause of shock results from disease of the heart itself. This is called cardiogenic shock, and its main cause is an extensive heart attack. The heart muscle is partly destroyed by the heart attack, and the more that is destroyed the more severe the effects of the attack will be. When more than 30 percent has been destroyed, shock is likely to develop because the remaining heart muscle simply lacks the power to pump enough blood.

Neurogenic shock

This occurs when the brain is starved of oxygen, causing a collapse of the nervous system and a complete loss of control over the circulation.

Anaphylactic shock

Another type of shock is a very rare and sometimes fatal allergic reaction. Common allergens that can cause such extreme reactions include insect stings, drugs, and some common foods such as nuts.

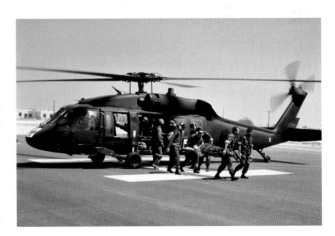

▲ *Early skilled assistance, in this case the replacement of lost body fluids with clear plasma, can be lifesaving to the shock victim. Many lives can now be saved on the battlefield by early treatment and rapid transport to a base hospital.*

Symptoms of shock

People with shock tend to have a similar appearance. They are pale and often cold and clammy to the touch; when the blood pressure is measured, it is found to be critically low. One exception to this, however, is during septic shock, where, despite the low blood pressure, the patient is warm to the touch.

The pallor is caused by lack of blood in the skin: blood has been forced from the skin by the vasoconstriction. The coldness is because the blood, which carries body heat, is sent back into the body's core.

It might seem strange that people are sweaty and cold at the same time, but the autonomic nervous system, which is responsible for running the body's unconscious functions, not only causes the vasoconstriction but also causes the adrenal glands to release epinephrine, which in turn makes the sweat glands work.

Effects of shock

As well as the immediate, dangerous effects of shock, it can create other, long-term problems. The two most important of these affect the kidneys and the lungs. When shock develops and there is insufficient blood passing through the kidneys, acute renal failure can develop. The kidneys stop passing urine, and waste products, particularly urea (a breakdown product of protein), start to build up in the blood. If the shock is dealt with fairly quickly, the kidneys are likely to recover speedily. However, the process can be slow and dialysis may be required for days or even weeks.

If shock has stopped the kidneys from working, the situation may deteriorate even further. The blood supply to the brain may become inadequate, and, as a consequence, confusion and then unconsciousness may set in. The skin can sometimes progress from being cold and clammy to a gangrenous condition resulting from the poor blood flow. When it has gone this far, there is very little hope for the patient.

The effect of shock on the lungs is a comparatively newly recognized condition. The effect, called shock lung, can occur even in apparently fit young people who have had large-volume blood transfusions after an accident. Patients who have this complication become breathless, and the level of oxygen in the blood starts to fall. There is also extensive shadowing on chest X rays.

What happens is this: the lung acts as a filter to any abnormal substances circulating in the blood, and, because it is common for transfused blood to contain a few little clumps of cells, these get caught up in the fine capillaries in the lungs and cause a blockage. The basis of most treatment is to take over the function of the lungs by placing the patient on a respirator.

Treatment of shock

The aim of treatment for shock in all its forms is to try to return the volume of blood in the circulation to normal so that the heart can pump normally and an adequate amount of blood flows to the tissues. When blood loss has been the cause of shock, then the

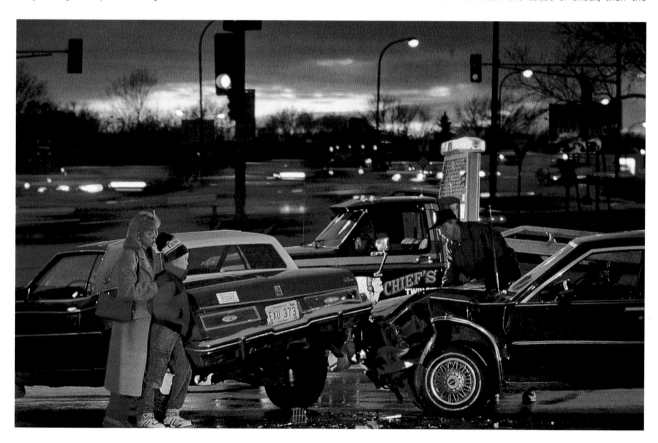

▲ *Car accidents are a major cause of injury and shock. Patients suffering from shock need constant attention, as their condition can change dramatically at any moment. They should be kept cool to conserve blood vital for the heart and brain.*

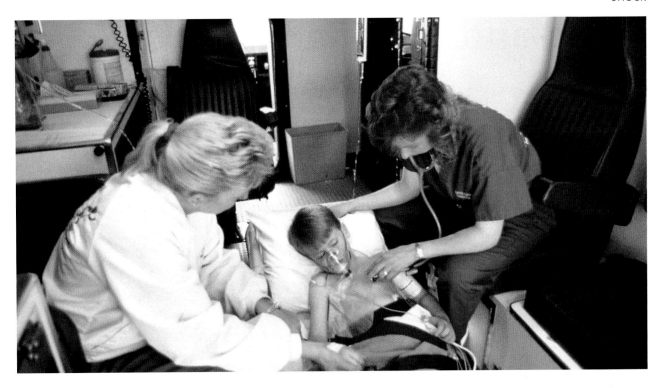

▲ *Paramedics care for an injured child in a large ambulance van immediately after a traffic accident.*

treatment is simply a transfusion of the correct amount of blood to bring the volume back to normal. When the shock is due to septicemia, the body still needs fluid even though the blood is pooled in the blood vessels. In this instance, clear fluids in the form of salt or sugar solutions or protein fluids such as plasma are used.

However, there can be problems in giving large amounts of blood or fluid to older patients, since these additional fluids can overload the heart and lead to heart failure. Doctors have to get around this problem, and to do this they have to keep a balance between having too much and too little fluid in the circulation. They measure fluid by checking the pressure in the right atrium of the heart.

This pressure measurement is called the central venous pressure (CVP). To take the pressure, a fine tube is passed into a vein in the leg or neck and the pressure is measured outside the body using a simple column of water. If the pressure is too high there is too much fluid; if it is too low there is not enough.

Shock caused by a heart attack (cardiogenic shock) cannot, however, be treated by a blood transfusion. Common forms of treatment include drugs that make the heart work harder (inotropic drugs such as digoxin) and drugs that reduce the amount of work it has to do. Drugs that make it work harder, however, can place a great strain on a weakened heart.

One technique that gets around some of these problems is a device called a balloon pump. A long sausage-shaped balloon is inserted at the top of the aorta, the biggest artery from the heart, and connected by a tube to a pump outside the body. The balloon is inflated between heartbeats to help force blood out along the arteries, reducing the amount of work the heart has to do and raising the blood pressure. When the balloon deflates, it allows more blood to be pumped from the heart into the aorta; when it inflates, it forces the blood around.

First aid for shock

In giving first aid for shock, it is important to diagnose and treat the cause of shock, rather than to diagnose and treat the shock itself. Very often the cause of shock is obvious: in a traffic accident, for example, the cause is generally major blood loss. The victim will often be dizzy; he or she may vomit or completely lose consciousness. The skin color will be very pale and the pulse rapid.

The victim should be laid flat with his or her legs slightly raised; this stimulates blood flow to the brain. He or she should be kept cool to ensure that blood continues to circulate to the heart and brain. Giving him or her liquids should be avoided, as these may make surgery difficult once the patient has reached the hospital. Above all, it is important to make sure that an ambulance is called promptly.

Outlook

The outlook for the patient with shock depends a lot on the fitness of the person before the condition developed and on what was the cause of the shock.

A fit person who loses a lot of blood in a traffic accident but whose injuries are not too serious should do well after a blood transfusion and treatment for the physical damage. However, an older patient who gets shock caused by infection after surgery is at much greater risk. Also, someone who develops kidney failure or shock lung is in a much more risky situation. The outlook for the person with cardiogenic shock is at present very poor.

See also: **Allergies; Bites and stings; Burns; Counseling; Heart attack; Infection and infectious diseases; Ulcers**

Sleep and sleep problems

Why can some people wake up and leap out of bed early, while I find getting up a real problem?

Patterns of sleeping and wakefulness are based on the way people's personal internal clocks work. Some people normally wake and get up early, whereas others go on feeling lively late into the night, but have trouble getting going in the morning—the night owls. Each group, in fact, has about the same amount of sleep, but it occurs at different times.

Why do babies spend so much time asleep?

Babies need to do a lot of growing in size and weight during their first few months of life, and sleep both conserves their energy and is a time when growth processes function best. Many people think that infants ought to spend virtually the whole of the 24 hours asleep, but this is not necessary. Other people think that most babies actually do spend almost all their time asleep. A few may, but if infants are observed around the clock, their total daily sleeping time turns out to be about 14 hours.

Are there aids to natural sleep?

Yes, several. A tired body and a quiet mind are important, so physical exercise, and mental relaxation in the form of reading, music, or television, can all help.

Is it possible to learn from tape-recorded information while asleep?

No. While you are asleep, your brain is not active enough to take in new material. The first half of the day, when your mind is rested, fresh, and uncluttered, is the best time to study and retain information, though of course many students study late at night.

People spend more of their lives asleep than in any other single activity. Difficulties in sleeping are very trying but can usually be overcome without recourse to sleeping pills, which should be regarded as only a last resort.

During a normal day people use up energy and tire themselves both physically and mentally. If people try to do without regular periods of rest they become exhausted. The most complete form of rest is sleep: for body and mind to be fresh and healthy, and to work efficiently, everyone needs to spend a part of every 24 hours sleeping. The body and mind do not stop working altogether during sleep; breathing continues and the heart continues to beat. Indeed, many parts of the body never rest; the eyelids flicker, people usually turn over several times

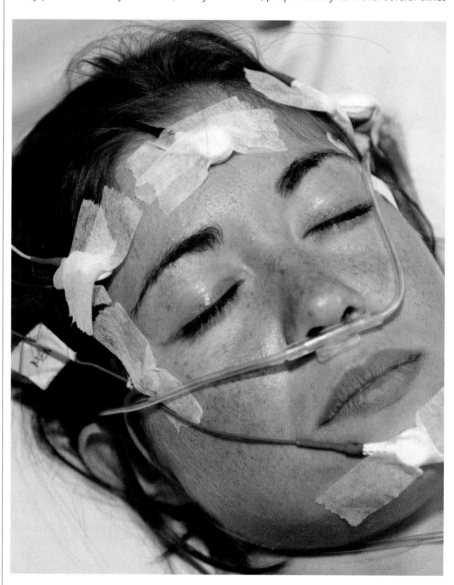

▲ *A woman is investigated for insomnia in a sleep observation laboratory.*

and kick about, and some people talk and even walk about while they are asleep. Even though vital processes, like respiration and the circulation of blood, continue while people are asleep, they do so at a much slower rate.

Brain activity

The sleep-wakefulness controls are located in the brain stem. Unless the brain cortex of the cerebral hemisphere, the thinking part of the brain, is activated by the brain stem, it is too torpid for conscious intellectual activity and it is said to be asleep. When someone is awake, the cerebral hemispheres are at a high pitch of activity, enabling the person to understand and respond to the things he or she sees and hears. The spinal cord is also highly tuned; it receives instructions from the brain to fire off carefully adjusted nerve messages that travel from the spinal cord cells along nerves to the muscles, which make the limbs move. Responsiveness in the cerebral cortex and in the spinal cord is brought about by electrical influences from the brain stem. When someone is awake the brain stem pours these currents along nerve channels and activates the cerebral hemispheres and spinal cord; the person then wakes up.

Several factors cause the brain stem sleep-wakefulness center to bring about wakefulness or sleep. What could be called a chemical clock induces sleep every 24 to 26 hours. The setting of the chemical

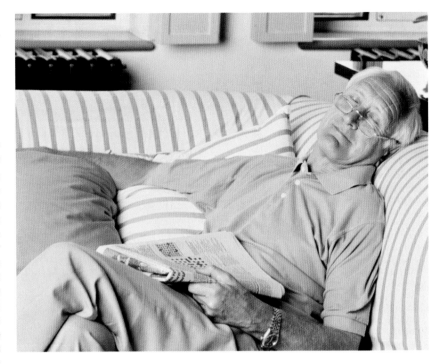

▲ *Relaxing in a comfortable, warm environment is enough to induce sleep.*

clock is quite difficult to change, as becomes evident after a long flight to a country in a different time zone—France, for example, where clocks are set five to eight hours ahead of those in America. For the first week in a different time zone people sleep very late in the morning but feel wide awake when most inhabitants are going to bed. The sleep-wakefulness center is also much affected by lack of sleep. Of most importance are events taking place and their significance. No matter how sleepy a person feels, if a disturbance occurs, he or she will almost certainly wake up. The brain stem centers are stimulated by physical sensations, and especially by a change of sensation, but it is not only nerve messages from the body's sense organs that are stimulating during sleep. The sleep-wakefulness center also receives messages from the cortex of the cerebral hemispheres, so that any anxiety present in the mind bombards the brain stem with stimulating messages that induce wakefulness.

Another factor in keeping someone awake is new sensations. If the sights and sounds in the environment are monotonous and a person is immobile, there is nothing new to stimulate the brain stem, and sleep comes easily. A continuous rhythm, such as the clattering of train wheels, will add to the effect. A warm temperature and a comfortable chair will also help to bring about relaxation and sleep.

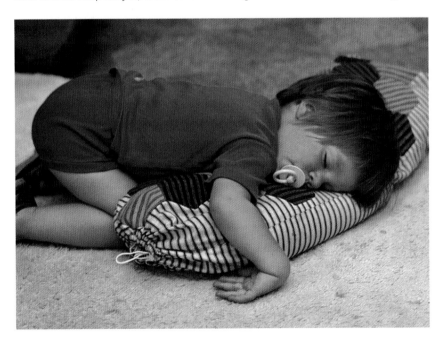

▲ *Young children sometimes resist daytime rests, but a comforter such as a special cushion or a pacifier can help a child relax enough to fall asleep.*

Questions and Answers

What is the best way to deal with children's nightmares?

Just as adults have nightmares, children have night terrors that they find frightening and distressing. The child may be temporarily disoriented during these episodes but usually the horror subsides and the child falls asleep again. However, the memory of the fear may linger, making the child fearful of going to bed or being left alone. Reprimanding or pleading with a child in this state is ineffectual; the child may feel rejected, and this will make the situation worse. The child finds nightly terror very real, so stay and read some stories, stroking the child's hair until he or she has fallen asleep. Keep a night-light on as well.

What are the dangers of taking sleeping pills on a regular basis?

It is undesirable to rely on drugs for a natural function like sleep. One problem is that some of the drugs have prolonged action and cause drowsiness the next day. It is often thought that since barbiturates were replaced by benzodiazepines, addiction to sleeping pills is less common. This is not so; drug dependence occurs with prolonged normal dosage of the newer drugs, and withdrawal symptoms—anxiety, agitation, irritability, and confusion—can be expected. Benzodiazepine drugs should be withdrawn gradually. Withdrawal symptoms will settle in three to four weeks depending on the personality of the patient.

Can prolonged sleeplessness make someone sick?

After about 60 hours without sleep a person will start seeing things that aren't there, or will fail to notice things that are. It becomes difficult to concentrate for more than a minute or so, and by 90 hours a person may suffer hallucinations. By 100 hours there may be signs of delirium. However, these symptoms persist only while sleep deprivation lasts.

HOW THE BRAIN CONTROLS SLEEP

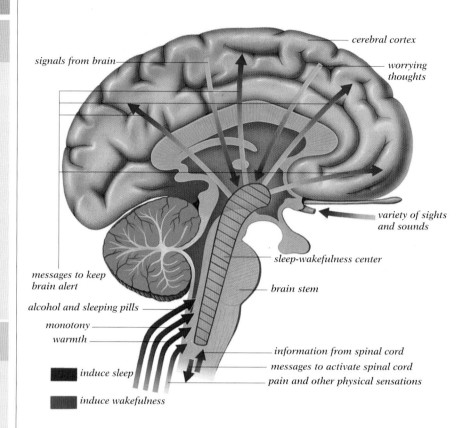

▲ *The sleep-wakefulness center is located in the brain stem. Stimulated by information, including physical sensations, it passes messages to the cerebral cortex, which determines whether we fall asleep or stay awake. It also responds to signals from the cerebral cortex, so that a worrying thought can keep us awake. Equally, a quiet mind, warmth, certain drugs, and even monotony will induce sleep. The brain waves change as we become drowsy, sleep, and subsequently wake up refreshed.*

The brain stem centers are also affected by chemicals and drugs. Some, such as amphetamines, will prevent sleep whereas others, such as alcohol or sleeping pills, will have the opposite effect and cause drowsiness.

How much sleep do we need?

There are rare people who regularly devote less than three hours to sleep, and others who demand more than nine hours—everyone is different. The majority of adults average just under eight hours, while children sleep longer and older people sleep less than average.

Over a short period of time, a sleep debt can accumulate and, if someone is forced to make do with just a few hours of sleep for a period of days or weeks, it will take more than an average eight hours at the weekend or on vacation to compensate. Although at times someone may manage to keep going on a reduced sleep ration, he or she probably does not feel really well and almost certainly are not as efficient, nor so attentive to detail in daily tasks.

Dreaming

No one can do without sleep; and everyone needs two different kinds of sleep. A definite pattern of events occurs during prolonged sleep; there will be increased restlessness, changes in the electrical brain waves, and spells of rapid eye movement which happen about every one and a half hours, and which last for 20 minutes each time. If people are deliberately woken during the

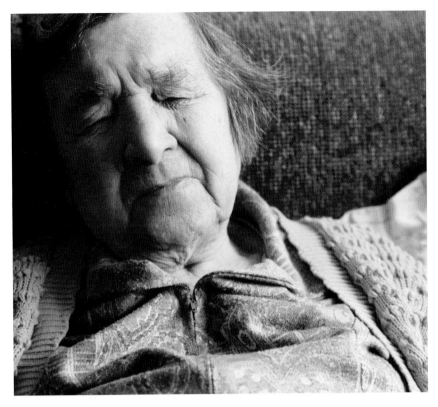

▲ *Elderly people like this woman often find it very easy to slip into a light sleep or doze, and can awake from it just as easily.*

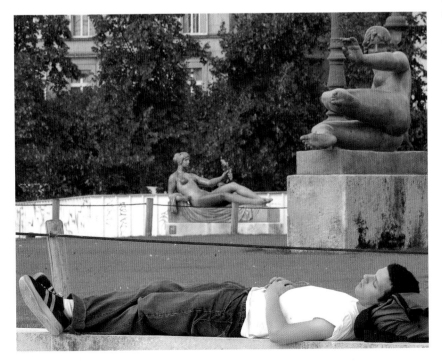

▲ *After eating or drinking, fresh air and sunshine can induce relaxation and then sleep—even on a rather uncomfortable bed.*

rapid eye movement periods, they usually say they have just been dreaming. If woken at other times they usually say they have not been dreaming and, indeed, have apparently forgotten the dream that presumably accompanied the previous rapid eye movement period. They may say they had been reviewing the day's events; not colorful, adventurous dreaming, but nevertheless not a total absence of mental life. Mental activity therefore seems to continue, often at a low ebb, throughout the whole period of sleep, although most people scarcely remember it.

REM sleep

The rapid eye movement phase of sleep is known as REM, or paradoxical, sleep. In these phases the electrical brain waves are faster than in the orthodox, non-rapid eye movement or NREM phases. The heart rate, breathing, and blood pressure undergo rapid fluctuations during paradoxical sleep, especially at the time of a sudden flurry of eye movements. Most bodily muscles are completely relaxed, the usual reflexes are absent, in men the penis is often erect, the blood flows more rapidly through the brain, and less flows through the muscles. At these times there is dreaming.

Mental activity during REM sleep is concerned with sorting out and making sense of disconnected items of memorized material. In the orthodox phase of sleep into which we always pass for an hour or so before moving into the paradoxical phase, brain waves are large and slow. Electrical activity of most individual brain cells is reduced, but at this time growth hormone is poured into the blood.

Adults do not grow taller, but growth, repair, and the renewal of many tissues, such as skin, liver, or blood-forming cells in the bone marrow, must continue. At some unknown signal from the chemical clock, these cells start to divide as the usual time for sleep approaches. Then, during the orthodox sleep phase, growth hormone is released. It is this hormone that helps the newly divided cells of the body to grow into complete new cells.

Adults do not grow new brain cells, although they do still need to renew the cells' constituents. It seems that the paradoxical phase of sleep, with plenty of blood flowing through the brain, is a time when this renewal is most active. When the brain is actually growing, at the time of birth, the paradoxical phase takes up twice the proportion of sleep it does a few months later, when brain growth has slowed down.

Babies and sleep

A favorite remark of many child care experts is that young babies do not suffer from sleep problems—but their parents do. In general a baby will sleep when, and for as long as, it needs. Problems arise only when a baby does not seem to need the amount of sleep that its parents think appropriate. At this stage a baby cannot inhibit sleep or wake up on purpose. It makes no difference to a baby if it sleeps all day and plays all night, but its parents cannot afford to follow a similar pattern. A baby has to be gradually persuaded to accept the usual daily rhythm of sleeping at night. Most people surface several times in the night, and babies are no exception. If each of a baby's brief awakenings brings a hovering, anxious parent to its side, a baby will not ignore an opportunity for sociability. An overattentive mother can prevent her baby from learning to settle back to sleep by itself, and therefore reinforces a pattern of disturbed sleep.

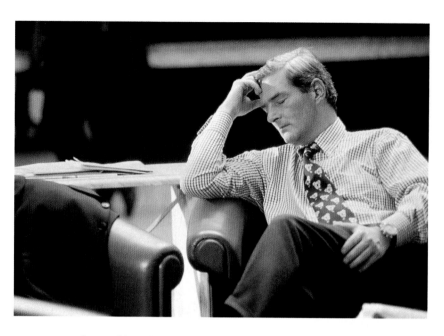

▲ *Some people are able to function after only three hours of sleep a night. Many people can catnap during their working day and wake completely refreshed.*

While slight rustlings and grumbles are probably best ignored, loud crying demands prompt attention. Toward the second year of life, nightmares begin to be common, although in a child not yet talking we cannot know much about such night fears. A child wakes suddenly, usually with a scream, and gives every appearance of being terrified. Usually all that is needed is a reassuring hug to settle the child back to sleep.

Problems in persuading a child to fall asleep in the first place can also arise around this time. Often it seems that what a baby resents is not sleep itself but the separation from its mother that sleep entails. Parents have to try to get a child to understand that there is no need to cry because there is no danger of being abandoned, and that there is no point in crying because it is now time to sleep. Visiting a child every five minutes or so while he or she continues to fuss, but staying just long enough to smile and repeat good night can often help a child to settle. If left alone to cry, a child will eventually exhaust itself and fall asleep, but he or she may be quicker to make a fuss the following night.

Insomnia

Difficulties in sleeping are a common and disturbing adult complaint. Insomnia may manifest itself as difficulty in getting to sleep, interrupted sleep, or waking too early. Worry, tension, and depression are by far the most common causes, but pain, uncomfortable surroundings, fever, breathing difficulties on lying down (orthopnea), a need to pass urine frequently, and dyspepsia that is worse on lying down—for example, if someone has a hiatus hernia—may also give rise to insomnia.

Persistent sleeplessness soon begins to cause daytime problems such as drowsiness, lack of concentration, and irritability. There are many ways people can help themselves if they suffer from sleeplessness. It is important to make sure that no unresolved tensions are left over from the day, because tension and stress are common causes of sleep problems. If possible, family arguments should be settled before it is time to sleep. An exercise that can help is for someone, once in bed, to go over all the events of the day from the time of awakening. Events happen so fast during the day that the mind cannot digest them properly, and this can disturb sleep.

The environment for sleeping is important. Quietness, warmth, and a firm mattress are good investments. Adequate physical fatigue can be important; it helps if the body is tired as well as the mind. If a person does not get much exercise at work, a late-night walk can be a successful way of dealing with insomnia. When someone is trying to resolve a problem in the mind that prevents relaxation and sleep, spending half an hour reading a good book or listening to music is much less stressful, and more effective, than being wakeful in bed.

Any difficulty in sleeping that goes on for more than two weeks should be referred to a doctor. By this time the cause needs to be identified and treated. Sleeping pills and tranquilizers should be regarded as a last resort; they are addictive and have the effect of changing someone into a person who is less alert, less aware, and less alive. However, there are times of exceptional stress and upset in most people's lives when they may have to resort to pills or tranquilizers for short periods. If such drugs are prescribed, a doctor's advice must be followed on how to take them, but a recommended way is to take an adequate dose about half an hour before bedtime in order to ensure sleep.

This regimen should be followed for three, four, or five nights; then the dose should be halved on the succeeding three nights; after that, a person should take the pills only if he or she is still feeling restless an hour after going to bed.

See also: **Stress**

Slipped disk

A slipped, or prolapsed, disk can cause a lot of pain and temporarily restrict normal movement. In a large majority of cases, however, letting nature take its course results in a patient's full recovery.

Questions and Answers

Does sleeping with a board under the mattress help to prevent a slipped disk?

No, it won't prevent a slipped disk from occurring. Many people with back problems find that a firm mattress helps their back because it is more comfortable. A soft mattress can sag in the middle so that lying on the bed bends the back. This is an uncomfortable position; you would not like to walk about all day with a bent back. Putting a hard board under a soft mattress is an inexpensive and effective way of making a bed more comfortable.

Are women more prone to slipped disks than men?

No. Two to three times as many men as women suffer from a slipped disk. The reasons for this are not clear, and, contrary to popular belief, heavy physical work is not associated with a greater risk of a slipped disk. However, a slipped disk is obviously more troublesome to a heavy manual worker than to someone with a sedentary lifestyle. Pregnant women are much more likely to develop a slipped disk. The increase in weight puts an additional strain on the back. Hormones secreted during pregnancy may also cause a general softening of the ligaments and the muscles.

What causes a slipped disk to rupture and what happens?

All slipped disks are in fact ruptured disks. The disk is made of a tough outer ring and a soft inner core. A slipped disk occurs when the tough outer ring weakens, so the soft inner material bulges out and presses on the nerves of the spinal cord. If the outer ring cracks, the inner material can escape into the area of the spinal cord.

CLASSIC SLIPPED DISK

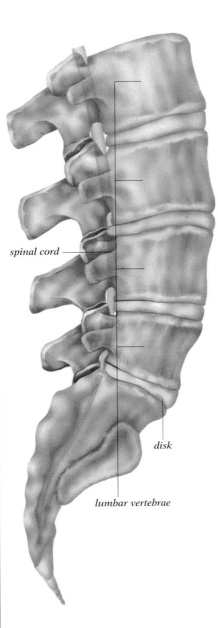

spinal cord

disk

lumbar vertebrae

▲ *A slipped disk usually occurs in the lower spine (the lumbar region).*

Back problems are an extremely common cause of pain and suffering, and many days of work are lost in the United States through backache. There are many causes of back problems, of which a slipped disk is only one of a range of possibilities. Although many cases of backache improve with time, medical treatment should be sought if the pain is persistent or particularly severe.

What is a slipped disk?

The disks are pads of tissue situated between each of the vertebrae that make up the spinal column. Each disk consists of a tough, fibrous outer ring called the annulus fibrosus and a softer, jellylike inner layer called the nucleus pulposus. The function of the disk is to act as both a strong connection between the vertebrae and a cushion to absorb weight on the spinal column.

A slipped disk does not really slip; the tough outer fibrous ring (annulus) cracks open and the softer inner layer protrudes (prolapses) through the crack, like toothpaste

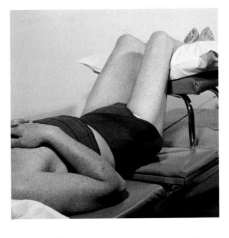

▲ *More than 90 percent of people with a slipped disk recover after just a short period of bed rest. If the symptoms persist, patients may have to spend time in the hospital with their legs supported in such a way that pressure on the nerves can be relieved.*

coming out through a crack in a toothpaste tube. For this reason doctors prefer to speak of a disk prolapse rather than a slipped disk.

The nucleus of a disk is softest and most jellylike during childhood. Over the years the nucleus gradually dries out so that by middle age it has a consistency similar to crabmeat. As someone gets older, the nucleus becomes even firmer. In elderly people the disk is mainly a section of scar tissue; this accounts for the fact that old people lose height. Disk protrusion occurs less frequently as people get older; it is a disorder affecting young adults and people in early middle-age. Disk protrusion occurs where the outer layer of the disk is weakest; that is, just in front of the nerve roots, which emerge from the spinal cord at each vertebral level. There is very little free space within the spinal canal, and the protruding disk material presses on the nerve root at that level and causes the painful symptoms of a slipped disk.

The area of the spine most likely to be affected is the lowermost part of the back. Here the greatest strains occur, and it is not surprising that most disks that fail are at this level. However, it is possible for disks to prolapse at any level along the length of the spinal column—in the back or the neck.

Causes

The disk begins to prolapse when a crack develops in its tough outer ring. This is usually the effect of wear and tear in the back as a result of normal aging. One particularly heavy or awkward lift, a fall, or even a sudden cough or sneeze may force some of the soft disk nucleus to prolapse, leading to sudden symptoms.

Symptoms

When a prolapsing disk presses on a nerve root, symptoms occur both in the back and in the area that the nerve root supplies. For example, a slipped disk in the lower back can cause pain in the legs.

Symptoms in the back can include severe backache. Often the sufferer will not be able to localize the pain with any accuracy. He or she may also develop painful spasms in the muscles that lie along each side of the spine, particularly in the early stages. The patient will feel more pain when moving about and some relief when lying flat. Coughing or sneezing can cause the prolapsing disk material to bulge out suddenly, causing a sharp pain in the back or legs. In addition there may be a curvature of the spine—the patient unconsciously leans away from the side of the disk prolapse to try to relieve the pressure from the nerve root that is involved.

If the pressure on the nerve root is not too severe, the nerve will continue to work but will be painful. The brain cannot tell that the painful pressure is coming from the area of the disk, but instead interprets the information as pain originating in the nerve end. In a lower-back disk protrusion the sciatic nerve can be irritated, and the individual may feel pain in the thigh, calf, ankle, or foot. This pain can shoot down a leg and is then called sciatica.

More severe pressure on the nerve root may cause the nerve to stop functioning altogether. Areas of skin that the nerve supplies will become numb, so that a light touch or even a pinprick cannot be felt. Muscles supplied by the nerve will become weak or even completely paralyzed. Reflexes such as the knee-jerk reflex may disappear. If only one nerve root is involved this is not too serious, because each nerve supplies only a small area of skin, or a limited number of muscles. If the nerves to the bladder or genitals are affected, however, their function can be permanently lost.

Urgent medical attention is needed to relieve the pressure on these nerves.

Treatment

Well over 90 percent of people with acute disk protrusions get better simply by resting in bed. The soft inner disk material tends to dry up and shrink once it has prolapsed, thus relieving the pressure on the nerve root. The main form of treatment is rest. Once the doctor has examined the individual and confirmed that there is a straightforward disk prolapse, he or she will advise the patient to rest as much as possible by lying flat in bed. In the horizontal position the pressure within the disk (acting in order to force out the soft inner material) is minimal. In the standing position this pressure is higher, and when the back is bent—for example, when a person is sitting or bending over—the pressure is much higher. A soft bed also bends the back, so it is best to put boards under the mattress or even to put the mattress on the floor.

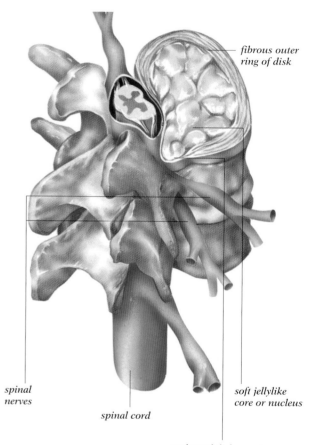

fibrous outer ring of disk

spinal nerves

spinal cord

soft jellylike core or nucleus

prolapsed disk pressing on a spinal nerve

▲ *A slipped disk most frequently occurs in the lower spine. The tough outer layer of the disk weakens, allowing the soft inner core, or nucleus, to bulge out, causing pain and muscle weakness. When the protrusion presses on a nearby spinal nerve, feeling may be lost in the lower part of the body.*

I strained my back when lifting a heavy chair. Does this mean I had a slipped disk?

The back consists of a series of bones, ligaments, disks, and muscles. Injury to any of these may occur in lifting heavy objects incorrectly. This can cause acute pain in the back, which may extend to the legs. Get your doctor to establish if the pain was caused by a slipped disk.

Is it possible to cure a slipped disk by surgery?

Yes. Although 90 percent of people suffering from a slipped disk recover within two months, a small number of patients will need surgery. Such operations are used for patients whose slipped disk has shown up clearly on a special X ray and who have not responded to other treatment. Occasionally a patient with a severe slipped disk, which is pressing on the nerves to the bladder, will need emergency treatment to relieve the pressure. Surgery for slipped disks is successful in the vast majority of cases. Around 85 percent of patients recover from their back pain, or else their condition is greatly improved.

My doctor thinks that I may have a slipped disk, and she is sending me to the hospital to have a spinal X ray. Can you tell me what will happen?

The X ray your doctor has recommended is called a myelogram. A dye is injected into the membranes surrounding the nerves in the spinal cord. This dye is opaque to X rays. If you have a slipped disk, the disk will protrude and this will show up as an indentation in the column of dye. If an emerging nerve is not outlined by the dye, this shows that the nerve has been compressed.

An operation, called a laminectomy, may then be performed to push aside the spinal cord and nerve roots in order to remove the disk material.

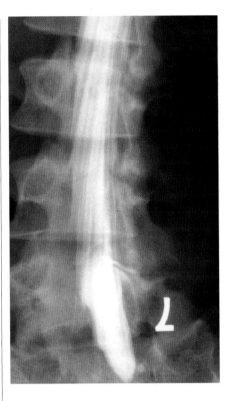

▲ *A special X ray, a myelogram (above), is used to diagnose a slipped disk.*

Painkilling drugs are of help in alleviating the pain in acute disk prolapse, although they will probably not take it away altogether. Drugs that relax the muscles, such as diazepam (Valium), help to settle painful muscle spasm.

Most patients with a slipped disk will get better after a short period of bed rest followed by a controlled exercise program. However, great patience is needed. Getting up too soon or exercising too strenuously will often result in a relapse.

Patients who fail to make a recovery after a proper course of bed rest may require further treatment. This may entail a period of hospitalization, perhaps with traction to the legs to help relieve the pain.

A magnetic resonance scan may be useful to determine whether the disk has prolapsed. If this fails, a special X ray may be necessary. X rays show only the bones of the spine—the disk itself shows only as a space between the bones. This space is altered in an acute disk prolapse. The special X ray is called a myelogram or radiculogram. A dye that shows up on X rays is injected into the space just outside the spinal canal; if the disk has in fact prolapsed, it will show as an indentation in the column of dye.

BACK STRAIN AND PRESSURE

The vertebrae in the small of the back (lumbar vertebrae) take most strain. This chart assumes that when you are standing the pressure on your lumbar vertebrae is normal, or 1.00. Pressure is reduced to 0.25, or a quarter, when you are lying flat, but increases threefold if you are sitting while holding weights.

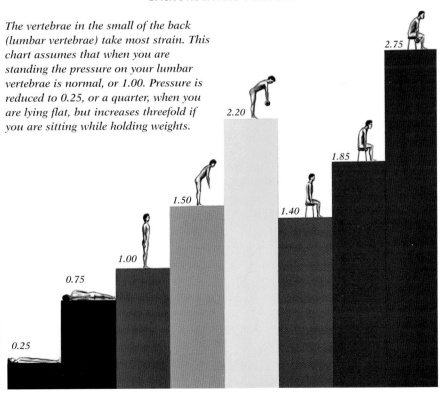

Surgery to remove prolapsed disk material may be necessary if bed rest fails to improve the symptoms, if there are signs of rapidly worsening function of nerve roots, or if the nerves to the bladder or the genitals are involved.

The operation (a laminectomy) involves making a small opening in the bones surrounding the spinal cord and gently pushing them aside, along with the nerve roots, to remove the disk material. Patients can usually become mobile within two weeks of this surgery.

Surgery for prolapsed disk has developed a bad reputation among the public, probably because in the past diagnosis was not always accurate and careful selection of those patients most likely to benefit from surgery was not always undertaken. With modern methods the success rate of surgery is high.

Many people suffering from disk prolapse receive other forms of treatment such as physical therapy and manipulation. Physical therapy may consist of heat treatment, which temporarily lessens the pain, and traction exercises. Traction helps to relieve pain by decreasing muscle spasm. Exercises help to strengthen the muscles of the back and stomach so that they can take strain off the bones and joints in the spine.

Manipulation is practiced by many physical therapists, some doctors, and all osteopaths. The aim is to move the protruding disk material away from its point of contact with the nerve root and to free the nerve from any inflammation. There is no evidence to show that the soft prolapsing disk material can actually be returned to the firm outer casing—this would be like trying to put toothpaste back into its tube—but enough movement to take some pressure off the nerve root may be achieved. Manipulation is probably more useful in other types of back disorders, although some individuals receive excellent results for prolapsed disk.

Another useful treatment is to administer an epidural injection. A quantity of local anesthesia mixed with steroids is injected into the space just outside the spinal canal, so that it reaches the nerve roots where they emerge from the spinal cord. This is often combined with manipulation of the legs in order to move the sciatic nerve and to break down any small pieces of scar tissue that have formed around the nerve roots. This treatment is used when sciatica persists after the other signs of an acute disk prolapse have settled. It often gives immediate relief from pain.

Other aids

Back supports, corsets, and plaster jackets are used by some doctors to prevent patients from bending their backs during the recovery period after a disk prolapse. Long-term use of a corset tends to weaken the back muscles so that the patient becomes uncomfortable when not wearing the support.

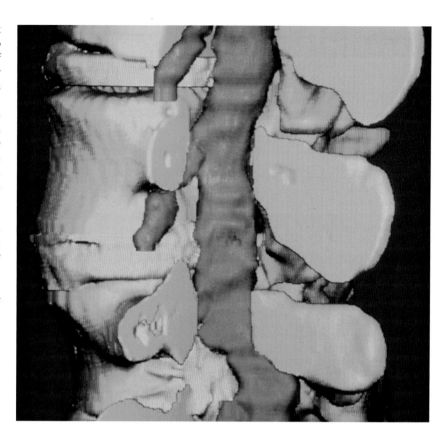

▲ *A CT scan clearly shows a slipped disk (yellow; lower center) pressing against the spinal cord (dark blue). The vertebrae (light blue) have been revealed in cross section by computer image manipulation.*

Prevention

People who have suffered from a disk prolapse and those who are at risk of a prolapse because of their occupation must learn to look after their backs. Proper lifting procedures such as keeping the back straight, bending at the knees rather than bending the back when picking things up from the floor, and avoiding lifting too much weight are important. It is also vital to keep body weight under control. Extra weight puts additional strain on the back. Regular exercise will increase the efficiency of the back muscles. Swimming is a particularly beneficial form of exercise, since the effects of gravity are eliminated and the back is not placed under undue strain.

Outlook

Some individuals fail to make a full recovery even after they have received adequate treatment. It may be necessary for people in strenuous occupations to find a less demanding job. The sufferer may have to change to a less active lifestyle and also recognize factors that affect the back. The sympathetic understanding of employers, relatives, and friends is important for such people.

The large majority of people who suffer from disk prolapse recover completely and are able to return to their previous activities. The recovery process may take several months, but patience is usually rewarded with a good result.

See also: Exercise; Physical therapy; X rays

Smoking

Questions and Answers

Will nicotine chewing gum or patches help me quit smoking?

Yes. Trials have shown that nicotine chewing gum and transdermal patches do reduce the craving for a cigarette, which is a common cause of failure in the first weeks of trying to give up smoking. They are effective antismoking aids worth trying.

I have tried, but I cannot give up smoking. Can I do anything to reduce the risk of getting a smoking-related disease?

Yes, there are several things that are worth doing. First, move down the scale of tar content step by step from high, to middle to high, to middle, and so on until you are smoking low-tar cigarettes. Second, on no account smoke any more cigarettes than your daily minimum. Use filter-tipped cigarettes; the benefit is not dramatic but it's enough to make some difference. Third, try not to inhale. Even though some of the nicotine is absorbed through the mouth and throat there are still advantages. Try to smoke less by gradually increasing the interval between cigarettes, leaving very long stubs, taking the cigarette out of your mouth between puffs, and increasing the interval between puffs.

My five-year-old daughter has asthma. I smoked very heavily during pregnancy. Did this cause her condition?

Children of mothers who smoke during pregnancy do have health disadvantages. They have a lower level of resistance that makes them more prone to infectious diseases, and they are usually slower to develop both physically and mentally. However, there is no evidence that asthma in children is caused by the mother smoking when pregnant.

The phrase "dying for a cigarette" is brutally apt. Fatal smoking-related diseases constitute a genuine epidemic and, unusually, it is one that is solely in the hands of the potential victims to eradicate.

Smoking the dried leaves of the tobacco plant in the form of cigarettes or cigars or in pipes was introduced into England around the middle of the 16th century by explorers and adventurers who had found the practice established in the New World. Consumption of tobacco in industrialized countries continued to increase until 1973, and then began to fall, but it remains among the most common habits in the Western world. It is an extremely dangerous habit with no less than lethal consequences for a very large proportion of those who indulge in it. And it is an addiction that is difficult to break.

Why do people smoke?

People smoke for a wide variety of reasons. Once they have smoked their first few experimental cigarettes, which can cause coughing, nausea, and sometimes vomiting, most smokers get pleasure from the taste and aroma of tobacco and tobacco smoke. They may also get pleasure from the whole ritual of lighting up: from handling cigarettes, a lighter, or matches; from the action of inhaling; and from watching the smoke curl upward.

Smokers make two claims for their habit: first, that smoking sedates them, or settles their nerves, when they need sedating; second, that it acts as a stimulant when they need to work. Evidence has shown that these effects are due to nicotine and that both these claims are true, depending on the dose, on what the smoker is doing, and on his or her particular psychological and physical makeup. There is also a true physical addiction to nicotine so that when deprived of the drug the person concerned suffers from unpleasant physical withdrawal symptoms which

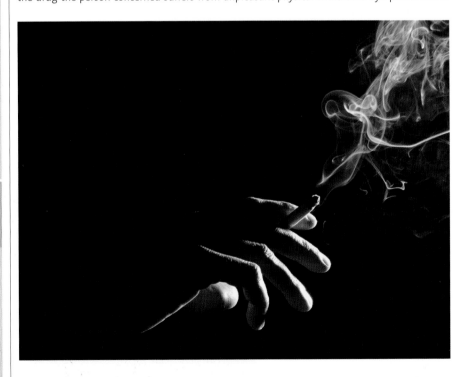

▲ *The sight and smell of cigarettes is unpleasant, but far more important than these aesthetic considerations, cigarettes are dangerous to health.*

Questions and Answers

How efficient are filters in actually removing harmful substances from cigarette smoke?

Putting a filter on a cigarette certainly reduces the tar and nicotine your body absorbs. In addition, there is evidence that people who smoke filter-tipped cigarettes are at less risk of getting lung cancer. So there certainly is some advantage. However, the benefit is certainly not so great that it is safe to smoke filter cigarettes. Probably the best that can be said for them is that if you cannot give up altogether, they are a little less dangerous than nonfilter brands.

Why do doctors tell you that if you must smoke, smoke only the first half of the cigarette?

For two reasons. The first is that the tar concentration in the bottom half of the cigarette, and particularly in the stub, is very much greater than in the top half. If you smoke only the top half of the cigarette, or at least leave a long stub, you are doing yourself a favor. The second reason is that any change in your habit which has the effect of decreasing the total amount that you actually smoke will benefit you by a similar amount. That is why those who have not been able to give up are strongly encouraged to at least try to make do with only half a cigarette at a time.

I stopped smoking five years ago. Will my lungs have returned to a normally healthy state?

That really depends on how long and how heavily you smoked before you gave up the habit. What is certain is that further damage to your lungs—and other parts of your body—stops from the time you give it up. It is clear that there is an improvement in lung capacity and your chances of getting either lung cancer or bronchitis drop. After 12 to 15 years of not smoking, the risk of developing lung cancer is the same as if you had never smoked.

are relieved only by a further dose. Dependence on smoking may be psychological as well as physical; smokers miss whatever enjoyment they get from smoking but do not really need it. Often, too, smoking has become such an ingrained habit that the smoker has a cigarette almost without being aware of it.

Some people smoke because they associate smoking with sociability. To offer and to take cigarettes establishes a bond between people. To the shy and introverted, it offers something for them to do with their hands and makes them appear self-confident. The smoker may smoke as much to be one of the company as to get pleasure from smoking. The pleasure comes from being with others and not from the cigarette.

The climate of opinion prevailing is an important factor in determining smoking, and over the last few years much has been done to try to discourage smokers. In more and more countries, smoking is now banned in public places such as movie theaters and subways. Many restaurants, bars, and places of work have adopted a no-smoking policy and it is no longer assumed that everyone wishes to be in

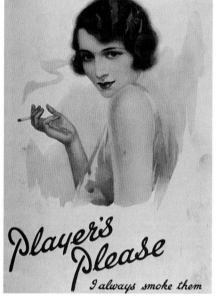

Player's Please

I always smoke them

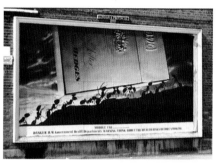

▼▲ *In the past, cigarette advertisers freely promoted the image of smoking as a sophisticated, and even, by associating it with the rigors of outdoor life, healthy activity. Now that there is evidence of the risks smokers run, and strict curbs have been placed on cigarette advertising, things are not so simple for the tobacco companies. They now have to advertise their products more obliquely, and with health warnings attached that sometimes loom larger than the advertisement itself. The sponsorship of sport is one of the principal means the industry uses to promote its product, although there are now moves to ban the practice.*

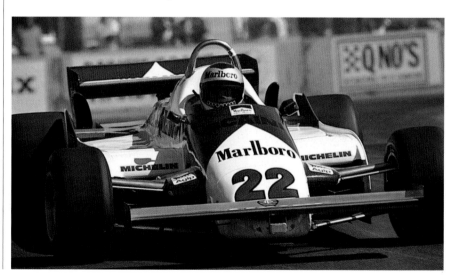

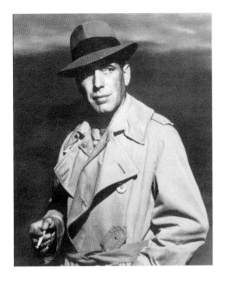

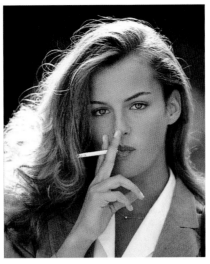

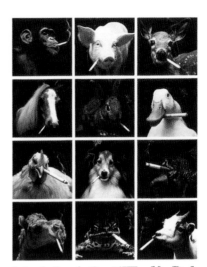

It Looks Just As Stupid When You Do It.

The glamorous image that smoking developed in film and fashion concealed the cost in health. Humphrey Bogart died from throat cancer.

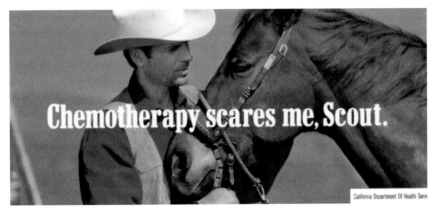

Chemotherapy scares me, Scout.

California Department Of Health Serv

▲ *Showing animals smoking and looking rather silly was meant to appeal to young people to make them realize how uncool smoking can appear to other people.*

◄ *This controversial billboard advertisement attempts to inspire fear in would-be smokers by using well-known images and twisting the text to get the message across.*

▼ *Antitobacco advertising is aimed at teens, who are most vulnerable to starting smoking. This stained-glass image was part of an antismoking campaign in 2003.*

smoke-filled environments. Some states are now pressing, and winning, claims for damages against the tobacco industry (which is worth billions of dollars) in order to finance the growing costs of health care resulting from smoking-related diseases.

Factors in starting smoking

There are strong connections between children's smoking and the smoking habits of their parents and older brothers and sisters. This is not surprising when the strength of family bonds and the desire of small children to be like their elders is taken into account. Children in the early years at school usually disapprove of the tobacco habit intensely. By the early teens, however, they are ready to experiment with smoking, and this is because of the strong identification formed at an earlier stage between drinking and smoking and being and acting like an adult.

What's wrong with smoking?

In Britain, shortly after the end of World War II, Professor A. Bradford Hill and Dr. Richard Doll published the first of a series of papers leading to the inescapable conclusion that cigarette smoking was the major factor in the rising incidence of lung cancer. They began with a retrospective study, in which they investigated a large number of patients with cancer of the lung and compared them with a carefully matched control group who did not have this form of cancer. After they compared a number of factors that might have a bearing on the cause of this disease, the only great difference to emerge was that the

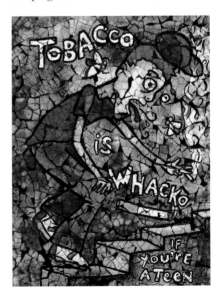

TOBACCO IS WHACKO IF YOU'RE A TEEN

Chemical contents of a typical cigarette

A cigarette is much more than tobacco and a filter wrapped in paper. A typical cigarette is a cocktail of chemicals. The following is a description of what is really in a cigarette.

PAPER

The white part of the paper is made up of cellulose that is bleached and dyed using unknown chemical agents. The paper is treated with various chemicals, such as titanium, to keep the cigarette burning, to give the ash a more pleasant appearance, and to add aroma. The dyed paper covering the filter of the cigarette is called the tipping paper, which is coated with a substance to keep it from sticking to the smoker's lips. Add to this the glue that holds the paper together and the ink in which the brand name is printed. All of these substances are being inhaled with the smoke.

FILTER

Filters were added to cigarettes in the 1950s in response to growing concerns about the health risks associated with smoking. The truth is that they do little to prevent the smoker from inhaling the particulates, or tar, or the vapor chemicals.

The cigarette filter is made up of about 12,000 cellulose acetate fibers, a type of plastic used in photographic prints. These fibers are bonded together with a plastic glue called triacetin. Some filters also contain charcoal, which is supposed to reduce some of the toxic chemicals in the smoke. However, fiber fragments caused by the machine cutting of the filter to length, or charcoal dust in the charcoal filters, can come loose while a smoker is puffing on the cigarette, and the fibers or particles can be inhaled.

TOBACCO

The majority of the tobacco used to manufacture cigarettes in the United States is not from the leaf of the plant but is a manufactured product called "reconstituted tobacco" in which the stems and ribs of the leaves are ground up with various chemicals and colorants, then dried in sheets, like paper. The paper is then shredded to make it smokable. Some manufacturers also use tobacco that is chemically bulked up to lower the cost of production.

Between 6 and 10 percent of the tobacco in a cigarette manufactured in the United States is a chemical additive. The manufacturers can add hundreds of ingredients to the tobacco to enhance the taste, moisture content, burnability, or pH of the cigarette. Although all of the additive ingredients listed on the package are generally considered to be safe when used in food products that are eaten, there is no indication that these are safe when burned and inhaled into the lungs. Indeed, glycerin, an ingredient added to keep the tobacco moist, becomes acrolein when burned, a known cancer-causing agent.

Burning tobacco produces as many as 500 individual gaseous compounds. These gaseous compounds have nitrogen, oxygen, and carbon dioxide as their major constituents, but they also contain the following toxic or tumor-causing agents: carbon monoxide, benzene, formaldehyde, hydrogen cyanide, and others.

---

smoking habits of the two groups varied. Only one in 200 male lung cancer patients were nonsmokers, indicating smoking as the cause. The same type of statistics appeared among studies of women. Furthermore, there appeared to be a relationship between the risk of getting lung cancer and the number of cigarettes a person smoked.

The problem with this kind of retrospective investigation is that people's memory, especially if they are sick, is inclined to be faulty. Bradford Hill and Doll therefore set up an investigation that would study the prospective health of smokers. They had 25,000 British doctors give details of their smoking habits as well as a variety of other relevant information. All the doctors were apparently well and had no reason to lie, and gave details of present smoking habits rather than the sometimes faulty recollections of past smoking. As the years passed, some of these doctors died; Doll and Bradford Hill investigated the cause of death in each case. Some of the deaths were from lung cancer and two facts emerged quite clearly. First, there was a very clear relationship between cigarette smoking and lung

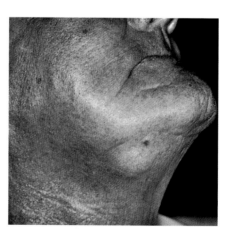

▲ *Simple and quick treatment is not possible to remove a smoking-related cancer of the jaw.*

cancer. Second, the chances of dying from the disease increased with increasing cigarette consumption.

Since then a mass of evidence confirming these results has poured in from all over the world. It also soon became clear that cigarette smoking was an important factor in causing other diseases, of which the most important are chronic bronchitis and coronary heart disease. The end result was the demonstration of two important facts: first, cigarette smokers live, on average, shorter lives than nonsmokers; and second, giving up smoking removes this excess risk in proportion to the amount of time that has elapsed since giving up.

In addition to the main diseases already mentioned above, there is evidence that cigarette smoking can cause other types of pulmonary disorders; delays the healing of gastric ulcers; is a major cause of various cancers of the mouth, voice box, esophagus, and bladder; and leads to a degree of skin wrinkling appropriate to nonsmokers who are 20 years older. It may not be widely appreciated that it is not nicotine that causes the harm from smoking. Smoking is dangerous because of the toxic substances in the vaporized tar.

Nicotine addiction and dependence

According to the American Psychiatric Association's *Diagnostic and Statistical Manual of Mental Disorders*, fourth edition (DSM-IV), there are seven dependence criteria associated with smoking behavior. Individuals are classified as dependent or addicted to nicotine if they experience at least three of the seven criteria.

CRITERIA

1. Tolerance is defined by either of the following:
   (a) A need for markedly increased amounts to achieve intoxication or the desired effect.
   (b) A markedly diminished effect with continued use of the same amount of nicotine.
2. Withdrawal, as manifested by either of the following (a) or (b):
   (a) Characteristic withdrawal syndrome; both (c) and (d).
   (b) The same or closely related substance taken to relieve or avoid withdrawal symptoms.
   (c) Daily use of nicotine for at least several weeks.

(d) Abrupt cessation or reduction in the amount of nicotine use, followed within 24 hours by four or more of the following signs: dysphoric or depressed mood, insomnia, irritability, frustration or anger, anxiety, difficulty concentrating, restlessness, decreased heart rate, increased appetite or weight gain.

3. The substance is often taken in larger amounts or over a longer period than was intended.
4. There is a persistent desire or unsuccessful attempts to cut down or control substance use.
5. A great deal of time is spent in activities necessary to obtain the substance or recover from its effects.
6. Social, occupational, or recreational activities are given up or reduced because of substance use.
7. The substance use is continued despite knowledge of having a persistent or recurrent physical or psychological problem that is likely to have been caused or exacerbated by the substance.

Cigarette tars contain some 3,000 different chemical substances of which several are carcinogenic and several cause other forms of damage to the body.

There are other factors about smoking that are worth knowing. Among nonsmokers, only about one in five will not reach retirement age; but for smokers of over 25 cigarettes a day, two in five will not reach retirement age. The death rate for smokers is much higher among those who inhale than among those who do not; the earlier you start smoking the greater the risk; and the more you smoke the greater the risk. According to findings in the United States, the use of filter-tipped cigarettes does slightly reduce the risk of lung cancer. For pipe (only) and cigar (only) smokers the risk of getting lung cancer is small, provided they do not inhale, although the chance is greater than for nonsmokers.

Effects on nonsmokers

There is an increasing amount of evidence that smoke inhaled by nonsmokers is harmful to their health. It has been shown that the smoke drifting up from the burning end of the cigarette contains twice as much tar as that inhaled by the smoker.

Concern about the effects of second-hand smoke and the rights of nonsmokers has led to changes in attitudes and even in the law in some cases. Nonsmoking areas are now common in public places and in the workplace; and many theaters, restaurants, and public transport facilities ban smoking altogether. There is also an increasing awareness about the risks to an unborn baby if a woman smokes during pregnancy. Smoking mothers have higher rates of miscarriages, stillbirths, and infant deaths than nonsmoking mothers.

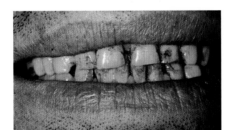

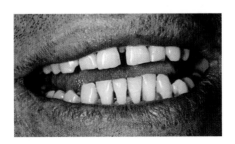

▲ *Nicotine badly stains the teeth, but if you stop smoking, your teeth can once again be sparkling clean.*

How to stop smoking

Giving up is not easy. There are no miracle cures, no magic methods, no shortcuts, and no foolproof formulas. Nevertheless it is a battle that can be won and several million people quit smoking every year.

For a person to give up something that he or she enjoys and has come to rely on is painful. The temptation to have just one cigarette, especially if a person is stressed, is extremely difficult to resist, but resisting a cigarette is crucial. Many people have given up smoking time and again, yet continue to return to it. To quit smoking permanently, determination is required. A halfhearted attempt, or a strategy based on gradual cutting down, is almost certain to fail. It is almost better for someone not to make the attempt until he or she has firmly decided to finally quit the habit.

Most smokers who try to quit find it difficult, not only because of the physical addiction to nicotine, but also because of the psychological addiction to behaviors such as smoking after meals or while talking on the telephone. These behaviors lead to urges to smoke, even when the brain does not need the nicotine

A person should be aware of and avoid the times and places when he or she most enjoyed smoking and break those routines. Some people also find a nicotine patch, Wellbutrin, or other medications to be helpful. However, it can take three weeks or longer before quitting is less of a struggle.

See also: Cancer; Heart attack; Heart disease; Ulcers

Sore throat

I always seem to get sore throats. What should I do about them?

People have persistent or chronic sore throats for many different reasons. Smoking is one of the most common, and quitting may be all that's necessary. However, your doctor may refer you to an otolaryngologist for investigation. Your complaint must be properly treated; don't rely on gargling or throat lozenges.

What is the best type of lozenge to suck?

Lozenges can only ease or soothe the soreness. They have no curative effect on the condition because most of the germs responsible for a sore throat are not on the surface of the throat but are in the tissues below, where the chemicals in the lozenge cannot reach. These strong antiseptic chemicals may actually worsen the condition by causing a chemical inflammation as well as the inflammation that is already present. By killing off many of the normal organisms of the throat, lozenges may disturb the natural balance so that other problems, such as the growth of fungi, are encouraged. For these reasons many doctors advise against using lozenges. If you do want to suck them, opt for something simple rather than for antiseptic lozenges. If your sore throat persists, see your doctor.

What is the difference between a sore throat and tonsillitis?

Sore throat is a symptom that can have many causes and can result from inflammation in any of the tissues that surround the throat. The tonsils are part of these tissues, and tonsillitis is a medical term which refers specifically to inflammation of the tonsils. Thus tonsillitis is only one possible cause of sore throats.

This common symptom results from inflammation of the throat or the surrounding tissues. In most cases very simple treatment is all that is needed to ease the pain and make a patient more comfortable.

The throat is one of the major passages of the body. Air constantly passes up and down from the nose and mouth to the lungs. Food and drink pass through the throat on their way from the mouth to the stomach. Because the throat is the only entry into the lungs or the stomach, all the air that is breathed in and all the food and drink that are taken in have to pass through the throat. The throat is exposed to any material coughed up from the lungs and bronchial passage or vomited up from the stomach.

The tissues that make up and surround the throat (the back of the tongue, the tonsils, the pharynx, and the space at the back of the nose) are constantly exposed to the risk of infection, making a sore throat a common human ailment.

Causes

Sore throat is not a disease in itself. The basic feeling of soreness in the throat may be the result of inflammation of any of the surrounding tissues. In addition, a sore throat is not necessarily caused by one particular germ, since a wide range of bacteria, viruses, and other microorganisms (such as fungi in the case of sore throat due to oral thrush) can attack the throat. In some cases the soreness is due not to infection, but to damage from other sources:

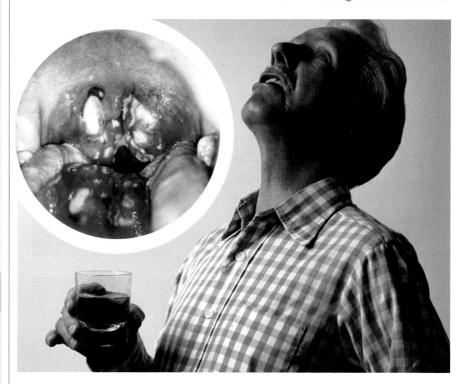

▲ *Gargling, even with something as simple as ordinary salt and water or a mixture of aspirin and water, is an effective way of soothing the symptoms of a sore throat. In a streptococcal throat (inset) the tissues of the throat and neighboring organs have been infected with streptococcus bacteria. This is what the infected area would look like to a doctor examining the patient's throat.*

THROAT AND SURROUNDING TISSUE

Three different views of the throat. Inflammation of many of the tissues shown here may result in a sore throat.

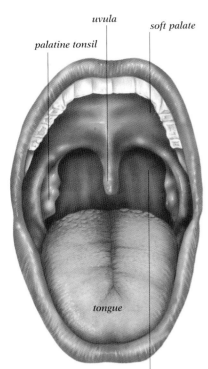

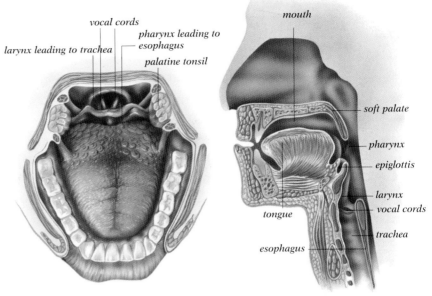

palatine tonsil
uvula
soft palate
tongue
back wall of pharynx

vocal cords
larynx leading to trachea
pharynx leading to esophagus
palatine tonsil
Cross section through the mouth

mouth
soft palate
pharynx
epiglottis
larynx
vocal cords
trachea
esophagus
tongue

swallowing foods and drinks that are too hot, discharge running down from the back of the nose, excessive smoking, or sucking too many strong sweets.

In some diseases (for example, influenza, scarlet fever, measles, and diphtheria), a sore throat is only the first, and relatively unimportant, symptom of a disease that develops into a condition much more widespread and serious. In most cases of sore throat, however, the trouble is confined to the throat.

The most common cause of sore throat is acute inflammation of the pharynx, or pharyngitis. Inflammation of the pharynx usually occurs suddenly, with a feeling of dryness, irritation, and soreness. There is a constant desire to clear the throat, pain on swallowing, a persistent dry cough, and often headache and fever. Pharyngitis is usually due to infection by a virus rather than by bacteria, and taking antibiotics not only is ineffective (they do not combat viruses) but may actually make things worse because of unwanted side effects. Like most viral conditions, the infection clears up of its own accord in a few days, and the only worthwhile treatment is to try to relieve the symptoms by means of hot drinks or appropriate gargles, such as aspirin or salt water.

Chronic pharyngitis may be the result of repeated attacks of acute pharyngitis, heavy smoking, working in dust or fumes, infected adenoids or tonsils, or discharge from the back of the nose or sinuses. It is important to find out exactly what is causing the chronic pharyngitis in order to resolve it.

Tonsillitis

Infections which start with a sore throat or pharyngitis often spread to nearby tissues and involve them too. The most commonly affected neighboring organ is the tonsil. This is likely to be affected if the sore throat is due to infection with streptococcus bacteria: the septic, or strep, throat. In sore throat associated with tonsillitis the pain becomes more severe and swallowing is almost impossible. The affected tonsils are enlarged and red, the glands are swollen and tender, and the patient develops a high temperature. If the tonsillitis is not treated, quinsy (a peritonsillar abscess) may develop.

Another serious complication of a sore throat occurs when infection spreads from the pharynx upward to the eustachian tube, which leads to the inside of the ear. This causes otitis media, which is characterized by earache as well as a sore throat. Infection may also spread downward from the pharynx into the voice box, or larynx, leading to laryngitis.

Diphtheria, which is much less common than it used to be, is yet another infection that involves a sore throat. This is characterized by the development of a membrane which is dirty gray in color and a sweetish smell to the breath, as well as the sore throat. Diphtheria was once a common cause of death in children and was feared by parents. The germs that cause it secrete a powerful poison, an exotoxin that gets into the bloodstream and is carried to all parts of the body, damaging the heart and other organs. Many children who survived the infection were often left with severely damaged hearts and nervous systems.

The sharp decline in the prevalence of diphtheria has nothing to do with antibiotics; it was the result of almost universal immunization against the disease. Public health authorities in countries in which this is not mandatory are constantly concerned that parents who have never known the disease may become casual about immunization. Regulations in the United States for

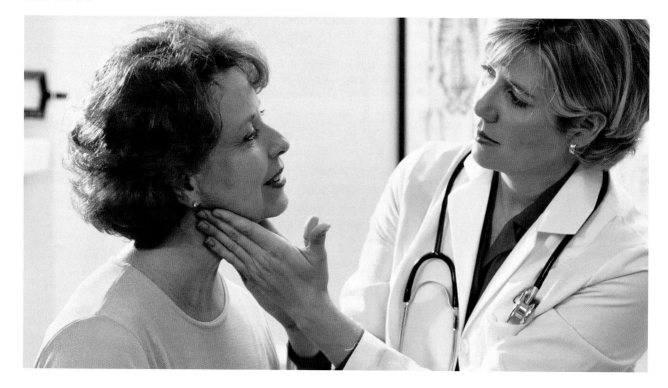

▲ *A doctor examining a sore throat will look down the patient's throat, often with the help of a flashlight, to identify any inflammation that may be present. He or she may also take a throat swab to be sent to a laboratory for identification of the germ involved.*

schoolchildren make it very unlikely that vaccination levels will drop, but it is important that adults are aware of the danger.

Throat abscess

One of the most acute and alarming complications of tonsillitis is peritonsillar abscess, or quinsy. This starts with a simple sore throat with tonsillitis, which seems to settle down. However, after a few days of comfort the affected person begins to suffer increasing difficulty in swallowing. Pain recurs and usually spreads to the ear on one side. It becomes difficult to open the mouth because of spasm of the chewing muscles, and the speech becomes thick and indistinct. Pain rapidly increases to a level that prevents eating. There is strong pressure in the neck and the head is tilted to the affected side. Rapid head movements are avoided. There is excessive salivation and bad breath. The temperature rises to 101°F (38°C) and the person becomes obviously ill. There may be partial obstruction to the airway by obstruction to the inlet of the voice box (larynx). This will produce difficulty in breathing.

Peritonsillar abscess is caused by a spread of infection from the tonsil to the tissues around and behind it. Occasionally it may arise from an infected and impacted wisdom tooth (third molar). If the inside of the mouth is inspected (which may be difficult because of the difficulty in opening the mouth wide) a distinct, red swelling will be seen, with marked protrusion of the tonsil, on one side.

The uvula (the soft, floppy flap of mucous membrane hanging from the center of the soft palate) is pushed across to the healthy side. The tongue is usually coated and the lymph nodes behind the angle of the jaw on the affected side will be enlarged and tender. Rarely, there may be an abscess on both sides.

Once any abscess, here or elsewhere, is fully developed, antibiotics are useless. This is because the center of an abscess is cut off from the general blood supply and no antibiotics can get to the germs. If severe tonsillitis is treated at an early stage with antibiotics, quinsy will be avoided; and if high-dosage antibiotics are given at an early stage of abscess formation, it may be prevented from becoming established. Painkiller drugs are given, an ice pack is applied to the neck, mouthwashes are prescribed, and a cold liquid or semisolid diet is taken. Gargling is useless and, in the presence of partial airway obstruction, dangerous. An established abscess is full of pus, and the only effective treatment is to drain the pus through an incision. This is done under local anesthesia and produces an almost immediate and profound relief of pain and other symptoms. In addition to surgery, antibiotics are normally given to cope with the infection that caused the problem.

The surgeon has two options. The first is to open and drain the abscess at the site of maximum protrusion, using a long scalpel which is wrapped in sterile tape so that only the tip is exposed. This is to prevent the danger of injury to the large blood vessels of the neck by too deep penetration. This procedure is followed by removal of the tonsils under general anesthesia (tonsillectomy) three or four days later. Alternatively, tonsillectomy may be done under general anesthesia as the initial procedure. Once the infected tonsils have been removed there is no longer any danger of developing any further quinsies.

Tonsillectomy is almost always done under general anesthesia. The head is tilted back and the mouth is propped open by a ratchet instrument called a gag. Each tonsil in turn is grasped with toothed forceps and is separated from its bed with minimal cutting. This is called blunt dissection. Bleeding from the raw areas left is sometimes brisk, and it is occasionally necessary to secure and close a small bleeding artery by tying it off. In rare cases, severe bleeding occurs some hours after the operation. This will require a return to the operating room for control of the hemorrhage. After tonsillectomy there is severe local discomfort, especially on swallowing, for about two weeks.

Consulting your doctor

Most sore throats are more of a nuisance than an illness, they clear up quickly on their own, and require neither medical advice nor treatment. Nevertheless, some do not clear up, and people should know when it becomes necessary to consult a doctor. If a person has ever had rheumatic fever or nephritis, or a rash develops, or the person is running a fever of 102°F (38.9°C), or if the throat has a gray or yellow coating, he or she may need medical help. He or she should also see a doctor if a sore throat shows no signs of improving by the third day.

The doctor will probably look down the throat with a flashlight. He or she may wipe the back of the throat with a swab and send it to a laboratory for testing, so that the germ that causes the sore throat can be identified and appropriate treatment given. The doctor will also feel the neck for enlarged glands, and examine the nose, ears, and chest to see if they are involved too. If a patient has had a lot of sore throats a doctor may consider it necessary to refer the person to an otolaryngologist for a more conclusive diagnosis.

Self-help

Sore throat is one of those conditions for which people can do a great deal to help themselves. Hot drinks are soothing for a painful throat, and it is worth trying a semisolid food diet so that swallowing is as free from pain as possible. Gargling is also helpful, though probably the relief is due more to the effect of the heat of the gargle than to what is chosen as the gargle. Ordinary salt and water or a mixture of aspirin and water will be effective. A salt gargle can be made simply by putting two teaspoonful of ordinary

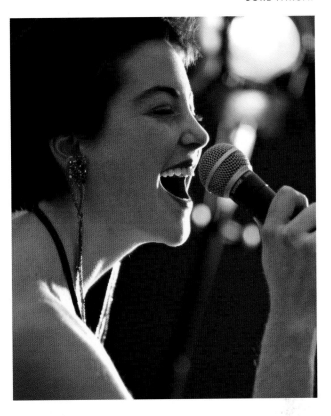

▲ *Singers who use the voice excessively can irritate the larynx to such an extent that the voice is lost and a painful sore throat develops. Rest of the voice is the only treatment.*

household salt in a cup of hot, but not too hot, water and stirring until it is completely dissolved.

Similarly, an aspirin gargle is made by dissolving two soluble aspirin in a cup of hot water. It should be swallowed rather than discarded when gargling is finished so that the aspirin can take effect internally as well by its painkilling and fever-reducing action.

In between gargling it may be helpful to suck a soothing lozenge; fruit pastilles or mentholated lozenges are traditional and effective. If the soreness and irritation in the throat cause coughing, old-fashioned lozenges, sucked as far back in the throat as possible, are safe and soothing. It should be pointed out, however, that the most lozenges will do is soothe a sore throat. Not even the so-called antiseptic lozenges have a specific medicinal property apart from their soothing effect.

▼ *Corynebacterium diphtheriae is the organism that causes diphtheria—a potentially fatal infectious disease that is now rarely contracted.*

▼ *The micrograph shows streptococcus bacteria which, by inflaming the tissues of the throat and surrounding organs, often cause sore throats.*

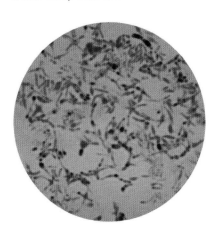

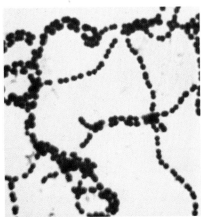

See also: **Bacteria; Burns; Fevers; Immunization; Infection and infectious diseases; Measles; Pain; Rheumatic fever; Scarlet fever; Smoking**

Speech

My son does not speak very clearly, and we can't even make out what he is saying at times. Should we be worried or is he just going through a lazy phase?

If you think your son has a speech problem, take him to your doctor. The doctor may be unable to find out the exact nature of the problem but will be able to refer him to a specialist for further tests and diagnosis if necessary. It is unlikely that his poor speech is caused by laziness, particularly if the defect is bad enough to make him hard to understand. A child may grow out of a genuine speech problem but as time goes on the problem could get worse, so it is essential that he sees a doctor.

My son is two years old and has not made any attempts at speech. All my friends' children of a similar age started speaking some time ago; should I be concerned?

It is not unusual for children, especially boys, not to speak until around the age of two. After this time they usually make excellent progress and catch up quickly. As a precaution, take your son to your doctor, who will be able to assess him and, if need be, send him to a speech therapist for further examinations. If there is a genuine reason for his slow speech development, the cause can be any number of things, from the purely physical (an abnormality of the voice box) to a deep-seated psychological problem. Whatever the cause, early diagnosis is vital, because if there is a defect, the earlier it is corrected the better the outcome. If the delay in developing language is marked, there can be an associated problem in learning the rules of syntax and grammar. Dyslexia or word blindness, for instance, can be associated with problems of speech development; some people believe that dyslexia is more common than was previously thought.

Anyone who has ever lost his or her voice for some reason will know how extremely frustrating it can be not to be able to communicate. Speech, one of humans' most essential and flexible abilities, is indeed a precious faculty.

Speech is one of the most complex and delicate operations that the body is asked to undertake. Ultimately all speech, talking, and comprehension are controlled and coordinated by the brain, and it is in the cerebral cortex that there are areas called the speech centers where words are deciphered and signals and instructions are sent out to the many muscles in the face, throat, and mouth that are involved in producing speech. All this complex control is something that people are born with the ability to do, but the actual way people speak and the sounds they make are learned from their parents and the people around them as they grow up.

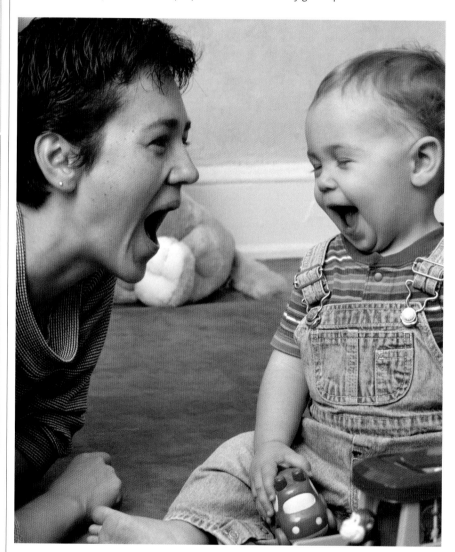

▲ *This 16-month-old child is learning to talk by imitating the physical movements of his mother's mouth and the sounds that come from it.*

Thinking and speaking

The cerebral cortex of the brain is divided into left and right sections called hemispheres. Speech and its associated functions are usually concentrated in one hemisphere; in a right-handed person this is usually in the left hemisphere, and in a left-handed person it is usually in the right hemisphere. This area of the brain is divided into the motor speech center, which controls the muscles of the mouth and throat; and the sensory speech center, which interprets the incoming sound signals coming along the nerve from the ears. Also nearby are the parts of the brain that coordinate hearing (by which people comprehend what others are saying), vision (by which they decipher the written word), and the complex hand movements used in writing, playing an instrument, and so on.

Conversation is a very complicated procedure, and the first thing that happens when a person hears another person speaking is that the hearing centers, in the cerebral cortex, recognize the jumble of incoming auditory signals from the ears. The sensory speech center decodes the words so that the other parts of the brain involved in the process can then recognize the words and formulate an answer. Once a reply has been thought up, the motor speech center and another part of the brain, called the brain stem, come into operation. The brain stem controls both the intercostal muscles, between the ribs, which inflate the lungs; and the abdominal muscles, which determine the pressure of the incoming and outgoing air. As air is expelled from the lungs, the motor speech area signals the vocal cords simultaneously to move into the stream of air in the throat, causing the cords to vibrate and produce a simple sound. This is called phonation.

The amount of pressure applied to the lungs during exhalation governs the speed with which the air passes over the vocal cords, and the faster the air, the louder the sound produced. During whispering the vocal cords are set wide apart so that they do not actually vibrate as the air passes between them, they merely act as friction surfaces. For the most part, however, the shaping of words is performed by movements of the lips, tongue, and soft palate—controlled by the cortex.

Producing words

To turn the simple sounds produced by the vocal cords into intelligible words, the lips,

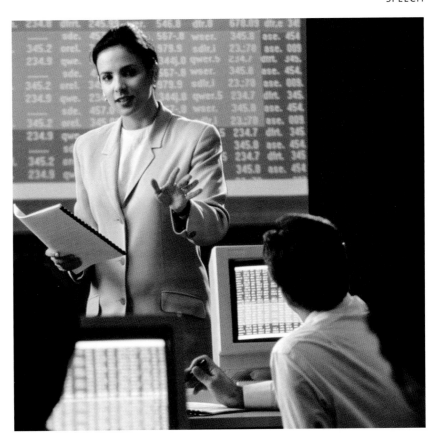

▲ *In job training sessions, the instructor must be articulate, and be able to speak clearly and directly to trainees.*

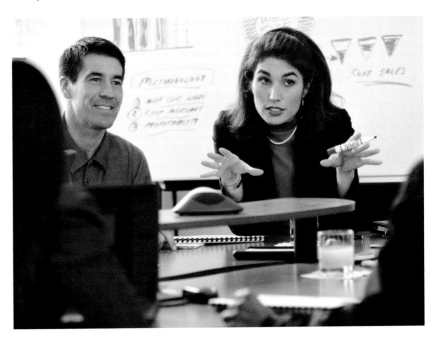

▲ *This woman is chairing a business meeting. Her ability to structure her speech and be articulate and concise with words will affect her success in the business world.*

Questions and Answers

My husband suffered a stroke some time ago which left him partially paralyzed. This also made him lose his powers of speech. What can be done to overcome his problem?

Loss of the power of speech (aphasia) may be due to the inability to understand words or the inability to express them, or both. Some degree of spontaneous recovery is common, but if this does not occur within a matter of weeks it is unlikely that speech therapy will help. It should always be tried, however. The method that might be used to retrain your husband would involve laboriously repeating words and phrases and the rules of grammar, just as a child would when initially learning the language. This would be supervised by a speech therapist.

I have been told that the only way to cure my child's speech problem is to send him to a special school. Is this really necessary?

Treatment of some speech defects can be a long and subtle process and is often most effective under confined and controlled conditions available at a special school. Treatment at a special school could last about three years, after which time the child may be able to return to a regular school. The length of time that the treatment lasts varies, however, depending on the cause of the child's problem.

What can be done for someone with a cleft palate, and is treatment effective?

A cleft palate is a gap or a cleft in the roof of the mouth or upper jaw. This condition is usually treated in babies immediately, or soon, after birth. The fissure is closed by surgery. If a cleft palate is not treated until after the person begins speaking, speech therapy is used to clear up any language defects that may have developed. Today, a cleft palate does not have any real effect on the way a person speaks, since the surgery available mends the damage completely.

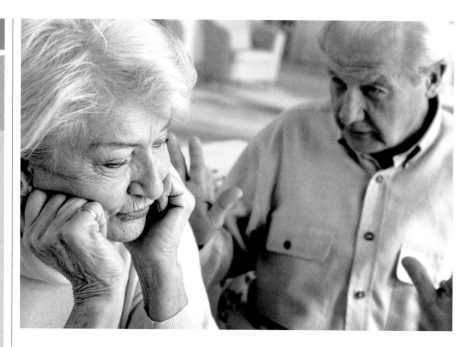

▲ *Arguments are another area in which the ability to present one's thoughts and feelings reasonably and precisely can help other people to understand the problems at hand.*

the tongue, the soft palate, and the chambers, which give resonance to the voice, all play a part. The resonating chambers include the whole mouth chamber, the nose, the pharynx (the part of the throat between the mouth and the esophagus), and to a lesser degree the chest cavity. The control of these structures is achieved by many muscles that work very closely together and at incredible speed. Put simply, speech is made up of vowels and consonants; vowels are all phonated sounds.

The resonant qualities of the various chambers of the mouth and respiratory system provide people with the individuality of their voices. For instance, the so-called nasal sounds like "m," "n," and "ng" depend for their correct vocalization on free resonance in the nose; if a person pinches his or her nose when speaking, the comic effect shows how the airspace of the nose gives the speech roundness and clarity. Everyone has a differently shaped nose, chest, and mouth; therefore different people have different-sounding voices.

The skull also resonates when people speak, and people hear part of what other people say transmitted through the bones of the skull, as well as what is picked up by the ears. This not only provides a person with vital feedback about what he or she is saying, but also explains why the voice sounds so strange when played back through a tape recorder—the sounds a person then hears being only those transmitted through air.

Learning to speak

The rate at which children acquire the power of speech varies from one individual to another, but the same landmarks in speech development normally occur in all growing children. For up to three or four months after birth, most of the sounds a baby makes are those used in crying. After this the baby starts to make speechlike sounds when gurgling and babbling. These noises are thought to be common to babies of all different nationalities, and are even found in babies who are deaf. This has led many people to conclude that the capability for language is inherent in all people.

At around four months of age the baby starts to coo and chuckle, and toward 10 months sounds heard around the infant may be repeated. From 10 to 12 months the first audible words are usually produced. These words are often nouns naming the things that the infant sees around him or her or mean that the baby is asking for something with one word.

From 12 to 18 months the child jabbers tunefully while at play and uses between six and 20 recognizable words; the child also understands many more words. From the age of two the

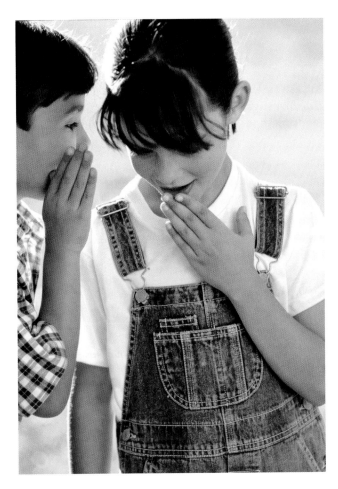

▲ *As children develop their speech as they grow older, they are increasingly able to control their speech volumes as appropriate, from shouting to whispering.*

structuring of language begins and more than two or so words are strung together at one time. Also, the child starts to pick up the idiomatic meaning of groups of words. From three to five years, sentences become longer and convey a more exact meaning, and basic grammar is gradually mastered. From school age, development of speech becomes more structured as vocabulary and grammar are learned in a more systematic manner.

One great asset that people possess is inquisitiveness, and this is nowhere more evident than in a child who is learning new words and phrases every day.

Speech defects

Because of the great complexity of the whole speech process, involving as it does many areas of the brain, the control of breathing, and all the many muscles that manipulate the sound-producing and sound-modifying apparatus, speech problems can be very complicated.

The disorders can be divided into several types: problems of the voice (disorders of the larynx and its parts); problems of voice development; problems caused by damage to the various speech areas of the brain; abnormalities of the mouth; and problems

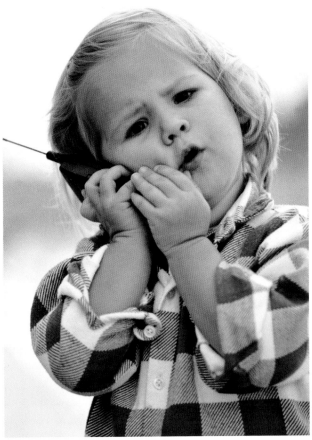

▲ *Toddlers will sometimes practice their speech by pretending to talk to other people on the telephone.*

brought on by or associated with deafness. Basically, anything that gets in the way of the ability either to formulate speech (in the brain), communicate the commands to the bodily parts (along the nerve network), or execute the commands (in the muscles) can cause some kind of speech disorder.

Some disorders caused by problems with the nervous system are called dysarthria. In this category are diseases such as cerebral palsy, shaking palsy, and chorea. Deafness can cause mutism because a deaf child will not be able to pick up the language being spoken around him. If the patient is deaf at birth, concentrated speech therapy must be undertaken using visual means to stimulate the correct vocalization of words.

These are some of the areas where there are problems with speech, and treatment depends on the actual cause of the disturbance. The determination of the cause can involve consultation with neurologists, psychologists, or any of the other specialists involved with the speech-producing mechanisms. Any eventual treatment may involve doctors and therapists from many specialties.

See also: Body structure; Child development; Stroke

Sports medicine

Should my daughter continue her sports training during her period?

The effects of menstruation vary considerably from one woman to another. Some women are virtually incapacitated during this time; others experience little or no discomfort. Exercise can improve a woman's capacity to cope with the changes that occur during menstruation, so if your daughter is comfortable training during her period, let her continue to do so. Many women athletes find that their sporting performance varies over the menstrual cycle, usually deteriorating in the days preceding their period and picking up in midcycle, though some find that they actually perform best during their periods. Many women athletes don't menstruate at all.

What is the value of high altitude training?

The air at high altitudes is at a much lower pressure, so less passes to the blood than at sea level. The body compensates by increasing the concentration of hemoglobin in the blood. This allows the body to use what available oxygen there is more efficiently. This increased oxygen-carrying capacity should also help an athlete's performance when he or she returns to sea level.

My son insists on wearing low-cut cleats when playing football. Wouldn't he be safer wearing cleats with better ankle protection?

Ankle injuries are more common with low-cut shoes. Heavier shoes give more protection, but may cause some loss of speed and agility, and may be tiring. If your son plays in midfield, where the chance of being kicked on the ankle are higher, a heavier shoe could be used. If he plays in a rear position, in which speed and agility are more important, a lighter-weight shoe might be better.

Virtually every sport involves some risk of injury, from the trivial to the disastrous. Sports medicine investigates the causes, determines the treatment, and recommends methods of preventing sports injuries.

One of the most important applications of sports medicine is to study the factors that can affect fitness—including strength, speed, skill, stamina, agility, and personality—and to suggest ways in which performance can be improved through diet, training, and lifestyle. Medical research and opinion may also make a valuable contribution to the design of sports equipment and protective clothing, and sporting authorities may turn to doctors for advice about the drugs that athletes can use without side effects. Generally, however, sports medicine is concerned with the causes, treatment, and prevention of sports injuries at all levels of participation.

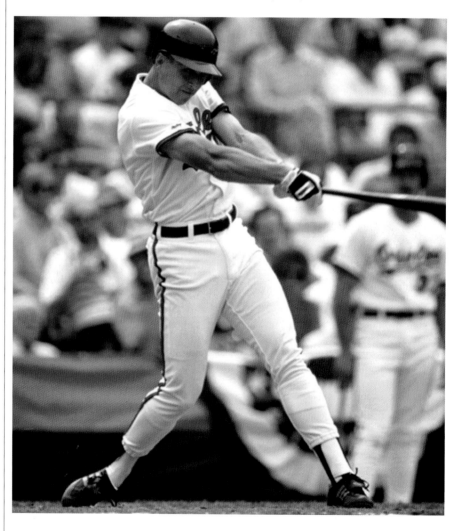

▲ *Injuries in highly competitive sports such as baseball are widespread. Protective clothing and equipment are vital to help prevent serious physical damage. Baseball players wear shin guards, padded gloves, thigh pads, and helmets to protect them from the very hard ball and from other players.*

▶ *Skiing injuries are very common. Before a ski outing, special exercises that condition and strengthen the main muscles used in skiing are advised to help prevent the most common injuries.*

Types of sports injury

Virtually every sport involves some risk of injury, although the pattern of injury varies considerably from one sport to another. Perhaps the most hazardous sports are those involving high speed, such as motor racing and skiing; or those that involve special environmental hazards, such as scuba diving and mountaineering.

Body-contact sports, such as football, basketball, and boxing, can also pose significant dangers. In football, for example, there is the chance of an injury to virtually any part of the legs, as well as the head and collarbone, as a result of the collisions that are so commonplace. In basketball, risks include breaking an arm or leg, or being injured in a collision. Continuous heavy blows to the head in boxing may cause serious lasting damage to the brain as it is knocked around inside the skull. Cut eyes, cut mouth, cauliflower ears, broken nose, and damaged hands are also common injuries in contact sports.

In noncontact sports, physical danger may come from the equipment used. Being hit on the head by a baseball and being spiked by a fellow athlete's track shoes are common examples. More often, injury is self-inflicted or it follows the overuse of some part of the body. Examples are strained elbows and damaged knee joints of tennis players, pulled muscles of sprinters or

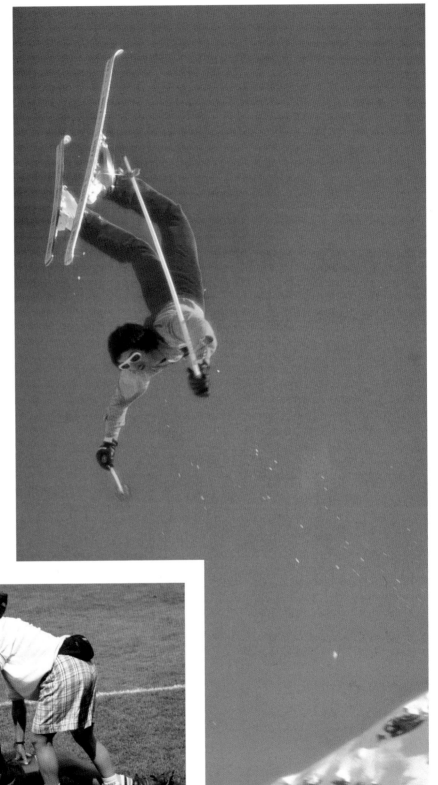

◀ *A football coach helps an injured player.*

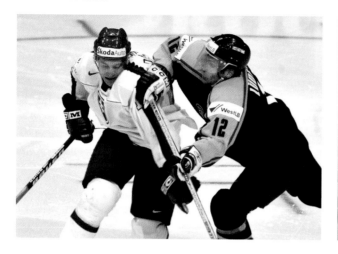

▲ *The bone-crushing sport of ice hockey makes extensive protective gear essential.*

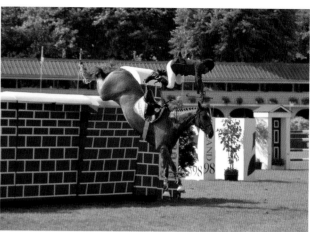

▲ *A show jumper falls from his mount. Riding helmets are essential safety gear, since falls often result in head injuries.*

throwers who have not warmed up properly before a competition, and stress fractures that sometimes affect long-distance runners in training.

Fractures

Sports fractures may occur as the result of a direct blow, and common types of fractures include the broken legs of footballers and skiers, broken collarbones among many ballplayers, and broken finger bones, arms, and ribs in baseball players. Small finger and foot bones usually heal up completely after four or five weeks, but leg fractures may require immobilization for a much longer period.

Stress fractures are overuse injuries caused by repetitive loading of a bone during training or playing. Athletes who train over very long distances each week are the most prone to this type of injury, particularly if they run mainly on roads or other hard surfaces and wear shoes without sufficient cushioned support. The bones most commonly affected are those in the middle part of the foot and the lower leg bones. Symptoms usually begin with pain in the affected area that occurs regularly during training and increases in severity

▼ *Thrills and spills of speed and power: racetrack driving is made safer by the use of helmets and leather suits.*

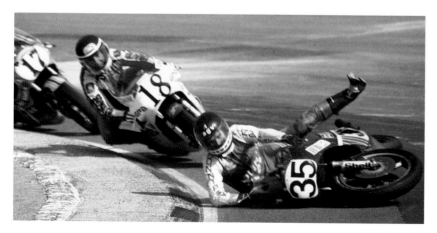

with each training session. At this point, the fracture may consist of a crack or a weakness in the bone structure. If the athlete rests from the activity for around four to six weeks, the injury will gradually start to heal, but to continue training in defiance of the pain could cause the bone to shatter suddenly with much more serious consequences.

Muscle and tendon injuries

Muscle injuries are very common in sports and usually involve a rupture of some of the muscle's fibers, variously described as a pull, a tear, or a strain. The thigh and calf muscles are the most commonly injured among footballers and the hamstrings at the back of the thigh among sprinters.

The usual cause of muscle strain is an excessive demand made on the muscle before it has been warmed up properly. Cold muscles contract in a jerky fashion, which can produce too great a load on some of the fibers. When they tear, the usual symptom is a sudden stabbing ache. Such pain may continue for a week or more, but it is a good idea to continue exercising gently during this time to speed the return to full activity.

Muscle stiffness is very common the morning after some unaccustomed effort, but it gradually disappears over a day or two. The stiffness is probably due to the combined effects of a number of very small tears in the muscle.

Tendons are the fibrous cords that join muscles to bone. They can be ruptured or torn by a direct blow or by excessive strain, or they may become inflamed through overuse. Tennis players, hockey players, and rowers often develop an inflammation of the tendons in the wrist due to a persistent tight grip on racket, stick, bat, or oar. A few days' rest usually relieves the condition.

Joint ligament injuries

Joint injury may involve damage to the bone ends that make up the joint; to the cartilage

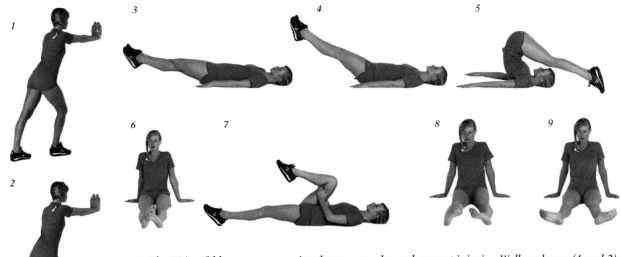

◄▲ The Weisenfeld warm-up exercises loosen muscles and prevent injuries. Wall push-ups (1 and 2) stretch calf and soleus muscles. The three-level leg lift (3, 4, and 5) builds up abdominal and thigh muscles. The foot press exercise (6) strengthens the thigh muscles and can be used for the treatment and prevention of "runner's knee." Knee-press exercises stretch both hamstrings and lower-back muscles, preventing pulled hamstrings and lower-back pain (7). By tensing the thigh muscles, turning the feet in or out, and holding for 10 seconds (8 and 9), the thigh muscles can be strengthened.

that coats each bone end; to the ligaments that determine the range of movement of the joint; or to a variety of other structures around and within the many different joints.

Sprains can arise when a joint is forcibly moved beyond its normal range and may involve the tearing or rupturing of a ligament; knee and ankle sprains are the most common.

Dislocations occur when one of the bone ends is completely displaced from its normal position, thus damaging the ligaments and rendering the joint either immobile or unstable. A doctor, or some other qualified person, must quickly reposition the bone before the tissues swell.

Following a sprain or a dislocation, a joint may need to be immobilized for several weeks so that the damaged ligaments can heal and regain their full strength.

Apart from sprains and dislocations, one of the most common injuries to the knee joint is a torn cartilage, which is painful and may considerably limit any knee movement. It is quite common for damaged cartilage to require surgical removal.

Rehabilitation

Initial treatment of most sports injuries consists of measures aimed at reducing pain and swelling in the area affected, together with the resetting of fractured bones and dislocated joints, and any other first-aid measures. Although the injured part of the body often has to be immobilized for some weeks to allow damaged tissues to heal, in many cases an early return to light exercise is encouraged to prevent muscle wasting or the formation of scar tissue that might delay full recovery.

A graded exercise program is worked out by doctor and physical therapist with the aim of rebuilding muscle, tendon, and bone strength or joint stability, and restoring a full range of movement. The temptation to return to full participation in a sport before obtaining the doctor's permission should be resisted. This is likely to lead to a recurrence of the injury, followed by a further, and usually longer, spell on the sidelines.

Avoiding injury

Most sports injuries could be avoided through a mixture of common sense, fitness training, expert supervision, and adequate preparation for the particular activity in question, which includes selecting and using the right equipment.

If a person has not had any exercise for several months, strenuous activities should be avoided until he or she has built up an appropriate level of fitness by taking part in a more moderate activity. Thorough stretching and warming up before a game will help protect the muscles and joints from injury when the game begins.

Protective clothing—such as helmets, pads, gloves, and boxes to safeguard the genitals for ice hockey and football players; shin pads for baseball players; and gum shields for boxers—should be worn wherever possible. Wearing the correct footwear is also particularly important for all types of sport. Training shoes should be comfortable and well padded with shock-absorbent material, and should have treads that provide an adequate grip on the training surface. For sports that involve rapid changes in direction, the shoe must provide adequate support to the side of the foot in order to prevent the ankle from turning.

Any persistent pain that occurs during training sessions should be dealt with by refraining from the activity for a few days. Even better, the injured person should pay a visit to the doctor. Ignoring the discomfort of a sports injury is likely to aggravate any persistent problem and also invites disaster. A person should take note and act on what his or her body is saying.

> *See also:* Diet; Dislocation; Exercise; Fractures; Pain; Physical fitness; Physical therapy; Pulled muscles; Sprains; Tennis elbow

Sprains

A sprain is one of the most common of all injuries, and the majority of people have sprained a wrist or ankle at some time in their life. The damage almost always heals by itself, with the help of simple home treatment.

A sprain chiefly affects the tissues around a joint, and it generally rates as more serious than a strain, but considerably less serious than a dislocation or fracture. Virtually any joint can be involved in a sprain, but some joints are far more likely to be affected than others because of their position and the strains they frequently have to bear. The ankle is particularly vulnerable because it bears much of the body's weight and is often involved in potentially hazardous activities.

Causes

Sprains are usually the result of the sharp twisting or wrenching of a joint beyond its natural limits. If the force involved is very great there may, in addition, be dislocation or even a fracture. Most commonly, however, the ligaments are affected. These are very tough bands of

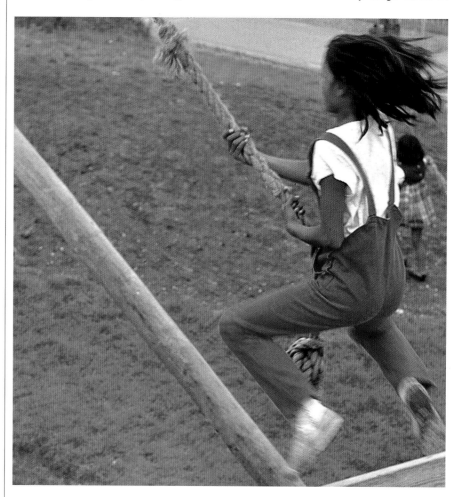

▲ *Accidents will happen when children become adventurous in their play; and a fall may result in a sprained wrist or ankle.*

Questions and Answers

What is the best type of bandage to use in treating a sprain?

The aim is to give the joint firm support while it heals, but it should not be completely immobilized as a fracture has to be. Some form of elasticized bandage is therefore required. An ordinary cotton bandage gives too little support, but crepe, webbing, and elastic bandages are all suitable. The bandage must be put on tightly enough to be effective, but not so tightly that it interferes with the circulation; the patient may then be in danger of getting gangrene. If the extremities (the toes in the case of a sprained ankle, and the fingers in a sprained wrist) go white, become numb, or get pins and needles, then the bandage is too tight. If this is the case, you must take it off and start again, bandaging a little more loosely.

How are cold compresses used in the treatment of sprains?

Very much as the name suggests. You take something like a piece of old linen, a handkerchief, a dish towel, or a roll of bandage and thoroughly soak it in cold, but not iced, water. You then wring it out so that it no longer drips, lay it on the sprained area, and bandage it in place. As soon as it begins to dry or get warm, take it off, soak it in cold water again, and repeat the process.

To have any effect on the pain and swelling of a sprain, the cold compress must be applied within the first few minutes.

Can massage help to treat sprains?

Perhaps. Gentle massage can be started when the immediate effects of the injury have worn off, usually on the second or third day. The area will be very tender, so only light pressure should be applied. The massage can become gradually more strenuous as the injury heals.

fibroelastic tissue that hold the joint firmly in the correct position and protect it from dislocation. In trying to resist the force that is suddenly exerted on them, the ligaments may become stretched and some of the fibers may even be torn. It is rare, however, for the whole ligament to be pulled apart or ripped away from the bone. Any tendons (the thin, tough tails of muscle) may be similarly affected. Blood vessels in the tissues surrounding the joint are likely to be torn, causing bleeding and the bluish discoloration which is characteristic of many sprains.

Any accident may bring about a sprain. People may sprain their ankles when tripping on the stairs or falling off a ladder. Wrist sprains are also a common consequence of falls. The larger joints, such as the knee and hip, may be sprained in the course of a strenuous sport, and neck sprains may result from whiplash injuries when an automobile is brought to a sudden, violent halt.

Symptoms

There are several changes in the joint that indicate it has been sprained. The most obvious is sudden, severe pain in the affected area. This comes from two sources: from the stretched or torn strands of ligament, and from distention of the surrounding tissue. This is brought about by bleeding and the secretion of fluid, which is part of the repair process.

The pain becomes dramatically worse if any attempt is made to move the joint or to make it bear any weight. As a result, there is also disability in the sense that the joint is put temporarily out of use. Any movement that is possible will be slight and of little practical value.

The swelling over the ligament usually develops quickly, and any bleeding into the underlying tissue will give it a blue or bruised appearance. As well as pain there will be tenderness. Even light pressure on the side of the joint will cause pain, but the actual site of the damage will be particularly sensitive. This is known as pinpoint tenderness, and it helps to indicate where the damage is in a swollen joint.

Treatment and outlook

Distinguishing between a sprain and more serious damage, such as a fracture, can be very difficult, but it is essential. It should be remembered that the two types of damage are really different stages in the same process, and that both involve pain, tenderness, swelling, and loss of use of the joint. Apparent sprains, unless they are obviously very minor, must therefore be treated with great caution until a doctor's opinion has been obtained. In this way, any aggravation of a possible fracture will be avoided. An X ray may even be needed to confirm the diagnosis.

The treatment of sprains has undergone considerable changes over the last decades. Not all doctors, however, are in complete agreement with the newer approach, which recommends using the joint rather than resting it.

Immediate treatments, nevertheless, remain fairly standard. If a doctor is available when the sprain occurs (as may happen with a sports injury), he or she may inject the area with local anesthesia to minimize the reaction. A cold, but not ice, compress may be used for the same purpose, but not with such dramatic effect. The affected joint should then be firmly bandaged to limit the swelling and provide support.

Heat should never be applied to a new sprain, though it may well be helpful in restoring function from the second day onward.

Bandaging a sprained ankle

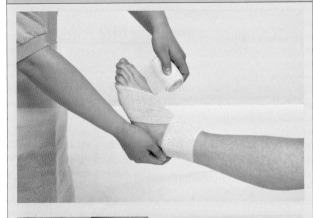

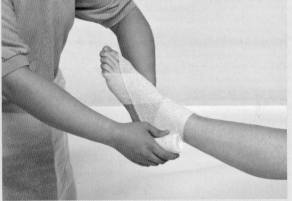

Stand in front of the patient and position the injured foot at a right angle to the shin.

Use an elasticized bandage, unrolling it as you work and holding the remainder so that it faces upward.

Starting well up on the ankle, make a "U" shape with the bandage, taking it down under the heel and up again, so that the foot is pulled up firmly to the leg.

Then take the strap around the back of the lower leg and down again to form a second "U."

Start off with a couple of firm turns to make sure it does not slip, then apply the rest evenly and firmly. Each successive turn should cover two-thirds of the previous one.

Secure with a safety pin through the two outermost layers. If it works loose through wear, remove and reapply.

The patient may then start to use the joint gradually, perhaps with the help of a crutch. In most cases, however, healing will be rapid.

See also: **Bruises; Dislocation; Fractures; Sports medicine; Whiplash injury; X rays**

Staphylococcus

My son had a staphylococcal infection. How does a germ come to have a name like that?

When the early bacteriologists first observed germs under a microscope, they noticed that many of them were spherical like tiny berries. The Greek word for a berry is *kokkos* so each one was called a coccus (plural cocci). Some cocci tended to form clusters resembling bunches of grapes. The Greek for a bunch of grapes is *staphyle,* so this variety of cocci were called staphylococci. When pure cultures of certain virulent staphylococci were grown on suitable media they were seen to be of a golden yellow color. The Latin for golden is *aureus,* so this species was named *Staphylococcus aureus. S. aureus* is a bacterium of great importance in medicine.

What makes staphylococci stick together in clumps?

It is what makes them prone to cause disease. *S. aureus* have on their surfaces special chemical receptors for a protein clumping factor, fibrinogen, that is present in the blood, and for proteins called fibronectins that are present on the surface membranes of body cells. The elements that cause staphylococci to stick together also cause them to stick to body cells so that they can proceed to damage or kill these cells.

Is it true that staphylococci cause food poisoning?

Yes. A food handler with a staphylococcal skin infection, such as a boil, especially on the hands, can contaminate the food with toxins that cause an explosive attack of illness within a few hours after the food is eaten. Infected food handlers should not have any access to food served to the public.

The staphylococcus is one of the most common disease-producing germs and although at one time, soon after the discovery of penicillin, it was thought that this germ had been conquered, it is now causing doctors more problems than any other bacterium.

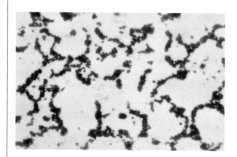

▲ Staphylococcus aureus *bacteria magnified 320 times; they cause both minor, and sometimes fatal, infections.*

Staphylococci of medical importance are spherical germs about one-thousandth of a millimeter in diameter. In the body they group into clusters like grapes. Under standard bacterial staining methods (Gram's stain) they take a dark blue color and are said to be gram-positive. The most important species is *Staphlococcus aureus.*

S. aureus are pus-forming organisms. They cause a range of skin infections such as boils, carbuncles, abscesses, impetigo, and the dangerous scalded skin syndrome in which the layers of the skin separate from each other. They can also cause toxic shock syndrome, food poisoning, sore throat (pharyngitis), pneumonia, and an infection of the inner heart lining called endocarditis. These germs are everywhere and it is almost impossible to prevent any raw surface from becoming infected with staphylococci. They commonly infect severe burns and postoperative surgical incisions. The most dangerous aspect of staphylococci is the emergence of a strain known as MRSA that is resistant to almost all antibiotics.

How do staphylococci cause disease?

Like many other germs, staphylococci do harm by producing a wide range of damaging factors and specific poisons (toxins) that can kill cells. Their DNA contains genes that code for adhesion factors so that they can bind on to living cells, enzymes that break down proteins, enzymes that break down the fat molecules that form cell membranes, and virulent poisons that can kill tissue cells, kill the white cells of the immune system, and break down the red cells of the blood.

S. aureus has shown a remarkable capacity to change so as to survive under different environmental conditions. Almost from the time antibiotics were first produced, it has developed the ability to resist destruction by one new antibiotic after another. This evolutionary process has been assisted by a tendency for doctors to prescribe antibiotics unnecessarily for trivial conditions and for patients to fail to complete full courses of antibiotic treatment.

MRSA

After *S. aureus* became resistant to many antibiotics, a stage was reached at which infections with certain stains of it could be treated effectively only with the antibiotic methicillin. When methicillin-resistant strains began to appear, the drug was withdrawn from general use. Today, over 90 percent of hospital strains of *S. aureus* are penicillin-resistant. This is a matter of great concern, as MRSA (methicillin-resistant *Staphylococcus aureus*) are responsible for many deaths. Initially MRSA infections occurred mainly in hospitals where the environment was suitable for the rapid evolution of bacterial antibiotic resistance, but infections have now spread into the community and are becoming common there. The DNA in MRSA now codes for an enzyme that allows these strains to continue to synthesize their cell walls even if their normal penicillin-binding proteins have been inactivated by methicillin. The structure of this enzyme was recently determined, providing scientists with the hope that there may be a solution to the MRSA threat.

See also: Antibiotics; Bacteria

Starch

Questions and Answers

Starch is a complex carbohydrate that functions as a source of energy for the body. Starch is considered to be a very fattening part of our diet, but this is only the case when people consume more starch than their bodies require.

Carbohydrates provide the body with energy, which it requires for movement, breathing, and all internal metabolic functions. People's main source of carbohydrates is starch—a complex of many molecules of sugar that must be released from it by digestive enzymes before the body can assimilate them. Sugar taken in excess of energy requirements is converted to fat and deposited under the skin and elsewhere.

Starch in the diet

People tend to eat a large amount of starch in their diets because foods rich in starch are usually cheaper and more readily available than proteins. In itself, starch will not make a person fat; it simply provides a ready supply of glucose that the body requires for its metabolism to work.

Many weight-loss diets stress cutting down on the eating of starchy foods. However, a person who does enough aerobic exercise on a regular basis has little to fear from gaining weight by consuming starchy foods.

Sources of starch

Plants manufacture carbohydrates by the process of photosynthesis, whereby they

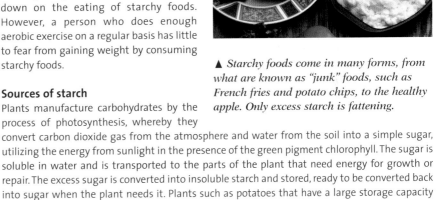

▲ *Starchy foods come in many forms, from what are known as "junk" foods, such as French fries and potato chips, to the healthy apple. Only excess starch is fattening.*

convert carbon dioxide gas from the atmosphere and water from the soil into a simple sugar, utilizing the energy from sunlight in the presence of the green pigment chlorophyll. The sugar is soluble in water and is transported to the parts of the plant that need energy for growth or repair. The excess sugar is converted into insoluble starch and stored, ready to be converted back into sugar when the plant needs it. Plants such as potatoes that have a large storage capacity therefore contain a large quantity of starch.

The digestion of starch

The process of digesting starchy foods begins in the mouth. Food is first broken into manageable pieces by the teeth and mixed with the saliva produced by the salivary glands in the mouth. The saliva contains a starch-digesting enzyme called ptyalin, or amylase, which is capable of breaking down the starch into simpler sugars. There is, however, little time for the starch-digesting enzyme to act before the food is swallowed and passed into the stomach. In the stomach there is no digestion of carbohydrates.

When the stomach contents are passed into the duodenum, or small intestine, enzymes from the pancreas continue to break down all carbohydrates into the simple sugars like glucose that make them up. This end product of digestion is absorbed into the body, enters the hepatic portal vein, and is transported to the liver before entering the bloodstream.

STARCH METABOLISM

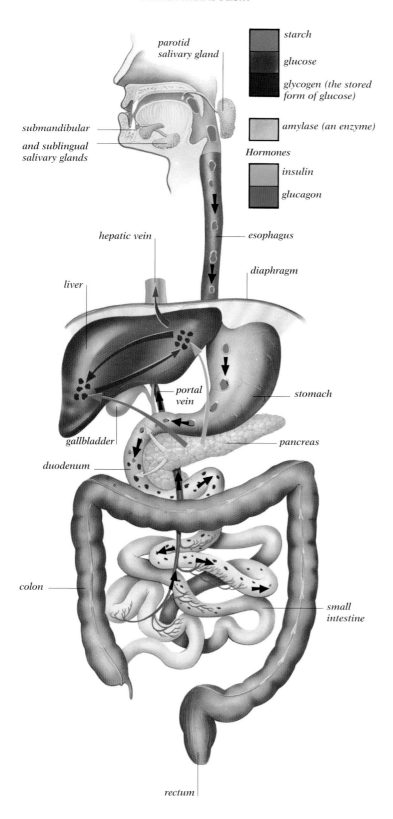

starch

glucose

glycogen (the stored form of glucose)

amylase (an enzyme)

Hormones

insulin

glucagon

parotid salivary gland

submandibular and sublingual salivary glands

hepatic vein

esophagus

diaphragm

liver

portal vein

stomach

gallbladder

pancreas

duodenum

colon

small intestine

rectum

◄ *During digestion, starch is broken down into glucose by the enzyme amylase. Glucose is carried by the blood to the liver. If the level of glucose is high, insulin, a hormone from the pancreas, causes the free glucose to be converted into glycogen, which is stored in the liver. When blood glucose levels become low, the pancreas releases another hormone, glucagon, which causes the stored glycogen to be released as glucose. The body uses glucose as a fuel to provide the energy it needs for movement.*

The liver and glycogen

In the same way as plants store starch for use when sugar supplies are low, so the body also stores a small reserve of a form of starch called glycogen, or animal starch.

Glucose absorbed in the small intestine can be converted to glycogen in the liver, which usually holds about 3.5 ounces (100 g). The muscles also contain substantial quantities. As glucose is used up in the body to provide energy, so the equivalent amount of stored glycogen is broken down by enzymes to glucose. In this way the concentrations of glucose in the blood and body fluids can be kept within limits.

The deposition of glycogen and its reconversion to sugar are controlled by hormones, most importantly insulin from the pancreas. When people eat meals that contain a lot of starch and sugar, the amount of sugar in the blood can double within a matter of minutes. This rapid increase causes the pancreas to pour out insulin, which acts on the muscles and the liver and instructs them to withdraw sugar from the blood before it is lost in the urine, and to store it as the starch glycogen. However, the muscles and liver can store only a limited amount of starch; the excess is converted to fat and laid down in fatty tissue. Weight for weight, fats can store almost three times as much energy as starch. Obesity is the result of excess intake over energy expenditure.

Epinephrine and thyroid hormones are also related to glycogen breakdown and storage. These hormones accelerate the conversion of glycogen to glucose and tend to act when the body is active.

See also: Diet; Dieting; Fats; Glucose; Obesity; Protein; Sugars; Weight

Streptococcus

Of the many different streptococcal species, only a few cause disease in humans. Those that do can be very dangerous, causing serious illness or even death, but most, if diagnosed early, can be effectively treated with antibiotics.

A coccus is a roughly spherical germ named after the Greek word *kokkos*, meaning "a berry." Germs reproduce by growing longer and then splitting into two. When streptococci do this, the daughter cells tend to stick together to form a chain like a string of beads. When this appearance was first noted under the microscope by the German surgeon Albert Billroth, he decided to call them after the Greek word for "a chain." However, he was mistaken as to the meaning of the word, since *strepto* means "twisted," but no one objected, so the name stuck.

Yes, billions, but most of these are species that do not cause serious disease and many of them are entirely harmless. *Streptococcus mutans* in tooth plaque, however, is one of the principal causes of tooth decay, and *Streptococcus viridans* can cause serious infections of the heart lining and valves (bacterial endocarditis) in people who have had rheumatic fever if these germs get into the bloodstream during dental treatment.

Most of the germs that cause sore throat are of reasonably low virulence, but *Streptococcus pyogenes*, which is the principal disease-causing streptococcus, can cause a dangerous infection. The danger is not so much to the throat itself as to the body generally in the aftermath of the infection. Strep throat may lead to a potentially serious kidney disorder called glomerulonephritis and to a joint and heart disorder called rheumatic fever.

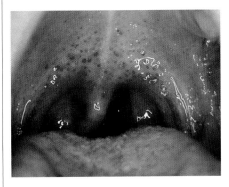

▲ *The streptococcus bacterium causes small red spots to form on the soft palate at the back of the mouth in the condition known as strep throat.*

A streptococcus is a spherical or ovoid bacterium about a thousandth of a millimeter in diameter. Under a microscope, individual streptococci look the same as staphylococci, but when they have been reproducing, streptococci remain in pairs or form characteristic short or long chains. Unlike many bacteria, they are incapable of independent movement and do not form spores. Streptococci stain deep blue with standard Gram's stain; they are said to be "gram-positive." Streptococci are found normally in the mouth and intestines of humans. They also occur in dairy products and other foods, and in fermenting plant juices. There are at least 85 different species of streptococci but only a few cause disease.

Streptococcal species

Streptococcus pyogenes is a pus-forming bacterium and the most dangerous of all the streptococcal species. It causes impetigo, acute tonsillitis, scarlet fever, the spreading skin infection erysipelas, septic abortion, puerperal fever, necrotizing fasciitis, muscle infection (myositis), and urinary infections. It produces many powerful toxins, some of the most important being hemolysins, which attack and destroy red blood cells. For this reason *S. pyogenes* is also known as a hemolytic streptococcus, or a group A streptococcus.

Streptococcus mutans acts on sugar in the mouth to convert it to lactic acid, which, in turn, demineralizes the enamel of the teeth. The bacterium also secretes a high-molecular-weight complex sugar (polysaccharide) that binds streptococci with other materials to form plaque.

Streptococcus fecalis is present in large numbers in the lower bowel and contaminates the skin around the anus. It is a common cause of urinary infections, especially in women, whose short urethra allows the streptococci to reach the bladder more easily than in men.

Streptococcus pneumoniae, also known as the pneumococcus, is the most common cause, worldwide, of lung inflammation (pneumonia) and infection of the brain coverings (meningitis). This species of streptococcus, however, has a polysaccharide capsule that allows an effective vaccine to be made against it.

Secondary effects of streptococci

The infections caused by *S. pyogenes* are often serious, but will almost always respond to antibiotic treatment. However, infection is not the only damage streptococci can cause: when they enter the body the immune system mounts a defense by producing antibodies against them. These are effective in immobilizing and destroying the invading streptococci, but they also have a dangerous secondary effect. Certain tissues in the large joints, in the heart lining, and in the kidneys have features in common with streptococci, so the antibodies, as well as attacking the bacteria, may attack these tissues. This is how rheumatic fever and glomerulonephritis are caused. These are not infections by streptococci, but autoimmune reactions caused by the antibodies provoked by the streptococcal infection.

> *See also:* Antibiotics; Bacteria; Pneumonia; Rheumatic fever; Sore throat; Staphylococcus

Stress

Questions and Answers

Does everyone suffer from feelings of stress?

Yes. Stress is an integral part of life. However, you have to be clear about what you mean by stress; it is not always unpleasant. For example, participating in, or even watching, competitive games involves considerable stress.

Is there good stress and bad stress?

Yes, in a way, but what you call bad stress might be very important to you. It might, for example, result in a lifesaving level of arousal and physical capability. In acute emergencies, people can perform amazing feats of strength or agility that would be impossible without stress.

Can stress be pleasurable?

A young stockbroker, tennis player, or champion skier would no doubt say "yes." Many occupations and activities involve pleasurable stress. Stress can be necessary to achieve a certain standard of performance.

But if stress is damaging, how come all these people don't die from heart attacks?

Stress can be damaging to some people, but others can withstand enormous strain without suffering any harm. The idea that a lot of stress will inevitably cause heart attacks, ulcers, skin disease, or cancer isn't borne out by the facts.

So is there no scientific evidence that stress is harmful?

Yes, severe, acute stress, such as life-threatening situations, can be harmful. Post-traumatic stress disorder is a real medical entity. However, the occasional stresses of minor emergencies are things we can't do without. We need them.

The popular view is that many diseases are caused by stress and, although this view is not universally accepted by doctors, the medical profession is now beginning to acknowledge that some stress can result in sickness.

The popular medical media have had a wonderful time with stress. For years, writers of books and articles for lay consumption have been stating or implying that almost any organic disorder can be attributed to stress. Such claims have met with a ready public response. Nearly all people are familiar with the unpleasant feeling of being stressed, and it is not surprising that they therefore fear that it may be doing them harm.

One of the reasons for the appeal of the early writing on the subject in the 1960s and 1970s was that it seemed to be new. The term "stress" was unfamiliar. In those days, people were accustomed to talking about strain, and suddenly everyone started to talk about stress instead. These terms come from the field of engineering; they are not widely understood and they are often confused. Stress is the force exerted on a body that tends to cause it to deform. Strain is a measure of the extent to which a body actually is deformed when it is subjected to stress. The terms can, of course, be applied to human bodies in exactly this mechanical way, but when people talk about biological stress they are usually speaking metaphorically, if not always logically.

The theory of biological stress

The man who brought stress into the limelight was the Austrian-born Canadian physician Hans Selye (1907–1982), whose initial papers on what he called the stress-adaptation syndrome were produced in the early 1950s. Selye was a well-qualified man who studied medicine in Prague, Paris, and Rome before working at McGill University in Montreal, Canada. In 1945 he became director of the Institute for Experimental Medicine and Surgery at the University of Montreal, an institute which he had founded. From then on Selye produced book after book: *The Story of the Adaptation Syndrome* (1952); *The Stress of Life* (1956); *From Dream to Discovery* (1965); *The Case for Supramolecular Biology* (1967); *Stress without Distress* (1974). These books were directed at the general public, and they made Selye and his ideas famous.

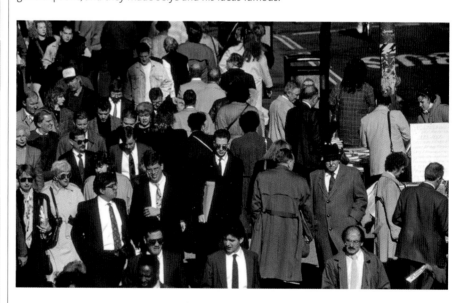

▲ *The hectic yet often monotonous life many people are forced to lead makes a certain amount of stress unavoidable. What can be done, however, is take positive steps, whenever possible, to ensure that these pressures of life are kept to a minimum.*

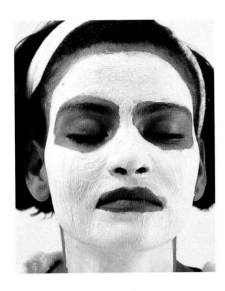

▲ *Physical exercise and pampering of the body, such as indulging in beauty treatments or massage, can help to alleviate the stresses of everyday life.*

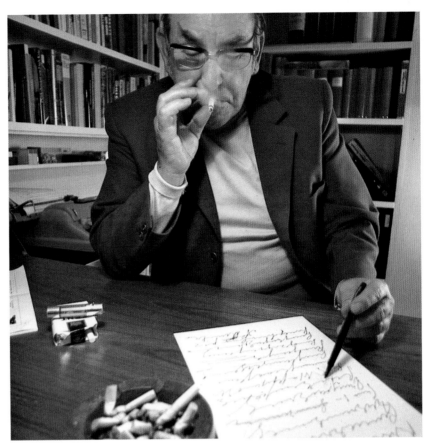

▲ *Different people have different ways of alleviating stress. Some methods, such as excessive smoking or alcohol consumption, are very destructive to the health. Exercise, whether it be jogging, yoga, or even dancing, is a healthier way to combat stress.*

Selye was a physiologist who knew all about the hormonal changes that occur in the body under conditions of anxiety. The production of epinephrine and the steroid hormone cortisol was known to be necessary for survival in fight-or-flight situations. Without these aids to alertness and sudden physical exertion, few primitive humans would have survived to take part in the evolutionary process. So, by natural selection, they became part of people's physical and physiological makeup. None of this was controversial.

Selye first thought of the idea of biological stress when he was a medical student. It occurred to him that all sick patients, however diverse their conditions and symptoms, had this in common: they looked and felt sick. His professor dismissed this idea as childish nonsense. Ten years later, while working at McGill, Selye discovered that rats who were given various damaging injections, or who were kept cold or persistently overworked, developed enlargement of their adrenal glands, the glands that produce epinephrine and cortisol, and often developed stomach ulcers. These rats were showing a general, and identical, reaction to various stress-producing events (stressors). Was this, he wondered, the thing that all sick people had in common?

His further research and thought led him to propose what he called the general adaptation syndrome. Stressors, whatever their nature—physical threat, actual injury, bacterial infection, social or marital problems, perceived danger of any kind—all caused, Selye claimed, much the same effects. The adaptation syndrome was divided into three parts: the alarm stage (previously described as the fight-or-flight reaction); the resistance, or adaptation, stage; and the exhaustion stage.

The alarm stage features secretion of epinephrine, a rise in the pulse rate and in blood pressure, rapid breathing, tense muscles, trembling, a feeling of butterflies in the stomach, slowed digestive processes, reduced blood supply to the skin, release of sugar fuel into the blood, and an increase in the clotting power of the blood.

Stressors, Selye suggested, may force the alarm stage to persist for long periods, even for months. If the stressor persists, the level of arousal drops a little but remains high, and in the resistance stage the body tries to repair damage caused in the alarm stage. Eventually, if the stressor persists, the person enters the stage of exhaustion in which he or she becomes highly vulnerable to bodily damage.

Selye was convinced that this mechanism was an important element in the production of such disorders as hardening of the arteries, heart disease, high blood pressure, strokes, stomach and duodenal ulcers, colitis, premenstrual syndrome, diabetes, and arthritis. Selye called these disorders diseases of adaptation.

Stressors

Many of these stressors are obvious, and many people feel that they can rate them by the strength of the physiological effects they produce, often by the amount of muscle tension felt in the upper part of the abdomen. These stressors include anxiety, frustration, discomfort, conflict, alarm, excessive ambition—all the things people have come to think of as the stresses of modern life. They also include physical insult to the body, whether from infection,

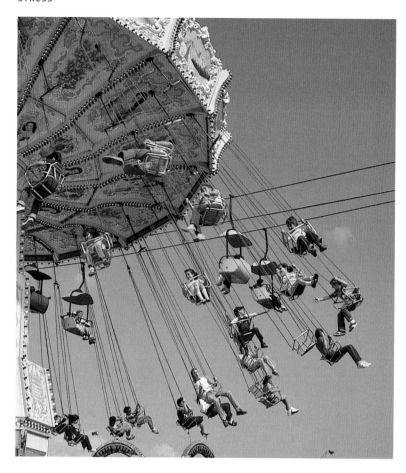

▲ *It is important for people to relax and to get away from their stresses. A trip to the amusement park may be one way of doing this—this activity may look hair-raising, but it will take a person's mind off his or her problems, and this level of fear is considered to be a healthy, invigorating form of stress.*

▼ *Some people let the demands of their job spill into their work breaks. This should be avoided whenever possible, because time to unwind can be vital.*

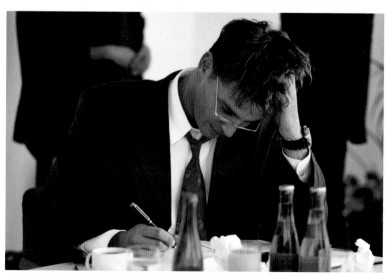

mechanical trauma, burns, radiation, intake of toxic substances, side effects of drugs, exposure to allergens (substances provoking allergic reactions), overcrowding, atmospheric pollution, and so on. There is a real distinction between acute (short and sharp) stress, such as a severe physical assault or a major psychological trauma, and chronic (long-term and less intense) stress, such as being disabled.

One of the most potently perceived stressors is frustration. People's motivation, or goal seeking, is central to their success and satisfaction, and when this is thwarted they are apt to suffer a strong emotional reaction that is felt as frustration. Motivation encompasses the whole spectrum of people's desires, and no one is free from frustration. Thwarting of major motivation may be an almost lifelong process, but people are also beset by numerous small frustrations related to different minor matters. Many people set their goals higher than is appropriate to their innate abilities. In such cases, frustration is likely to be prolonged and may be very severe, causing stress.

In 1967, inspired partly by Selye's work, the psychologists Thomas Holmes and Richard Rahe, working at the University of Washington, came up with a new set of stressors relating to life changes. Selye had already decided that stress was caused by both bad events (distress) and good events (eustress) and that both kinds could cause disease. He postulated that bad stress was usually the more serious because it was nearly always more severe and more persistent than eustress. Holmes and Rahe now came up with a table of events graded in terms of their severity in causing harm. They arbitrarily allotted the figure of 100 to what they considered the most stressful life event—the death of a spouse—and smaller numbers for less severe stressors, such as moving house, going on vacation, or financial troubles.

It is easy to criticize this scheme on the grounds that, for different people, different events can have widely varied significance and, consequently, different stress values. Moreover, most of these events can be quantified over a considerably wide range. Trouble with the boss, for example, might range from a minor disagreement to a major, livelihood-threatening row. Some of the categories actually involve clusters of other changes. Even so, tables of this kind have won a fair measure of acceptance as a guide to the totality of stress suffered by a person.

Conclusions

What is significant about all this research is that Holmes and Rahe claimed to have found that about 80 percent of people whose total stress events added up to more than 300 points in one year developed serious illness. This compared with about 30 percent of those whose totals were less then 150 in a year.

It has to be said, however, that the ability to withstand stress varies enormously with the person. Some people thrive on stress; other people break down under a minor level. The reasons for this variation remain obscure but may have something to do with personality types.

A-type and B-type personalities

In 1974, the heart specialists Meyer Friedman and Ray H. Rosenman, while studying the causes of heart disease, suggested that many people create their own stress. These are the A-type people: impatient, competitive, driven, and constantly under pressure. A-type people do everything in a hurry. They are always early for appointments, go crazy in traffic jams, and demand perfection of themselves in everything they undertake. The cardiologists concluded that A-type behavior was a more accurate predictor of heart attacks than almost any other combination of factors. B-type people are laid-back, relaxed, patient, easygoing, and are much less prone to heart attacks.

This concept aroused much interest and, for a time, it featured strongly in the medical literature. There were, however, some strong medical criticisms of it, and the initial enthusiasm for the idea was not sustained. Most doctors, however, would admit that there are certainly A-type people around, and that they are more susceptible to certain diseases, especially heart attacks.

Public and scientific response

Selye's ideas, and those of his followers, have aroused enormous public interest. The response of the medical profession, however, has been muted. Some doctors have accepted the ideas without question. Many who are cautious about adopting new ideas without strong scientific evidence have been more critical. Some voiced strong skepticism; many ignored it in their books and papers or explicitly stated that it was all nonsense.

Selye's assertions have never gained the unequivocal support of the scientific establishment. Even today, when stress has become a household word, his name is conspicuously absent from biographical dictionaries of scientists. There are some reasons for this that are not necessarily related to the intrinsic merit of his ideas. His habit of passing his ideas direct to the public by way of books that ordinary people could understand, for example, did not always endear him to the medical profession, and this may have been the origin of some of the prejudice against him. Doctors like to announce medical advances by way of the medical press, where they are subjected to the criticism

Scale of life event units	
Death of a spouse	100
Divorce	73
Marital separation	65
Jail term	63
Marriage	50
Being fired	47
Retirement	45
Pregnancy	40
New baby	39
Death of a close friend	37
Large mortgage	31
Son or daughter leaving home	29
In-law trouble	29
Trouble with employer	23
Change of residence	20
Change of school	20
Vacation	13
Minor law violation	11

of their colleagues. This is called peer review. They are not happy when this process is bypassed by those who appeal directly to the public. Selye died without ever having gained full medical acceptance of his ideas.

What is stress?

The real basis for medical doubts, however, arose from the nature of the subject. For a start, there is the question of definition. What, in short, is stress? It is, of course, entirely subjective. Stress is what people feel, and one person's stress is another person's challenge. What is painfully stressful to one person may be excitingly gratifying to another. Stressors are not, in themselves, stressful. It is the interaction of the stressor and the individual that creates the stress, and people are different in their responses. These points have not always been adequately appreciated, and there has been considerable confusion between cause and effect. Selye himself admitted that his English was not quite good enough for him to appreciate the difference between stress and strain and that he got his terms the wrong way around.

Critics of Holmes's and Rahe's life-event stress factors have pointed out that the results of the research might equally be explained on the hypothesis that people predisposed to physical or psychological disease may be just the kind of people whose lives involve a greater number of stressful changes. Spouses and long-term partners share influences that commonly lead to the development of similar disorders. Also, people with a predisposition to certain types of illness have a higher than average history of being fired from work.

As to the question of the A-type and B-type personality, critics remind us that most people do not fall into these clear-cut categories. Certainly there are people at both extremes of the spectrum. There are some people who are obvious A types, and others who are obvious B types, just as there are obvious introverts and extroverts. However, the number who are in either of the extreme groups is a small proportion of the whole. This makes the entire concept open to debate. Nearly all the evidence for linking A-type personalities with heart disease is in the popular literature.

Current medical views

Although doctors are still arguing about stress, the term, perhaps significantly, is cropping up far more frequently in textbooks and medical papers than ever before. A search on the word "stress" in any medical database will turn up thousands of examples. This is partly because the word has become so fashionable that it is used in all kinds of contexts and with a range of meanings.

Many diseases are now believed to have at least some basis in stress. Typical is the state of opinion on stress and peptic ulceration of the lining of the stomach and the first part of the small intestine. Most of the research into this question has been in the form of retrospective studies looking back to see whether people with peptic ulceration were people who had been stressed. This is not considered the ideal method, and too much is left to the opinion of either the patient or the doctor.

Prospective studies to see whether stressed people later develop ulcers are better. One 13-year prospective study of over 4,000 people with no history of ulcers showed that those who were aware of stress in their lives were more likely to develop peptic ulcers than those who were not. Again, however, the assessment of stress has to be subjective, and this makes convincing research difficult to organize. Only objective evidence is fully acceptable to science. One study, however, found many more personality disturbances in people with peptic ulcers than in those with kidney stones or gallstones. Currently it is agreed that more prospective studies are needed to determine the role of emotional stress in peptic ulceration.

These doubts have not prevented many scientific doctors from trying to produce theories to explain the relationship between stress and the processes that lead to disease. New models of how stress might operate appear regularly in the medical and psychological journals. A review of the medical literature indicates some support for the opinion that stress operates on the immune system. There is an awareness of the link between the immune system and brain processes concerned with thought, environmental perception, behavior, appreciation of stress, and so on. The immune system does not work in isolation in its defense against infection, tumors, and foreign material. A new branch of medical science, called psychoneuroimmunology, is concerned with the study of interactions between the mind and the immune system.

Psychoneuroimmunology

Doctors are now gaining a clearer understanding of the ways in which hormones can affect the immune system. They are also discovering that immune system regulation can be mediated by direct nerve connections to the lymphoid tissue of the system. These advances begin to explain much that was previously obscure about the way in which the body can respond to stress. This research also promises to advance people's understanding of how human behavior can control the function of the immune system and how psychosocial factors and emotional states can affect the development of diseases such as infections and cancers.

The science of psychoneuroimmunology is still in its infancy, but remarkable advances in our knowledge of both neurologic and immunologic control mechanisms are making it increasingly clear that there are previously unsuspected ways in which stress can cause various diseases.

Post-traumatic stress disorder

For those who respond badly to stress, there are certain warning signs suggesting danger. These include increasing irritability, loss of appetite, sleeping difficulties, loss of concentration, greater difficulty in making decisions, inability to relax, short fuse, and anger over trivial matters. All these are commonplace.

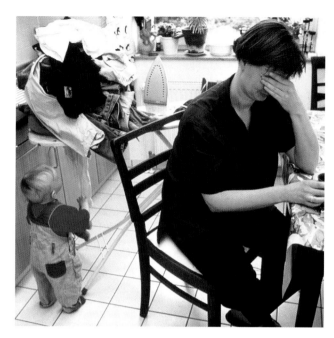

▲ *Some people find child rearing particularly stressful. The anxiety and worry of keeping a young child in good health and away from danger can take its toll of stress on a parent.*

Less common is the acute stress reaction which relates obviously to a particular event, and which is followed within about an hour by obvious symptoms. These may include anger, despair, aggression, withdrawal, or excessive grief. The outlook in this condition is good, but time is required for recovery. No one would try to deny that there are levels of stress so severe that many people exposed to them would suffer psychological damage. Again, the outcome in such cases varies with the personality. When people are involved in major disasters, such as train or plane crashes or earthquakes, many come through the experience apparently unharmed; others react very badly.

In World War I, soldiers were exposed to appalling stress from long periods of intense artillery or mortar bombardment and small arms fire. These unfortunates were frequently required to get up out of their trenches and run across open terrain in the face of machine gun fire and almost certain death. Those who broke down were said to suffer from lack of moral fiber. Those who ran away were tried for cowardice and shot. Thousands who survived these ordeals subsequently suffered from what was then called shell shock, and what is now called post-traumatic stress disorder.

This disorder features a repetitive reliving of the stressful event or events, with intrusive flashback memories and nightmares. Any event or circumstance that reminds the sufferer of the stressor event causes serious distress. The features of stress listed above are often present, and there may be loss of memory (amnesia) of the event. If not treated, the disorder can become permanent.

See also: **Arthritis; Cancer; Exercise; Heart attack; Heart disease; Infection and infectious diseases; Personality; Sleep and sleep problems; Stroke; Sugars; Ulcers**

Stroke

Questions and Answers

My mother had a serious stroke when she was 53. Does this put me at risk of having one too?

Not necessarily. Your chances of having a stroke depend to some extent on what caused your mother's disease. If high blood pressure was the cause, then it may be advisable to have your blood pressure checked so that, if high blood pressure is found, suitable treatment can be given. If there is a long history of strokes in your family, then it is important that you do not add to the risk by smoking.

Does taking the Pill increase the risk of having a stroke?

In a tiny number of women, strokes have occurred while they were on the Pill. For this reason doctors try to discourage women who are over 40 from taking the Pill. There is far less risk in women who are under 40. However, doctors will try to dissuade women under 40 from continuing with the Pill if they have a history of migraine, as it does slightly increase the chances of having a stroke at a younger age.

Is there any surgery that can treat people who have had a stroke?

Strokes from leaking berry aneurysms can sometimes be treated surgically to stop the bleeding and prevent further hemorrhage. Occasionally, one of the larger arteries in the neck may be narrowed or roughened inside, and surgery to correct this may prevent further damaging strokes.

My father has just had a stroke and can't speak. Will his speech return?

Yes, it is very likely that his ability to speak will come back, at least to some extent. Sometimes people are not able to speak at all in the first few days after a stroke, but later recover almost completely.

With little or no warning a stroke can cause sudden weakness, paralysis, or even death. Nevertheless, however fearsome this common affliction may be, rehabilitation can help survivors overcome any resulting disability.

Strokes often (though not exclusively) attack older people and are one of the most common causes of death throughout the Western world. However, present advances in medical research, particularly in connection with the role of high blood pressure, have helped doctors' understanding of this illness. Many strokes are now preventable through early identification and treatment of those at risk.

What is a stroke?

Most people have some idea of what a stroke is; such knowledge is a testament to how often the disease occurs. The common factor in all strokes is that, owing to a disease of the blood vessel that supplies a particular part of the brain, a section of the brain suddenly stops working. The person involved often has little or no warning that something is wrong before he or she is struck down, most often with weakness or paralysis down one side of the body. This condition may be accompanied by aphasia (loss of speech) or by other problems in higher brain functions. A small number of strokes occur in parts of the brain that do not control the body's movement, so that paralysis does not occur.

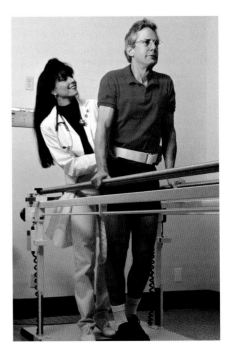

▲ *A stroke need not signal the end to a person's active life. With physical therapy, it is often possible to restore the function of affected limbs to varying degrees.*

What causes a stroke?

Like the rest of the body, the brain must have a constant supply of blood reaching it through its arteries. If one of these arteries becomes blocked, the part of the brain that it feeds will die because of the lack of oxygen. There are many cross-connections in the brain between neighboring blood vessels, so that the area of damage is generally restricted. However, even the part of the brain that does not die may swell and damage the rest of the brain. The other way in which strokes may be caused is that blood vessels in the brain burst. When this happens, the blood rushes into the brain under pressure, severely damaging nerve fibers.

These two basic mechanisms, cerebral infarction (when the artery is blocked) and cerebral hemorrhage (when there is bleeding into the brain), can be brought about by a variety of disorders.

Obstruction of an artery in the brain can result from a disease that produces a blockage in the artery itself (a cerebral thrombosis), or when a blood clot passes up the blood supply to the brain artery and gets stuck there. This is called a cerebral embolism.

Thrombosis (or blood clotting) generally occurs when an artery of the brain becomes narrowed: fatty material accumulates in the walls of the artery. This is what happens in the disease called atherosclerosis, which also causes the heart's blood vessels to clot, resulting in heart attacks. Occasionally, other problems in the arteries can cause thrombosis. These include inflammation of the artery, which can occur on its own or as a result of some serious infections.

Embolisms can be caused by heart diseases or by disorders in the main arteries in the neck from which the blood enters the brain. Heart disease and strokes are thus linked, not only

Does everyone who has had a stroke have to be hospitalized?

This would depend on the severity of the stroke, and whether or not the facilities available in the stroke patient's home enable him or her to be properly looked after. In some areas, special teams of physical therapists are available to treat people in their own homes. However, people with strokes often need to remain in the hospital while they are very disabled so that their stroke can be properly assessed, in terms of treatment and of prevention of further strokes.

Is there any point in having someone's blood pressure treated after a stroke, or is this like shutting the stable door after the horse has bolted?

Immediately after a stroke, the blood pressure is usually left alone for a few days, since a sudden drop may impair the flow of blood to the damaged areas in the brain. However, careful studies have shown that it is important to treat the blood pressure vigorously to prevent further strokes, which might cause further disability.

My uncle had a bad heart attack and a few weeks later had a stroke that paralyzed his left side. Was this connected with his heart attack, and why did this happen?

After a heart attack, blood clots may form on the inside wall of the chamber of the heart. Occasionally, part of a clot can become dislodged and fly upward to block off one of the brain's blood vessels, thus producing a stroke. Patients who have had very serious heart attacks can be given anticoagulant drugs to help prevent this.

Is it possible to prevent strokes?

Yes, in some cases. If patients who have high blood pressure are identified and treated early, this can greatly reduce the risk of a stroke.

because the same disease of the arteries can cause trouble in both the heart and the brain, but also because in many diseases of the heart, blood clots form on the valves or on the damaged inside walls of the heart and these then fly off as emboli.

Cerebral hemorrhages (in which the blood vessels in the brain burst) also have a number of causes. The most common cause is that there are weak places (called aneurysms) in the walls of the brain's arteries which then burst, often because they have been weakened by atherosclerosis. In the larger brain arteries at the base of the skull these aneurysms may be congenital, though they may not rupture until late in life, if at all. Less common causes of cerebral hemorrhage can occur as a result of the presence of small, abnormally formed blood vessels in the brain, rather like the strawberry marks that are a similar abnormality of the blood vessels in the skin. This is called arteriovenous anomaly, and again this condition is congenital.

Who is at risk?

Certain people have a higher risk of having strokes than others. The main conditions that predispose a person toward a stroke are atherosclerosis, high blood pressure, having high serum

DAMAGE CAUSED BY A STROKE

▲ A stroke can be caused by a blockage in any of the four pairs of cerebral arteries. Each type has different results, depending on the area of the brain that is affected. A blockage in an anterior artery is common, and one in the basilar is usually fatal.

MAJOR CAUSES OF STROKES

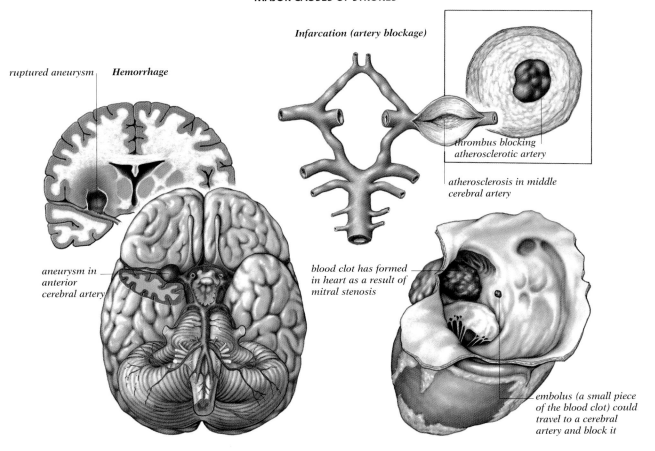

Infarction (artery blockage)

ruptured aneurysm   **Hemorrhage**

thrombus blocking atherosclerotic artery

atherosclerosis in middle cerebral artery

aneurysm in anterior cerebral artery

blood clot has formed in heart as a result of mitral stenosis

embolus (a small piece of the blood clot) could travel to a cerebral artery and block it

▲ *Strokes can be caused by hemorrhages or blockages (infarctions) in the brain. Many hemorrhages are caused by the rupturing of weakened arteries (aneurysms). Infarctions are caused either when a blood clot forms in a diseased cerebral artery (thrombus), or when a clot travels from another area of the body, such as the damaged walls of the heart, and lodges in the brain (embolus).*

cholesterol, having diabetes, and smoking cigarettes. In addition, strokes seem to run in some families, though because the condition is so common, this is difficult to prove. Finally, there are people with heart diseases that can cause a stroke by embolism. Therefore, people with a high risk can often be identified, and preventive measures can be taken to reduce the chances of a stroke.

Symptoms

Many stroke patients have a warning attack in the weeks or months before a major stroke. These warning attacks take the form of short-lived episodes of weakness down one side, or transient blacking out of vision in one eye—a sign of blockage in one of the blood vessels to the retina. These warnings are called transient ischemic attacks (TIAs) and they must never be ignored. Medical attention at the stage of the TIA can save life. In most cases, disabilities such as loss of function on one side of the body or loss of speech reach their maximum within minutes, though occasionally it may take hours. In

the following days and weeks, there will be an improvement as some of the brain cells recover. After six months the disabilities will be considerably less than they were at the onset of the stroke.

Other symptoms may include loss of vision in the right- or left-hand half of the visual field of both eyes, difficulty in dressing or finding the way around familiar surroundings, and various other subtle difficulties in brain function. If a large area of the brain was damaged at the start of the stroke, the patient may not have a clear awareness of what has happened, or may ignore everything that happens on one side of his or her body. As the damaged brain swells, he or she may become drowsy or lose consciousness. This may happen much more quickly in brain hemorrhages, since the surge of blood into the brain causes damage to the mechanisms that maintain alertness.

Treatment

Initial treatment consists of limiting the amount of damage that may be caused by swelling spreading to the unaffected parts of the brain. This is done by paying close attention to the blood pressure and administering certain drugs, particularly steroids. Very seldom can surgeons remove the blood clots that are causing pressure, since they are often situated in inaccessible parts of the brain.

However, the main care of patients who have had strokes lies in the hands of the nursing staff, physical therapists, speech therapists, and occupational therapists. Careful nursing is very important to prevent the emergence of bedsores and chest troubles, which can

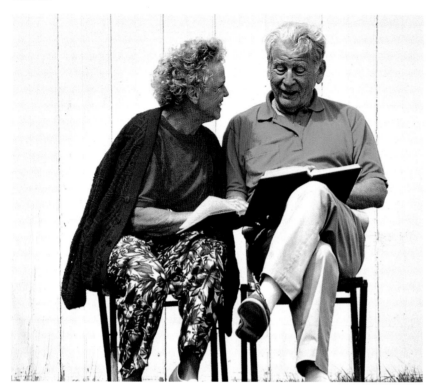

▲ *One of the most important stages in the recovery of a stroke patient takes place at home, where the support of family and friends becomes vital.*

▼ *Communication boards are available for stroke victims with speech impairment. This patient can point to words and illustrations that express his thoughts or needs.*

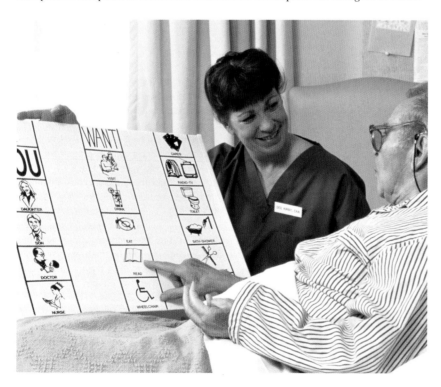

seriously impair a patient's recovery from a stroke. During this vulnerable period when the stroke patient is often unable to undertake his or her own care, good nursing can literally save a life.

Physical therapists maximize the effect of movement as it returns to affected limbs. Later they become even more vital because the therapy they suggest may make the difference between a patient's becoming seriously disabled or able to fend for himself or herself despite residual disabilities.

Treatment is in two stages. First, physical therapists ensure that the unused limbs remain supple and that unnecessary stiffness does not set in. Later, when the patient is ambulant (and this happens early, since prolonged periods in bed can be dangerous), the physical therapist concentrates on overcoming the abnormal reflex movements that interfere with the return of more useful muscle power.

Speech therapy plays an important role when the stroke has affected the power of speech. Speech therapists will be able to identify the difficulties the patient has and will work to encourage the return of speech, which often does happen to a greater or lesser extent. Further treatment by speech therapists consists of retraining patients with aphasia to make the best of the speech faculties that are left.

Occupational therapists try to prepare the patient for a return to as normal a life as possible. The therapist assesses the patient, and works out ways of overcoming problems that resist physical therapy.

The stroke patient at home

Many stroke patients are hospitalized while they are physically dependent (often in special stroke units), and then further recovery can be looked for when they go home. The patient's family will need a lot of support and guidance to make sure that they are not so overprotective that they slow his or her recovery. Therefore, the work of the physical and occupational therapists often extends to the home, where they can continue to supervise the patient's recovery. Special aids are available for facilitating such everyday tasks as taking a shower, cooking, and eating, which often present difficulties.

Preventing a stroke

The recent advances in stroke research have been concerned with prevention. The fact that in recent years in the United States the

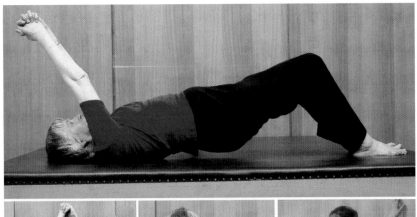

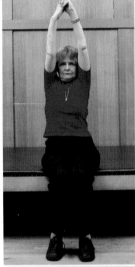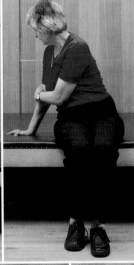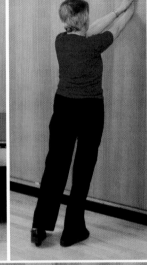

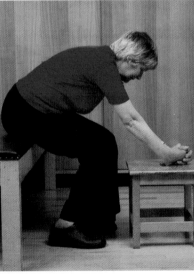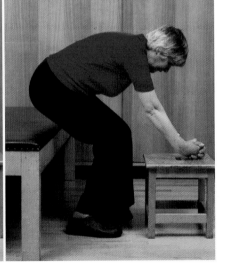

number of strokes has declined is indicative of the effectiveness of the research. This is due to the recognition of the importance of transient ischemic attacks (TIAs) and the identification and treatment of high blood pressure. TIAs cause temporary failure of part of the brain, owing to reduced blood supply. They often herald a stroke; awareness of this has provided doctors with the opportunity for positive intervention to avoid strokes.

Most people with high blood pressure feel well and may need convincing to take their pills regularly to keep it down. Generally, the doctor will take the blood pressure as a matter of routine when they consult him or her and will be able to detect high blood pressure before it leads to trouble.

After minor strokes from which the patient may have recovered, it is an important part of treatment to try to prevent another more serious episode from occurring. Surgery can sometimes be performed on the large blood vessels in the neck. This may be done if the blood vessels have roughened parts in their lining from which clots fly off as emboli.

Small doses of aspirin are also being tried for stroke prevention. It has been found that small amounts of the drug can affect the clotting ability of the blood to a degree sufficient to prevent the brain's blood vessels from becoming obstructed. Anticoagulant drugs reduce the blood's liability to clot, and these are used to prevent a stroke when one of the predisposing heart conditions is identified. Many other drugs that can prevent a stroke in those at risk are now undergoing trials.

Outlook

Although a stroke can be fatal, most victims recover to some degree. At least half of those who have had a stroke progress to a point where they can look after themselves, and most people paralyzed by strokes learn to walk again. Only about 5 percent of patients require long-term institutional care. While the remainder of stroke sufferers may have to depend on relatives to look after them at home, they or their caregivers should make full use of the variety of home aids and of the hospital and therapeutic treatments available to them to help patients overcome or live with their disabilities.

▲ *Stroke patients can exercise in their own homes. Exercises include using the strong arm to support the weak arm (top left) or paralyzed side (top right) by pulling it up. Additional strengthening can be achieved by doing swiveling (middle left) or pressing exercises (middle right), which require propping up the weak arm. Better balance can be gained by raising the body to a half-sitting position (above).*

See also: **Aspirin and analgesics; Cholesterol; Heart attack; Heart disease; Paralysis; Physical therapy; Speech**

Sugars

Sugar has other uses as well as sweetening foods and drinks. In various forms, sugar plays a vital role in providing energy for the body—and the body's preferred source of energy is the sugar glucose.

Do glucose tablets and drinks provide instant energy?

No. Glucose is the fuel that gives the body energy, but it does not instantly provide energy. Glucose is absorbed into the body and stored in the liver and muscles as glycogen until it is required. The amount of glucose found in the blood is small (0.1 percent of the blood is glucose), and more is added from the glycogen store when blood sugar levels drop. All carbohydrates convert to glucose, so there is no need to take glucose tablets and drinks.

Why do diabetics have to restrict their sugar intake?

A diabetic diet consists of a controlled amount of all carbohydrates. Diabetes is caused by the inability of the body to control the amount of sugar in the blood, so the diet aims to provide the patient with the exact amount of carbohydrates needed.

My children eat lots of candy. Will it affect their teeth?

Yes. Sugary and starchy foods provide a breeding ground for bacteria; they tend to produce acid substances that attack the protective enamel of the teeth. Once the enamel barrier is breached, the problem becomes worse. Encourage your children not to eat so much candy, and make sure they brush their teeth to get rid of the bacteria.

Is brown sugar better for you than ordinary white sugar?

Brown sugar is virtually the same as white sugar, but it has not had all the impurities removed. White sugar is produced by chemical processing. The basic constituent of sugar is sucrose. Brown sugar is almost pure sucrose.

The major part of a balanced diet consists of carbohydrates, which are sugars and starches. Carbohydrates contain atoms of carbon, hydrogen, and oxygen in varying configurations and it is the arrangements of these atoms that give the different carbohydrates their specific properties and names. Single sugar units or simple sugars are called monosaccharides, such as glucose. Disaccharides such as sucrose, lactose, and maltose are formed from two single saccharide molecules bonded together; they are the sugars normally found in foods. Polysaccharides, such as starches and glycogen, are long chains of glucose molecules.

Sugar and digestion

During digestion, carbohydrates are broken down into simple sugars, especially glucose, which can be absorbed into the body and used as fuel to provide energy for all metabolic processes. The glucose absorbed into the body is not all poured into the bloodstream after being digested; a certain amount is diverted to the liver where it is converted into glycogen, or animal starch. The liver acts as an energy store for the body. When instant energy is required, the liver converts some of the stored glycogen into glucose and releases it into the bloodstream. Thus, a high-glucose meal has no special energy-giving properties, because the excess is simply stored. Even if there is a temporary lack of carbohydrate, the liver is able to synthesize glucose from fats and proteins.

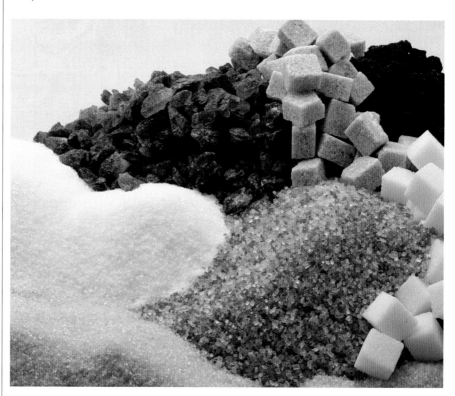

▲ *White sugar is pure sucrose and brown sugars are virtually the same. It is their impurities that give brown sugars their color.*

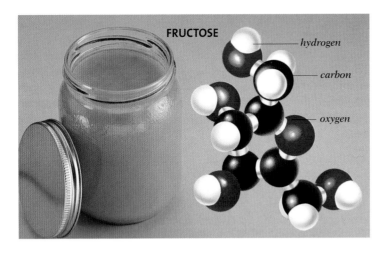

▲ *The simple sugars (monosaccharides) are commonly found in natural foods. Fructose, found in honey, is a prime example.*

uneasiness, and sweating; it may even lead to epileptic fits or unconsciousness. Usually, people who suffer from hypoglycemia learn to recognize the symptoms and eat a sugar-rich food to arrest the problem.

Sugars and health

Although a certain amount of sugar is useful in that it contributes to providing energy for the body, an excess of sugar can also lead to harmful effects. These include obesity and tooth decay. In addition, sugar is thought by some to be a contributory factor in hardening of the arteries.

There is a certain amount of evidence that an excess of sugar in the diet, along with smoking and a high fat intake, can contribute to atherosclerosis. Also, sugar is a very potent source of calories, and people with a tendency to obesity should avoid pure sugar. Although all the starchy food that is eaten is converted to simple sugar in the body, for a steady supply of energy it is best to eat complex carbohydrates, such as brown rice, grains, and other whole

Blood sugar

The blood contains about 0.1 percent glucose, and this continuously supplies the energy needs of the body tissues. It is particularly important to the brain, which has no means of storing fuel. For this reason, it is crucial that the concentration of sugar in the blood is monitored and regulated. Several hormones, of which insulin is the most important, are involved in the fine control necessary to attain the correct balance between the instant availability and storage of glucose. When the level of sugar in the blood rises, the pancreas releases insulin to the bloodstream and this enables glucose to be stored or used by the tissues. Too little insulin, or a total lack of it, leads to high concentrations of blood sugar; this condition is called diabetes mellitus, or sugar diabetes.

On the other hand, an overproduction of insulin leads to a condition called hypoglycemia, which results from too little sugar in the blood. This condition quickly impairs brain function, leading to such symptoms as hunger,

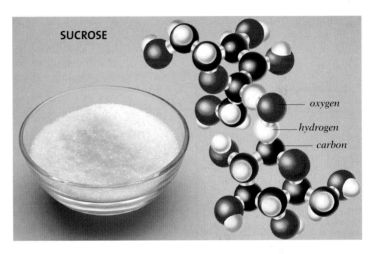

▲ *When two simple sugar molecules join together a disaccharide is formed. Ordinary table sugar (sucrose) is the best-known.*

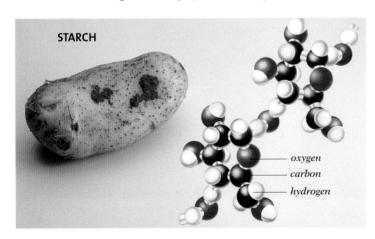

▲ *When many sugar molecules join up, polysaccharides are formed. These are the starches found in vegetables.*

foods. Digestion of these foods takes longer and the slow absorption of sugars provides a constant supply of energy and limits the amount of sugar converted into fat and thereby stored. This helps to guard against atherosclerosis. In general, a healthy diet should contain more starch, less fat, and little refined sugar.

Sugary foods are thought to cause dental caries. In fact, sugars can have an effect on dental health, but indirectly. The mouth is a breeding ground for bacteria, which will feed off sugars or starches left clinging to the teeth and produce acid waste products that attack and etch the teeth, producing cavities.

Finally, carbohydrates do not require oxygen to convert them to energy, so they fuel exercises involving muscular contractions.

See also: **Bacteria; Diabetes; Diet; Fats; Glucose; Obesity; Smoking; Starch; Weight**

Suicide

Most people have moments of despair and self-hatred, but only a small number of them will actually attempt or commit suicide. What drives people to it, and what help is available for people who have reached the breaking point?

Questions and Answers

My sister is frequently depressed and often threatens suicide, but so far she has never attempted it. Should I take her threats seriously?

It is a common error to think that those who talk about suicide never do it. Her suicidal threats are an expression of her obvious distress, and treatment for her depression should be sought before she does something drastic. Ask your doctor to recommend professional help.

Is it true that the suicide rate is higher among artists and writers?

There is a high rate of suicide in all jobs that place a lot of pressure on the achievement of the individual. However, the majority of suicides occur among older people, the less well off, the unemployed, and the physically ill.

My friend's son committed suicide, and later it was learned that he was bullied in school. Could his suicide have been prevented?

Possibly. Many suicides would not take place if the distressed person had been able to talk about his or her problems. However, many factors usually contribute to drive an individual to suicide, and although the bullying may have been an important one, it may not have been the only one.

Why do many women make repeated suicide attempts?

It is thought that more women survive an attempted suicide because of their tendency to use less violent methods than men (poisoning, for example), leaving a chance of survival. It has also been suggested that women use the appeal effect of a suicide attempt more because other methods of exerting pressure or displaying aggression are not in their nature.

Many factors can contribute to causing the depression, despair, or low self-esteem that drive a person to suicide. Suicidal individuals are now recognized as either being ill or in great distress, and should receive help and treatment before it is too late.

Who commits suicide?

More men commit suicide than women, but a far greater number of women make unsuccessful attempts to kill themselves. Studies show that virtually no children below the age of 15 commit suicide, but the rate tends to increase steadily as people get older. Divorced and widowed people are far more likely to kill themselves than married or single people. People with strong family, community, or religious ties are less prone to suicide.

Suicide is more frequent among the professional classes (managers, executives, doctors, and businessmen) and among low-status unskilled workers than among the skilled workers who form the middle group of the population. People living in small country towns are among the least likely to kill themselves. Those living in big cities, especially in the city center rather than in the suburbs, are most at risk.

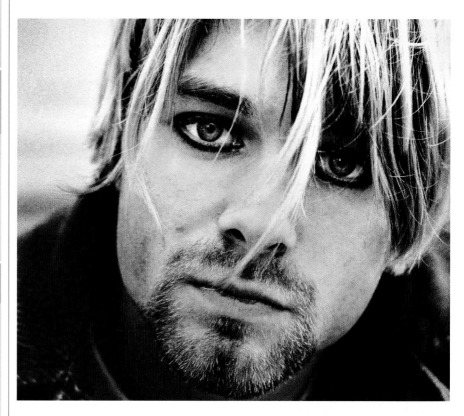

▲ *Nirvana frontman Kurt Cobain committed suicide in 1994. As with many suicides, there was a clear warning of the approaching tragedy. Six weeks before he fatally shot himself in his Seattle home, Cobain went into a coma after overdosing on a cocktail of painkillers and champagne while in Rome, Italy, on tour.*

More people commit suicide in spring and early summer than at any other time of the year, and there are often more deaths during public holidays, when the lonely feel even lonelier. The low rate of suicide in wartime has been explained by the closer involvement of the individual with the group, family, or community during that time.

Why?

Contrary to popular belief, suicide is not generally the result of a rational weighing of the pros and cons of living. Though an individual may have had suicidal thoughts, the final decision to kill him- or herself is usually made impulsively under severe emotional stress.

Usually there is a combination of factors that drives an otherwise stable person over the edge into the desperate act of suicide. A major misfortune or life change, such as the end of a marriage or relationship, the death of a loved one, or the loss of a job, may trigger the despair that precedes suicide. Social factors have been found to contribute to suicide in two-thirds of cases; in one-third of suicides they were the principal cause.

Nearly a third of those who kill themselves are physically ill. It has been estimated that for one in five of all suicide cases poor physical

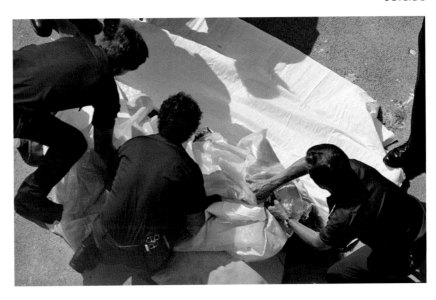

▲ *For every person who commits suicide there are 25 who attempt suicide but survive, because the method chosen is not effective or they are rescued in time.*

health was the primary reason for the action. An unhappy love affair appears to be the motivation for suicide in only one out of 20 cases, and failed examinations or pregnancy out of wedlock are even less common as a cause.

Loneliness and alienation from the community are an important cause of suicide. The person who kills him- or herself is likely to experience a high degree of isolation and separation from the society he or she lives in. High rates of suicide are found where communities have disintegrated and are unstable, and where the needs of the individual are not satisfied.

The majority of those who kill themselves are severely depressed, and indeed a similar psychological state underlies depression and suicide. In both cases, the individual turns against him- or herself hostile impulses that were originally meant for other people. If he or she is unable to express angry or aggressive feelings externally, they may turn into self-aggression, which is expressed as self-criticism and self-hatred, or in the more extreme actions of self-injury and self-destruction in the case of a potential suicide.

Alongside the urge toward self-destruction, there is frequently a contrasting urge toward human contact and communication with other people. Suicides know their act will affect others, and usually they give warning before or during a suicide attempt. Sometimes an individual may use the act of suicide as a means of forcing others to express their love and concern for him or her.

The aged, the poor, and the physically sick make up a large proportion of those who kill themselves, and who are particularly vulnerable. Those living away from their family group are also more likely to commit suicide than others. The rate of suicide increases with age and the peak age for suicide is over 84 years.

Marriage and a big family have been linked with a lower rate of suicide but a higher rate of homicide, often a family crime. The impersonal life of the big city has been blamed for the large number of suicides, especially among immigrants and those living alone. Poor areas with a highly mobile population show the highest rates of all worldwide.

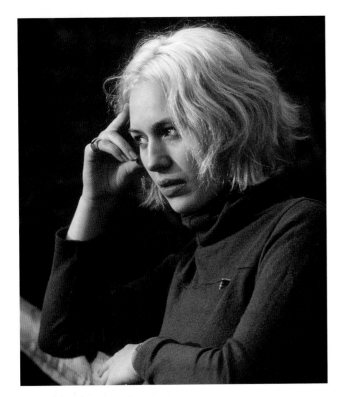

▲ *Suicide is very often preceded by depression. Young women are the most likely to attempt a suicide that is unsuccessful.*

Questions and Answers

Someone I knew committed suicide last month after he lost his job. Is there really any link between unemployment and suicide?

The change of life that occurs when a person loses a job, and the consequent loss of self-esteem, disorientation, and isolation from the community, may trigger a depression that leads to suicide. However, it is not possible to generalize from this and say that there is a close relationship between economic climate and levels of suicide. Many other factors will always come into play.

Why do some people make suicide pacts?

Most people who make suicide pacts are not young unhappy lovers but older married couples, particularly when one may have a serious illness. Pacts, which are extremely rare, are illegal, and a survivor may be charged with the criminal offense of aiding and abetting the suicide of the other.

A friend recently took an overdose of pills, but it was not fatal. Will she do it again?

Those who have attempted suicide are more at risk of suicide than any other members of the population, especially during the first four years after the attempt. The likelihood of a second attempt depends on whether the situation that caused the first attempt has improved.

Does a person's religion or cultural background play any part in determining whether he or she might commit suicide?

In some cultures suicide has been admired: for example, some Eastern religions have honored people choosing to free themselves from their bodies. In contrast, the Jewish and Christian religions condemned suicide as sinful. However, modern attitudes in many countries have moved toward seeing suicide as a psychological and social problem.

Substance abuse and suicide

Most studies support the view that substance abuse is associated with a risk of suicide, particularly in young people. The substances most often implicated in suicide are alcohol, stimulants, and opiates. Studies disagree on whether there is a link between extreme cannabis use and suicide.

ALCOHOL
Evidence suggests that alcoholics and drug abusers may drink to reduce feelings of depression, but that the initial state of well-being is replaced within hours by anxiety, depression, and increased suicidal thoughts. No cause-and-effect relationship between alcoholism or drug abuse and suicide has been established, but it may be that such substances reduce inhibitions and affect judgment to the extent that any suicidal thoughts are more likely to be acted on.

ANTIDEPRESSANTS
It is not only illicit drugs that have been linked with suicide. The antidepressant Paxil, known in Europe as Seroxat, was withdrawn as a prescription drug for young adults in European Union countries after surveys linked its use among this group with a possible increased risk of suicide. The European regulatory agency covering such drugs, the European Agency for the Evaluation of Medicinal Products, issued an advisory to member states suggesting that it be prescribed "with caution" to anyone under 30. The drug is a member of a group of drugs known as SSRIs, or selective serotonin reuptake inhibitors. The U.S. Food and Drug Administration has also warned that taking the drug could increase suicidal impulses.

STEROIDS
Withdrawal from the use of steroids—taken by some athletes to enhance performance—has also been linked to an increased risk of suicide. Depression is one of the major risks when ending use of these drugs. Among former users, researchers note feelings of "paranoid jealousy, extreme irritability, delusions, and impaired judgment stemming from feelings of invincibility." Left untreated, depressive symptoms can last up to a year.

The suicide rate is much higher among the unemployed than among the employed. Heavy drinkers are also particularly vulnerable to attempts at suicide. Among people suffering depression, those individuals most at risk are likely to be those undergoing prolonged bouts of insomnia, those who come from a broken home, and those who have already made a previous suicide attempt. They are probably not receiving any psychiatric help.

Methods
Few suicides or attempted suicides are carefully planned. The method used depends on what is available to the individual. In the United States, where guns are relatively easy to obtain, shooting is the most common means of suicide—the majority of gun-related deaths are suicides. In Great Britain, by contrast, where many kinds of gun are illegal, poisoning accounts for most deaths. Other common methods are hanging and drowning.

Those who survive a suicide attempt may suffer some lasting aftereffects, depending on the method used. Aspirin and acetaminophen can sometimes cause permanent damage to the kidney and liver. Some drugs taken in large quantities cause permanent brain damage. Survivors of more violent attempts may be left with a physical disability, or may spend some painful days or weeks in a hospital before dying from an indirectly caused ailment such as pneumonia.

Attempted suicide
For every person who kills him- or herself, there are many more who attempt suicide and survive. A large number of cases of attempted suicide are never brought to a hospital, either because the injuries are small or because the individual or the individual's family feels ashamed.

While the majority of actual suicides are older men, women attempt suicide two to three times as often as men. There has also been a rise in the number of suicide attempts by young people, with the standard profile of an adolescent suicide being a male who dies of a gunshot

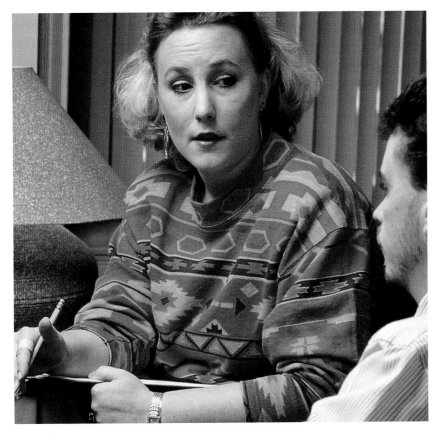

▲ *For many people who survive a suicide attempt, sympathetic counseling may be all they need to help them come to terms with their problems.*

are vital if the patient is to feel secure, loved, and valued.

A suicide attempt sometimes reveals problems that can then be remedied. The impact that it creates may lead to an improvement in family relations or to the individual's being removed from a socially isolated situation. In many cases, it highlights an emotional or physical illness that can be treated. Sometimes the social services of the community can give practical help and advice.

Prevention of suicide

In recent years much valuable work in suicide prevention has been done by organizations such as the Samaritans and Lifeline. People in distress can call them at any time and speak in complete confidence to a sympathetic layperson. If appropriate, they may be referred to a doctor. In cities where these organizations operate, surveys have shown a reduction in the suicide rates.

Living wills and assisted suicides

For many people the right to die is an important part of human dignity. Some people who are terminally ill, for example, believe they have a right to end their own life if the quality of life sinks below what they consider bearable. Others argue, often from a religious viewpoint, that every life is sacred and that no one has the right to take it away. Doctors can sometimes find themselves caught between, on the one hand, their professional duty to preserve a patient's life and, on the other, their respect for a patient's right of self-determination and compassion for his or her suffering.

It is against this background that the phenomenon of the living will has developed. The living will is a document by which individuals let it be known what they would like to happen to them should they no longer be in a position to determine their future—for example, if they were to be permanently brain-damaged or in a coma. Those who have living wills elect not to be kept alive by artificial means if the chances of recovery seem very slight. Living wills have proved ethical and legal minefields, and in some states they are illegal. Before anyone makes a living will, it is important to check with the district attorney's office to find out what position his or her state takes on this issue.

The related issue of assisted suicide (providing help to end the life of somebody who cannot end it himself or herself) is even more contentious. While under strictly defined circumstances it is legal in the Netherlands, it remains illegal throughout the United States. Any person who assists another to commit suicide can be indicted on a charge of homicide.

wound and the standard profile of an adolescent nonfatal suicide attempter being a female who took pills. For many students in high school and college, these are emotionally stressful years, when unhappy love affairs and failure to make friends or to pass examinations can seem like major tragedies to which suicide is the only solution.

In the past, those who attempted suicide were often branded as attention seekers who were making a gesture to manipulate others without any genuine intention of killing themselves. However, research has shown that apparently harmless acts are often followed by more dangerous acts. It is now recognized that the cry for help of the attempted suicide generally represents a sincere statement of distress.

Treatment

Although many doctors will prescribe antidepressant drugs to tide an individual over a period of crisis, the only long-term cure is for the patient to receive some kind of psychotherapy. He or she will then be able to discuss any problems and come to terms with painful or aggressive feelings whose suppression may be responsible for the self-injury.

The doctor or therapist may enlist the cooperation of sympathetic relatives or friends, who can very often contribute a great deal to the success of recovery, either providing insights into the patient's problems or giving the routine care and support that

See also: **Alcoholism; Aspirin and analgesics; Depression; Family relationships; Poisoning; Stress**

Sunburn

Deliberately exposing the skin to the sun can be a risky activity. To limit skin damage, common sense and forethought will help prevent not only the discomfort of sunburn but also the danger of developing serious conditions such as skin cancer.

The sun has traditionally played a beneficent role in human civilization and has been seen in many cultures as a life giver. Attitudes are beginning to change, however. The discovery in the mid-1980s that the ozone layer—the part of the Earth's atmosphere that protects the planet from the sun's harmful ultraviolet radiation—was under assault from synthetic pollutants and that, as a consequence, people increasingly run the risk of developing skin cancer and possibly cataracts from overexposure to the sun's rays, has made people view the sun with more wariness.

How sunburn occurs

Sunburn is the result of immediate sun damage to the skin. Sunburn is a form of radiation burn rather than heat burn. Unlike a burn caused by heat, sunburn does not completely develop and is not felt until a few hours after it happens.

The sun is really a small star and its energy can be compared with a continuous and enormous atomic explosion. Some of its rays are deadly, but these are filtered out by the Earth's atmosphere and never reach the Earth itself. The rays that do pass through the atmosphere are part of the sun's spectrum, which consists of visible rays that are seen as light; infrared rays that

Questions and Answers

I am fair-skinned and my friend is dark. Why can she spend a long time in the sun without burning while I have to be very careful?

Being fair-skinned means that you have little pigment in your skin. Your friend has more pigment, and can also manufacture more than you when exposed to sunlight. She has a natural barrier to the sun's harmful rays, and is capable of developing even greater protection. You will burn easily because your skin cannot produce enough protective pigment and no amount of sunbathing will alter this.

Can some drugs make you more sensitive to the sun?

Yes. Examples are the tranquilizer chlorpromazine and the antibiotic oxytetracycline. This abnormal reaction is called photosensitivity. A rash like sunburn develops on areas exposed to the sun, but if the drug is stopped, the rash fades.

I have very sensitive skin. Is there any treatment I can have before going on vacation this year?

You could have a course of ultraviolet ray therapy beforehand, to increase your pigmentation. Or you could use a sunscreen preparation that filters out the sun's stronger rays, allowing a slow tan to develop.

I have fair hair that becomes lighter in the sun while my skin becomes darker. Why is this?

The pigment in hair is already present, while that in skin appears only when the pigment-producing cells are activated by sunlight. Fair hair has a different sort of pigment from dark hair and, unlike dark hair, light hair becomes bleached on exposure to strong sunlight.

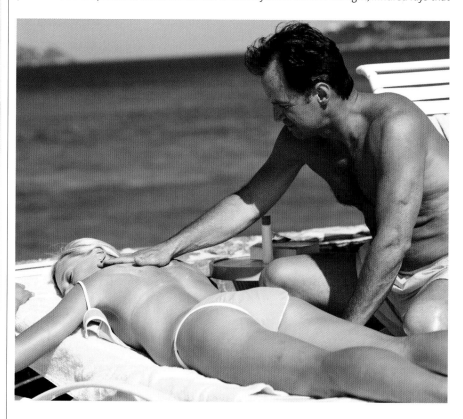

▲ *Although sunbathing on the beach is a relaxing activity, in reality the sun's rays reflecting off water can be extremely damaging to the skin.*

can be felt as heat; and the ultraviolet rays, which cause sunburn. The rays are called ultraviolet because they are positioned beyond the violet end of the visible spectrum.

Both ultraviolet and infrared rays are capable of causing damage to the body. However, infrared rays do not cause a problem, since they are registered as heat, and an exposed area can be withdrawn before any harm is done. It is the ultraviolet rays that cause problems because they can penetrate and damage the skin without giving an immediate feeling of warmth; this results in sunburn.

Ultraviolet rays produce their effect by transferring energy to molecules in the skin, causing a photochemical reaction. The amount of energy released depends on the wavelength of the rays. The shorter wavelengths carry and release more energy than the longer ones, and are more penetrating.

Effects on the skin

The skin is made up of two layers. In the outer layer (the epidermis), cells are continuously being shed from the surface and replaced by new cells, which are formed in the lowest level of the epidermis. It is in this outer layer that the effects of sunburn occur.

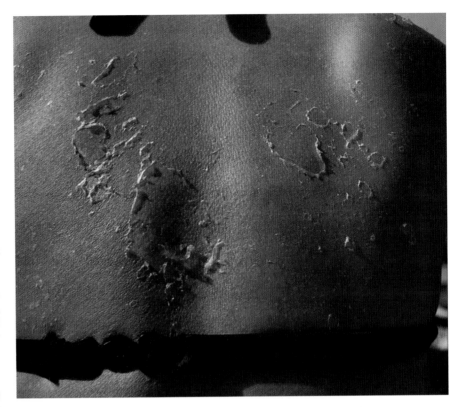

▲ *A tan does not prevent sunburn. Once the pigment-producing skin cells have been saturated with ultraviolet light, further exposure results in radiation burn.*

The bottom (basal) layer of the epidermis contains pigment-producing cells or melanocytes. These are stimulated by ultraviolet light to produce the pigment melanin, which acts as a very efficient filter of the ultraviolet rays. The new pigmentation (which is seen as a suntan) begins soon after exposure to the sun and builds gradually during continual exposure. After a period of exposure, the pigmentation will fade at varying rates, and is likely to disappear within nine months. Sunburn occurs when there is not enough pigment filter present.

Sunburn cells

There are two types of sun damage: immediate and delayed. The immediate type of damage is sunburn, but, as with other radiation burns, its effects do not show for some hours. The first signs are redness and a sensation of burning caused by an increase in the blood supply to the skin. This may happen anytime up to 24 hours after exposure. Later, small blisters may develop.

More severe damage produces larger blisters and can actually damage some of the cells in the epidermis. These damaged cells are called sunburn cells. The degree of sunburn depends on the strength of the ultraviolet rays.

Long-term sun damage

Sunburn itself is not as serious as the long-term damage to the skin. This is caused by repeated sun damage to the cells at the skin's surface and to the supporting tissues below. It takes years to develop, but once it has happened it is irreversible.

The changes are similar to those of aging, and the obvious effects can be seen in a sailor's or land worker's face, where there is marked wrinkling and a leathery thickening of the skin. Other effects can be very localized, such as patchy increases in the pigmentation and a thickening of the horny covering of the skin. This can give rise to wartlike lumps, called solar keratoses, which are common in the middle-aged and elderly. Widening of the blood vessels of the face and dryness and cracking of the skin are part of the aging process but are more marked in people who have spent their lives outdoors exposed to weather and to the sun.

Skin cancer

The most serious risk that can result from repeated overexposure to the sun is skin cancer. The high incidence in the 21st century of skin cancer among people of northern European descent can be directly related to the fact that for the first time they live in areas of bright sunshine. By contrast, skin cancer was very uncommon in the Victorian era, when there was little exposure of the skin. Today, it occurs frequently in sun-worshiping regions like California or Australia. Australia currently has the highest incidence of skin cancer in the world.

People who have had several episodes of sunburn are much more likely to develop skin cancer than those who have never suffered sunburn. However, skin cancer occurs also in people with long-term sun exposure who have never suffered sunburn.

► *In the Victorian era, a pale skin was considered a sign of refinement and, in women, of beauty. This, and concealment of the body, almost certainly explains the low incidence of skin cancer over the general population.*

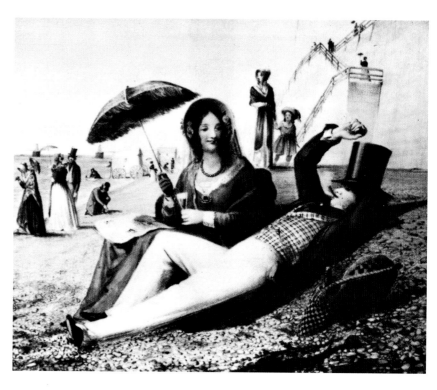

Fair-skinned people who can produce enough melanin pigment to get a good tan are still vulnerable to skin cancer. There is a limit to the number of harmful rays that can be absorbed by the pigment filter, and once this has been saturated these rays can then cause damage. It is therefore not impossible for a tanned person to develop sunburn from excessive exposure. Dark-skinned people can also suffer the same effects but to a much lesser degree.

Children are at particular risk from sunburn. Repeated exposures to sunburn during childhood increase the likelihood of skin cancer during adulthood.

Treatment

Once sunburn has occurred, the most important factor in treatment is to prevent further damage by avoiding further exposure. In mild burns the redness and burning usually resolve in a few days, and are often followed by peeling. Soothing lotions such as calamine are most effective, and if sleep is disturbed antihistamines may be prescribed. These are mildly sedative but have no effect on the skin.

In more severe burns, the symptoms are usually most acute on the second day when blisters may form on the affected areas.

Steroid ointments reduce inflammation as well as the intensity and duration of the skin reaction.

Prevention

Most people quickly learn how much sun they can take without burning. The body's natural protection is, of course, a tan built up every day by gradually increasing the periods of exposure.

The intensity of the sun must also be taken into account. The most accurate way of gauging this is not by the degree of heat or light, but by the angle of the sun above the horizon. This determines the amount of ultraviolet light that reaches the skin. At midday, the sun is directly overhead and the rays pass through less of the Earth's atmosphere. When the sun is low, in the morning and evening, the strength of the ultraviolet rays is considerably reduced. People are therefore less likely to get sunburned in the early morning or after midafternoon. The danger period is thus roughly 10 A.M. to 3 P.M., when exposure should be kept to a minimum.

Particular care should be taken in swimming, sailing, or skiing. Water absorbs the heat rays but the ultraviolet rays are still being directed onto the skin; and snow gives a feeling of coolness but actually reflects the ultraviolet rays.

There are many sunscreen creams and lotions available that can help to prevent sunburn. Both the American Academy of

Recommendations of the American Academy of Dermatology and the Skin Cancer Foundation to help reduce the risk of skin cancer and sunburn
Keep exposure to the sun to a minimum at midday and between 10 A.M. and 3 P.M.
Apply sunscreen with at least a skin protection factor (SPF) of 15, or higher, to all areas of the body that are exposed to the sun. Reapply the sunscreen every two hours, even on cloudy days, and after swimming or perspiring.
Wear clothing that covers the body. Hats should have wide brims to shade both the face and the neck.
Avoid exposure to ultraviolet radiation from sunlamps.
Children should be protected from excessive exposure to the sun when radiation is strongest (10 A.M. to 3 P.M.). Sunscreen should be applied liberally and frequently to children aged six months or older. Sunscreen should not, however, be used on babies under six months.
For babies under six months, keep exposure to sunlight to an absolute minimum, and apply sunscreen.

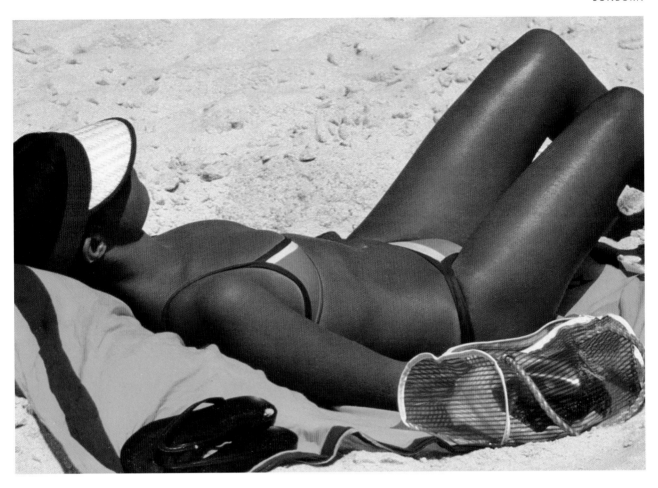

▲ *For much of the 20th century, there was a fashion for gaining a highly prized tan, often at the expense of health. We are now turning full circle: pale skin is becoming acceptable, even fashionable, again.*

Dermatology, and the Skin Cancer Foundation, advise that sunscreen preparations should be applied frequently, and especially just before and after swimming. They protect mainly against the sun's rays but, depending on their strength (sunscreen factor), will let through enough of the longer ultraviolet waves to produce a gradual tan. The tan is, however, no deeper than one obtained simply by gradual exposure without a sunscreen. Some sunscreens give almost total protection by stopping all the ultraviolet and visible rays, so that prolonged exposure without skin damage is possible.

Some parts of the body are more prone to sunburn than others because they are exposed the most. A bald head and the face, nose, tops of the ears, forearms, and backs of the hands are particularly at risk. A hat should always be worn when the hair is thin, and this will also protect the nose and tops of the ears. Otherwise, a sunscreen should be used on these small areas. Clothing is an efficient filter of the sun's harmful rays, if it is opaque.

Children should be protected and must always wear a hat when they are playing out in the sun, and sunblock should be applied liberally and frequently to exposed areas of skin. If possible, children should not be allowed to stay out in the sun for prolonged periods between 10 A.M. and 3 P.M. However, sunscreen should not be used on babies of six months or less, who should rather be kept out of strong sunlight altogether.

Outlook

In the future people will increasingly have to become more sun-conscious and protect themselves and their children against the possible negative effects of sunburn. However, it is important to remember that not all the effects of ultraviolet light are harmful. Sunlight is essential for health, and perhaps even emotional well-being. A healthy glowing skin can make someone feel lively and happy, whereas dull, gloomy weather has a depressant effect.

Photosensitivity

Some people have excessive sensitivity to the sun which can cause a red, painful rash, scaly skin, and itchy blisters. In severe cases, the person has to avoid going outdoors in daylight. Treatment is with steroids or antihistamines and with desensitization to ultraviolet light, and the sufferer has to wear a high-factor sunblock.

See also: **Blisters; Burns; Cancer; Pain; Sunstroke**

Sunstroke

Sunstroke is a dangerous condition that occurs when the body's thermostat breaks down from overheating. Care must be taken in extreme heat, since, even with treatment, sunstroke can be fatal or cause permanent damage.

Questions and Answers

If you go to a hot country, do you get acclimatized so that you are at less risk of sunstroke?

Yes, you do. However, it takes several weeks or even months for someone to get acclimatized to the heat. To a large extent, this depends on the amount of physical effort that is required in the heat. It is going to take much longer to be able to carry out strenuous work in the heat than it is if you are just going to take it easy. It is not clear exactly what changes are going on in the body during the period of acclimatization, although there is probably some increase in the efficiency of the sweat glands. Research suggests that a newcomer to the heat loses more salt in sweat than someone who has become used to the heat.

Is there any difference between sunstroke and heatstroke?

No. Both terms describe the serious and potentially fatal condition that can occur if the body is excessively heated, resulting in the total breakdown of the temperature-regulating mechanism in the body. Heatstroke, however, is a more accurate name because you can suffer from its effects away from the sun. Heatstroke is a serious problem in some South African mines. If the temperature is high enough, you can get heatstroke even if you're not in direct sun.

Does prickly heat make you more prone to sunstroke?

Prickly heat occurs when the skin becomes so hot that the skin cells swell and block the sweat glands, resulting in an itchy rash of tiny, red blisters. Prickly heat is actually very common, and doesn't really indicate any serious trouble. There is one form of heat exhaustion that is often preceded by an episode of prickly heat, but it is nowhere near as severe as heatstroke itself.

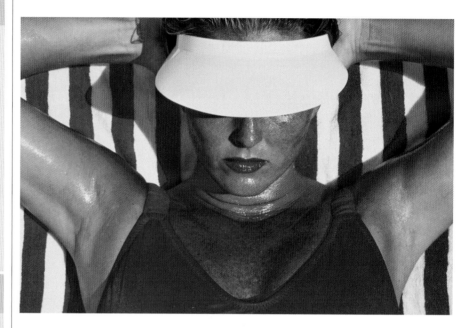

▲ *Sunstroke is often caused by lengthy exposure to the sun's heat. Someone who is unused to the heat, such as a person from a cold climate who goes to a hot climate and spends long hours sunbathing, is more at risk than a person who lives in a hot climate.*

Most people are used to thinking of the extremely serious heat disorder called sunstroke as something that happens only to people who stay out too long in the hot sun. However, the real cause of the condition is not the sun's rays but the intense heat that the sun produces. For this reason, doctors prefer to talk about heatstroke rather than sunstroke.

Any environment that gets hot can be dangerous. For instance, people who find themselves in very hot places such as engine rooms and steelworks can suffer the severe effects of sunstroke without ever being exposed to the sun.

The body's reaction to heat
The body has two main mechanisms for losing heat. First, the blood vessels to the skin are dilated so that more blood flows to the surface, allowing it to lose heat through the skin into the air. Second, the sweat glands pour out salty fluid onto the surface of the skin, where it evaporates and heat is lost by the latent heat of vaporization. It takes more than 500 times the amount of heat to turn 0.04 ounce (1 gr) of water 1.8°F (1°C) into vapor.

Overheating
There are many ways in which the environment can intensify the effects of heat on the body. It is not, therefore, just a question of reading the degrees on the thermometer. If the air is humid, then this reduces the ease with which the sweat evaporates, so that it becomes more difficult to lose heat. Similarly, if the air is very still, less heat is lost from the surface of the body by convection.

People doing hard physical work in a hot environment are, of course, producing a lot of heat of their own. They may be losing up to 1 quart (0.9 l) of sweat every hour, compared with the 1 quart (0.9 l) per day of the sedentary worker in a temperate climate. This loss of salt and water can contribute to a condition known as heat exhaustion, which, unless checked, can lead to the eventual breakdown of the body's temperature-regulating mechanisms. However, as the body gets used to working in a hot environment, it adapts, and the loss of salts decreases, making the body less vulnerable to heat disorders.

Additional risk factors

The very young and the very aged are most at risk from heat disorders, and consequently from heatstroke. This is because their temperature-regulating mechanisms are not very efficient. And because of this deficiency, older people also tend to wear heavy clothes even on sunny days, thereby increasing the risk of overheating still further.

There are several other predisposing factors. People who are unused to heat, who are very overweight, who drink heavily, or who are suffering from a feverish illness may also be at a greater risk from heatstroke.

Symptoms and dangers

The three basic signs of heatstroke are: a high temperature (more than 106°F [41°C]); a total absence of sweating; and, most seriously, problems of the nervous system that may lead to coma. Disturbances of mood, disorientation, and headache, often

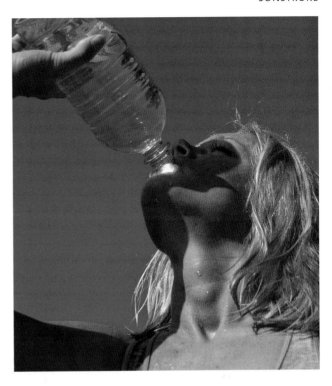

▲ *Drinking plenty of water in hot environments, especially if undergoing much physical exertion, helps prevent sunstroke.*

accompanied by dizziness and difficulty in walking, all happen in the early stages of heatstroke until consciousness is lost.

Fully developed heatstroke is an extremely dangerous condition and over 20 percent of sufferers may die, even with treatment. Even those who do recover may have persistent trouble in the nervous system and their balance and coordination may take months to return to normal. However, if treatment is prompt (at the first sign of symptoms and before consciousness is lost) then the chances of recovery are good.

Treatment and prevention

As soon as any of the symptoms of heatstroke appear, it is essential to call a doctor immediately. Meanwhile, cool the patient down as quickly as possible. The temperature needs to be brought down to about 102°F (39°C), but no lower, as the patient's circulation may go into shock. Remove the patient's clothes and cover him or her with a thin cotton blanket, which should be continually doused in cold water. If possible, the best way to cool the patient down is in a tub of cold water. In a hospital, special slatted beds on which sufferers can be doused with water and cooled by fans are used.

The most sensible and effective way to fight sunstroke is, of course, prevention. This can be done simply by ensuring that the body is not overheated. This entails not staying out too long in the sun; wearing cool, loose clothing in the heat; and taking salt tablets and drinking plenty of liquids when doing physical work in very hot environments.

See also: **Alcoholism; Obesity; Salt**

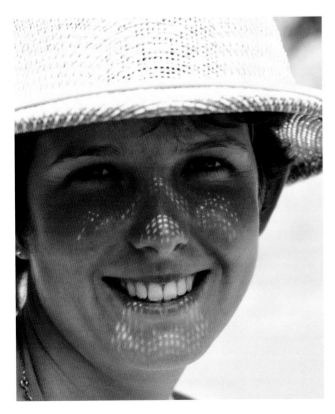

▲ *Wearing a hat, especially at midday when the sun is beating down directly, helps to keep the body from overheating.*

Tennis elbow

This painful muscle condition deserves its graphic name. Although athletes suffer from it, it can also be brought on by mundane activities such as wringing out wet clothing.

If I had tennis elbow, how would I recognize it?

You would have a dull ache around the elbow area and upper side of the forearm, with a particular tender spot on or near the bump that can be felt on the upper side of the elbow when the forearm is placed across the chest. Typing, using a squash or tennis racquet, or even picking up heavy objects may be painful.

How soon can one resume playing tennis after tennis elbow?

That depends on how serious the injury was; you should seek your doctor's advice. The symptoms vary from person to person. In mild cases, you may have to wait only a few days until the pain and stiffness subside, and resume the sport gradually. More serious cases may take longer. If you find that the tenderness returns whenever you play, consult your doctor as soon as possible.

I am due to play in a tennis tournament, but now have tennis elbow. What can I do?

Ask your doctor for a painkilling injection, but he or she may not be willing to give it. The danger is that you could seriously aggravate the injury and delay full healing for weeks or even months. As an alternative wear an elasticized bandage around the affected forearm to provide relief and reduce the chance of aggravating the injury. Ideally you should rest the arm for a few days.

Do you get tennis elbow only from playing tennis?

No. The injury is common in many sports, especially racquet sports, and also occurs as a result of doing other repetitive tasks, such as those involved in carpentry.

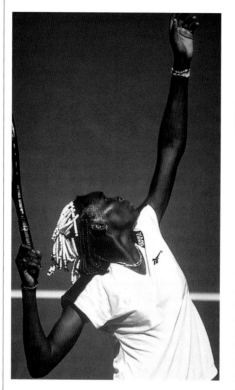

▲ *The flamboyant tennis star Venus Williams demonstrates her fluid service action, which requires healthy muscles.*

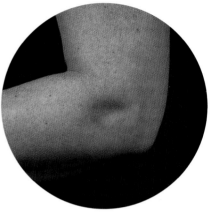

▲ *A case of tennis elbow.*

Tennis elbow is a common arm injury. Although it often develops during a game of tennis, it can also occur in other sports, and even as a result of nonsporting activities. The injury is not in fact to the elbow itself, but an inflammation of the tendon that attaches the muscles of the forearm to the bones of the upper arm. The muscles control movements of the wrist and fingers; that is why it is such a common injury among racket players. The elbow joint forms a pivot between the bone in the upper arm (humerus) and the two bones in the forearm. At the lower end of the humerus are two projections (epicondyles) to which forearm muscles are attached. The pain is due to small tears where the muscles join the lateral epicondyle.

The cause of the injury is vigorous or prolonged use of the forearm muscles, especially during sports such as tennis, squash, racquetball, and athletic throwing events. It can also be caused by wringing out wet clothing or using a carpentry tool such as a screwdriver.

Symptoms and treatment

Tennis elbow comes on gradually, and is made worse by activities that involve gripping something or picking up a heavy object such as a full kettle. A very tender spot can usually be felt at the site of the injury where the forearm muscles are attached to the lateral epicondyle, but pain and stiffness may sometimes extend over the whole of the upper side of the forearm.

Rest and a pain-relieving drug usually permit use of the affected arm within a few days. More persistent tennis elbow may be treated with a corticosteroid injection containing an anesthetic to reduce pain and tenderness during healing.

When the injury is severe and persistent, heat treatment and physical therapy are used. Some have found acupuncture helpful.

See also: Sports medicine

Tetanus

A rusty nail, a clumsy step, and the resulting wound could be the ideal breeding ground for the virulent bacterium that causes tetanus. The disease can be fatal, so adequate immunization is of the utmost importance.

Tetanus is a frightening and dangerous disease that can be fatal, even with the best medical care. However, all the techniques of intensive care can be brought to bear on sufferers in developed countries, and there is no doubt that modern treatment does significantly reduce the number of deaths from this disease.

Cause

Tetanus is caused by a bacterium called *Clostridium tetani*. The organism is found freely in soil, and is even more common in manured and cultivated soil, since it is very common in animal dung. However, the organism is not confined to soil; street dust from the center of a town certainly contains the spores of the bacteria, and spores can even be found inside buildings in large amounts.

The bacterium has one very important characteristic that controls the way the disease behaves; it is killed by oxygen and grows only in oxygen-free surroundings. That is why the bacteria have to be introduced into the body through a wound, such as a cut, since the blood supply, and therefore the oxygen supply, is cut off as a result of the tissue damage. The deeper and more contaminated a wound, the higher the risk of tetanus.

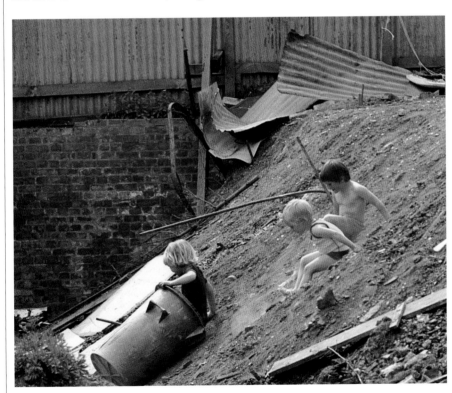

▲ *It is not uncommon for tetanus to be picked up in cities. The bacterium makes spores that are resistant to the effects of drying and heat, and can survive for long periods in dust. These children, if not immunized, would therefore be at risk, simply because they are playing in a dusty area where they are exposed to injury.*

The toxin made by the bacterium is a deadly substance, exceeded in potency only by the toxin responsible for botulism. Only one-tenth of a milligram is a fatal dose for an adult. The toxin is produced in the site of a wound that has been contaminated by the bacterium; from there, the toxin passes into the spinal cord and the brain. It is thought that it travels through the nerves, although transmission in the bloodstream could also be important. Once in the nervous system the toxin cannot be neutralized by antibodies, either produced by the body after immunization or given as antitoxin.

Symptoms

The incubation period is six to 10 days as a rule, although in rare cases it may be several months. In some cases, symptoms can occur extremely quickly, in 24 hours.

There is a short vague illness with headache, general illness, and fever, but the important first signs are due to the generalized muscle rigidity that is one of the two classic symptoms of the disease. This especially affects the jaw muscles—giving rise to lockjaw, by which name the disease is sometimes known—the muscles of the abdomen, which are found to be rigid on examination, and the muscles of the back. Eventually, the back may be arched over and the neck bent back.

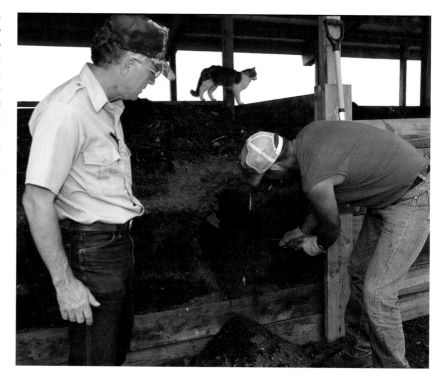

▲ *People who work on the land—such as gardeners and farmers—are most likely to catch tetanus. The bacterium is commonly found in animal dung, a normal component of fertilized and cultivated soil.*

Spasms develop later and can be brought on by any stimulus. Minor spasms may simply affect the face, with contraction of the facial muscles into a ghastly grin, known by the chilling Latin title *risus sardonicus*, meaning sardonic smile. Breathing can be affected by these spasms and when they become more generalized they lead to even more exaggerated arching of the back and neck.

The difficulty in caring for tetanus patients really becomes marked when the disease interferes with the way that the brain controls vital functions. The heart may be affected, leading to abnormalities of rhythm and either very low or very high blood pressure. Sometimes the temperature may increase very rapidly.

Treatment

The aim of treatment is to maintain the patient over the period of his or her illness and prevent a possibly fatal outcome from occurring. Problems that can occur include exhaustion due to spasm, asphyxia during spasm, pneumonia due to stomach contents entering the lungs, and death due to disorders of control of vital functions, such as the heartbeat and blood pressure.

In milder cases, simple sedation and the avoidance of all types of disturbance will

▲ *Once in the body, the bacterium may grow in an area with no blood supply, making it difficult for antibiotics to reach.*

prevent spasms, but in the more severe cases a tracheotomy is performed to make an opening in the windpipe (tracheostomy), and the patient is totally paralyzed using curare (a paralyzing drug), while breathing is taken over by a respirator. The disease is likely to be most severe when the incubation period has been short and when there has been less than 48 hours between the first symptom and the first spasm.

Prevention

Immunization with tetanus toxoid is given with a baby's first immunization, and boosters are given when children start school and on leaving. After that, a booster should be given every 10 years—or more often if you are at special risk, for example, if you work on the land. In people who have not been immunized it is necessary to give an antitoxin after any serious wound.

The risk of contracting tetanus can be reduced by immediately cleansing all wounds, even minor wounds, and the use of large doses of penicillin. Adequate immunization, however, is the best option, as it can eliminate the risk completely.

See also: **Bacteria; Immunization**

Tropical diseases

Questions and Answers

I am planning a trip to India, and know that rabies is common there. Should I be vaccinated before I go?

There is now a safe and effective—though expensive—vaccine against rabies. Rabies is spread by animal bites. The risk to ordinary travelers is usually so small, however, that vaccination is not routinely advised before a vacation.

Last time I went to Tunisia I had a terrible attack of diarrhea that ruined my visit. Can I take anything with me next time to prevent this from happening again?

Your doctor may be able to give you some tablets to relieve the symptoms in case it should happen again. However, travelers' diarrhea is nearly always due to eating or drinking contaminated food or water, and strict hygiene is the best preventive measure. Diarrhea is nature's way of eliminating noxious agents from the body, so treatment should focus on replacing lost fluids and salts—this is of vital importance in hot climates. If diarrhea does not get better within a short time, contains blood or mucus, or is associated with fever, consult a doctor at once.

I'm planning a trip to South America, and am scared of poisonous snakes. Is there anything that I should take with me in case I get bitten?

Snakes bite in self-defense, so always wear boots when walking outdoors in snake-infested areas. Snakebites are very uncommon and, usually, little or no venom is injected, but it is still important to get to a hospital without delay. Dramatic measures such as cutting into bites or using tourniquets are unnecessary and can cause harm. Reassurance is the most important part of treatment. Antivenin can be dangerous, and should be administered only by medics.

The grim backdrop to most tropical diseases is the shocking conditions in which so many people live. Governments and medical teams are waging war against the havoc wreaked by these resilient enemies of humanity.

In spite of all the progress that has been made in modern medicine, large numbers of people around the world still die from tropical diseases. Although the medical profession now understands a great deal about how these diseases spread, and how they can be treated, they still maim, blind, disable, and cause suffering on a massive scale.

What are tropical diseases?

Tropical diseases include not only strange parasitic disorders like elephantiasis, but also rare and deadly fevers like Lassa fever or Marburg fever. Relatively few diseases occur only within the tropics. Diseases such as leprosy (now referred to as Hansen's disease) and plague, which most people now

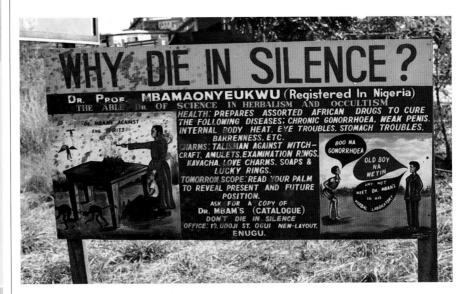

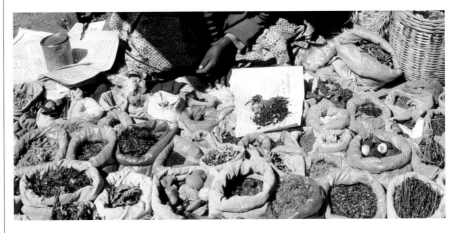

▲ *An African sign (top) promises bizarre cures for many complaints. A Peruvian herbalist displays his colorful herbal cure-alls for sale (above).*

think of as tropical, were once widespread in Europe. Likewise, diseases now familiar in Europe, such as measles or tuberculosis, are much more dangerous in developing countries. For example, more than 95 percent of deaths from measles occur in countries with low per capita incomes and weak health infrastructures.

Fighting tropical diseases

Smallpox is the only disease totally eradicated by humans. The campaign against smallpox began in 1967, lasted 10 years, and cost $200 million.

Although the World Health Organization (WHO) has a campaign to eradicate polio and leprosy from the world within a relatively short time, it is not likely that humankind will be able to eradicate many other tropical diseases in the foreseeable future, and much more money for research is necessary. However, the World Health Organization has determined that the following diseases should be singled out for particular attention.

Malaria: The disease affects up to 250 million people each year and causes up to a million deaths. It is one of the world's greatest killers. Control of the disease depends largely on control of the insect that spreads it—the anopheles mosquito. Public health measures to remove mosquito breeding areas, and public knowledge of how the disease is spread, can help. For travelers, malaria can be prevented through chemoprophylaxis, which suppresses the blood stage of malaria infections, thereby preventing malaria disease.

Schistosomiasis: Also called bilharzia, this is an unpleasant and sometimes fatal disease caused by small worms in the liver, intestine, and bladder. Eggs passed out in the urine and feces hatch

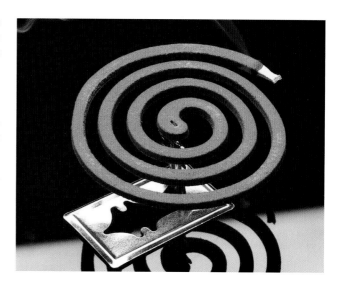

▲ *A pyrethrum mosquito coil should be burned at night to keep mosquitoes at bay in countries where malaria is rife.*

in water and produce organisms that infect certain types of snails. These produce other types of organisms, which penetrate human skin and then pass in the bloodstream to the liver. The disease is usually caused by contact with water that has been contaminated by human sewage.

Sleeping sickness: Spread by the tsetse fly, this has made vast areas of Africa uninhabitable. The disease is caused by a tiny, single-celled parasite that lives in the blood and the brain, and causes serious damage to the nervous system.

◄▼ *The spectacular wildlife of the Masai Mara game reserve attracts thousands of tourists to Kenya every year. However, such an area is home to the tsetse fly (below), which spreads sleeping sickness to both humans and animals. Mosquito coils should be standard travelers' equipment because they repel such unwanted visitors.*

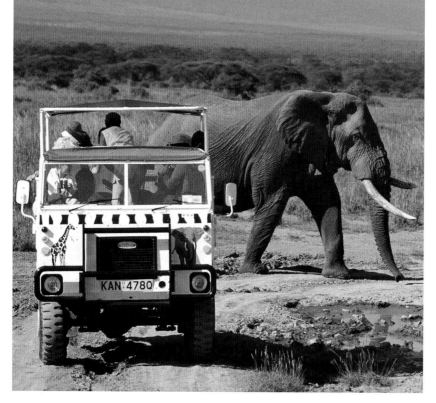

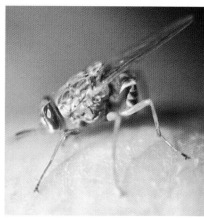

I've heard that cholera vaccination does not always work. Is there any other treatment for cholera?

A better vaccine is needed to fight cholera. At present, the vaccine protects in only 50 percent of cases for only a few months. Thus the best way to avoid cholera is to avoid food and water that might be contaminated. Cholera causes severe diarrhea, with salt and fluid loss. Prompt rehydration is vital in order to save a person's life.

My sister-in-law has just returned from a trip to Jamaica, where she became ill with dengue fever. What is dengue fever, and is there any chance that she could infect someone else?

Dengue is due to a virus. It is spread by certain types of mosquito, so you could not catch it directly from her. It causes fever, painful muscles and joints, headaches, and a rash, but complete recovery usually occurs.

Is it true that malnutrition can be caused by worms?

Intestinal parasites do not, on their own, cause malnutrition, although hookworms often cause anemia. However, in the tropics worm infestation in undernourished children is common, and often leads to severe malnutrition.

I am going to be touring the Middle East and I have heard that there is a disease there that causes blindness. Is there any chance that I might catch it?

The disease you are worried about is known as trachoma, an infection of the conjunctiva and cornea of the eye. Trachoma causes blindness on a massive scale: around 84 million people have the disease, of whom 8 million are now visually impaired. Repeated infection is necessary for damage to occur, and treatment with antibiotic ointment is highly effective. Travelers are most unlikely to be affected by it.

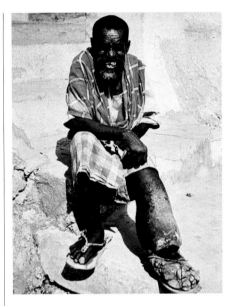

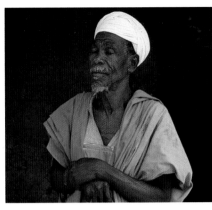

▲ *Blindness is a widespread tropical condition; in fact, one million people suffer from river blindness in West Africa alone.*

◄ *Elephantiasis is common in the tropics.*

Treatment is difficult and there is no vaccine. The disease is a risk to visitors to African game parks, who should therefore take special precautions to avoid insect bites.

Hansen's disease: This disease still affects millions of people around the world. If the disease is diagnosed promptly, it can be treated effectively and disability can be prevented. However, if it is neglected, blindness, paralysis, and deformity result. Almost more terrible than the disease

Basic precautions

At present, many tropical diseases cannot be prevented by drugs or vaccines, so travelers should take a few basic precautions:

Biting insects spread diseases in different countries. In some parts of Africa, tsetse flies spread sleeping sickness; in others, insects spread viral diseases or filariasis. Minimize exposure to biting insects, and wear sensible clothes. Use insect repellents containing diethyltoluamide (DEET), and at night use a mosquito net or burn pyrethrum mosquito coils. Electronic insect repellents do not work.

Don't eat food that has been exposed to flies. Always eat food that has been freshly cooked to kill all parasites and bacteria. Wash hands before handling food.

Check that drinking water is safe; if in doubt, drink boiled water, or use purifying tablets containing chlorine or iodine.

Wash fruit and vegetables with detergent or a dilute solution of potassium permanganate.

Never walk around barefoot.

Cleanse and dress all wounds.

Do not swim in canals or rivers.

If you develop a fever, severe diarrhea, or blood in the feces, consult a doctor.

Have a medical checkup when you return home.

itself is the social stigma of the disease due to the ancient and irrational fear of infection. The disease can be treated with a course of multidrug therapy that lasts six to twelve months. The treatment, which is highly effective, has few side-effects and low relapse rates.

Filariasis: This disease is caused by a variety of small worms that enter the body through the bites of mosquitoes and flies. These worms also cause elephantiasis by blocking the lymph passages in the body. African river blindness is another form of filariasis. This can cause blindness by infestation with a worm that enters the body through a blackfly bite. Filariasis can be treated with drugs.

Leishmaniasis: Spread by sandflies, and caused by a parasite that attacks the skin, liver, and spleen, the disease takes many forms and is not adequately understood.

Immunization schemes

Measles, diphtheria, polio, tetanus, tuberculosis, and whooping cough (medically known as pertussis) kill millions of children in developing countries each year. The World Health Organization set itself the huge task of immunizing all the children in the world against these diseases. Although the target has not yet been met, progress has been made and positive results have been observed. The practical problems are enormous, since 80 percent of the world's population live in remote areas. Even when vaccines arrive, their effectiveness cannot be guaranteed; vaccines are quickly inactivated by tropical heat.

Problems

Poverty, overpopulation, overcrowding, bad housing, inadequate nutrition, poor sanitation, and lack of education are a few of the factors that facilitate the spread of tropical diseases in the developing world, and make them more difficult to bring under control. A billion people have no access to a safe water supply within 220 yards (200 m) of their home.

Ironically, many aid projects aimed at improving the quality of life have actually made things worse. In Egypt, for example, the construction of the Aswān high dam controlled the floods of the Nile and permitted much better

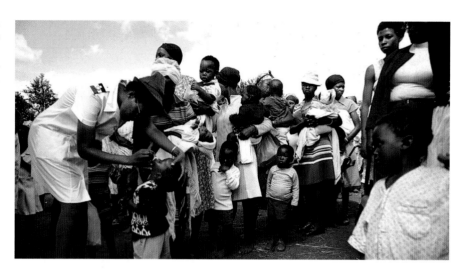

▲ *Massive vaccination programs are taking place in Africa.*

Facts about tropical diseases
CHOLERA: Cholera is an acute diarrheal disease that can kill within hours if untreated.
ELEPHANTIASIS: Elephantiasis most often affects the legs.
HANSEN'S DISEASE: Hansen's disease is curable, and treatment provided in the early stages averts disability.
HEPATITIS: Hepatitis A and E are typically caused by contaminated food or water.
LASSA FEVER: The incubation period of Lassa fever ranges from 6 to 21 days.
LEISHMANIASIS: The sandflies that spread leishmaniasis breed in forest areas, caves, or the burrows of small rodents.
MALARIA: Growing resistance to medicines has undermined efforts to control malaria.
POLIO: Polio cases have decreased by more than 99 percent since 1988.
SCHISTOSOMIASIS: The symptoms of schistosomiasis are caused by a body's reaction to the worms' eggs, not by the worms themselves.
SLEEPING SICKNESS: Sleeping sickness occurs only where there are tsetse flies.
SMALLPOX: Routine vaccination against smallpox was stopped in all countries by 1986.
TYPHOID: Vaccines against typhoid fever are not completely effective.
YELLOW FEVER: The "yellow" in the name of yellow fever refers to jaundice.

irrigation and crop yields. Although this was a benefit, it also, however, allowed the snails that transmit bilharzia to flourish. It is estimated that more than 200 million people are affected by bilharzia worldwide and that more than 85 percent of those people live in Africa.

Why do babies who are suffering from malnutrition have such enormous abdomens when the rest of their bodies seem to be just skin and bones?

The swollen abdomen of the malnourished child is due to wasting and weakening of the abdominal muscles, fluid collecting in the abdomen, gas distending the intestines, and an enlarged liver. This type of malnutrition, called kwashiorkor, results from a diet containing little or no protein, and carries a high mortality rate.

Is it true that there is resistance to various antimalarial drugs among certain malaria strains, rendering these drugs ineffective?

In some parts of Africa, Asia, and South America, resistance to some of the drugs used to prevent malaria is now increasing. Check with your doctor before you travel, explaining exactly which countries you plan to visit, so that he or she can select the most suitable treatment. Don't forget that even the shortest stopover in a tropical zone may expose you to malaria.

Is vaccination against certain tropical diseases dangerous during pregnancy?

If there is a significant risk of exposure to disease, vaccination is usually the safest option. Ask your doctor for his or her advise.

I thought that leprosy was found only in underdeveloped countries, but I read recently that it still occurs in Europe and the United States. Is this true?

It is true, but it is nothing for you to worry about. Leprosy (Hansen's disease) has never been eradicated completely from Europe or the United States. There are millions of sufferers from the disease in the world. However, contrary to commonly held beliefs, Hansen's disease does not spread easily, and most people are not at all susceptible to the disease.

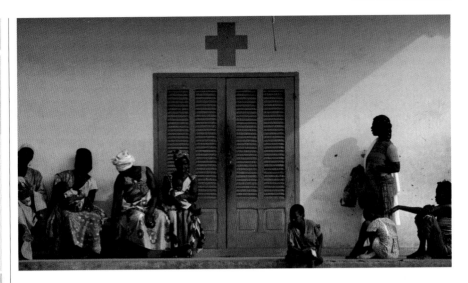

▲ *Women and children from an Ivory Coast village await treatment in the local community hospital.*

The countries in which tropical diseases are most common are those least able to conduct the intensive research that is essential if new drugs and vaccines to combat these diseases are to be found. They simply do not have the financial and technological resources.

It costs many millions of dollars to research and test each new drug, and developing countries can barely afford the drugs that are already available.

Travel

Jet travel has made it possible for a disease acquired in one country to produce symptoms only after the traveler has arrived in another country, often many thousands of miles away. Yellow fever, for example, which is a dangerous viral illness occurring in Africa and South America, is transmitted by mosquitoes, and the symptoms do not appear until six days after a mosquito

▼ *Attempts to control the spread of river blindness have included the introduction of public showers in India.*

▼ *With the help of better health education and medical care, African children have real hope of a longer, healthier life.*

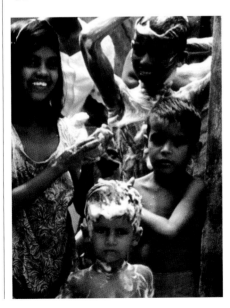

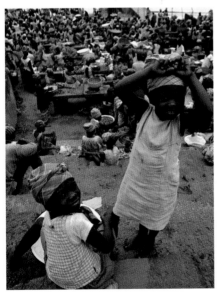

Travel precautions

If you are planning to visit a country where tropical diseases are present, see your doctor well in advance to allow plenty of time for any immunizations you may need. You will probably require specific protection against the diseases listed below.

DISEASE	PROTECTIVE MEASURES	DOSAGE	DURATION OF PROTECTION	EFFECTS OF DISEASE	ROUTE OF DISEASE SPREAD
Cholera	Immunization Hygiene	2 doses, 1–4 weeks apart	6 months	Severe diarrhea, fluid loss, and dehydration	Unhygienic food handling, and contaminated water
Hepatitis	Gammaglobulin injection Vaccine for hepatitis B	Single dose 3 doses	2–6 months Life	Fever, jaundice, viral liver infection	Contact with infected cases, unhygienic food handling, contaminated water
Malaria	Antimalarial drugs Mosquito nets Mosquito repellents	Start drug treatment before arrival, continue for at least 6 weeks after leaving	During period of exposure	Fevers and chills	Mosquito bites
Polio	Oral polio vaccine Hygiene	Single booster dose, if previously immunized with inactive polio not live vaccine	5 years	Paralysis	Unhygienic food handling, and contaminated water
Smallpox	Vaccination is no longer required or advised. The disease has been eradicated.				
Tetanus	Immunization. Careful cleansing of cuts and wounds.	2 doses, 4–6 weeks apart. 1st booster dose 1 year later; then every 5 years	5–10 years	Severe muscle spasms and rigidity	Contamination of a wound or wounds
Typhoid	Immunization Hygiene	2 doses, 4 weeks apart	3 years	Fever; intestinal infection	Unhygienic food handling, and contaminated water
Yellow fever	Immunization	Single dose	10 years	Fever, also jaundice, bleeding	Mosquito bites

bite. International health regulations ensure that all travelers arriving in Asia from Africa or South America have been vaccinated against yellow fever for their own safety, and to prevent the spread of the disease. There is, at present, no yellow fever in Asia, although there are plenty of mosquitoes that would be able to spread the disease rapidly.

Only a few tropical diseases can be prevented specifically by drug treatment or by vaccination, so travelers to regions where diseases are endemic must accept that they are at an increased risk of picking up a disease against which they have no natural immunity.

An additional hazard is that when particular symptoms develop after a traveler has returned home, they may not be recognized immediately as symptoms of a tropical disease. Cases of malaria are imported into the West each year, but the symptoms are easily confused with those of influenza and the diagnosis is often delayed.

Travelers should, therefore, always tell their doctor where they have been when they return home, and should have a full checkup.

Outlook

Many tropical diseases are on the increase, and are a long way from eradication or control. Improved health education and public health services are the most urgent measures that must be taken to limit the spread of tropical diseases. New vaccines, new drugs, and more research are essential if the fight against tropical diseases is to succeed.

See also: Bites and stings; Hygiene; Immunization; Infection and infectious diseases; Measles; Parasites; Tuberculosis; Vaccinations; Viruses

Tuberculosis

Questions and Answers

Can I get TB from milk?

Two strains of the TB bacterium are important causes of the disease in humans. The first is the human strain, and the second is the bovine strain that can be passed on in milk. However, because cattle are now tested for infection—so-called tuberculin-tested herds—the bovine strain is no longer passed on in milk.

My grandfather had several ribs cut away because of TB, and was left with a deformed chest. Why?

Before antibiotics became available, surgery was one of the few ways of fighting TB. One method was to cut out the affected parts of the lung, although this was a major operation, and the disease was likely to affect both lungs. Another approach was to reduce the volume of areas of affected lung, since the disease caused cavities, particularly in the upper parts of the lung. If the cavities were removed there seemed to be a better chance of curing the disease. This sort of surgery is no longer necessary, since drugs can now cure the disease.

Can I be vaccinated against tuberculosis?

Yes you can. There is a vaccine called BCG, which is a modified form of the TB bacterium. This can fire the immune system against the disease but does not cause serious disease. Children at special risk are tested for evidence of previous contact with the disease (primary TB) and, if they are negative to testing, they are given BCG. Children who react are known as tuberculin-positive and are immune. People at risk from the disease, such as medics, are tested and revaccinated as necessary. Mass vaccination is not carried out in the United States.

Thanks to improved nutrition and living conditions, tuberculosis is no longer prevalent in the developed West, although in recent years there has been a resurgence of a resistant form of the disease in inner-city areas.

Tuberculosis—or TB as it is more commonly known—remains one of the most serious infectious diseases in the world. Although improved standards of living conditions have made the disease less prevalent in the West, it remains a killer in the developing world.

TB is caused by a bacterium called *Mycobacterium tuberculosis*, and there are two main strains of this particular organism that cause disease in humans; a human strain and a bovine strain, which primarily infects cattle, but which is also capable of causing human disease. The incidence of this chronic infection and the problems it can cause vary from country to country. In the United States, infection of the lungs—pulmonary TB—is the most usual form of the disease, whereas in Africa abdominal TB is very common.

How TB develops

At one time most people growing up in a country like the United States would have been in contact with tuberculosis at an early age. Such early contact with the disease leads to an infection called primary TB, which often, but not always, has no significant symptoms. The disease is contracted by contact with someone who has sufficiently severe disease in the lungs to cough up sputum containing TB bacteria. If the amount of bacteria inhaled is relatively small, then the primary TB will be a minor infection that will help build up a partial immunity to the development of full-blown TB later on.

The more serious forms of the disease that occur in later life are called reactivation disease. It seems that the usual cause of these infections is that the immunity to the original infection has broken down and the TB bacteria have broken out of their original site. Although this is probably the usual mechanism of development of the disease, it is also likely that some people who develop TB later in life do so because they are exposed to a very high infecting dose of bacteria. The reasons immunity breaks down are not clear. In most cases it seems that social rather than medical factors are of significance, since there is little doubt that TB these days is a disease most common among vagrants and alcoholics, although it may still occur in an apparently fit person who is well fed and lives in good housing. Because of the loss of immunity, the World Health Organization (WHO) estimates that one-third of people who are HIV-positive are infected with *M. tuberculosis* and will develop overt TB. TB rates in the United States, which had been falling steadily, showed a rise again around 1987, largely because of AIDS but also because of growing social deprivation.

Complications of primary TB

Although primary TB is often a relatively minor infection with no symptoms, it can develop into a serious disease in young children or in children who have another debilitating disease. The site of infection is nearly always the lungs, although in some parts of the world it may be the abdomen. The original infection causes a small area of

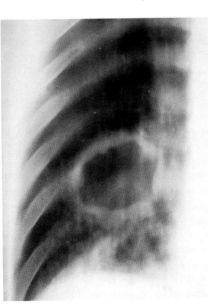

▲ *This X ray of a lung shows a large cavity created by a primary TB infection; bacilli are still contained inside it.*

Questions and Answers

Is it true that you have to be hospitalized for months to be cured of TB?

No. If you are found to have TB these days, you won't necessarily have to be in the hospital at all. In the past there was no effective cure, and it was found that rest in a sanitarium was beneficial. People who could afford it were sent away to mountain resorts where the purer air was thought to be helpful. Today the drug treatment is so efficient that you are no longer infectious after about 10 days. However, the standard length of treatment for pulmonary TB is still six months.

My friend had TB which affected the liver and abdomen. Isn't TB usually a chest disease?

You are right in thinking that the disease normally affects the chest. However, disease outside the chest does occur, although it is not very common in the United States. One of the most interesting things about TB is the way it presents itself in different ways in different groups of people. Immigrants to the United States from Africa or India are much more likely to have TB in areas other than the chest than someone who was born here. This does not seem to be due to racial differences, since the children of immigrant parents who are born and raised in this country seem to get TB in the lungs if they do happen to develop it.

Is it true that modern drugs are so effective that TB is no longer a common problem?

It is true that the disease is much less common than it used to be, and that the drugs to treat the disease are very effective. However, there is little evidence that the two facts are related. TB was on the decline before the drugs were widely available. It is thought that the combination of improved housing and improved nutrition is the main reason for the reduced incidence of TB.

inflammation in one of the lungs, and this produces a reaction in the lymph nodes that drain lymphatic fluids from that part of the lung. This patch of inflammation and enlargement of some of the lymph nodes at the root of the lung is called the primary complex.

In most cases, the TB bacteria in the primary complex are contained by the lymph nodes and spread no farther, but in a few children and adolescents with primary TB the defense mechanism breaks down soon after infection. This allows the bacteria to spread throughout the body, leading to a serious condition called miliary TB, which causes general illness, with loss of weight and a high fever. Diagnosis is by X-ray examination of the chest, which shows that both lungs are full of tiny nodules, each of which represents an area of tuberculous infection. Sometimes the general spread of the disease soon after the primary infection leads

PROGRESS OF PULMONARY TUBERCULOSIS

Advanced TB usually results when a dormant primary infection is reactivated and the bacteria spread to cause extensive cavitation in both lungs (below). The blood vessels then become congested and are likely to rupture, causing hemorrhage.

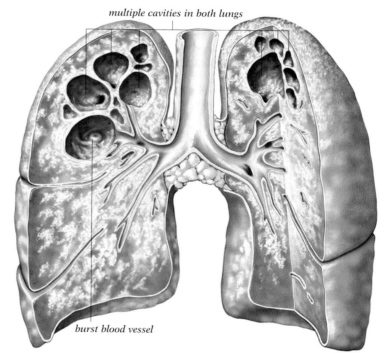

multiple cavities in both lungs

burst blood vessel

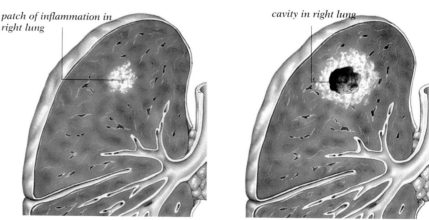

patch of inflammation in right lung

cavity in right lung

▲ *TB begins as a small inflamed area in one lung (above left), which turns into a cavity (above right).*

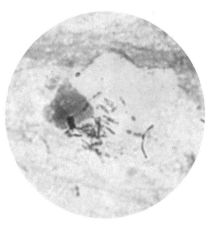
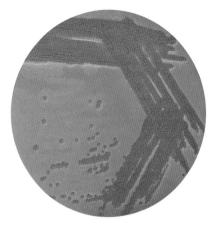

▲ *Untreated TB can lead to infection of the pleura (the membranes encasing the lungs) and then to pleural fibrosis (above left). This is usually very rigid, being full of calcium, and will impede breathing. When stained, any bacteria will appear as thin red rods (above center). If the diagnosis is unclear, a bacterial culture is grown on a plate (above right).*

to an infection in the nervous system called TB meningitis. Unlike the more common types of meningitis that develop within a day or so of infection, TB meningitis may take some weeks to develop. The first symptoms are general ill health, a slight fever, headaches (a very unusual complaint in a child), and, occasionally, fits. At a later stage, the fever rises and signs of drowsiness and neck stiffness appear. Finally, the temperature rises even higher and obvious problems with individual nerves, such as those controlling the eyes, will occur. This is a very dangerous condition, and it is important to start treatment as soon as the diagnosis is made. The diagnosis is confirmed by performing a lumbar puncture, which enables doctors to examine the cerebrospinal fluid that bathes the brain and spinal cord. One of the findings that indicate TB meningitis is a level of sugar in the fluid that is very much lower than that in the blood. This finding is almost unique to this particular condition.

Pulmonary TB

Although the primary focus of pulmonary TB occurs in the lungs, it is not until the postprimary stage of infection that there are any problems in the lungs. In a few cases of primary TB, the lymph nodes at the root of the lung may break down and liberate the bacteria into one of the main tubes (bronchi) supplying a particular lobe of the lung. This in turn will lead to lobar pneumonia soon after the original infection.

Most cases of tuberculous lung disease, however, happen many years after the original infection with the disease. The primary focus has a tendency to attack the lower lobes of the lungs, whereas the postprimary infection is much more likely to occur in the highest segments of the upper lobes of the lungs. It seems that the large amounts of oxygen that are available there, together with the relatively poor supply of blood, create particularly suitable incubators for the lung disease.

When the disease has become established in the upper part of the lungs, it may cause cavities to form there. Once this has happened, large numbers of TB bacteria may be present in the sputum, and this means that the sufferer becomes a serious source of infection until he or she is treated. The sufferer is most likely to

infect young children, giving them primary TB, TB meningitis, or TB bronchopneumonia. It is even possible that someone spreading large numbers of TB bacteria is able to rekindle the disease in people in older age groups who have already suffered from the primary form of the illness.

Left untreated, pulmonary TB can lead to the formation of fluid in the pleural space that surrounds the lungs, to infection of the pleura (lining membrane), and subsequently to pleural thickening and fibrosis. A particular characteristic of TB is that the fibrosis it leaves behind is often full of calcium and is therefore very rigid. Obviously, a lung surrounded by a hard wrapping of bonelike fibrosis is not going to be able to move freely, and breathing will be seriously impaired.

Sometimes the same sequence of events will happen to the pericardium—the membranous sac that surrounds the heart. This has even more serious effects, since tuberculous pericarditis may restrict the activity of the heart and stop it from pumping enough blood to the rest of the body.

Diagnosis

It is usually easy to diagnose a case of pulmonary TB. In a well-developed infection there will be marked changes on the chest X ray, particularly in the upper parts of the two upper lobes. One of the difficulties in diagnosing from an X ray, however, is identifying whether the changes represent a new infection of tuberculosis or an old infection. The fibrosis caused by an early episode of TB will persist for life, and the changes in the lungs will be visible on any chest X-ray for the remainder of the patient's life.

In a case of suspected tuberculosis, the first laboratory test will be to inspect the patient's sputum under a microscope. When there is a heavy infection, the sputum will contain a lot of bacteria. These will show up as thin red rods when stained with a special stain called Ziehl-Neelsen stain. The presence or absence of bacteria on direct staining of the sputum is of great relevance, since if there are no bacteria the patient cannot be infectious, even if he or she does turn out to have TB at a later stage. Infection with the presence of bacteria on direct staining is called open TB, and this is the only type that can possibly be infectious.

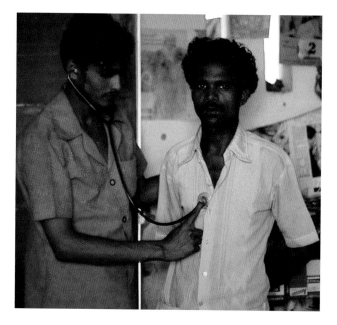

▲ *TB is a pervasive problem in India, but there are now clinics set up where people can be diagnosed and treated.*

Other forms of TB

Although pulmonary TB is the most common form of the disease, there are many other areas of the body that it may attack, such as the uterus, genitals, kidney, skin, and spine.

Abdominal TB

Abdominal TB is a common problem, particularly in Africa and India. It can be difficult to make a confident diagnosis, since there is no convenient test, such as a chest X ray, that confirms the disease. Sufferers simply appear to be generally rather sick, and will have a raised temperature. A simple way to make a diagnosis is by performing a liver biopsy: that is, surgically removing a small piece of liver and examining it under a microscope to see if any TB bacteria are present.

TB may also attack the lymph glands in the neck, and cause an abscess to form, which sometimes involves the overlying skin. This condition is called scrofula.

Treatment

Prior to the 1950s, when there was no effective drug treatment available, TB was often fatal. The cure for pulmonary TB, for instance, relied on building up the patient's resistance with rest and nourishment. However, this care often came too late. The clarity of the air and the relative lack of oxygen at great heights were also thought to be helpful, and there were many sanitariums in mountain resorts where wealthy TB sufferers went to recover.

Surgery was also routinely performed to remove severely infected areas of the lungs. This reduced the volume of the lungs and obliterated the cavities, thereby halting the spread of the disease through the lungs.

However, before antibiotics were introduced as a treatment for TB, attempts to achieve a cure were frustrated by the fact that the disease was often widespread before treatment was started. This often resulted in very intense fibrous scarring of the lung tissue, which prevented it from fulfilling the function of transferring oxygen from the air into the blood. Even today, if cases of TB are left untreated for too long, fibrosis will occur and this condition cannot be helped by antibiotics.

With modern treatment, however, it is possible to stop the progress of TB within a few days of starting treatment, although it can take as many as nine months to achieve a complete cure. There are now a selection of drugs that can be used to treat the TB infection. The first of these was streptomycin and, although still used, it is somewhat limited by the fact that it has to be given by injection. The usual drugs used today include rifampin, isoniazid, ethambutol, and pyrazinamide.

In order to prevent the organism from becoming resistant to any one drug, it is customary to use a combination of drugs during the early stages of the infection. Once the organism has grown—and this may take three months—it is possible to show that it is sensitive to at least two of the drugs and one is then withdrawn. The length of time it takes to cure TB varies depending on the particular type of infection, but it takes at least six months in the case of pulmonary TB.

Prevention

It is possible to test the population for immunity to TB using a preparation of TB-derived protein called tuberculin. People with a partial immunity to the disease as a result of a primary TB infection in the past will show a reaction when tuberculin is injected into the skin. In cases of established postprimary TB the extent of the reaction will be greater. If a child between the ages of 11 and 13 has not yet come into contact with the disease, then it is well worth vaccinating him or her with BCG (bacille Calmette-Guérin), a vaccine that is a modified form of the TB bacterium. The vaccine produces the same effect as a minor primary infection, and gives a certain amount of immunity against the disease. It is also worthwhile having younger children vaccinated when there is a risk of contact with the disease.

However, the most effective prevention is to improve risk factors such as living conditions and poor diet. This advancement has reduced the incidence of TB in countries like the United States. Although the introduction of curative drugs was undoubtedly important, the number of people suffering from the disease had actually started to decline before these drugs became available. Today, TB is very uncommon in well-nourished, well-housed communities, and it is likely that TB would disappear altogether if everyone lived under such conditions.

Reported cases of tuberculosis in United States	
Data estimated by the Centers for Disease Control and Prevention	
YEAR	CASES
1980	28,000
1985	22,000
1990	26,000
1995	23,000
1996	21,000
1997	20,000
1998	18,000
1999	17,500
2000	16,000
2005	14,000
2009	11,500

See also: **Antibiotics; Bacteria; Infection and infectious diseases; Vaccinations**

Ulcers

Questions and Answers

My teenage daughter keeps getting ulcers on her forearm, and our doctor says that he believes she is inflicting the injuries on herself. How can this be?

The doctor probably suspects that your daughter is suffering from a psychological condition, the symptom of which is self-mutilation. Self-inflicted injury may be performed to gain attention or avoid some anxiety-producing situation at home or school and she may be unaware that she is injuring herself. Ask your doctor about taking her to have psychiatric counseling.

I have an embarrassing ulcer in my groin region. What could this be due to?

There are a number of possible causes of an ulcer in the groin, ranging from mild irritation or injury to more serious sexually transmitted diseases. See your doctor as soon as possible to have the cause of the ulcer diagnosed.

My father is bedridden and suffers from bedsores. How can these be prevented?

A special air mattress, which has sections that can be alternately inflated and deflated to change the pressure-bearing areas, will help considerably. Also, always ensure that his position in bed is changed at frequent intervals.

Do ulcers in the mouth indicate that one is run-down or unhealthy?

Not necessarily. Mouth ulcers can be caused by a number of different factors. Recurrent ulcers caused by herpes are particularly common and often appear following any emotional stress or during illness. However, mouth ulcers may also be a symptom of anemia, and if this is the case, one would feel run-down.

Although commonly affecting the stomach or duodenum, ulcers also occur elsewhere on the body. Caused by a variety of factors, from disease to injury, they can range from a mild irritation to a serious condition.

An ulcer is a localized area of loss of tissue on the surface of the skin or on any other surface in the body, such as the wet lining of the digestive tract and other internal surfaces. The result of such loss is an open sore. An ulcer heals slowly because its edges are separated, and healing can occur only by growth of tissue in from the edges. Ulcers are usually associated with inflammation somewhere in the body. Loss of surface tissue as a result of a wound from injury is not primarily an ulcer, but if infection occurs such a wound may become ulcerated.

Ulcers are often circular or oval in shape and sometimes irregular in outline. Ulcers on the surface of the body vary considerably in their depth, some involving skin loss only, but others extending deep into the muscle or bone beneath the skin. The causes of ulcers are numerous and range from a mild irritation or injury to a serious disease.

Mouth and lip ulcers

Mouth ulcers are a common problem, and occur either as a onetime condition or as a recurrent disease. Almost everyone has at some time or other suffered the discomfort of the nonrecurrent type of mouth ulcers. They are brought on by a variety of factors but are usually due to some identifiable physical, chemical, or biological cause or are a symptom of some underlying condition.

Physical causes of mouth ulceration include irritation from jagged teeth, compulsive cheek-chewing, too vigorous use of a toothbrush, and burning from hot foods or drinks. Chemical causes

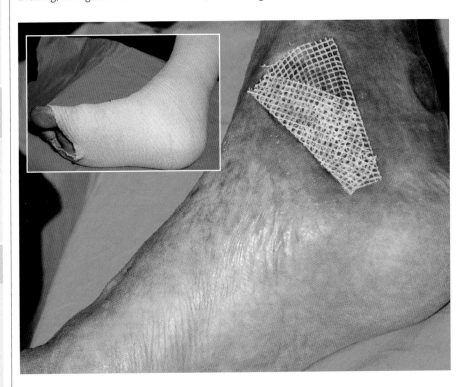

▲ *A leg ulcer is first cleaned, covered with a sterile gauze pad cut to fit, padded for protection, and then bandaged so that even pressure is applied to the wound.*

include caustic drugs, tablets, and sweets that are allowed to dissolve in the mouth; strong antiseptics; and mouthwashes and chemicals used in dental treatment.

Biological causes of ulcers include the syphilis bacterium, various fungi, and the herpes simplex virus. A syphilitic chancre in the mouth is rare but, like a chancre anywhere, is very serious. It is sexually acquired, consisting of a single round, button-sized, painless ulcer on the tongue or lip.

By contrast, an acute herpes infection in the mouth consists of numerous smaller, painful ulcers on the gums, tongue, and membranes that line the inside of the cheeks or the inside of the lips.

Nonrecurrent, but persistent, mouth ulcers may also be a symptom of diabetes, blood diseases, or tuberculosis. Cancer of the lip, though uncommon, often makes its first appearance as an ulcer.

Aphthous ulcers

"Aphthous ulcer" is the medical term given to a condition of mouth inflammation characterized by intermittent episodes of painful mouth ulcers on the internal mucous membrane. Aphthous ulcers are

▲ The aphthous ulcer, seen here on the tongue, is the most common of all single mouth ulcers and can be caused by broken teeth or spicy food.

also known as canker sores, aphthous stomatitis, or ulcerative stomatitis. These ulcers are covered with a grayish discharge. They are surrounded by a red halo, and occur singly or in groups. Even without treatment aphthous ulcers will heal spontaneously in one to two weeks.

Recurrent mouth ulcers affect about one person in three. They usually consist of numerous small, painful ulcers on or inside the lips,

or on the tongue, throat, or roof of the mouth, and may persist for a week or two, disappear, and then appear again some weeks or months later. The causes of recurrent mouth ulcers are not so well understood, but it is known that those confined to the lips are nearly always due to the herpes simplex virus. Those inside the mouth may also be caused by herpes, but are more likely due to an allergy, a nutritional deficiency, anemia, or celiac disease.

▼ Habitual cheek-biting can become so self-destructive as to cause a line of tissue breakdown that soon leads to an ulcer.

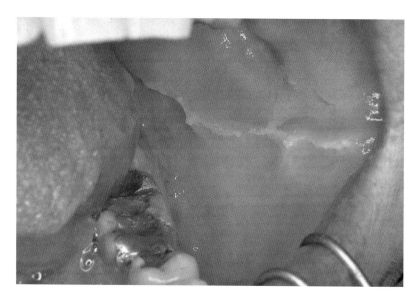

Mouth ulcers and general disease

Mouth ulcers may provide clues to the presence of many other general diseases. They are, for instance, regular features of several important and potentially dangerous disorders such as ulcerative colitis, Behçet's disease, and Reiter's syndrome.

Ulcerative colitis is an inflammatory disease of unknown cause affecting the lower part of the large intestine and the rectum. There is extensive ulceration of the inner lining of the intestine, leading to the passage of blood and mucus in the stools and episodes of constipation.

Behçet's disease is characterized by recurrent simultaneous or successive attacks of mouth and genital ulcers and an internal and inflammatory disorder of the eyes known as uveitis. The disease affects men more often than women, and occurs most often in adolescence. The uveitis is by far the more serious aspect of the disorder. This calls for skilled ophthalmic management if permanent impairment to the eyesight is to be avoided.

My mother has a leg ulcer, and the doctor has told her that she should sleep with the foot of her bed raised up. Why is this necessary?

Your mother is almost certainly suffering from a type of leg ulcer that develops from varicose veins. In this condition, blood tends to pool in the lower legs. Fluid collects and eventually the skin in the area becomes thinned and breaks down to form an ulcer. During treatment it helps for the person to keep the leg raised above the body during sleep or rest, thereby encouraging normal blood circulation.

Is it possible to have a stomach ulcer without knowing it?

Certainly. Many people accept that a small amount of indigestion is normal. A fair proportion of these people would be found to have an active ulcer, or the signs of an old ulcer, if they had a gastroscopy. If the ulcer is asymptomatic (without any symptoms) and does not have any complications, then it is really not a great concern.

I've been told that I have to eat frequently because of a stomach ulcer. Now I'm putting on a lot of weight. What can I do about this?

The trick is to eat frequent small meals. The idea is that frequent small meals do not allow the level of acid to build up, since the acid is continually being neutralized by the food. Obviously, you do risk putting on weight, and you should aim to eat a normal amount of food, but split it into a greater number of smaller meals.

Does surgery for a stomach ulcer leave a huge, ugly scar?

No, because minimally invasive surgery is increasingly used. This type of surgery leaves four or five tiny scars which are barely visible after a few months. Other advantages are a shorter hospital stay, less postoperative pain, and reduced recovery time.

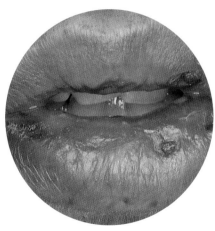

▲ *Herpes is often the cause of clusters of small ulcers on the lips, a condition that is also known as gingivostomatitis.*

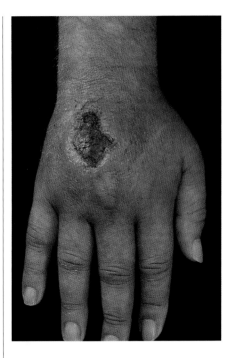

◄ *This ulcer was caused by a faulty IV drip attached to the hand. An anticancer drug accidentally leaked out onto the skin.*

Reiter's syndrome is also associated with internal eye inflammation. The syndrome consists of mouth and genital ulcers, and inflammation of the urine outlet tube with discharge, uveitis, and joint inflammation. Many cases may also involve persistent diarrhea. These different elements may occur together or separately at intervals of months or years, but once the arthritis is established it is often continuously present.

The treatment of any mouth ulcer depends greatly on the cause; for example, dental therapy for jagged or decayed teeth, surgery for lip cancer, and a gluten-free diet for celiac disease. In many cases of recurrent ulceration, when the exact cause cannot be found, mouthwashes, tablets, and analgesic creams and jellies are often prescribed by the doctor to help soothe the pain. Herpetic ulcers are treated with the drug aciclovir (Zovirax) formulated as a cream, which should be applied at the earliest indication of symptoms and repeated about five times a day.

When an ulcer becomes persistent, or when there are repeated bouts of ulcers, it is extremely important for a person to visit his or her doctor to have the cause diagnosed. A strong mouthwash or gargle may seem the most likely method of treating a mouth ulcer, but the solution of the mouthwash may be strong enough to aggravate the condition. In addition, the underlying cause will remain untreated. So it is essential to seek medical advice immediately.

Leg ulcers

Like mouth ulcers, leg ulcers are quite common and have a number of different causes: injury, infection, blood disease (such as sickle-cell anemia), and cancer are frequent causes. The most common cause, however, is disease of the blood vessels in the legs.

Blocked or narrow arteries diminish the blood supply to the tissues, causing the tissues to die and break down, thereby producing an ulcer. Ulcers of this type tend to occur on the lower leg or foot, and have a regular appearance. They may be several inches wide, may be quite deep, and are extremely painful.

Defective valves in the veins not only cause varicose veins, but can also bring about ulcers in the legs through the slow circulation of blood. In this case, the tissues break down to form large, shallow ulcers over the inside of the lower leg and ankle. The ulcers are not particularly painful but may ache considerably.

The immediate treatment for leg ulcers is aimed at keeping the area as free from infection as possible. This includes frequent cleaning, the use of antiseptic ointments or soaks, the application of a sterile foam pad, and firm bandaging. Painkilling drugs may also be prescribed. Long-term treatment is also necessary to tackle the underlying cause. This may range from antibiotic therapy to surgery in order to remove or to seal off the defective veins.

Peptic ulcers

The term "peptic" refers to ulcers of the lining of the stomach and of the first part of the small intestine, called the duodenum. These are known, respectively, as gastric and duodenal ulcers, the latter being the more common. Peptic ulceration also includes ulcers forming at the lower end of the esophagus (gullet). The whole of the intestine is lined with a wet membrane called a mucous membrane, and peptic ulcers involve local loss of this membrane, with some penetration into the underlying muscular layer of the big intestine. The condition is common, affecting about 10 percent of all adult males and 2 to 5 percent of women. Cigarette smoking interferes with the healing of ulcers and contributes to their causation.

Some of the cells of the stomach lining secrete a powerful hydrochloric acid. This is necessary to help break down food as a preliminary to digestion and to activate an enzyme called pepsin that digests proteins. Ulcers result when the mechanisms that protect the stomach lining from its own juices have become ineffective and when stomach acid is ejected into the duodenum. In effect, a peptic ulcer is a local partial digestion of the inside of the intestine wall. Normally this does not occur, because the acid and pepsin are present in insufficient quantity and because the linings are protected by mucus and by neutralizing bicarbonate of soda that is secreted by the lining cells.

Various factors interfere with the ability of the lining to resist digestion. These include the taking of certain drugs, especially aspirin and alcohol, the reflux of bile, and secretions from the duodenum into the stomach. In recent years it has become apparent that the germ *Helicobacter pylori* is also important in bringing about peptic ulceration. Severe head injury, burns, major surgery, and severe infections can also promote peptic ulcers. Ulceration of the lower esophagus occurs when there is considerable upward reflux of acid and pepsin from the stomach.

Duodenal ulcers

The duodenum is the C-shaped first part of the small intestine. The name comes from its dimensions, said to be equal to the width of 12 fingers. Because the stomach contents empty directly into the duodenum, the first inch or so takes the brunt of this highly irritating mixture, and it is here that duodenal ulcers occur. However, the acid is quickly neutralized by the alkaline digestive juices secreted by the pancreas, the duct of which enters the duodenum at about its midpoint. Duodenal ulcers are local areas in which the intestine wall is being digested by the acid and the pepsin. They do not occur in people who do not secrete stomach acid.

Duodenal ulcers are usually single, but two or more may occur simultaneously. Those that occur on areas of the intestine wall in contact are called kissing ulcers. They are usually about half an inch in diameter (1.3 cm) and penetrate the mucous membrane to erode the muscular coat immediately under the lining. In severe cases, both gastric and duodenal ulcers may pass right through. These are called perforating ulcers and they leave a hole through which the contents of the intestine can escape into the sterile peritoneal cavity of the abdomen surrounding the intestine. This causes a serious condition, peritonitis. Another serious complication of peptic ulceration is severe bleeding caused by the digestion of an artery in the wall of the intestine.

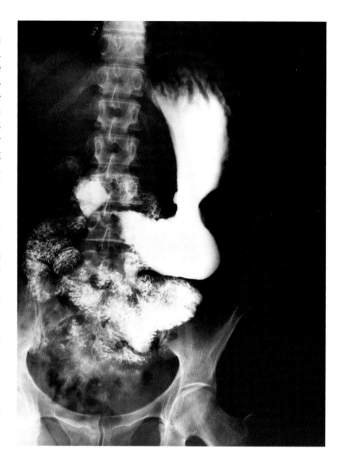

▲ *This X ray shows a gastric ulcer—the small white bulge on the left side of the large white mass (the stomach) to the right of the spinal cord.*

As in gastric ulceration, causal factors of duodenal ulceration include the amount of acid secreted, the efficiency of the mucus secreted by the lining in protecting its own surface from digestion, and the presence of *Helicobacter pylori*. To what extent, and by what means, these and other factors are influenced by the psychological or emotional state of the affected person, or by stress, is not entirely clear, but it is common experience that some forms of stress make symptoms worse.

Symptoms of peptic ulcers

Peptic ulceration causes a burning, gnawing pain high in the abdomen in the angle between the ribs. The pain usually comes on about two hours after a meal.

Duodenal ulcer pain is characteristically relieved by taking a small amount of food. This causes the stomach outlet to close, temporarily, so that the new food can be retained for digestion. The pain is not present on waking but tends to come on around the middle of the morning. It is also common for duodenal ulcer pain to wake the sufferer two or three hours after falling asleep. The diagnosis is often apparent from the history but may be confirmed by barium meal X-ray or by direct examination through a flexible illuminating and viewing tube. Most gastric and duodenal ulcers heal in four to six weeks.

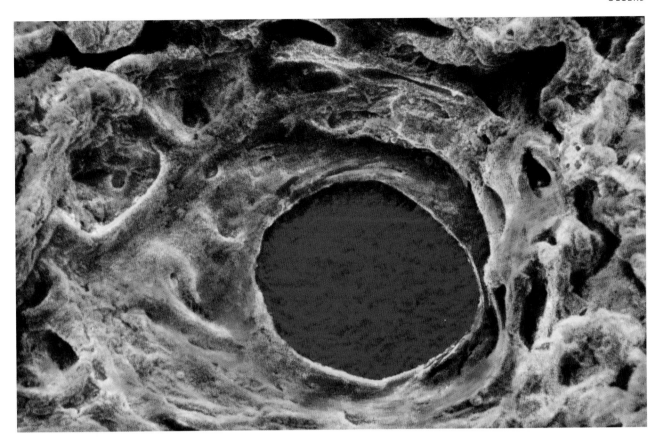

▲ *A micrograph of a gastric ulcer. The round, granular wound is surrounded by a smooth border of cells—the body's attempt to repair the injury—and then the rough texture of healthy gastric mucosa.*

Treatment of peptic ulcer

A wide range of treatments are used. Antibiotics are used to eradicate *Helicobacter pylori* organisms, and bismuth antacid drugs to neutralize stomach acid. Histamine H-2 blockers are used to reduce acid secretion, whereas proton pump inhibitor drugs such as omeprazole (Losec) interfere directly with the chemical mechanism by which the acid is formed. Other drugs are used to form a protective coating on the base of the ulcer and promote healing. Prostaglandin drugs are also used, since they have a wide range of actions on cells, some of which can be exploited to cut acid secretion.

In some cases, surgical treatment, such as bypassing the duodenum (gastroenterostomy), reshaping the stomach outlet (pyloroplasty), removing an affected part of the stomach (partial gastrectomy), or cutting some of the nerves to the stomach that promote acid secretion (selective or truncal vagotomy) may be helpful. In addition, treatment with tranquilizing drugs may help by relieving anxiety or depression.

In spite of treatment, chronic peptic ulceration often persists for life, with relapses every two years or so. The condition is virtually prevented if *Helicobacter pylori* organisms are eliminated. In all cases the outlook will be greatly improved if the patient quits smoking, stops taking aspirin, drinks alcohol only in moderation and in reasonable dilution, and reduces dietary intake. Strict diets are not needed; patients need only avoid items known to cause symptoms.

Other ulcers

Pressure sores (which are known medically as decubitus ulcers) commonly affect older, bedridden, and long-term patients. These are caused by constant pressure that impairs the blood circulation through an area of skin and underlying tissue, and commonly occur on the hips, heels, and base of the spine.

The rodent ulcer is a particularly nasty ulcer that occurs on the face. This is actually a type of skin cancer, starting as a red lump that grows and breaks down to form a circular ulcer. Without treatment this continues to grow and spread, but surgical removal or radiation therapy can result in a complete cure. Ulcers can occur in the groin region for many reasons, including sexually acquired herpes or syphilis. Any groin ulcer should be investigated immediately by a doctor, as there is a chance that it may be due to syphilis, which is a very serious disease if it is left untreated.

Any persistent, suspicious, or spreading ulcer should always be taken seriously and brought to the attention of a doctor.

See also: **Alcoholism; Allergies; Anemia; Antibiotics; Arthritis; Burns; Cancer; Depression; Diabetes; Sexually transmitted diseases; Smoking; Stress; Tuberculosis**

Vaccinations

Questions and Answers

After he was given a measles shot, my son got a rash and a mild cold. Are these the usual symptoms of measles?

Yes. The measles vaccine, like many of the really successful vaccines, consists of an attenuated (weakened) strain of the virus itself, which is given as an injection of live virus. This is likely to produce the minor reaction that your son had; a mini-attack of the disease. Anyone who has seen the misery of a young child with measles would be the first to agree that the mild reaction to a measles shot is preferable to suffering the disease.

When my daughter was due to get a TB vaccination, the hospital ran a test and said that she didn't need the vaccine at all. Why not?

Tuberculosis is an unusual infection. It is common for people to acquire the illness toward the end of childhood. When this happens, a child may show no symptoms, and build up an immunity that keeps the disease in check. A child in this situation will not need the vaccination, since he or she already has immunity. The original test injection is an extract of the cell wall of the bacteria, and it is read two days later. A red welt on the site of the injection is evidence of a previous tuberculosis infection.

How is a vaccine weakened so that the germs build up immunity and yet do not cause the disease?

Antivirus vaccines are used in a live form, that is, living viruses are injected into the patient, so they must belong to a strain that gives immunity without causing serious disease. The strains are produced by growing repeated cultures of the virus or by infecting and reinfecting a series of animals until the virus has lost virulence.

Like many medical advances, vaccination developed almost by accident—when a doctor discovered that inoculation with cowpox virus prevented smallpox. Now vaccines offer complete protection against many diseases.

The development and use of vaccines have revolutionized treatment of many serious diseases. For example, with the help of an effective vaccine one killer disease—smallpox—has been eradicated worldwide, and another potentially fatal disease, diphtheria, has all but disappeared from developed areas of the world.

The body's defense system

The body's first line of defense is the skin, which cannot be crossed unless it is broken. The lining membrane of the gut and the lungs are also constantly assaulted by organisms, and their main protection lies in mucus-secreting glands. The final line of defense is the complex, blood-based immune system, which comes into action if the skin or a mucous membrane is breached by a foreign organism.

One of the main functions of the immune system is the activity of antibodies, which are protein molecules that are carried in a dissolved form in the blood. The function of antibodies is to help to control and bind infecting organisms, which can then be attacked by phagocytes. Lymphocytes also play a role: they are white blood cells involved in making antibodies and include cells that attack organisms directly, giving rise to cellular immunity.

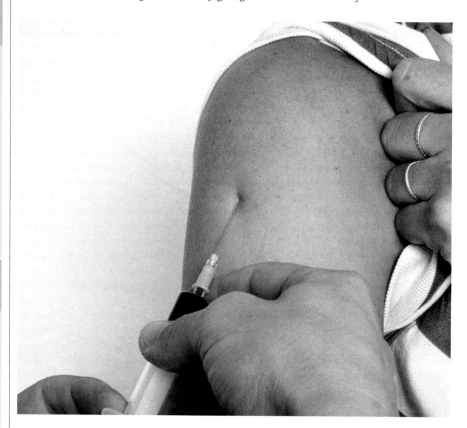

▲ *Vaccination introduces an infectious organism into the body. Although the organism is harmless it stimulates the production of antibodies against the organism.*

Cellular immunity is an important process for dealing with organisms that are capable of infiltrating the cells; one example of such an organism is the tuberculosis bacillus.

Vaccines work by priming the immune system for invasion by an infecting organism so that the body's defenses are prepared for an actual attack by the disease. Generally vaccines are better at building up antibodies than they are at establishing cellular immunity.

The origin of vaccination

Like many of the great advances of medicine, vaccination was an accepted technique before its theoretical basis was understood. In the late 1700s, the English surgeon Edward Jenner heard that milkmaids who suffered from cowpox seemed to have a degree of immunity against smallpox, and he reasoned correctly that this might point to a way of preventing the latter disease. He proceeded to inject the fluid from the pustules of cowpox into

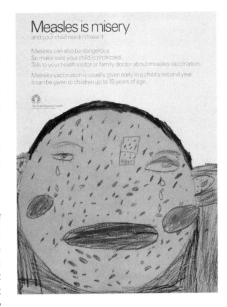

people who were at risk from smallpox. His reasoning was shown to be correct. (Cowpox is called vaccinia, hence "vaccination.")

The reason the cowpox fluid was effective was that the vaccinia virus is so similar to the smallpox virus that it creates effective antibodies to smallpox without giving rise to serious disease. Jenner's intuition occurred long before doctors were aware of antibodies.

Live vaccines

The vaccinia virus is alive, and in certain conditions it may cause serious disease. For example, people with eczema may contract a fatal infection from vaccinia if they have been vaccinated. In most cases, however, vaccinia is a virus that is attenuated for the average individual: that is, it does not normally cause serious

▲ *Variations on the theme of public health: the poster is part of a campaign to persuade parents to have their children inoculated against measles.*

▼ *A medical team vaccinates villagers in Democratic Republic of the Congo in an attempt to control diseases endemic in that part of the world.*

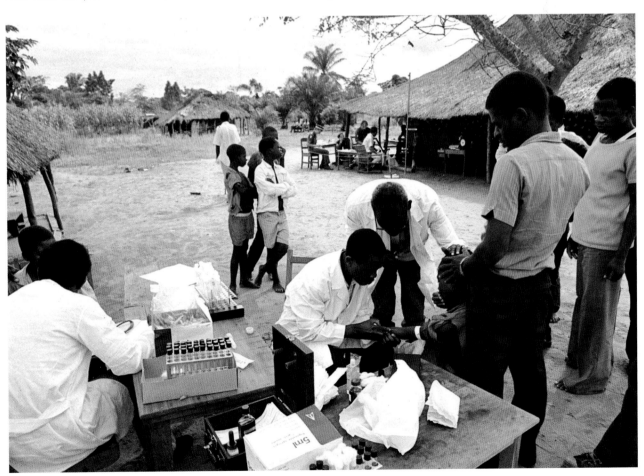

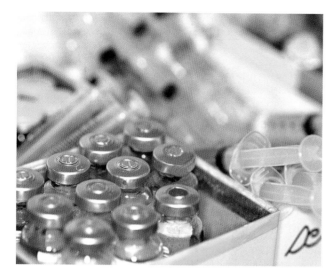

▲ *A supply of vaccine is ready to be used to provide protection against disease. Since the introduction of immunization programs, many diseases have declined.*

disease. In order to provide adequate protection in other serious diseases such as polio, rubella, yellow fever, and the like, the original virulent (disease-producing) virus has to be treated in the laboratory to reduce its virulence, while its capacity to create immunity is preserved. Virulence is reduced by growing repeated generations of viruses on a suitable medium, or infecting and reinfecting animals such as mice, until the virus loses its capacity to cause serious disease.

▼ *A flu shot is given to an elderly patient. The flu vaccination is recommended for those who are likely to become seriously ill if they develop influenza.*

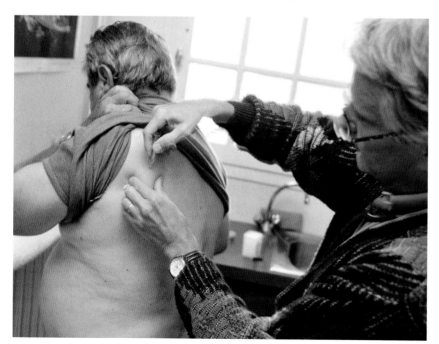

▲ *Some diseases may eventually be eradicated if a program of vaccination is implemented. Vaccination is often used to prevent disease from spreading in a community.*

Killed vaccines versus live vaccines

In some cases, particularly bacterial infections, it is not possible to produce live vaccines—dead bacterial extracts are used instead. Vaccines used against whooping cough and cholera are examples of killed vaccines.

Generally, however, live vaccines are superior to using extracts of killed organisms. In addition, a vaccine such as the polio vaccine can be administered by mouth, so that it goes straight to the normal port of entry of the disease, which is the intestine. As a result, local defenses of antibodies can be built up in the intestinal wall.

Vaccines in common use

In most developed countries, preschool children are offered protection against tetanus, diphtheria, and whooping cough in the form of a combined vaccine called a triple vaccine. Oral polio vaccine is also given at this time. A triple vaccine of measles, mumps, and rubella is given between the ages of 12 months and 15 months; a booster is given between four and six years. It may also be given later.

Travelers may be offered vaccines to prevent yellow fever, typhoid, and cholera. Some countries require certificates of immunization against these diseases; travelers should check with a consulate or travel agent.

> *See also:* Immunization; Infection and infectious diseases; Rubella; Tuberculosis

Vegetarianism

Is a vegetarian diet healthier than one that involves eating meat?

As far as diet goes, eating meat is not harmful in itself. However, eating anything to excess can be dangerous, and a heavily meat-centered diet can, for example, produce too high an intake of fats. However, meat is an excellent source of protein and iron, which the body needs. If these nutrients are not eaten in meat, they must be found elsewhere. The body also needs a certain proportion of fat, so avoiding meat without using careful supplements can be bad for you. However, a well-balanced vegetarian diet can be very healthy, and is prescribed for certain conditions that are caused or aggravated by a high intake of saturated fats or a low intake of fiber. A vegetarian diet is high in fiber and low in saturated fats.

I am newly a vegetarian. What should I eat when not at home?

The best approach is to have the courage of your convictions and tell your host in good time that you are vegetarian. No friend would feel inconvenienced, if you tell him or her early. You wouldn't think twice about stating dietary preferences if you were, say, a diabetic. Your vegetarianism is nothing to be ashamed of.

Will my children get the necessary vitamins on a vegetarian diet?

A vegetarian diet that is properly balanced will contain all the vitamins that you are ever likely to need, if it is carefully planned. However if you are vegan and do not eat meat or animal products of any kind you must give your children vitamin B12, vitamin B2, and vitamin D supplements if you want them to follow the same diet as you. Note that excess B12 is dangerous in children.

Just a few decades ago, vegetarianism was uncommon and considered to be unusual. However, there is now more much awareness of the advantages of eating a diet based on vegetables, fruits, and whole grains.

Vegetarianism is the adoption of a diet in which plant foods are eaten in preference to, or to the exclusion of, animal products. Knowledge of nutrition increased greatly in the 20th century. Led by such knowledge and by economic necessity, many Western societies moved away from heavy, meat-centered meals of 10 to 12 courses to a lighter, healthier, more balanced diet. The vegetarian movement started in the United States in the early 1970s, fueled by reasoning that growing livestock was uneconomical, and that human dentition was not suited to eating meat. Over the next two decades, other convincing arguments persuaded many people to adopt a vegetarian diet. One of these centered on health issues such as heart disease. In the 1990s the U.S. government introduced a food pyramid, suggesting that the ideal diet should be based on grains, vegetables, beans, and fruits, and that dairy products and saturated animal fats, which are linked to heart disease, should be limited. In 2011, the U.S. government put forward new guidelines in the form of MyPlate, which emphasizes fruits, vegetables, and whole grains. Detailed information on MyPlate is available online (www.choosemyplate.gov), as is information on the *Dietary Guidelines for Americans, 2010* (www.cnpp.usda.gov/dietaryguidelines.htm).

Another issue that persuaded many people to become vegetarians was poor animal welfare, such as factory farms, force-fed animals, and calves' being reared in crates to retain their white flesh for those who demanded veal.

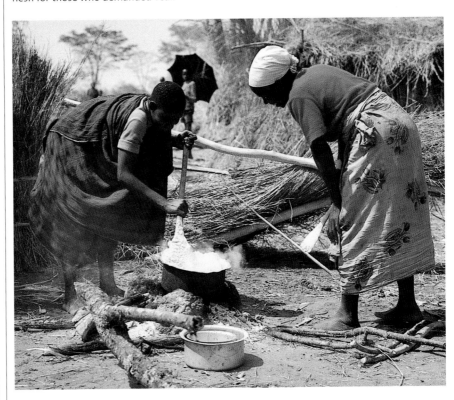

▲ *In the West, vegetarianism is a practice based on personal preference. In the poorer parts of the world, however, the economics of necessity are paramount: vegetables may be all that is available, or affordable.*

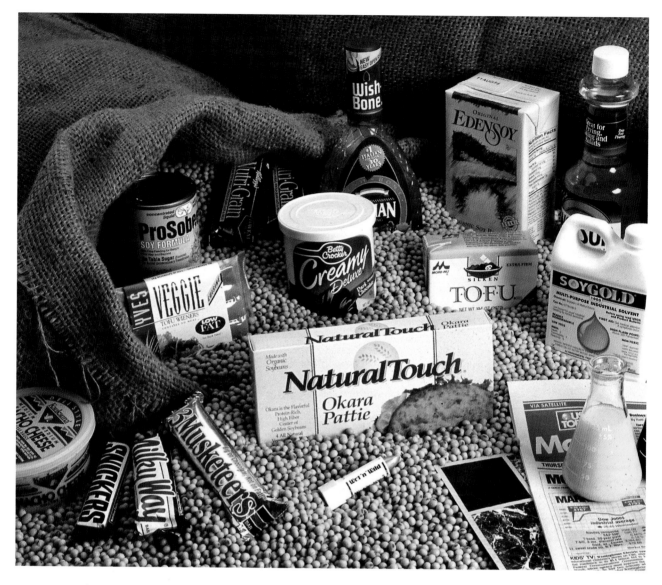

▲ *Soybeans are used to make myriad products; tofu, soy yogurt, soy milk, and soy sauce are just a small selection. Soy protein and soy oil appear in dozens of common foods.*

A way of life

For many people, vegetarianism is a complete way of life that involves more than just dietary rules. Naturism, homeopathy (natural medicine), spiritualism, and yoga all have links with vegetarianism.

There are many forms of vegetarianism, but most vegetarians fall into one of five main groups. First, demivegetarians at the least rigorous end of the scale are those who will eat white meat, such as chicken or fish, and animal products, such as cheese and eggs, but will avoid red meat. Second are the lacto-ovo (milk-egg) vegetarians, who avoid all forms of flesh, including fish and fowl, but will eat eggs and dairy products. Third are the lacto vegetarians, who avoid all flesh and also eggs, because they believe eggs are embryos and therefore flesh. Fourth, there are those who follow a macrobiotic

diet, part of a whole lifestyle based on hatha yoga, which concentrates on whole grains, cereals, and some vegetables, but also includes fish. Last, there are the vegans, who eat no flesh or animal products of any kind.

Why become a vegetarian?

There are probably almost as many reasons for becoming a vegetarian as there are vegetarians. The motive may be ethical, economic, ecological, social, emotional, spiritual, or medical. One obvious and widespread reason is a simple dislike of meat—its taste or appearance, or both. Other reasons are aesthetic: for example, one person became a vegetarian after seeing a particularly bloody automobile crash; she claimed that the mutilated bodies reminded her of a butcher's shop, and that she has been unable to eat meat ever since.

In early cultures, there were often cultural reasons for a vegetarian diet. Some Indian and African communities have no tradition of hunting, and therefore they have no source of fresh

ECONOMICS OF VEGETARIANISM

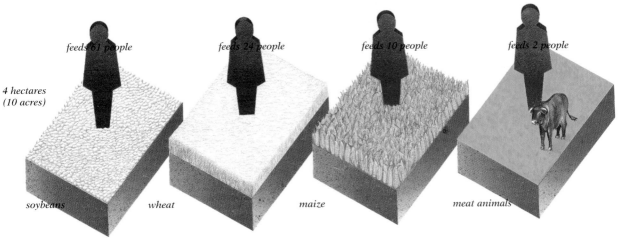

feeds 61 people   *feeds 24 people*   *feeds 10 people*   *feeds 2 people*

4 hectares
(10 acres)

soybeans   *wheat*   *maize*   *meat animals*

meat. Rather, they live on cereals and plants. Economic pressures may also be relevant, since with the rising cost of fish and meat, many people cannot afford to buy either.

Perhaps more commonly, there are ethical reasons for becoming a vegetarian. The Vegan Society was founded by vegetarians who felt that the methods used in dairy farming, especially the early separation of cow and calf, were in some ways more cruel than those of meat production. In protest, they refused to eat animal products of any kind.

Most vegetarians avoid meat and meat products because they are distressed by the idea of animals being slaughtered to provide their food, by the methods of slaughter, or by the treatment of the animals on the journey to a slaughterhouse.

There is also an ecological and economic argument that the starving people of the world could be better provided for if our diet were not so meat-centered. Fifty percent of the world cereal crop is fed to animals, and it takes 10 tons of vegetable protein fed to an animal to produce one ton of animal protein. The theory is that if less grain were used to raise fewer animals for slaughter, more grain would be available for humans.

Several religious and spiritual sects advocate vegetarianism as part of a pure, simple life. The macrobiotic lifestyle, for example, centers on the belief that pain and disease are the result of spiritual imbalance, and that concern for the origin of food is one way to restore the balance. A pure natural diet is thought to rid the body of harmful toxins. If a natural diet is eaten and, at the same time, yoga and prayer are practiced, spiritual well-being will be promoted.

Finally, some people become vegetarians for health reasons. Although a meat-free diet is not necessarily better for everyone, certain medical conditions—especially heart and digestive diseases—can be improved by eating a vegetarian diet which is low in saturated fat and high in fiber.

A balanced vegetarian diet

In the 1970s, it was believed that the quality of protein obtained from individual plant sources was low compared with animal protein, and that by combining certain plant proteins a high-quality

▲ *These diagrams represent how, in terms of land use, it is more economical to grow crops rather than graze animals destined for slaughter and the dinner table.*

▼ *Soybeans are used in many everyday products; for example, soy oil is the most widely used oil in the United States.*

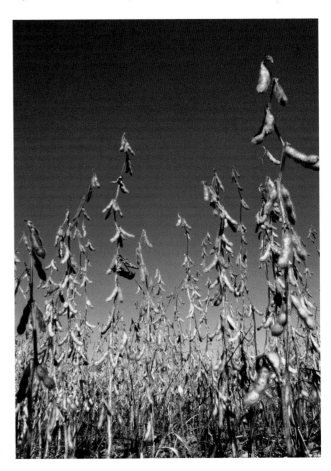

protein can be obtained. This theory has been disproved and it is now known that all the essential and nonessential amino acids are to be found in single unrefined starches such as rice, wheat, potatoes, and corn. If people eat enough calories, they are virtually certain of getting enough protein. After all, people were eating farm animals that ate nothing but plants yet remained healthy.

The original myth about complementary proteins seems to have originated from a study on rats. Rats, however, require 10 times as much protein as humans, because rat milk is 50 percent protein compared with 5 percent protein in human breast milk.

Vegans do not eat any dairy products or eggs; therefore, to ensure that their protein requirements are met, they should eat a diet of mixed protein sources, including cereals, nuts, legumes, potatoes, and oil seeds. A balanced vegetarian diet can have many health advantages. Vegans tend to weigh less than omnivores (those who eat many kinds of food—flesh and vegetable), and weighing less can be an advantage. Also, vegetarians eat a greater amount of fiber, which helps prevent constipation and intestinal diseases such as cancer and colitis.

Other conditions that a vegetarian diet has improved or even cured in some cases include infantile eczema, childhood asthma, acne, and, in adults, diabetes, hypertension, circulatory problems, blood clots, angina, and migraine. The most widely discussed argument for

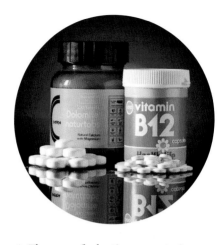

▲ *The crux of adopting a vegetarian diet is that it must be balanced, containing the vitamins your children are likely to need; vitamin supplements can provide reassurance.*

vegetarianism on health grounds, however, is the avoidance or alleviation of heart disease. One of the most common causes of heart attacks is the accumulation of fatty deposits along the walls of the coronary arteries, a condition called atheroma. Diets rich in fats—particularly saturated fats (fats with a high concentration of hydrogen atoms), which are found predominantly in animal products—appear to contribute to the disease.

Heart disease is almost unknown in nonindustrial vegetarian communities. The highest incidence of heart disease is in Russia, followed by countries in central Europe and eastern Europe. The United States is placed at about number 13 in a world table, near to the UK, New Zealand, and the Scandinavian countries. France and Japan are at the bottom of the table, with a much lower incidence of heart disease.

▼ *These soybean seeds show a wide range of colors, sizes, and shapes. Soybeans are grown in half of the United States, yet were virtually unheard of 100 years ago.*

▼ *A tempting lunch box for kids to take to school. What's special about this one is that the food in it is vegetarian and contains all the nutrients necessary for a well-balanced meal.*

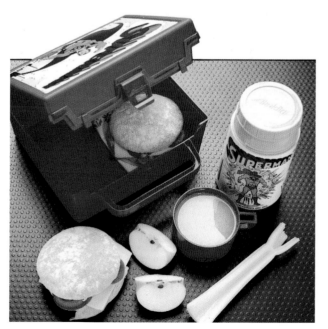

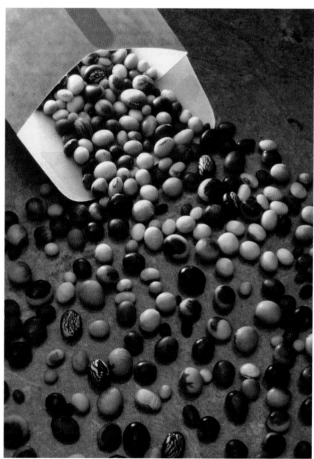

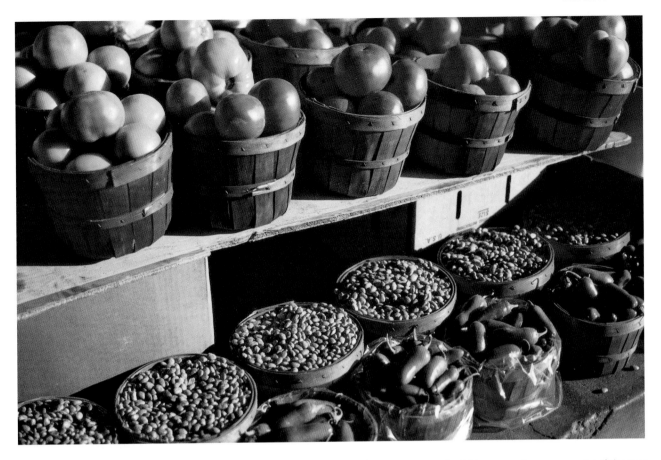

▲ *Fresh fruits and vegetables, and nuts and legumes are perfect ingredients for a vegetarian diet; they can be obtained at farmers' markets.*

A balanced vegetarian diet

A commitment to vegetarianism, and especially veganism, requires a sensible approach to diet, and factors that contribute to good health must not be neglected.

Weight loss, often accompanied by a loss of energy, is a common effect of changing over to a vegetarian diet. This can be serious in someone who is already underweight. More serious illnesses that are connected with veganism in particular are spinal ataxia, a condition causing an unsteady gait, stooped posture, and loss of balance and sensation in the legs; and megaloblastic anemia, a deficiency in the blood. Both of these conditions, caused by vitamin B12 deficiency, are quite rare, but deficiency of this vitamin is the major health risk for vegans.

Cobalt is a vital constituent of this vitamin; in a vegan diet, because vitamin B12 is found only in animal foods or microorganisms, it can be obtained naturally only by eating vegetables old enough to have a growth of mold on them. One way to avoid such a deficiency is to include a vitamin B12 supplement in the diet. There is vitamin B12 in eggs and cheese, so it is only vegans who are at risk of a deficiency.

Vitamin D is also absent from plant foods. However, individuals can make this vitamin by the action of sunlight on the skin. Vitamin D deficiency can occur in children reared on a vegan diet if they are not sufficiently exposed to sunlight. It would be a sensible precaution, especially in winter, to give children extra vitamin D in the form of drops.

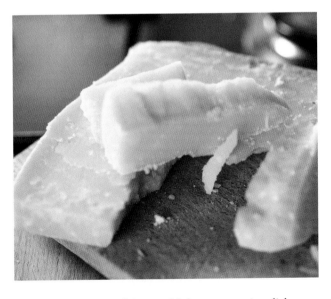

▲ *A small quantity of cheese added to a vegetarian dish enriches it with protein.*

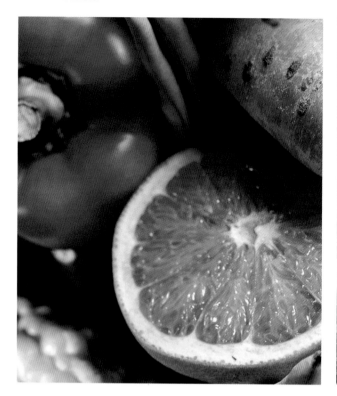

▲ *Citrus fruits are a good source of vitamin C and bioflavonoids, which have a beneficial effect on the body. They protect the nervous system and strengthen capillary walls.*

Ultimately, the choice of diet is a personal one, based on belief, preference, or circumstances. However, a properly balanced diet should consist of the correct proportions of fats, carbohydrates, proteins, vitamins, and minerals, and contain appropriate calories.

▼ *A diet rich in soy and whey protein, found in products such as soy milk and low-fat yogurt, has been shown to reduce the incidence of breast cancer in rats.*

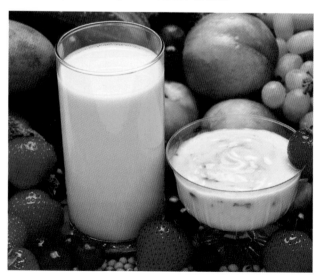

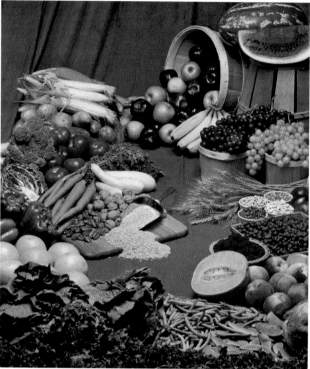

▲ *The U.S. government food guide pyramid recommends three to five servings of vegetables and two to four servings of fruit daily as part of a healthy diet.*

Changing one's diet should always be a slow and careful process, as any sudden change can be a shock to the system. A dietitian should be consulted before making any radical change in the amount or type of food eaten. A well-balanced diet and plenty of sensibly planned exercise are vital for health. Whether that diet is vegetarian depends on individual needs and preferences.

Daily vegetarian fare

A good daily intake of fresh vegetables and fruit is essential, particularly green leafy vegetables. Because cooking can destroy vitamins, minerals, and other nutrients, vegetables can be eaten raw or lightly steamed, baked, or microwaved.

Brown rice, oats, barley, corn, nuts and legumes, and seeds supply adequate amounts of dietary fiber. Because a range of health problems are associated with the consumption of saturated fats, butter and cheese should be eaten rarely. Monounsaturated oils such as canola oil or olive oil can be substituted. Soy products such as tofu supply protein and have the advantage that they do not contain cholesterol or saturated fat. Fats are made up of fatty acids; most are made by the body but two of the unsaturated fatty acids have to be supplied in the diet. A good source for vegetarians is flaxseed oil, which contains omega-3 fatty acids, and safflower oil and soybean oil are important sources of omega-6 fatty acids.

See also: **Alternative medicine; Anemia; Diet; Fats; Heart attack; Heart disease; Nutrition; Protein; Vitamin B; Vitamin D; Weight**

Viruses

Why is it that viruses cannot be treated with antibiotics?

Bacteria that respond to antibiotics are complicated organisms, although each consists of only one cell. Viruses, on the other hand, are very simple, consisting of a core of nucleic acid (genetic material) surrounded by a protein capsule. Antibiotics work by impeding the activity of the bacterial cell without harming human cells. However, virus metabolism and structure are quite different from those of bacteria, so antibiotics that attack bacterial structure and metabolism have no effect on viruses.

Is it likely that any new treatments will be able to affect the course of minor viral diseases like the common cold?

It seems unlikely that any form of direct treatment for minor viral diseases will be discovered in the near future, unless a sudden major breakthrough in the research of viruses occurs.

It has been very difficult to make a vaccine against the common cold because the common cold is caused by some 200 viruses and these are always mutating. The natural antiviral substances in the interferon range of drugs do have some useful effects against viruses, but the high expense of producing these drugs makes them impractical for general use. However, there are many different antiviral drugs currently in use—most of them acting to inhibit the synthesis of DNA or RNA in the viruses, or to inhibit viral uncoating—and the range of antiviral drugs is continually growing. Therefore, it seems likely that, eventually, effective treatments may be found for many minor viral infections. In the meantime, the best approach to minor viral diseases may be in prevention rather than cure.

Influenza, measles, and rabies are disparate diseases that have something in common: being caused by viruses. An increasing number of diseases caused by viruses can now be effectively treated by new antiviral drugs, and new drugs are constantly being developed.

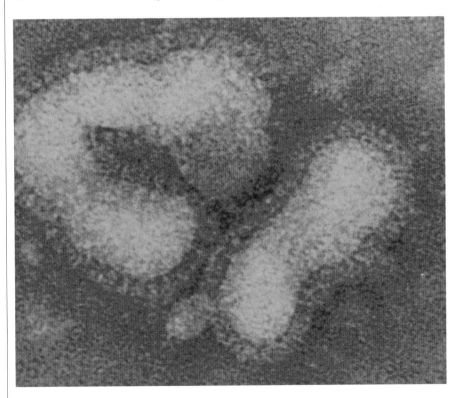

The work of great people like Louis Pasteur (1822–1895) led to the discovery of bacteria—the cause of many of the most serious illnesses. However, by the end of the 19th century there were still many diseases for which a bacterial cause was suspected but not found. Pasteur had demonstrated that rabies was an infection and had produced a vaccine against it, but he had not been able to find a bacterium that caused it. He rightly deduced that this was because the organism was too small to be seen under a microscope.

The first virus was found in 1892 and was identified as tobacco mosaic virus. This virus causes disease in plants rather than in humans. Following this discovery it was shown that

▲ *Viruses are extremely simple structures that usually consist of a thin protein membrane containing one of the nucleic acids, DNA or RNA. The influenza virus (above) is a typical example. It is also wrapped in an outer envelope, as shown in the model (top). The influenza virus can change its protein structure with each new infection in order to fool the body's immune system.*

391

HOW A VIRUS MULTIPLIES

Viruses are totally parasitic, since they multiply only in the cells of other organisms. When a virus invades a host cell (1) its genetic material mingles with that of the host cell (2), which then starts to produce more viral genetic material (3). Finally, the new viral particles (4) become enveloped again in a protein membrane and emerge from the cell (5) to invade other cells.

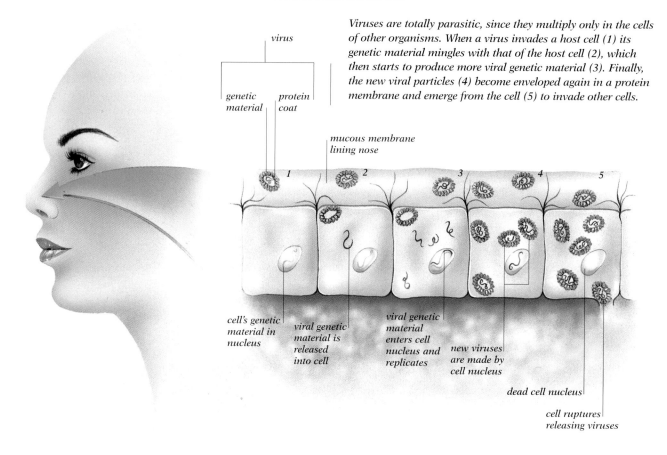

virus

genetic material   protein coat

mucous membrane lining nose

1   2   3   4   5

cell's genetic material in nucleus

viral genetic material is released into cell

viral genetic material enters cell nucleus and replicates

new viruses are made by cell nucleus

dead cell nucleus

cell ruptures releasing viruses

▼ *The hepatitis A virus is often found in food and water contaminated with fecal material. The infection thus occurs in areas with poor sanitation.*

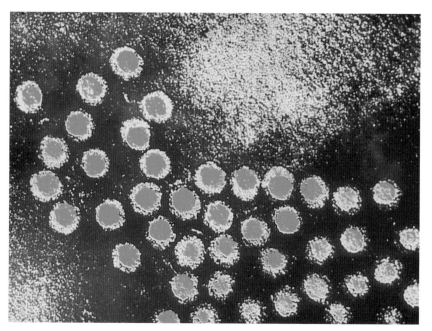

foot-and-mouth disease, which occurs in cattle, was caused by a similar tiny organism.

It was demonstrated that these viruses were able to travel from plant to plant or animal to animal after passing through a filter too fine to let a bacterium through.

Research was carried out in the light of knowledge at the time, but was impeded by the fact that it was still not possible to see viruses. It was the electron microscope that first revealed what viruses actually look like.

What are viruses?

Viruses are very tiny organisms. For example, a polio virus is 20 nanometers across (a nanometer is one-thousandth of a micrometer, which in turn is one-thousandth of a millimeter).

The basic structure of viruses is so simple that it is questionable whether they should be regarded as living matter at all. Essentially, they consist of no more than a capsule of protein that contains their genetic material in the form of one of the nucleic acids, DNA or RNA. These are the

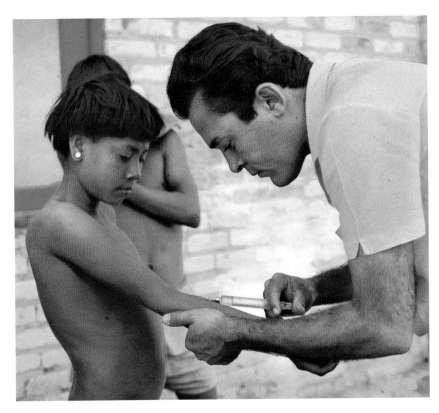

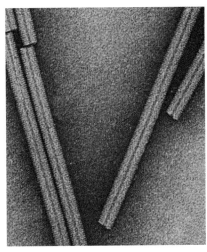

▲ *The first virus to be discovered was the tobacco mosaic virus. It is viewed here under the electron microscope, which enabled research to progress.*

◄ *Vaccination is vital for preventing the deadliest viral infections, especially in developing countries where so many other serious health problems are rife.*

substances that carry the genetic message from generation to generation in all living things. It is the DNA that is passed on in the process of reproduction and is contained in the nucleus of living cells. The DNA then sends messages to the chemical factories inside the cells, instructing them to make various types of protein. These messages are carried by the RNA.

Viruses work by invading the cells of the organism they are infecting. Once a virus is inside a cell, it inserts its DNA into the DNA of the cell, and the protein-producing apparatus of the cell starts to work for the virus instead of for the cell itself. Having taken control of a cell, the virus manufactures more viruses, so that more cells and finally other individuals can be infected.

Therefore, viruses are very lifelike in their ability to pass on their own characteristics from generation to generation by the use of genetic material. The two nucleic acids, DNA and RNA, are the basic stuff of life, and even if they are contained in only a thin capsule, they make up what is virtually a living organism.

Structure

Viruses are extremely small, the smallest being 20–30 nanometers across and the largest 10 times that size. Most viruses are more or less round in shape. Exceptions are the rabies virus and its related viruses, which are bullet-shaped; and the smallpox virus and its related viruses, which are brick-shaped.

Viruses are basically classified according to whether they carry the nucleic acid DNA or RNA. The nucleic acid core of a virus is called the genome and the protein capsule the capsid. The capsid is made up from many identical protein blocks called capsomeres. The way in which the capsomeres line up around the genome dictates the overall shape of the individual virus particle.

Different groups of viruses have different shapes, one of the most common being the icosahedron, a structure with 20 flat sides of equal size, effectively forming a sphere. The capsid of other viruses forms a hollow cylinder. These differences in structure can be determined only by pictures taken with an electron microscope (electron micrographs). Some viruses have another structure on top of their capsid, aptly called an envelope.

All these variations place a virus in a particular group. The viruses that cause human disease are now all classified. The five hepatitis B viruses are classified as hepadnaviruses (hepatitis DNA viruses), and the hepatitis A virus is classified as a picornavirus (pico RNA virus); "pico" means "very small."

Viruses and bacteria

There is an enormous difference in size between viruses and bacteria. For example, a streptococcus is 50 times greater in diameter than a polio virus.

An individual bacterium is able to reproduce itself by splitting in two, and it can live independently, having the apparatus to carry out many metabolic processes within its cell wall. All bacteria contain DNA and RNA. In contrast, although viruses can survive outside the cells of other organisms, they need these cells to supply them with building materials and enable them to reproduce. They do this by making exact copies of themselves according to instructions from their DNA or RNA, a process known as replication. They contain only one kind of nucleic acid.

How are viruses spread?

Viral diseases can be very infectious. A disease like measles is so infectious that until vaccination was introduced, it was certain that virtually every child in the United States would get it. A new epidemic used to occur about every two years.

The measles virus, like many others, is spread by droplet infection. A cough or sneeze from an infected person will carry the virus into the air to be inhaled by someone else.

The polio virus and enteroviruses (primarily infecting the intestines) enter the body via the digestive tract. Another group, the togaviruses, which are carried by insects, make their way into the body through the skin as the result of an insect bite. Rabies also enters via a bite from an animal that has been driven to distraction by the disease.

The rhinoviruses that are responsible for the common cold enter the cells of the mucous membrane joining the nose to create symptoms in the nose and upper airways.

Once inside the body, viruses invade the cells, usually selecting one particular type of body cell.

Viruses in the laboratory

Viruses not only are difficult to see but are very difficult to grow in the laboratory, since they depend on living cells for replication. In the early days of virology it was not possible to grow viruses at all; it was possible only to pass them from one laboratory animal to another.

The first advances in this field came with the realization that viruses could be grown inside fertilized chickens' eggs. The influenza, mumps, and herpes viruses can all be grown in this way by injecting infected tissue into the inside of the egg. This will produce a collection of tiny colonies just like those on a bacterial culture plate.

The next step was the development of tissue cultures, which are collections of mammalian cells grown in a test tube. Preparing a culture is not a routine technique of investigation, but it is vitally important in the making of vaccines that protect us against the most dangerous and widespread viral infections.

A particular viral infection is usually diagnosed by monitoring the levels of antibodies in a patient's blood over a period of two weeks.

Treatment of viral infections

The AIDS pandemic has resulted in an enormous expansion in research into viruses and the details of their life cycles and modes of reproduction. As new facts were discovered, it became possible to produce new drugs that interfered with various aspects of these reproductive processes. As a result, many antiviral drugs are now in general use. Diseases against which these agents are effective include AIDS, influenza A and B, herpes simplex infections, cytomegalovirus infections, hepatitis B and C, and Lassa fever. Combinations of antiviral drugs can reduce HIV replications to levels undetectable in the circulation and postpone the development of AIDS.

Antiviral drugs work in several different ways. Some replace substances that viruses build into their structure. Some replace chemicals that viruses need to produce the enzymes necessary for DNA replication (DNA polymerases). Some act to block the processes of virus uncoating so that the genome cannot be released. Antiretroviral agents, such as those used to kill HIV, act by inhibiting the viral enzyme (reverse transcriptase) that catalyzes the conversion of RNA into DNA. HIV protease inhibitor drugs block another essential viral enzyme.

Prevention

Many serious viral infections can be prevented. Smallpox was eradicated worldwide through a combination of vaccination and

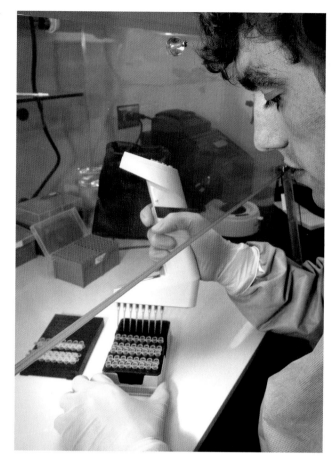

▲ *SARS virus tests are being done at the Viral and Rickettsial Diseases Division of Centers for Disease Control and Prevention.*

isolation of cases. Vaccinations also exist for measles, rubella (German measles), yellow fever, polio, and rabies.

There are some infections, however, against which it is more difficult to produce an effective vaccine. New viruses, such as SARS, need to be thoroughly studied before a vaccine can be attempted. Other viruses, such as influenza, have a remarkable ability to change their protein structure as they pass from person to person. These minor changes enable them to fool the body's immune system with each new infection. This explains why people get so many attacks of the same disease in a lifetime.

A vaccine will be effective if it is made from the current strain of a virus, but for this to be possible, a manufacturer would have to predict the strain accurately, which would be a very difficult proposition. The problem is multiplied in the case of the common cold, since it involves so many viral strains. Therefore, it is unlikely that prevention or treatments for the common cold will be available in the near future.

See also: AIDS; Bacteria; Common cold; Genetics; Hepatitis; Infection and infectious diseases; Influenza; Measles; Protein; Rabies; Rubella; Streptococcus; Vaccinations

Vitamin A

Questions and Answers

Deficiency in vitamin A is relatively rare in the West, but when it does occur, generally owing to malabsorption, serious health problems are the result, including eventual blindness.

Vitamin A is one of the vital groups of vitamins that the body needs to function properly. It enables people to see in a dim light, keeps the skin healthy, ensures normal growth, and renews the body tissue. With only a few exceptions, all the necessary vitamins are obtained from food, and the minute amounts the body requires mostly exist in their natural state in food. Vitamin A, however, is largely manufactured by the body from a food substance called carotene.

Sources of vitamin A

The vitamin A in food comes in two different forms from two different sources. The pure form, called retinol, is found in foods such as fish liver oils, liver, kidney, cheese, eggs, and butter, and has already been manufactured by the animal concerned. The second form is made in the body from carotene, which is found in such vegetables as carrots, spinach, cabbage, and tomatoes.

Vegetables are orange, yellow, or dark green in color because of carotene, and the darker the green, the greater the carotene content. Spinach and watercress contain more carotene in each pound than cabbage, and dark green cabbage provides more than lighter-colored vegetables. Carotene is converted into retinol in the liver and in the small intestine, and then some of the vitamin A in the form of converted carotene or retinol is absorbed into the bloodstream and circulated around the body to be used in its everyday functions, while the rest is stored in the liver.

Although vitamin A is not present in many foods, those that contain it are readily available. A fifth of people's average intake comes from vegetables, mainly carrots. Turnips and potatoes are no substitute, however, since they contain no carotene. Milk and butter are other common sources; margarine, to which vitamin A is added artificially, contains almost as much vitamin A as butter and is therefore nutritionally comparable.

Foods rich in vitamin A tend to retain their vitamin content, although prolonged exposure to light and air can reduce the amount. Cooking at normal temperatures has no serious

If halibut-liver oil is good for me, is a double dose twice as good?

Halibut-liver oil is a valuable source of vitamin A, but it is dangerous to exceed the recommended dose. Because vitamin A is stored in the body, excessive amounts can be toxic.

Does vitamin A prevent colds?

Vitamin A aids the body in producing mucus-secreting cells, and In this way the body protects itself from germs. It works by removing them from the body— by the nose in the case of a cold. A lack of vitamin A makes you more likely to catch colds.

Is it true that eating carrots will help me see in the dark?

There is no truth in this old wives' tale. Visual purple in the light-sensitive retinal cells needs vitamin A, but you would have to be severely deficient for its function to be affected. Taking more will not improve vision.

Is a poor diet the only cause of vitamin A deficiency?

No, not in developed countries. The usual cause is the failure of the intestine to absorb enough vitamin A, which may be due to malabsorption syndromes or other damage to the intestine. Deficiency can occur as a side effect of long-term treatment with anticholesterol drugs. Diets with low levels of fat and retinol can also cause a deficiency.

What are the symptoms of vitamin A deficiency?

A deficiency results in night blindness. The eyes become dry and inflamed, with eventual corneal damage.

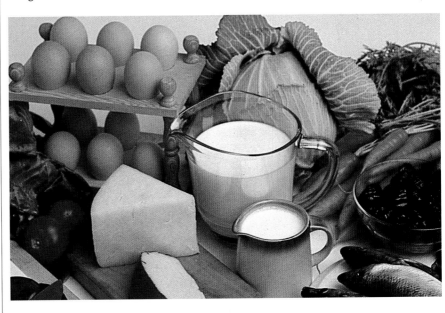

▲ *Dairy products, fish, liver, and certain vegetables contain high levels of Vitamin A.*

Vitamin A: Are you getting enough?

The daily requirement for different age groups and the vitamin A content in the foods listed are given in micrograms (1,000 micrograms = 1 milligram, or one-thousandth of a gram). If someone is unable to take the correct amount every day, it is necessary only for him or her to regulate the amount taken over a week and ensure that it gives the correct daily average.

Age group		Daily requirement
Babies	0–12 months	450
Children:	1–3 years	300
	4–8 years	400
	9–13 years	600
Adolescent and adult men (14+)		900
Adolescent and adult women (14+)		700
Expectant mothers:	14–18 years	750
	19+ years	770
Lactating mothers:	14–18 years	1,200
	19+ years	1,300

Vitamin A content of foods

Food	Vitamin A content
Apricots, dried, 2 oz. (57 g)	340
Butter, 1 oz. (28 g)	282
Cabbage, 4 oz. (114 g)	56
Carrots, 4 oz. (114 g)	2,267
Cheese, 2 oz. (57 g)	238
Cod-liver oil capsule, 1	180
Cream, heavy, 2 tbsp. (30 ml)	130
Egg, 1	80
Halibut-oil capsule, 1	1,200
Kidney, 4 o.z (114 g)	340
Fish, oily, 4 oz. (114 g)	52
Liver, cow, 4 oz. (114 g)	6,800
Margarine, 1 oz. (28 g)	255
Milk, whole, 7 fl. oz. (0.2 L)	80
Peas, frozen, 4 oz. (114 g)	56
Prunes, dried, 2 oz. (57 g)	90
Spinach, 4 oz. (114 g)	1,136
Tomato, 1½ oz. (42 g)	49
Watercress, 1 oz. (28 g)	142

effect, but frying at a high temperature will result in loss of vitamin content.

Vitamin A deficiency

A lack of vitamin A can cause itching, burning, and reddened eyelids, and a drastic deficiency can lead to blindness. Many children in developing countries are vulnerable as a result of early weaning onto an unsuitable food like skim milk, which contains little or no vitamin A. However, prepared baby foods usually have essential vitamins added to them. In more affluent societies the diet tends to be better balanced, and most people get as much vitamin A as they need; about two-thirds of it comes from retinol and one-third from carotene. Nevertheless, a deficiency of vitamin A can cause night blindness. Normally it takes about seven to 10 minutes for the eyes to become used to a dim light; so if someone cannot distinguish objects in the twilight, vitamin A deficiency may be the reason. Halibut-liver oil capsules can be taken, since this oil is one of the best sources of vitamin A. When people have a high- protein diet, they are at risk of deficiency because the body uses up the vitamin faster when converting protein into body tissue and energy. The body also uses up its store of vitamin A quickly during fevers. Certain drugs can cause a loss; a doctor will advise how much vitamin A is needed in any of these situations.

Because vitamin A is stored in the liver, daily intake is not essential, although regular supplies are needed. Too much vitamin A can be taken from an excess of halibut oil capsules. Symptoms include insomnia, weight loss, dryness of the lips, and aching limbs. Taking slightly more than is needed is unlikely to cause harm.

See also: Diet; Fevers; Nutrition; Vitamin B; Vitamin C; Vitamin D; Vitamin E; Vitamin K

Vitamin B

Vitamin B is essential for some of the body's biochemical processes. Unlike most other vitamins, it is not stored in the body and needs to be consumed daily. It is present in a wide variety of foods, however, and deficiency is unusual.

Vitamin B is a complex of at least eight separate water-soluble vitamins: B1 (thiamine), B2 (riboflavin), B3 (niacin), folic acid (folacin), B6 (pyridoxine), B12 (cyanocobalamin), biotin, and pantothenic acid. People can obtain the B vitamins in adequate supplies if they eat a well-balanced diet, since these vitamins are present in a wide variety of foods.

Nonetheless, B vitamins can be destroyed easily, and their absorption and use by the body are affected by drugs or excessive consumption of alcohol. If a deficiency occurs, disease can result.

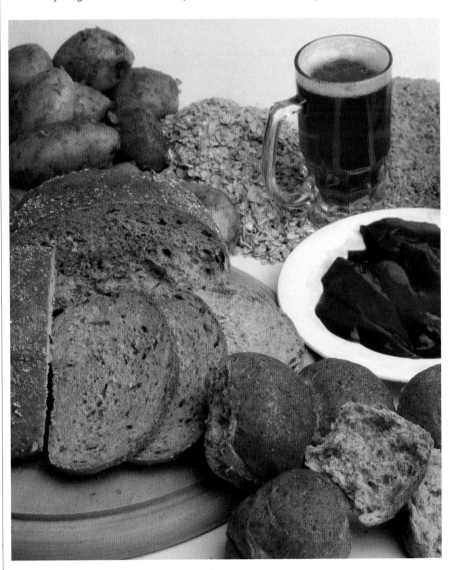

▲ *A good diet is the best guarantee of adequate vitamin B, which is present in a variety of foods such as whole-grain bread and cereals, liver, and root vegetables.*

Vitamin B How much vitamin B complex do you need in a day?			
AGE GROUP	**THIAMINE (MG)**	**RIBOFLAVIN (MG)**	**NIACIN (MG)**
Babies under 1 year	0.3 to 0.4	0.4 to 0.5	5 to 6
Children aged 1 to 6	0.7 to 0.9	0.8 to 1.1	9 to 12
Children aged 7 to 10	1.0	1.2	13
Male adolescents	1.3 to 1.5	1.5 to 1.8	17 to 20
Female adolescents	1.1	1.3	15
Men	1.2 to 1.5	1.4 to 1.7	15 to 19
Women	1.0 to 1.1	1.2 to 1.3	13 to 15
Pregnant women	1.5	1.6	17
Lactating women	1.6	1.7 to 1.8	20

Uses

The B vitamins are all coenzymes and have a number of uses in the body. They act with enzymes and in doing so allow many essential biochemical enzymes to work. These vitamins are involved in the process of providing the body with energy, basically by converting carbohydrates into glucose, and are vital in the digestion and use of fats and protein. The B vitamins are also necessary for the normal functioning of the nervous system, and for the maintenance of muscle tone in the gastrointestinal tract.

Pyridoxine (B6) assists in hormone production, and it must be present for the production of antibodies and red blood cells. Folic acid and B12 are also involved with red cell formation. Riboflavin maintains the skin, liver, and eyes. Other B vitamins also perform functions necessary to good health.

Sources

Almost all the vitamins in the group occur in brewer's yeast (the richest natural source), liver and other organs, and whole-grain cereals. Cow's milk, eggs, nuts, legumes, and green leafy vegetables are also rich in many of the B vitamins.

In addition, B vitamins, particularly biotin, are produced by bacteria in the human intestine. These bacteria grow best on milk, sugar, and small amounts of fat in the diet.

How vitamin B is lost

Since the human body does not store vitamin B, regular daily replenishment is vital. Also, because the B vitamins dissolve in water, much of their nutrient value can be lost in cooking. Premature harvesting and long and improper storage cause vitamin B loss, as well. Thiamine is most affected, and niacin the least.

Food processing also affects the B vitamins in foods. Milling wheat to produce white flour results in a lowering of the thiamine and niacin content. Milling and the extraction of bran and germ from rice mean that polished rice contains less thiamine. Generally, cereals that have been processed contain fewer vitamins.

Canned meats contain fewer vitamins than home-cooked meats. Light affects riboflavin in bottled milk.

Ideally, all vegetables and fruits should be ripened on the plant and eaten raw, with the skin still on, immediately after being harvested. Since such circumstances are impractical for most people, attempts should be made to buy fresh produce only in quantities that can be used promptly, and to cook it as little as possible (preferably by steaming rather than boiling in water). Often frozen vegetables and fruits contain more vitamin B than those that have been shipped and stored improperly.

Deficiency

Deficiency of vitamin B can occur both from low intake and from additional requirements, as in pregnancy or rapid growth. A lack of vitamin B can lead to various conditions, including beriberi, although this is found rarely in developed countries such as the United States.

Wet beriberi arises from a thiamine-free diet, and is characterized by edema (waterlogging and swelling of the body). Dry beriberi occurs through a thiamine deficiency, with a slower deterioration in health; edema may not appear in such cases. Both forms of beriberi affect nervous system function, but the brain is usually unimpaired.

Infantile beriberi is a disease that affects children breast-fed by thiamine-deficient mothers. Here, brain malfunction takes place together with convulsions, uneasiness, and loss of voice. In rare cases beriberi might arise following fever, pregnancy, or hard physical work.

In the United States, thiamine deficiency occurs almost exclusively in alcoholics, primarily owing to a poor dietary intake. However, it has also been demonstrated that severe alcoholism affects intestinal absorption of thiamine.

Pellagra is another vitamin B–related condition present in countries where poverty and famine exist. However, it also occurs in people whose diet consists mainly of fats and carbohydrates, or who suffer from alcoholism. Pellagra is a result of an inadequate supply of niacin, and symptoms include burning and itching, skin blotches, weakness, diarrhea, and depression.

Pernicious anemia is a disease that occurs in people who lack the ability to absorb and utilize vitamin B12. It may also occur in vegans, who choose not to consume any dairy products, eggs, meat, or fish. B12 can be taken in pill form or by injection; eating raw liver is also a cure for the condition.

Sores on the skin, often at the corner of the mouth, are caused usually by a deficiency of riboflavin. Riboflavin deficiency also causes lesions of the cornea. A deficiency of folacin is indicated by a very red tongue, diarrhea, and sometimes anemia, poor growth, and graying hair. Pyridoxine (vitamin B6) deficiency can cause anemia, irritability, kidney stones, and muscle twitching.

Lack of biotin can lead to tiredness, depression, nausea, skin problems, and aches and pains. A deficiency of pantothenic acid is rare because it is found in most foods.

Vitamin B in the diet

People need to eat a normal, balanced diet in order to satisfy their daily requirement of vitamin B. As can be seen from the chart below, a wide variety of foods contain vitamin B components. Vitamin amounts are given in micrograms (1,000 micrograms = 1 milligram). The quantities of pyridoxine, B12, folic acid, pantothenic acid, and biotin required for health are minuscule and are present in an everyday diet.

THIAMINE		RIBOFLAVIN		NIACIN	
1 large slice of whole wheat bread	150	4 oz. (114 g) cabbage	1000	small glass of milk	1800
4 oz. (114 g) cured, cooked ham	600	1 whole wheat bread roll	100	4 oz. (114 g) hard cheese	7000
4 oz. (114 g) wheat flakes cereal	600	4 oz. (114 g) liver	3500	4 oz. (114 g) beef	8000
½ cup (70 g) blackberries	200	1 egg	250	½ cup roasted peanuts	1200

Sources of vitamin B

	Milk	Tea/ coffee	Whole wheat bread	Cheese	Liver	Potatoes	Eggs	Peanuts	Whole-grain cereals	Chicken	Green vegetables	Kidney	Beef
Thiamine (B1)	x		x			x		x	x		x		x
Riboflavin (B2)	x			x	x	x	x		x	x	x	x	
Niacin (B3)	x	x		x		x	x	x	x		x		x
Folic acid			x		x			x	x		x	x	
Pyridoxine (B6)			x		x	x		x	x			x	x
B12	x				x							x	x
Biotin	x				x		x	x				x	
Pantothenic acid	x		x		x		x	x	x	x	x	x	x

When a supplement is necessary

The need for vitamin B increases if a person is suffering from an infection or stress, as well as during pregnancy and in the presence of certain pharmaceutical drugs. The contraceptive pill, for instance, creates a greater need for pyridoxine. Women on the Pill who experience headaches or depression may need to add a pyridoxine supplement to their diet.

Pregnant women can benefit from taking two B vitamins. If an expectant mother suffers from early signs of toxemia, such as swelling feet, ankles, and fingers, she can take an increased dose of pyridoxine; this supplement should be continued during breast-feeding. Vitamin B can also be used as an antisickness treatment in pregnancy.

Most important of all is the fact that the B vitamin folic acid has been found to be strongly protective against the development of neural tube defects such as spina bifida or absence of the brain in the developing fetus. The presence of the vitamin in adequate dosage is necessary at the time of conception to ensure this effect. Food supplementation with folic acid is required currently in the United States.

Folic acid is also involved in the making of red blood cells. The body has to produce more of these cells in pregnancy to help with the nourishment and development of the fetus. Without folic acid, a pregnant woman will risk such complications as toxemia, premature birth, and hemorrhaging. These possible risks are all the result of a condition called megaloblastic anemia, which causes symptoms such as tiredness and weakness. Breast-feeding mothers are also advised to increase their niacin intake.

Doctors recommend additional pyridoxine to alleviate the symptoms of premenstrual syndrome (PMS), such as headache, depression, and painful breasts.

Finally, the use of steroids, the hormone estrogen, and dieting all create a need for pyridoxine. This B vitamin can also be helpful for acne, and in helping to alleviate the side effects of menopause.

Toxicity

Overconsumption is rare with B vitamins, since they are not stored in the body. However, excessive amounts of niacin may cause flushing, headache, cramps, and nausea.

Too much folacin may mask the presence of pernicious anemia, and large supplements of vitamin B6 have been shown to cause sensory nerve damage.

Purported B vitamins

There are several other substances that are claimed by some to be B vitamins. B13 (orotic acid), for example, has been synthesized in Europe and is found in organically grown root vegetables, and B17 (laetrile) is the one B vitamin that does not occur naturally in brewer's yeast. Some of these substances are promoted as cures for various ailments. Scientific evidence is lacking, however, and a physician's advice should be sought before taking large doses of either these or other vitamins.

See also: **Alcoholism; Anemia; Diet; Vegetarianism**

Vitamin C

Vitamin C is considered to be one of the most vital vitamins. However, it is not enough just to eat the right foods—they must be properly prepared too, otherwise the vitamin content may be sharply reduced or lost altogether.

Vitamin C is probably the most controversial of all the vitamins. Great claims have been made for its healing and protective powers in connection with the common cold, aging, heart disease, and many other conditions. The official view remains skeptical, but no one denies that even in affluent societies people are more likely to be deficient in vitamin C than in any other nutrient.

Vitamin C is vital for maintenance of the body's connective tissue—the skin, fibers, membranes, and so on that literally hold it together. Collagen, a protein that is important for the formation of healthy skin, tendons, and bones, depends partly on vitamin C for its manufacture, and the vitamin is also needed for the release of hormones and the production of other chemical substances that play a part in human survival and resistance to infection.

Deficiency of vitamin C

The extreme form of vitamin C deficiency is a condition called scurvy, in which the connective tissue disintegrates so that blood vessels break down and there is bleeding into the skin and joints, and from the gums. Teeth are loosened, bruises appear, and resistance to infection is lowered.

Scurvy was one of the earliest deficiency diseases to be discovered. In 1497, the Portuguese navigator Vasco da Gama lost more than half his men through its effects, owing to the inevitable shortage of fresh fruit and vegetables on long voyages. In 1753, the British naval surgeon James Lind showed that scurvy could be prevented and cured by giving victims orange and lemon juice, although he was unaware of the reason for this.

Vitamin C was not actually identified as the curative agent until 1932. The name "ascorbic acid" (used to describe vitamin C when it is manufactured) comes from the term "antiscorbutic," meaning the ability to prevent and cure scurvy. This deficiency can be cured very quickly with high doses of vitamin C, but if the condition is neglected there could be permanent damage.

Vitamin C sources

Rose hips are the richest natural source of vitamin C available. Paprika is good, too, but neither of these sources of vitamin C is on everyone's daily menu, so other sources have to be relied on.

Vegetables such as potatoes, which do feature in most people's diets in the Western world, contain some vitamin C, as do brussels sprouts, cauliflower, and cabbage. Among fruits, black currants are best,

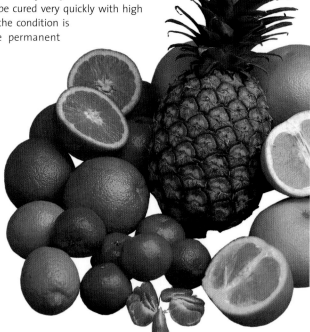

▲ *Fruit is rich in vitamin C, especially citrus fruits like oranges, lemons, and limes.*

People at risk from vitamin C deficiency

Older people	perhaps living alone, existing on canned and packaged foods
Young people	perhaps in college dormitories, living on junk foods
Food faddists	advocates of macro-cereal-based diets who do not understand the body's nutritional needs
Bottle-fed babies	given cow's milk formulas without vitamin supplements or orange juice

Vitamin C in the diet

FOOD	APPROXIMATE VITAMIN C CONTENT (MICROGRAMS)
4 oz. (114 g) fresh blackberries	220
4 oz. (114 g) fresh strawberries	70
4 oz. (114 g) lemon juice	60
1 fresh orange	60
4 oz. (114 g) canned orange juice	40
Half grapefruit	20
4 oz. (114 g) canned pineapple	12
4 oz. (114 g) boiled brussels sprouts	40
4 oz. (114 g) boiled cabbage	24
4 oz. (114 g) frozen peas	12
4 oz. (114 g) raw green peppers	112
4 oz. (114 g) boiled potatoes (according to season; new potatoes contain most)	4–20
1 fresh tomato	10

Daily vitamin C requirements

The requirements for different age groups is given in micrograms (1,000 micrograms = 1 milligram, or one-thousandth of a gram).

Babies under 12 months	30–35
Children 1–10 years	40–45
Adolescents 11–18 years	65–75
Adults	75–90
Expectant and lactating mothers/smokers	115

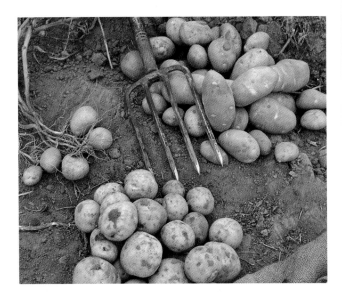

▲ *Potatoes are easy to prepare and packed with vitamin C.*

followed by strawberries. Further down on the list, but available all year round, are citrus fruits (oranges, lemons, limes, and grapefruit). Rose hip syrup is obviously brimming with vitamin C, and is available from most health food stores.

There is not much vitamin C in apples or pears, virtually none in milk (though it is sometimes added), and none in cereal grains, dried peas and beans, nuts, or dried fruit (the drying process rids fruit of any vitamin value). All green and root vegetables and fruit contain a certain amount, but this varies from season to season. For example, new potatoes contain three times as much vitamin C as old ones.

When extra vitamin C is needed

Some distinguished experts maintain that people need far more than the normally recommended daily allowances of vitamin C. It is generally acknowledged that the body requires additional vitamin C after a severe illness or injury, and there have been experiments showing that burns heal faster when a vitamin C solution has been applied to the skin in conjunction with injections or doses taken by mouth.

High doses of vitamin C have also been used successfully in experiments carried out to reduce levels of cholesterol in the arteries, and it is thought that the vitamin might offer protection against gastric bleeding in those who have to take large regular amounts of aspirin for such conditions as arthritis.

It is now known that many disease processes are ultimately mediated by what is ordinarily called oxidative stress. Highly active chemical groups called free radicals, generated by environmental processes such as toxic pollutants, radiation, and smoking, operate damagingly in many forms of pathology and can form dangerous chain reactions in tissues. Vitamin C, like vitamin E, is a strong antioxidant and has the power to "mop up" free radicals. Medical research has shown that high levels of vitamin C help reduce some of the major killing diseases, especially heart attacks and strokes.

Too much vitamin C

The body excretes any surplus of vitamin C and any massive dose that is not utilized by the body is flushed away in urine, so there is no possibility of an overdose. However, people seem to be able to function normally and healthily on small amounts.

See also: Antioxidants; Burns; Common cold; Diet; Environmental hazards; Nutrition; Protein; Smoking; Vitamin A; Vitamin B; Vitamin D; Vitamin E; Vitamin K

Vitamin D

The sunshine vitamin, vitamin D, helps the body to absorb calcium and so is essential for the normal growth and development of a child's bones, and for the maintenance of healthy bones in an adult.

No. You will get some vitamin D, but not as much as you need. Diet is much more important, and you must make sure that yours contains sufficient vitamin D. However, some people with seasonal affective disorder (SAD) claim that using a sunlamp is an effective treatment, and it is possible that SAD is related to a deficiency in vitamin D.

I sunbathe in the yard when the weather permits. Do I need to worry about getting enough vitamin D in my diet as well?

If you lived, say, in Hong Kong, you could afford not to worry about vitamin D in your diet. There, the average diet is low in vitamin D, but signs of deficiency are rare because of the higher-than-average annual amounts of sunshine. However, people who live in temperate climates get less sunshine, so diet is important. If you try to eat a helping of canned fish or oily fish such as herring once a week at least, you should get enough vitamin D.

My son is going on a trip to southern Europe in August. For how long will he benefit from the vitamin D he converts there?

The body can store vitamin D for several months. In the northern hemisphere, the highest rates are found in the blood in September. A survey of children who had spent some weeks at the coast in summer showed that they had much higher reserves of vitamin D as compared with children who had not; these reserves were still present the following February. While sunshine is good for you, you also need to be aware of the damage that can ensue from staying out too long in the hot sun without taking precautions.

Vitamin D is sometimes called the sunshine vitamin because humans derive part of their essential supplies from exposure to the sun. People also obtain it from food, but there is some danger of deficiency, since it does not occur in many foods. Humans need vitamin D so that they can get enough calcium to make healthy bones. Vitamin D helps the absorption of calcium and phosphorus from the intestinal wall and maintains correct levels in the bloodstream.

There are two main types of vitamin D. When people derive it from sunshine, ultraviolet rays hit the skin and convert cholesterol in the skin into cholecalciferol, or vitamin D3. The other main kind of vitamin D is called ergocalciferol, or D2, and is manufactured from plant materials such as yeasts.

Comparatively few foods contain vitamin D. Besides cod-liver oil, it is available most richly in herrings, kippers, canned salmon, and sardines. If a person thinks he or she is not taking a sufficient amount, supplies of vitamin D can be increased with a daily spoonful of cod-liver oil or a helping of canned fish once or twice a week. Margarine is required to have vitamin D added to it during production, and evaporated milk usually has extra, too. Butter and fresh milk have much

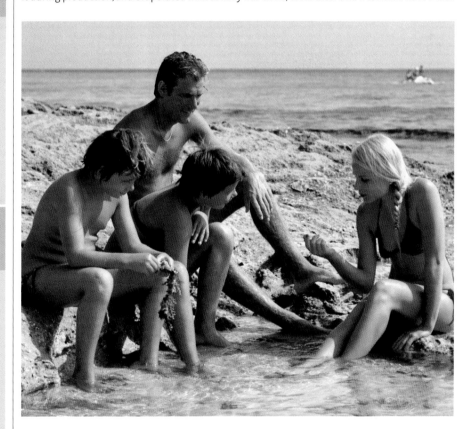

▲ *People need to be aware that the ultraviolet rays in sunlight can be both beneficial and harmful to health. Vitamin D is crucial to the body's production of vitamin D; at the same time, ultraviolet rays can cause serious long-term damage to the skin, including cancer. Exposure to the sun should always be regulated sensibly.*

Vitamin D: How much do you need?

It is not necessary to maintain the intake on a daily basis, but over a period of a week the intake should average out. The figures here are in micrograms (1,000 micrograms = 1 milligram or one-thousandth of a gram).

AGE RANGE	DAILY INTAKE
Children	10
Adults 19–50 years	5
Adults 51–69 years	10
Adults 70+ years	15
Pregnant and lactating women	10

Vitamin D content in foods

FOOD	VITAMIN D CONTENT
Glass of milk	0.16
Canned sardines in oil 4 oz. (114 g)	14.16
Hard cheese 2 oz. (50 g)	0.14
Cod-liver oil 1 tbsp. (15 ml)	60.00
1 egg	1.00
Fortified evaporated milk 4 fl. oz. (125 ml)	0.44
Fried liver 4 oz. (114 g)	0.44
Herring 4 oz. (114 g)	25.60
Kipper 4 oz. (114 g)	25.52
Margarine 2 oz. (50 g)	4.50

smaller amounts, but because of their use daily by most people, they are a good source. Eggs contain some vitamin D, as well.

Vitamin D deficiency

The main result of vitamin D deficiency is rickets in children. Rickets is a condition of defective bone growth. It causes bowlegs and knock-knees; the ribs also take on a distorted appearance and the chest and pelvis become narrowed.

Early symptoms of rickets include restlessness, sweating, lack of muscle tone, and softening of the bones of the skull.

The baby's teeth may be slow in appearing or may be soft and susceptible to decay. The bones are fragile and easily broken, and there may be muscle spasms and twitching. Extra vitamin D can reverse the effects if it is given early enough, but damage can be permanent. Rickets has now been virtually wiped out in the Western world.

An adult form of vitamin D deficiency is osteomalacia, which causes bone softening and breakage, muscular weakness, tenderness, and pain. The condition can affect older people if they live on a diet that is low in calcium and vitamin D. Osteomalacia is often associated with osteoporosis, which also increases risk of breakage.

Excessive vitamin D

Since vitamin D is stored in fat, any extra cannot be expelled easily from the body. Instead, it is stored in the liver and can lead to certain poisonous effects if the intake is too high. Early signs of excess vitamin D include appetite loss, nausea, and vomiting. Because vitamin D helps the absorption of calcium, too much vitamin D may cause unhealthily high concentrations of calcium in the blood, leading to brittle bones, hardening of the arteries, and growth failure in children.

In the West vitamin D, mainly in the form of D2, may be recommended for pregnant and breast-feeding women, and children under age five. Anyone taking a vitamin D supplement should follow the instructions and take no further D2 on top of the suggested dose.

See also: Calcium; Cholesterol; Diet; Nutrition; Osteoporosis; Vitamin A; Vitamin B; Vitamin C; Vitamin E; Vitamin K

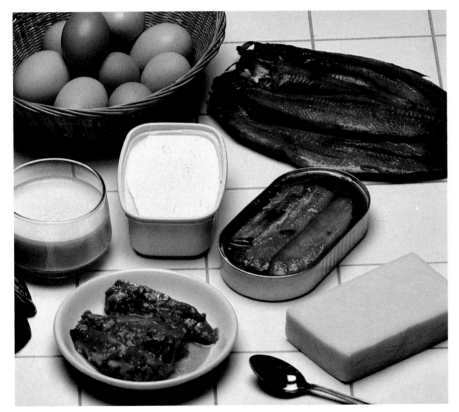

▲ *People living in temperate climates must get a proportion of the vitamin D they need in their diet. It can be found in foods such as oily fish, milk, eggs, and hard cheese.*

Vitamin E

Questions and Answers

Should I give my family muesli for breakfast? I have heard that it contains a lot of vitamin E.

It depends on the muesli. Look at the label on the packet to see if the contents include whole or rolled oats, nuts, and sesame seeds; all these contain vitamin E.

Does vitamin E improve sexual performance?

Vitamin E does have this reputation, but there has yet to be definite proof. Possibly the greatest benefit is psychological.

Could my iron pills interfere with my ability to absorb vitamin E?

Medications containing iron work against the absorption of vitamin E. Therefore, iron should be taken at a different time of day—in the morning if vitamin E is taken in any extra form in the evening. Mineral oils such as castor oil, taken as a laxative, impair absorption of vitamin E and other nutrients. Estrogen in the contraceptive pill and in hormone replacement therapy may impair absorption. Some people taking iron or estrogen have a daily teaspoon of wheat-germ oil, though this is probably not necessary.

Should I use vegetable oils in my cooking as a source of vitamin E?

In theory, yes, since these oils contain vitamin E, but a high intake of polyunsaturated vegetable oils creates an increased need for the vitamin. This is because the presence of other fats restricts the absorption of vitamin E. Polyunsaturated fats may be recommended for patients with high cholesterol levels, since the fats help reduce these levels, but more vitamin E is needed to maintain a balance.

Research into the benefits of vitamin E is still in progress, but some people claim that it has remarkable curative and rejuvenating powers. It is the antioxidant powers of vitamin E that are of particular interest.

Until the last few decades, vitamin E was not of any particular interest, largely because doctors have tended to be been mainly focused on the effects of vitamin deficiency; and vitamin E deficiency is very rare. However, a new and exciting role for this neglected vitamin has appeared.

It was believed that the fat-soluble vitamin E was unimportant. Some people have even gone so far as to say that vitamin E is of no medical relevance in humans. These views have now undergone a radical change.

History

In 1922, it was discovered that female rats required an unknown substance in their diets to sustain normal pregnancies. Without this substance, they could ovulate and conceive normally, but within about 10 days the fetus died and was absorbed. Male rats deficient in this substance were also found to have abnormalities in their testes.

The unknown substance turned out to be a new vitamin, and was given the designation "vitamin E." Fourteen years later it was chemically isolated from wheat-germ oil, and was found

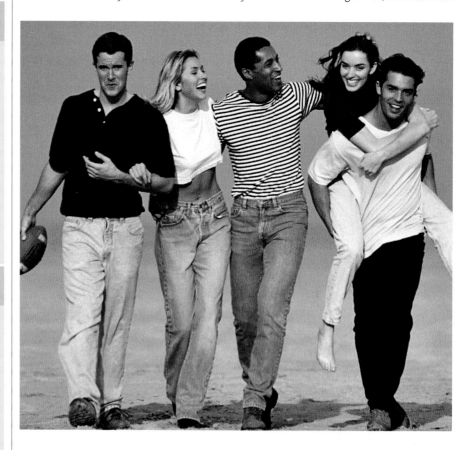

▲ *Vitamin E can help keep skin young and healthy-looking. Eating a sensible balanced diet should provide enough vitamin E, but supplements, in the form of either capsules or lotions, can also be taken.*

to be one of a range of eight very complicated but similar molecules known as tocopherols.

The news of the availability of the new vitamin was greeted with interest, and, for a time, vitamin E enjoyed a reputation as a vitamin that could be used to treat sterility. Doctors prescribed vitamin E freely as a treatment for infertility, although this was illogical: there was no reason to suppose that the people concerned were deficient in the vitamin.

Erroneous use

In the same way that other vitamins were used to treat deficiencies, vitamin E was used, but in the belief that it could benefit, in people who were not deficient in it, those conditions caused by its deficiency. By association, vitamin E was also used, quite mistakenly, to attempt to treat various menstrual disorders, inflammation of the vagina, and menopausal symptoms. Once it was found to be ineffective for these conditions, interest died down, and for many years the vitamin was largely forgotten.

Vitamin E deficiency

Human vitamin E deficiency is very rare because the vitamin occurs widely in many foods, and especially in vegetable oils, such as sunflower oil. Deficiency occurs only after many months on a severely restricted diet or in people who are artificially fed. A daily intake of 10 to 30 mg of the vitamin is sufficient to keep blood levels within normal limits, and this will be provided by any reasonable diet. Human milk contains enough to meet a baby's needs. In the unlikely event that deficiency does occur, however, the effects can be devastating.

Severe deficiency can cause myriad health problems: degenerative changes in the brain and nervous system, impairment of vision, double vision, problems with walking, anemia, an increased rate of destruction of red blood cells, fluid retention, and skin disorders.

Although deficiency effects are extremely uncommon, in the last few years the reason for such devastating effects has become known.

▼ *Eggs, nuts, sunflower oil, and whole grains are good natural sources of vitamin E. If supplements are taken, they should not exceed 150 international units (IU).*

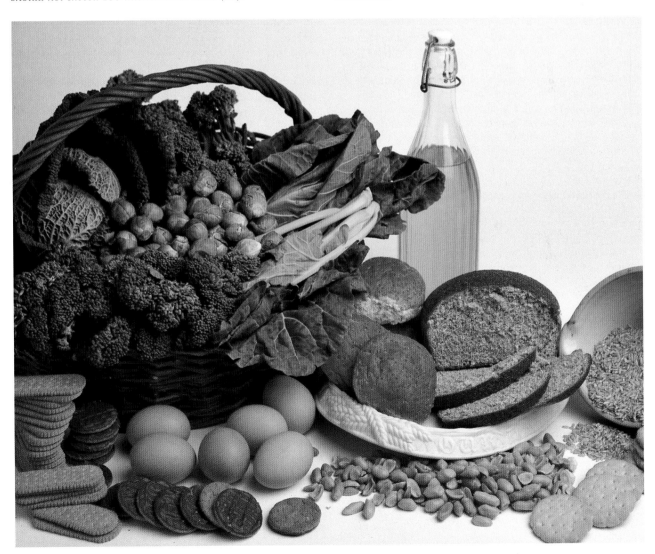

Free radicals

Chemists have known about free radicals for about 100 years, and gradually it has become apparent that they are implicated in disease. Free radicals are highly active, short-lived chemical groups that contain an atom with an unpaired outer orbital electron. The stable state is a pair of electrons, and if only one is present the atom will quickly capture an electron from a nearby atom, causing molecular damage or oxidation. When this happens the deprived atom forms a free radical. In this way a chain reaction can be set up that can quickly damage tissues. For many years, chemists have known that free radical oxidation action can be controlled, or even prevented, by a range of antioxidant substances. Antioxidants are used to prevent lubricating oils from drying up, and to protect plastics from free radical damage.

Foodstuffs have long been protected from free radical damage by antioxidants. When fat goes rancid it does so by a free radical oxidation reaction. This can be prevented by additives with antioxidant properties such as BHA (butylated hydroxyanisole), BHT (butylated hydroxytoluene), and tocopherol (vitamin E).

Natural body antioxidants

Medical interest in the possibility that free radicals were involved in disease processes was aroused when it was discovered that the body has its own natural antioxidants. One of the most effective of these is vitamin E. This vitamin is especially important because it is fat-soluble and much of the most significant free radical damage in the body is damage to the membranes of cells and to low-density lipoproteins. Vitamin C is also a powerful antioxidant, but it is soluble in water, not in fat. Therefore, it is distributed to all parts of the body. Vitamins C and E are highly efficient at mopping up free radicals, and work together to do this.

The tocopherols

Among the richest natural sources of the tocopherols are seed germ oils, alfalfa, and lettuce. They are widely distributed in plant materials. Tocopherols are almost insoluble in water but dissolve in oils, fats, alcohol, acetone, ether, and other fat solvents. Unlike vitamin C they are stable to heat and alkalis in the absence of oxygen, and are unaffected by acids at temperatures up to 212°F (100°C). Because vitamin E consists of so many slightly different tocopherols, worldwide standardization is difficult and a little arbitrary. The

Vitamin E—How much do you need?

United States recommended daily allowances are as follows.

AGE RANGE	mg
Babies up to 6 months	3–4
Children 6 months to 8 years	6–7
Children 9–13 years	11
Adolescents 14+ and adults	15
Lactating women	19

international unit of vitamin E is taken to be equal to 1 mg of alpha-tocopherol acetate. For practical purposes of dosage, however, 1.5 international units (IU) is considered to be equivalent to 1 mg.

Antioxidant properties

All the tocopherols have antioxidant properties and this appears to be the basis for all the biological effects of the vitamin. The effects of vitamin E deficiency are, it seems, the effects of inadequate antioxidant protection. Vitamin E is involved in many body processes, and, in conjunction with vitamin C, operates as a natural antioxidant, helping to protect important cell structures, especially cell membranes, from the damaging effects of free radicals. In animals, vitamin E supplements can protect against the effects of various drugs, chemicals, and metals that can promote free radical formation. In carrying out its function as an antioxidant in the body, vitamin E is, itself, converted to a radical. It is, however, soon regenerated to the active vitamin by a biochemical process that probably involves both vitamin C and another natural body antioxidant, glutathione.

Dangers of overdosage

Publicity about the antioxidant value of vitamins E and C has led many people to take these vitamins on a regular daily basis, sometimes as part of an organized therapy. Like vitamin C, vitamin E is generally regarded as a fairly innocuous substance and few if any warnings are heard of the dangers of overdosage. For adults, this is probably reasonable, but there are limits to the amounts that can be safely taken and recommended dosages should not be exceeded.

Vitamin E and babies

There is, however, a special caveat in the case of babies. Although free radicals are generally destructive, the body also uses them for beneficial purposes. They are, for instance, the mechanism by which phagocyte cells destroy bacteria. This action is unlikely to be interfered with in adults, but it is known that dangers have arisen from overdosage of vitamin E in premature babies. Large doses of vitamin E have been shown to interfere sufficiently with the action of the cells of the immune system to cause a dangerous form of intestinal infection. For this reason, doses of supplementary vitamin E should never be given to babies except under strict medical supervision.

Good sources of vitamin E

Figures are given as the number of micrograms in 100 grams (3.527 ounces)

Bran	2,000
Almonds, shelled	2,000
Butter	2,000
Cornflakes	400
Potato chips	6,100
Eggs	1,600
Hazelnuts, shelled	2,100
Peanuts, fresh or roasted	8,100
Muesli	3,200
Sunflower oil	1,800
Whole wheat bread	200

See also: Anemia; Antioxidants; Bacteria; Diet; Nutrition; Vitamin A; Vitamin B; Vitamin C; Vitamin D; Vitamin K

Vitamin K

By helping the blood to clot, vitamin K performs a vital function in the body. A balanced diet provides some of the vitamin K required by the body, and deficiencies are rare and usually easily treated.

Vitamin K consists of vitamin K1, a yellow oil found in a variety of vegetables; and vitamin K2, a yellow waxy substance produced by bacteria. Although vitamin K1 is abundant in leafy vegetables such as spinach and green cabbage, a normal diet will provide only a proportion of the daily requirement. The remainder of vitamin K2 is obtained from bacteria that live in the intestines, and this ensures that there is always a steady supply. In healthy people a deficiency resulting from an inadequate diet is rare.

Vitamin K deficiency

Vitamin K is used by the liver to produce three of the blood components known as the clotting factors. A deficiency results in a decreased production of these three factors. The most important clotting factor is prothrombin. When an injury occurs, the ability of the blood to coagulate will be impaired. Small cuts will bleed vigorously, and large bruises will form under the skin in response to even minor injuries. In severe cases of vitamin K deficiency, serious and even fatal hemorrhaging may occur. Because vitamins K1 and K2 are fat-soluble (they are dissolved and stored in fat), a

Questions and Answers

My young nephew is a hemophiliac. Would giving him vitamin K prevent him from bleeding if he is injured?

No. The abnormal bleeding tendency in hemophilia is due to an inherited deficiency of one of the clotting factors, factor 8. Factor 8 is not one of the three clotting factors that depend on vitamin K for their production. Your nephew must rely on conventional treatment.

Is it true that antibiotics kill the bacteria in the gut that produce vitamin K?

Only powerful antibiotics taken over long periods will kill the intestinal bacteria. A vitamin K deficiency would take about two weeks to appear. However, antibiotics in everyday use have little or no effect on the bacteria that produce vitamin K.

I am two months pregnant. Will I need extra vitamin K?

No. You do not need to take vitamin K in increased amounts during pregnancy.

I had gallstones, and had to have my gallbladder removed. Do I need to take extra vitamin K?

Bile, which is stored in the gallbladder, is necessary for the absorption of vitamin K from the intestines. Extra vitamin K would be needed only if the bile ducts were blocked and the bile failed to reach the intestines from the liver. Patients such as you hardly ever need extra vitamin K.

How can I be sure that I am getting enough vitamin K?

Your intestinal bacteria will supply an adequate amount.

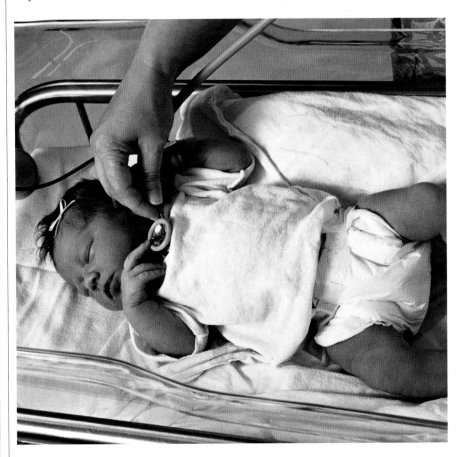

▲ *Babies may be given vitamin K at birth because they have no intestinal bacteria to produce it and the supply from the mother's bloodstream is quickly depleted.*

Vitamin K—How much do you need?

The figures below are only rough estimates. Daily requirement cannot be calculated accurately, because so much of Vitamin K intake is supplied by intestinal bacteria. The figures given below are in micrograms (1,000 micrograms = 1 milligram, or one-thousandth of a gram).

AGE GROUP	DAILY REQUIREMENT
Babies up to 1 year	5–10
Children under ten years	15–30
Adolescent men (11–18 years)	45–65
Adolescent women (11–18 years)	45–55
Adult men (19+)	70–80
Adult women (19+)	60–65

Vitamin K content of food

Figures given are micrograms per 100 gm (3.53 oz) of food.

Lean meat	100–200
Cows' liver	100–200
Pigs' liver	400–800
Eggs (each)	20
Cows' milk	2
Human breast milk	20
Potatoes	80
Spinach	4,200
Green cabbage	3,200
Carrots	100
Peas	100–300
Tomatoes	400

deficiency may occur in diseases that cause decreased digestion and absorption of fats and oils. These include an obstruction of the bile duct and celiac disease. This deficiency can easily be treated with vitamin K injections or with pills containing synthetic vitamin K. Some liver diseases, such as cirrhosis of the liver and hepatitis, interfere with the utilization of vitamin K, and vitamin supplements in large doses may then be required. A deficiency is sometimes difficult to treat and can be dangerous in patients with liver failure, who may develop uncontrollable internal bleeding.

Finally, vitamin K deficiency is often found in the newborn, and may cause serious damage both from blood loss and from bleeding into the brain and other vital organs. Intestinal bacteria are not present at birth; milk contains very little vitamin K; and the supply from the mother's bloodstream does not last long. To make up this deficiency, some newborn babies are given a small shot of vitamin K.

Excess vitamin K

Vitamin K is nontoxic (that is, not poisonous) if taken in excessive amounts because the liver controls the rate of production of the clotting factors. Some patients have an increased tendency to thrombosis, (formation of blood clots). These blood clots obstruct the healthy blood vessels in which they are first formed, and may also be carried around the body in the bloodstream to obstruct blood vessels elsewhere. The limbs, lungs, brain, and heart may suffer serious damage. Thrombosis is not caused by excess vitamin K, but in such patients, further blood clot formation can be prevented by taking drugs such as warfarin that stop the liver from using vitamin K to produce clotting factors.

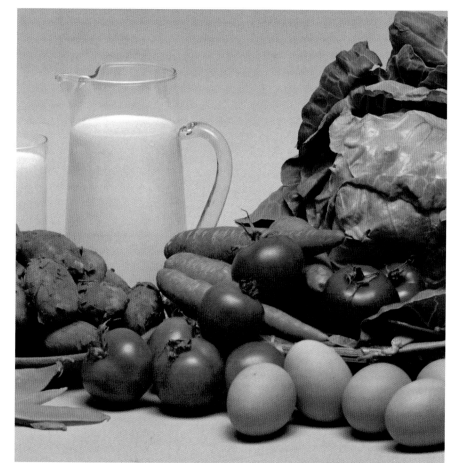

▼ *These foods supply some of the daily requirement of vitamin K, which is required to help blood to clot. The body also manufactures the vitamin to ensure a good supply.*

See also: **Diet; Fats; Hepatitis; Nutrition; Vitamin A; Vitamin B; Vitamin C; Vitamin D; Vitamin E**

Warts

Warts are unsightly but harmless growths that can make youth a time of embarrassment. They will disappear through medical treatment or, sometimes, on their own.

Questions and Answers

Why are warts more common among young people?

Warts are caused by a virus, to which it is possible to develop immunity so that reinfection is less likely. The strength of acquired immunity is not as great for warts as for other common childhood viral infections, such as measles or chicken pox, but because of immunity many people who had warts during childhood have a built-in defense against the infection as adults.

What is the difference between warts and verrucas?

The word "verruca" is the correct medical term for a wart, regardless of its appearance, location, or shape. "Verruca" is an abbreviation of the medical term "verruca plantaris" which means "wart on the sole." These warts are different from warts elsewhere on the body because they are pressed into the foot and usually surrounded or partly covered by a thick layer of skin.

Can warts be dangerous and do they lead to further complications?

Most warts are harmless, but warts in the genital area can obstruct the vagina, anus, or penile orifice, and wartlike growths in the throat may cause obstruction to breathing. Very rarely a wart may develop from a benign growth into a malignant or cancerous one which requires urgent surgical removal.

Is it true that childhood warts should not be treated?

Warts on the hands or knees are best left alone, since they may disappear within three years, and often within months, whereas treatment increases the risk that they will spread.

Warts are a very common, usually harmless, skin affliction that affect mainly children, and to a lesser extent adults and teenagers. They consist of small rounded growths that appear on the skin and can occur virtually anywhere on the skin surface, although they are most common on the hands, knees, face, and genitals. Rarely any cause for concern, warts are usually painless and can disappear within a few months or years. However, facial and genital warts may cause some embarrassment or discomfort. They should be treated, since they can persist for years.

A type of wart that appears on the sole of the foot, commonly but wrongly known as a verruca, is often painful and also requires treatment.

Causes and transmission

Warts are caused by a virus called papillomavirus, which can infiltrate and multiply within the outermost layer of the skin cells. When the virus infects the skin, it causes the skin cells to

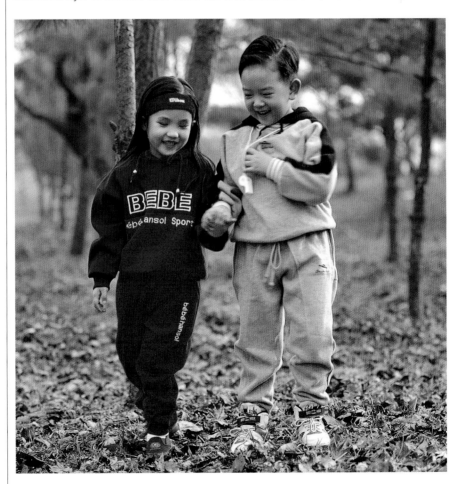

▲ *The virus that causes warts is contagious and can be passed on by holding hands with someone affected. This explains why children transmit it to each other.*

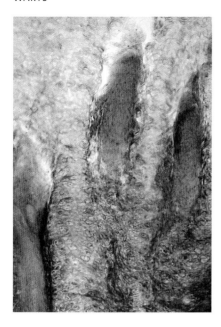

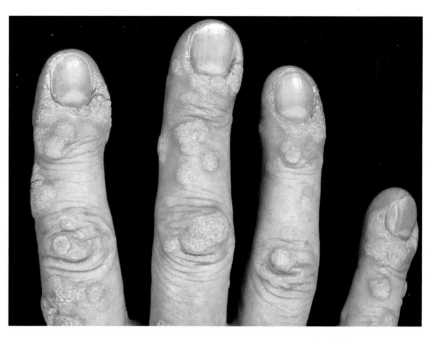

▲ *This photomicrograph of a slice of wart tissue shows the mass of active mutant cells (in purple) that are responsible for the growth of the wart.*

▲ *Clusters of warts on the hands can be unsightly and inhibiting. Either freezing or electrical burning techniques will remove them, in most cases, permanently. Sometimes they disappear spontaneously.*

proliferate in a disordered fashion, producing, in effect, a small, benign tumor. This is of interest to doctors, since warts are one of the few growths found in humans that are definitely known to be caused by a virus.

The wart virus is contagious and can thus be transmitted from one person to another or from one part of the body to another,

▼ *Troublesome adult warts on the face can be irritating and are best removed, especially if they obstruct vision.*

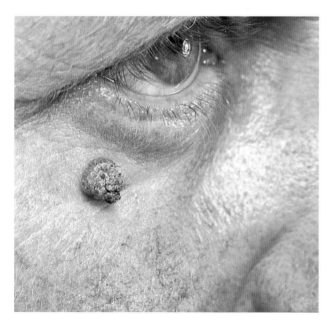

either by direct skin contact or indirectly by an intermediate object such as a towel. A break in the skin, such as a scratch, may facilitate entry of the virus.

Warts on the hand are most probably transmitted by hand-holding; genital warts are transmitted by sexual intercourse. The period between infection and the appearance of the warts may be weeks or months.

Warts on children are rarely transmitted to adults, probably because adults have acquired some immunity to the virus through infection during their own childhood. The viruses that cause common warts on the hand and genital warts are slightly different, so a person who was afflicted with hand warts during childhood is not immune to genital warts during adulthood.

Appearance

The appearance of warts varies a little according to where they occur on the body. Warts on the palms of the hands are usually solitary growths consisting of a hard, dome-shaped, raised area of skin with hundreds of tiny conical projections, which give the surface of the wart a velvetlike appearance.

The color of warts also varies from pink to brown. Warts on the hands, knees, or face are often numerous and sometimes have a flat, plateaulike surface. Another variety, called filiform warts, consists of fine, elongated outgrowths that appear on the face or neck.

Genital warts may occur in and around the folds of skin of the vulva in women or around the tip of the penis in men, or anywhere in the surrounding genital area. They often grow and spread profusely, creating clusters of cauliflower-like growths that, despite their rather unsightly appearance, cause little discomfort. Sometimes, however, they may obstruct normal sexual or excretory functions. The presence of genital warts should always be reported

"Magic" cures

The treatment of warts has a rich history of myth and magic, most of which probably originated in medieval days, when sufferers would have consulted the local healer for treatment. Herbs, chants, and incantations were the standard weapons against most ailments, and these treatments were effective in dealing with warts. Indeed, some of these methods are still used in rural districts. For no good medical reason, they sometimes appeared to have the desired result but it is probably more realistic to assume that the warts were about to disappear anyway.

However, some old wives' remedies may have some beneficial psychological effect, because if one is positively convinced that the remedy will work, then it is possible that this may promote the wart's disappearance.

Here are some improbable cures:

- Tape a cat's hair to each wart.

- Rub the leaves of a wartwort plant over the growth.

- Bury a piece of meat in the yard.

- Leave a bag of pebbles with a silver coin inside by the wayside; if the finder keeps the silver coin, he or she will get a wart, while the sufferer is cured.

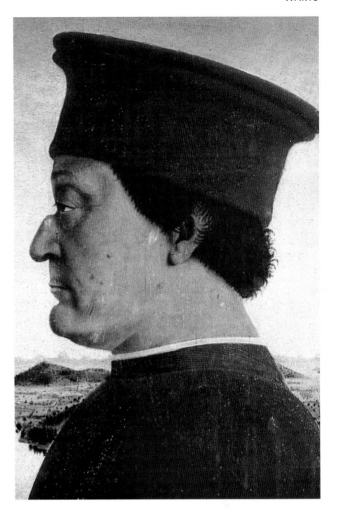

▲ *The famous Renaissance portrait of the duke of Urbino by Piero della Francesca is remarkable for its realism, showing hooked nose, warts and all.*

to a doctor, since they often accompany more serious sexually transmitted infections.

All warts have tiny blood capillaries, and if the surface of the wart is cut away, these appear as tiny bleeding points, or as black seeds, on the surface of the wart where the blood in the capillaries has coagulated. The presence or absence of these bleeding points or black filaments helps doctors to distinguish warts from other skin growths of similar appearance.

Treatment

Over the centuries a wide variety of folk remedies have been used in the treatment of warts, ranging from chants and incantations to rubbing the warts with plants or vegetables. A number of people have also claimed that they have special gifts or talents for charming warts away. Some people claim that hypnosis works and the warts just disappear afterward. Although these unconventional cures may sometimes appear to work, a visit to the doctor will probably have a more rewarding result.

There are a number of more conventional treatments for warts, but there are no specific drugs for combating the wart virus. However, the growths can be attacked with corrosive ointments, or by freezing, scraping, or electrically burning them off. All of these procedures are carried out by a doctor.

Common childhood warts on the hands and knees can be left to disappear in their own time, or they can be treated painlessly with an antiseptic acid paint. Applied twice a day, this usually causes the wart to disappear in two or three months.

Troublesome adult warts on the face or hands are sometimes treated by freezing with liquid nitrogen or solid carbon dioxide, which can be mildly painful but is very effective and causes little scarring. Electrically burning a wart off is more likely to cause a scar and is often followed by a recurrence of the infection, so this technique is less often used.

Genital warts are treated either by surgery or topically by applying a corrosive substance, such as podophyllin. This must be applied by a doctor or nurse, since careless application of the ointment causes soreness. It is important to wash the ointment off some four to six hours after it has been applied. Podophyllin is never used to treat genital warts during pregnancy, since it may be absorbed into the body and can have harmful effects on the fetus.

However, even though a wart has disappeared or been permanently removed, the wart virus sometimes lies dormant in the skin and may resume its activity some weeks or even months later.

See also: **Sexually transmitted diseases; Viruses**

Weight

Questions and Answers

I try to lose weight, with no success. Can my doctor give me drugs to stop me from overeating?

Weight loss involves balancing energy intake with energy use. In extreme cases, a doctor may give you appetite suppressing drugs, but many have side effects, including addiction. Increased exercise and cutting down high-calorie foods will help weight loss.

I have been very overweight for years. What should I do?

Surgery is possible in severe cases of obesity, but it is not always successful. The stomach can be stitched to reduce its size, however, nutritional advice should also be provided to prevent a relapse after surgery.

My daughter exercises too much and eats very little. How can I encourage her to increase her body weight?

She may have anorexia nervosa. It is an eating disorder that involves obsessive dieting, often accompanied by excessive exercise. Sufferers are usually obsessive in other ways as well, constantly cleaning and cooking for other members of the family, for example. They are often high achievers at school. The condition can have very harmful effects on the body and in some cases is fatal. It is essential to seek medical advice early if you suspect your daughter has anorexia nervosa. Your doctor will monitor her weight, and may advise counseling or other therapy. If you have difficulty in persuading your daughter to go to the doctor, try to find another pretext, such as brittle hair or a lack of periods (also symptoms of anorexia nervosa). Simply telling her to stop dieting and start exercising will not work. She needs professional help.

A person's weight in relation to his or her height is an indicator of fitness. For some people, weight watching is an obsession, whereas for others, food is an obsession; and the result is overweight and obesity.

Determining if a person is overweight is not as easy as looking at a scale. A scale measures how much a person weighs but does not indicate whether it is a healthy weight. In the 1980s, researchers developed a new gauge, the body mass index (BMI), to evaluate a person's weight in comparison with his or her height. BMI can be determined by using a formula, a chart, or an online calculator. For adults, a BMI of less than 18.5 is classified as "underweight," 18.5 to 24.9 is "normal," 25 to 29.9 is "overweight," 30 to 39.9 is "obese," and 40 or greater is "extremely obese." For teenagers and children, an individual's BMI is compared with the BMIs of people in the same age and gender groups. These BMIs are discussed in terms of percentiles.

Being overweight has been shown to increase the risk of death from a range of disorders, including high blood pressure; coronary heart disease; stroke; type II diabetes; gallbladder disease; osteoarthritis and respiratory disorders; and sleep apnea (cessation of breathing during sleep). Risks from certain cancers, including breast, prostate, and colon cancer are also greater in overweight people. Being underweight can also be bad for the health. Underweight people are prone to deficiencies of nutrients, anemia, osteoporosis, and heart problems.

Weight as a symptom of a disorder

Being underweight or overweight is not in itself an illness, but it may be a symptom of a disorder. Weight gain or weight loss, or both, may be a result of eating disorders and other psychological disorders such as depression. Many people eat for comfort in times of stress; other people find it difficult to eat when they are anxious.

Sudden weight gain often occurs at puberty when changing hormone levels affect the bulk of muscle in teenage bodies and increase the level of fat stores, particularly in girls. Weight gain is also a symptom of pregnancy. Such changes are normal, but must not be excessive. Weight gain or loss is also associated with contraceptive pill use. New users should monitor weight, and consult their clinic if symptoms persist after a few months of use.

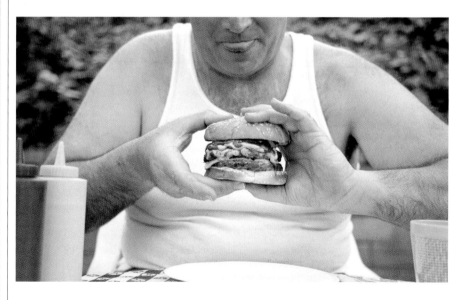

▲ *Taking little exercise, and getting into a habit of eating large meals that have a large amount of saturated fat, is a certain way to put on excess weight.*

BMI	20	22	24	26	28	30	32	34	36	38	40	42	44	46	48	50	52	53	54
Height (in.)								Body weight (lb.)											
58	96	105	115	126	134	143	153	162	172	181	191	201	210	220	229	239	248	253	258
59	99	109	119	128	138	148	158	168	178	188	198	208	217	227	237	247	257	262	267
60	102	112	123	133	143	153	163	174	184	194	204	215	225	235	245	255	266	271	276
61	106	116	127	137	148	158	169	180	190	201	211	222	232	243	254	264	275	280	285
62	109	120	131	142	153	164	175	186	196	207	218	229	240	251	262	273	284	289	295
63	113	124	135	146	152	169	180	191	203	214	225	237	248	259	270	282	293	299	304
64	116	128	140	151	163	174	186	197	209	221	232	244	256	267	279	291	302	308	314
65	120	132	144	156	168	180	192	204	216	228	240	252	264	276	288	500	312	318	324
66	124	136	148	161	173	186	198	210	223	235	247	260	272	284	297	309	322	328	334
67	127	140	153	166	178	191	204	217	230	242	255	268	280	293	306	319	331	338	344
68	131	144	158	171	184	187	219	223	230	236	249	276	289	302	315	328	341	348	354
69	135	149	162	176	189	203	216	230	243	257	270	284	297	311	324	338	351	358	365
70	139	153	167	181	195	209	222	236	250	264	278	292	306	320	334	348	362	369	376
71	143	157	172	186	200	215	229	243	257	272	286	301	315	329	343	358	372	379	386
72	147	162	177	191	206	221	235	250	265	279	294	309	324	338	353	368	383	390	397
73	151	166	182	197	212	227	242	257	272	288	302	318	333	348	363	378	393	401	408
74	155	171	186	202	218	233	249	264	280	295	311	326	342	358	373	389	404	412	420
75	160	176	192	208	224	240	256	272	287	303	319	335	351	367	383	399	415	423	431

▲ *Find height in the left-hand column. Read across row to find weight. The figure at the top of this column is the BMI.*

Weight gain may also be a symptom of edema—water retention, which can be caused by kidney and liver disorders. Edema can be treated by diuretic drugs prescribed by a doctor, but the underlying causes should be investigated and treated. Edema in pregnancy is a serious condition because it is one of the symptoms of the life-threatening disorder preeclampsia. Other symptoms are high blood pressure and protein in the urine. Regular checks for these symptoms are routine at prenatal clinics. Rest, and in severe cases, hospital bed rest, is the main form of treatment. Drugs to prevent convulsions may be prescribed, and early delivery may be necessary since the condition does not persist for long after labor.

Sudden weight loss may also be a symptom of an underlying disorder. If someone loses more than 10 pounds over a period of 10 weeks without being on a weight-reduction diet or taking increased exercise, he or she should check for other symptoms that might indicate a problem.

Unexplained weight loss

If weight loss is accompanied by a feeling of restlessness, sweating, weakness, and difficulty sleeping, the problem may be an overactive thyroid gland. If weight loss is accompanied by excessive thirst, a need to urinate frequently, and general tiredness, the cause may be diabetes or another hormone deficiency. Weight loss with persistent diarrhea may be a symptom of a disorder in the digestive tract, which prevents absorption of food. Any unusual bowel habits, such as watery, pale or dark-colored stools are cause for concern. Weight

Calculating BMI

To calculate a child's BMI divide weight (in kilograms) by height x height (in meters).

$$\text{BMI} = \frac{\text{weight (kg)}}{\text{height (m) x height (m)}}$$

If the metric equivalents are not known:

$$\text{BMI} = \frac{\text{weight (lb.) x 703}}{\text{height (in.) x height (in.)}}$$

Body mass index (males: ages 2 to 20 years)

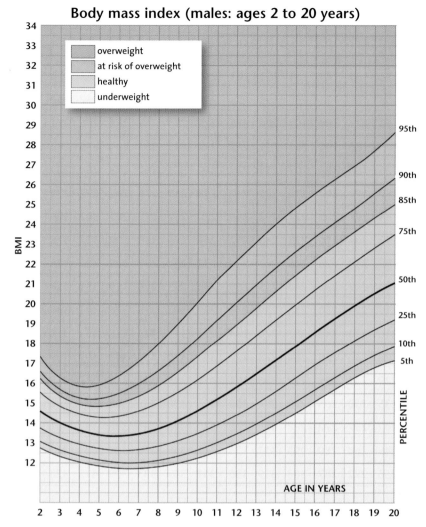

	overweight
	at risk of overweight
	healthy
	underweight

BMI

AGE IN YEARS

PERCENTILE

95th
90th
85th
75th
50th
25th
10th
5th

◄ *After calculating BMI, look on the graph to check that it is within acceptable limits for the person's age.*

Foods that are high in fats and carbohydrates (starch and particularly sugar) are higher in calories, and therefore more fattening. These are the first foods to cut out in a weight-reducing diet. A balanced, healthy diet is the best way to reduce weight, with at least five portions of fresh fruit and vegetables every day. White meat chicken and pork, fish, high-fiber bread, and pasta or rice may be consumed in moderation. Sauces and dressings often contain unwanted calories. The method of cooking is also important, for example, fried foods should be avoided in favor of grilled, steamed, or boiled dishes. Snacks such as salted nuts, chips, fries, candy, and cookies should be cut out and replaced with fresh fruit instead. Alcohol is high in unnecessary calories, sodas and sweetened coffee made with whole milk are also high in calories and should be avoided. Government agencies now put more emphasis on the type of food eaten, rather than on total caloric content, but calories charts are still a useful rule of thumb.

▼ *Young girls may perceive themselves to be fat when in reality they are very thin.*

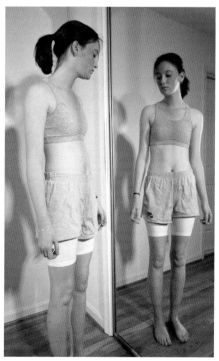

loss is a symptom of many infections, including tuberculosis, and disorders of the immune system, such as AIDS. It can also be the result of certain cancers. A doctor should be consulted about any unexplained weight loss.

BMI for children and teens

For children and teenagers, an individual's BMI is compared with the BMIs of a large group of young people of the same age and gender. BMIs are discussed in terms of percentiles. For example, if a teenager's BMI matches the BMI for the 5th percentile, 5 percent of teenagers of the same age and gender have a lower BMI and 95 percent have a higher BMI. A person with a BMI between the 85th and 95th percentiles is considered "at risk" of becoming overweight. A person with a BMI above the 95th percentile is classified as "overweight."

Teenagers who are very muscular and athletic can weigh a lot for their height because muscle is dense and heavy. Such individuals may seem to be overweight or obese according to their BMIs, even though they do not have a lot of body fat. A doctor can help determine whether a young person's BMI is in the healthy range.

A high BMI

If someone has a high BMI, they should lose weight. Weight depends on the amount of calories consumed and the amount of calories burned. If more calories are consumed than burned, the person will put on weight, so the amount eaten must be reduced or more exercise taken, or ideally, both.

Body mass index (females: ages 2 to 20 years)

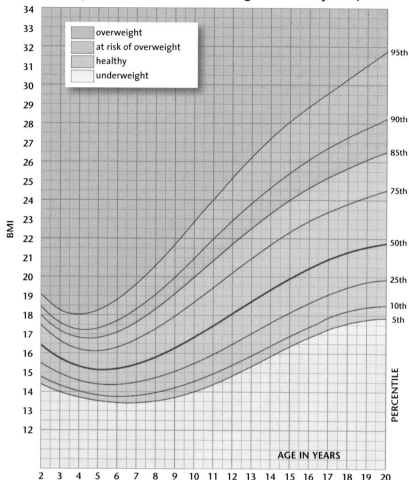

- overweight
- at risk of overweight
- healthy
- underweight

BMI (y-axis): 12–34

Percentile lines labeled: 95th, 90th, 85th, 75th, 50th, 25th, 10th, 5th

PERCENTILE

AGE IN YEARS (x-axis): 2 to 20

▼ *Monitor pregancy weight closely.*

▲ *Girls develop at different rates.*

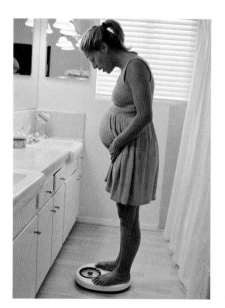

amount of body fat as a proportion of body weight affects the BMR because muscle cells burn up calories. For this reason, men usually have a greater BMR than women because they have greater muscle mass. BMR also increases with height and weight. The older people are, the lower their BMR becomes (growing children and teenagers have a high BMR). Body temperature also affects BMR: if someone has a fever, his or her BMR increases because the chemical reactions in the body happen faster. The outside temperature also affects BMR; in cold weather the BMR is higher because the body shivers in an attempt to keep warm. Extremely high temperatures over a long period can also raise BMR. An overactive thyroid gland will increase BMR, as well as excessive production of adrenaline in the body. Exercise is the most important factor controlling BMR; anyone who is physically active not only burns more energy during exercise, but also builds lean muscle tissue which burns up energy even when the body is resting. Finally, a sudden drop in caloric intake owing to dieting reduces BMR. The reduction in food consumption slows the use of energy in the body, which is why many people have difficulty losing weight when on low-calorie diets. It is essential to manage weight loss through a balanced diet and exercise.

Exercise

Exercise programs in overweight and obese people should be carefully monitored, since people in this condition are susceptible to heart problems. A sudden increase in exercise can put excessive strain on the heart. At least three sessions of 30 minutes of an aerobic exercise each week is recommended. (Aerobic exercise involves working out until someone feels slightly breathless.) Walking briskly to start tones up muscle, and the amount of exercise can gradually be increased. Swimming and exercise machines at gyms are useful forms of exercise, but exercise can also be easily introduced by taking the stairs instead of the elevator, and by mowing the lawn once a week. Even tackling housework in a vigorous way can be included as part of a daily exercise program.

The caloric content of prepared food can be checked and calorie charts consulted to assess total intake. For a person of average height and weight, the suggested caloric intake varies between 1,900 and 3,000 calories. The lower figure is for women over 50; men generally need more calories, and the higher figure is for boys aged 15 to 18. Women who are pregnant or breast-feeding require an extra 300 to 500 calories. Anyone overweight or obese should aim to reduce his or her total caloric intake by up to 500 calories each day to start with.

Metabolic rate

Metabolism (the rate at which calories are used) also affects the amount that people need to eat. The basal metabolic rate (BMR) can be affected by several factors. The

See also: **Anorexia and bulimia; Dieting; Heart attack; Nutrition; Obesity**

Whiplash injury

Questions and Answers

Will wearing a seat belt prevent a whiplash injury?

No. The injury occurs when the head snaps back suddenly if a vehicle is struck from behind. Properly adjusted headrests can prevent most of these injuries. Seat belts may lessen the severity of the injury by preventing the wearer from bouncing forward again once the initial blow is over, and may prevent other injuries when a driver or passenger could be flung against a windshield.

Is it true that a whiplash injury can occur when a baby is abused?

It is possible for a whiplash injury to occur in these circumstances. It may, however, be much more difficult to diagnose than more obvious injuries caused by child abuse because there are usually no outward signs of injury at all. Because a baby cannot complain, especially of neck pain, such an injury might never be detected.

Are whiplash injuries as common today as they were 25 years ago?

Whiplash injuries have become more common over the past 25 years. This may be partly due to the increased number of vehicles on the road, but may also reflect an increasing tendency for victims to file for damages, so that more cases come to public attention.

Is it possible to break your neck in a whiplash injury?

It is rare for the bones of the neck to fracture in a whiplash injury. In a whiplash injury the head is jerked back and the soft tissues of the neck are sprained. Broken bones in the neck are caused when the neck is loaded by an abnormal weight—for example, when diving into shallow water and cracking the head on the bottom.

With more vehicles on the road than ever before, the chances of a whiplash injury, or a sprained neck, have increased. How should a whiplash be treated, and are there any measures that prevent it from occurring?

The term "whiplash injury" conjures up images of devastating damage to the neck. In fact, whiplash refers to a single type of neck injury that is essentially a sprain. Like any sprain, it can vary greatly in severity, ranging from a few days of mild discomfort to months of pain, or even to permanent disability. In the majority of cases, however, recovery is complete within about a month.

Causes

Whiplash injury is nearly always caused by traffic accidents, usually when a stationary automobile is struck from behind by another moving vehicle. When this happens, the occupants of the stationary automobile are suddenly propelled forward, causing their heads to be momentarily left behind. The neck is bent violently backward, and the muscles and ligaments at the front of the neck and throat are placed under a sudden strain. This results in minor hemorrhage into these muscles and ligaments, which resolves within a short period of time. In severe cases there may be momentary dislocation of one or more small

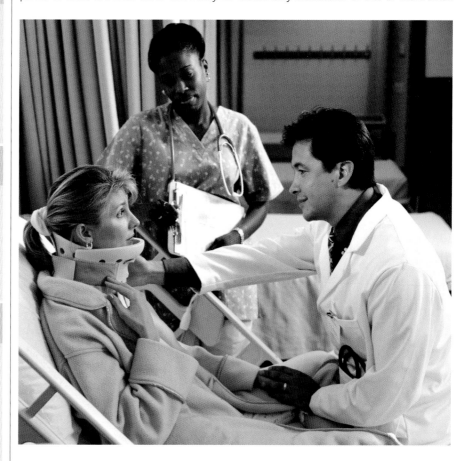

▲ *When a whiplash injury causes pain and stiffness, a neck brace supports the neck and allows the injured muscles time to recover.*

Preventing whiplash injuries

Use properly adjusted headrests: they will prevent the head from jerking back to an extreme degree in rear-end collisions.

Apply the hand or foot brake when the vehicle is stationary: if it is hit from behind, it won't accelerate rapidly, thereby avoiding any sudden jerking of the head.

Ensure that rear lights and brake lights are functioning, and that the rear fog spotlights are used in conditions of poor visibility. This will reduce the chances of a rear-end collision.

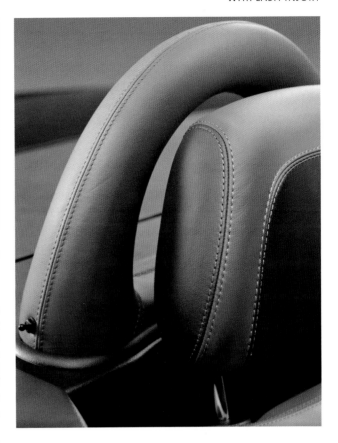

▲ *To protect someone from whiplash injury, a headrest must be high enough to prevent the head from snapping backward when the body is forced upward.*

joints in the neck, or rarely, there may even be fractures of the neck bones.

Symptoms and dangers

Often there is little pain immediately after the accident. The following day, however, there is an indistinct pain in the neck that may be difficult to pinpoint, and this may spread into the shoulders or upper arms. Neck movements may become restricted by muscle spasm. People with more severe injuries may complain of blurred eyesight, headaches, dizziness, or difficulty in swallowing because of bruising around the nerves and blood vessels in the neck. X rays are usually unhelpful, since the injuries are located in the soft tissues, which do not show on standard X rays.

In most cases, the symptoms settle down within a few days. However, people may develop persistent pain and stiffness, which may last for many months. Some of these pains may be due to underlying arthritis in the joints of the neck, which is triggered by the injury. In other cases, there is a vicious circle of pain and stiffness giving rise to muscle spasm, which in turn causes more pain and stiffness. In some cases there is a psychological element that keeps the pain going—often while an insurance claim is awaiting settlement. It has been observed that people rarely suffer from persistent problems from whiplash injuries suffered in sports, domestic accidents, or motor sport competitions, where the question of compensation does not arise.

The main danger of whiplash is that symptoms will become persistent. Serious injury to the neck is rare: fractures of the neck bones, slipped disk, dislocations of the joints, and spinal cord and nerve root injuries are more commonly caused by bending the neck forward or by direct force applied to the top of the head. Other complications may include pain so acute as to be immobilizing. Constant headaches and dizziness may require heavy medication.

Initial treatment

Initial treatment consists of resting the neck so that the neck muscles can relax and avoid going into spasm. This may be achieved by lying flat so that the neck muscles do not have to work to hold the neck upright. A more convenient method is to apply a collar or neck brace to support the neck: this takes over the function of the muscles and allows the person to remain fairly active. At this stage, painkillers are useful to prevent sore muscles from going into spasm and worsening the symptoms.

Long-term treatment

If pain persists much beyond a couple of weeks, physical therapy may be helpful. Gentle traction to the neck will relieve painful muscle spasm and reduce any pressure on the nerves leading to the shoulders and arms. Exercise to mobilize the neck, often combined with heat treatment, may also help to relax tense muscles. Some patients fail to respond to any form of treatment and it will take time to result in an improvement.

The associated symptoms of dizziness, blurred vision, and headaches can be difficult to treat. Drug treatment may help, but often the patient has to learn to live with these irritating symptoms and wait for them to subside. In the rare cases when dislocation or fracture occurs, the neck bones may have to be stabilized by surgery.

Outlook

Most patients will recover completely within a month. With those whose symptoms are more persistent, it may take as much as one to two years for them to resolve, although complete recovery generally occurs in time.

See also: **Arthritis; Bruises; Dislocation; Exercise; Fractures; Headache; Pain; Physical therapy; Slipped disk; Sprains; X rays**

Whooping cough

Highly infectious and very distressing for sufferers, whooping cough can be one of childhood's most dangerous illnesses. However, it can be effectively prevented by immunization in infancy.

Whooping cough, or pertussis as it is medically known, is a highly infectious bacterial disease caused by *Bordetella pertussis*. Anybody who has neither had, nor been immunized against, whooping cough can catch it. The disease is spread by droplets of bacteria that are in the air. The bacteria settle in the mucous lining of the respiratory tract, causing inflammation and production of a thick, sticky mucus.

Symptoms of whooping cough and their incidence

Whooping cough in the unprotected may be severe and dangerous, especially in very young children, and often requires admission to the hospital. More than half of infants under one year who develop whooping cough must be hospitalized. The younger the infants, the more likely treatment in the hospital will be needed. Of those infants who are hospitalized, 1 percent will have convulsions, 50 percent will have apnea (slowed or stopped breathing), and 20 percent will get pneumonia. Whooping cough is a common disease in the United States, where period epidemics occur every three to five years and there are frequent outbreaks. The number of whooping cough cases reported in the United States reached a peak in 2004 with more than 25,000 cases. However, after a subsequent drop, the number of cases began increasing again in 2007. There were nearly 17,000 cases of whooping cough reported in the United States in 2009.

Questions and Answers

Do most doctors now advise the whooping cough vaccine?

Yes, if there is no history of convulsions or brain damage in you or your children. The risks of severe illness are greater from whooping cough than from the vaccine.

Why is whooping cough such a dangerous illness in babies and small children?

Whooping cough produces very thick, sticky mucus in the air passages to the lungs, which can prevent air from getting to the lungs unless it is coughed away. Small children can be too weak to cough this up, so their lungs get blocked. Babies can suffer lack of oxygen, causing brain damage, and they are also prone to pneumonia.

Does a baby get natural immunity to whooping cough from his or her mother?

No. Pertussis antibodies, or the cells in the blood that fight the whooping cough infection, do not seem to pass across the placenta. Therefore, babies are born without any protection against whooping cough. They can get some immunity from the colostrum (the breast milk in the first days after birth) if they are breast-fed. However, because it is such a dangerous illness in small babies, they should be given antibiotics immediately if they come into contact with the bacterium.

My three-year-old son recently recovered from whooping cough but still has the whoop. How long will this last?

It can last three or four months, and the whoop may get worse if he gets a cold, but some whoops may be just a habit. The Chinese call the illness the 100-day cough because it can last that long.

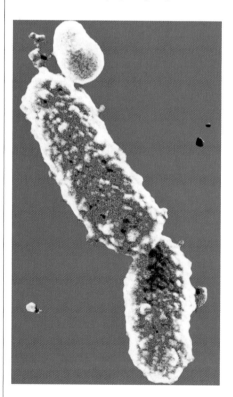

▲ *A scanning electron micrograph (SEM) of* Bordetella pertussis—*the bacterium that causes whooping cough.*

Course of the illness

The incubation period lasts six to 20 days from contact, with seven days as an average. The patient is infectious from the catarrhal phase and for about four weeks, and he or she should be isolated for a month or until the cough has stopped. Children under the age of one year in particular should be kept away from those who have the condition. The illness can be divided into three distinct stages: the catarrhal phase, the paroxysmal phase, and the convalescent phase.

The catarrhal phase lasts one or two weeks. Initially, the symptoms are rather like a cold: runny nose, red runny eyes, a slight cough, and fever. The paroxysmal phase lasts from two to four or more weeks, and in this stage there are episodes of coughing, becoming increasingly worse and more frequent, often up to around 40 bouts a day. The bouts consist of five to 10 quickly repeated coughs while breathing out, followed by a prolonged effort to breathe in, which in older children produces the characteristic whoop. The face turns red or blue, the eyes bulge, the tongue sticks out, both eyes and nose run, and the veins in the neck become more obvious. Episodes of this coughing occur until the patient manages to dislodge the plug of mucus. During this time, in severe attacks, young children may lack oxygen and stop breathing or have a convulsion.

At the end of the coughing bout the child will vomit. The vomiting is really more characteristic of whooping cough than the whoop. These episodes are extremely exhausting, and infants become tired and lose weight. Attacks can be triggered by movement, yawning, sneezing, eating, or drinking, or even by thinking about them. Between attacks, the patient appears relatively well.

During convalescence, the paroxysmal coughing, whooping, and vomiting gradually subside, although the cough and whoop may last for many weeks or months and they often recur if the child catches a cold or throat infection.

Diagnosis

The diagnosis is usually made on the clinical symptoms, but in older children and adults who suffer a milder attack this can be difficult. The best method is to take a swab from the back of the nose and do a culture. Blood tests are not very helpful, though the number of lymphocytes (a type of defensive blood cell) may be very high, aiding diagnosis. Otherwise, two samples of blood are needed, at the beginning and end of the illness, to show a rise in pertussis antibodies during that time. If the sample is not taken early enough, it will not show a large enough rise to make the diagnosis.

Complications

Most deaths from whooping cough are caused by complications such as pneumonia and brain damage. Usually pneumonia is due

▼ *These are some of the most common vaccines, including the DPT vaccine Infanrix (right), which is used to immunize against diphtheria, tetanus, and pertussis (whooping cough).*

not to pertussis bacteria, but to other invading bacteria that enter the affected lungs. Plugs of mucus may block off the bronchi (the tubes leading the air from the throat to the lungs), and cause the lung to collapse. It may then become infected by bacteria. Sometimes the lung collapse is permanent.

The most serious complications of the established disease in children who have not been protected by immunization are those affecting the brain. It must be remembered that the type of cough produced by this organism makes it almost impossible for the child to take a breath in the course of a paroxysm of coughing. One cough follows another so rapidly that there is not time to breathe in. It is only when the long paroxysm has passed that the child can inspire, and even then, obstruction to inspiration—the cause of the whoop—further impedes air intake. The thick mucus that forms in the bronchial tubes in whooping cough tends to obstruct the bronchi.

All this adds up to the risk that the child will fail to get enough oxygen. Since the brain has much higher oxygen requirements than any other organ of the body, this situation can lead to oxygen deprivation and brain damage. Although this is very rare, the effects can be disastrous. They include convulsions, blindness, deafness, movement disorders, paralysis, coma, and death.

Treatment

Antibiotics are not helpful once the illness has begun, but if the antibiotic erythromycin is given to a child who has been in contact with the disease before any symptoms appear, the severity of the illness may be reduced. The drug is given to children who have whooping cough because it makes these children less infectious to others.

Other treatment is symptomatic: avoiding stimuli that cause coughing; a warm room, especially at night; small and frequent

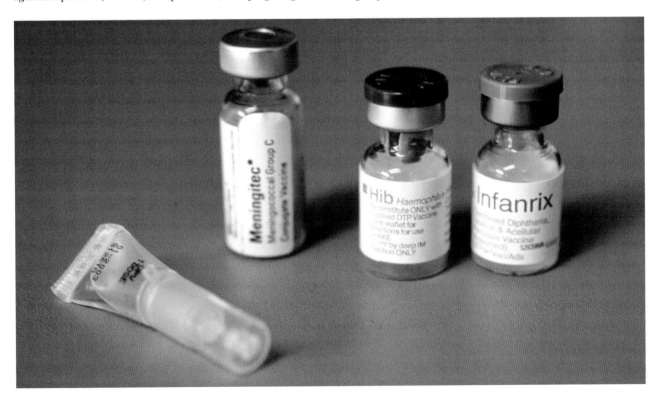

My daughter had whooping cough. Since then, she has had a series of coughs and colds. Is this because the illness has weakened her resistance to infection?

No. It's probably just bad luck. However, you should ask your doctor to check her over because sometimes part of the lung collapses after whooping cough and this may be her problem.

Is croup the same as whooping cough?

No. Croup arises from a viral infection that causes swelling of the larynx, so that when a child breathes in there is rather a harsh bark. It's not usually associated with a paroxysmal cough or vomiting, and it usually gets better in a few days.

My granddaughter has a bad cough that sounds very much like a whoop, and she sometimes vomits at the end of a coughing fit. Could this be whooping cough?

Yes. Although the phlegm in a bad cough can cause vomiting, it rarely causes a whoop. Take her to the doctor and keep her away from other children, particularly babies.

Is it possible to get whooping cough even after immunization?

Yes, but it's a much milder disease. It's more likely to recur in teenagers and adults who were immunized as babies, rather than in children.

My child has had convulsions, so the doctor won't give him whooping cough vaccine. Should my son also not have had the tetanus and diphtheria vaccine?

No. There is no evidence at all that the tetanus and diphtheria vaccine causes any neurological problems, and it is very important that he should have these and the polio vaccine that is usually given at the same time.

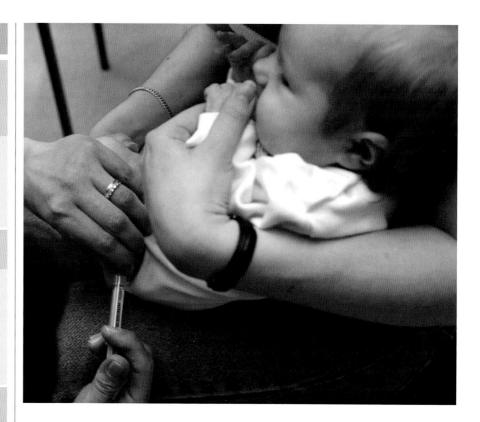

▲ *Whooping cough vaccine is most often given as part of a triple vaccine, the other two being diphtheria and tetanus, that is injected using a hypodermic syringe.*

drinks and meals; and no rushing about. Children who go blue during coughing bouts, or who cannot keep fluid down, need hospital admission for oxygen therapy, suction to remove mucus plugs, and replacement of fluids either by a tube through the nose into the stomach, or by injection into a vein. Some doctors give a mild sedative to reduce coughing spells.

Prevention

Lifelong prevention occurs only after an attack of whooping cough, so that pertussis can be prevented only by active immunization with the pertussis vaccine. The vaccine consists of a suspension of killed organisms of *Bordetella pertussis*. They stimulate the body to produce antibodies without actually giving rise to an attack of whooping cough.

The vaccine has to be given in three doses to give about 95 percent protection against the disease. The vaccine is more conveniently given at the same time as diphtheria and tetanus vaccine (hence the triple vaccine of diphtheria, tetanus, and pertussis—DPT or DPaT—given to most infants). According to the National Center for Health Statistics, in 2009, 84 percent of children between the ages of 19 months and 35 months received the vaccination.

The American Academy of Pediatrics recommends that a course of five whooping cough vaccinations be given to children at two months, four months, six months, 15 to 18 months, and four to six years. The fourth dose may actually be administered as early as 12 months, as long as at least six months have elapsed since the third dose. Immunity from whooping cough wanes steadily after immunization and an additional booster dose is necessary for adolescents and young adults.

The immunization controversy

Whooping cough was once common in the United States, but following the introduction of a vaccine in the 1940s and subsequent widespread immunization, its incidence declined. Since 1980, however, the incidence has been rising and there have been sporadic epidemics from time to time as a result of failure of immunization programs, usually because of the fear of side effects. Also, the

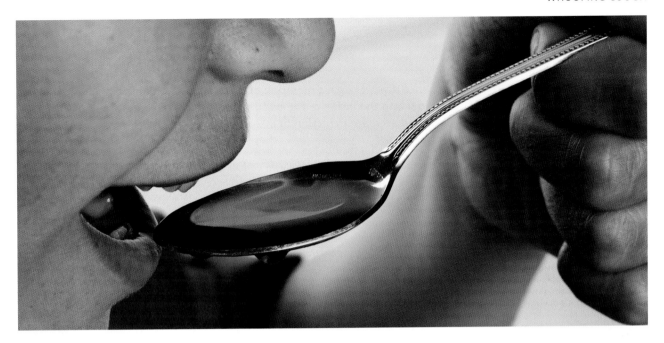

▲ *Suppressants such as cough syrups should be used only for dry, nonproductive coughs.*

incidence of whooping cough among adolescents and adults has increased substantially because immunity diminishes in many adolescents and adults. However, the death rate from whooping cough has been reduced by immunization to very low figures.

In view of these facts it is no longer acceptable that parents should be influenced by out-of-date information about the risks of immunization. In the mid-1970s, when vaccination against whooping cough had been widely used for about 16 years, reports began to appear about cases in which children had suffered convulsions and permanent brain damage attributed to such immunization. Because the same effects are a feature of the disease, there was no clear evidence that these cases were due to the immunization. However, severe anxiety among parents led to a widespread rejection of whooping cough immunization. The result was major whooping cough epidemics with the deaths of many young children.

Risks of immunization

The common adverse reactions from whooping cough vaccination consist mainly of swelling and redness at the site of the injection. A small, painless lump may form. This is of no consequence and will disappear in due course. Occasionally, the reaction takes the form of crying, screaming, and fever. Very occasionally, a child will become pale for a time and go limp. Convulsions sometimes occur, but these are not uncommon in children in the first year of life, whether they have been immunized or not.

In one major research study in Britain, the conclusion was that the number of cases was too small to provide conclusive evidence that the vaccine could cause permanent brain damage. Studies in the United States produced similar findings. In one of these a group of children who had seizures or floppy episodes within 38 hours of vaccination were checked six or seven years later. None of them showed serious brain damage or intellectual impairment.

When not to vaccinate

Because of the risk of complications, pertussis vaccine should not be given to any child who has a fever or feverish illness; who has had convulsions, or whose parents or siblings have had convulsions; who has late development; or who has a known disorder of the central nervous system. If there is any severe local or general reaction such as a very high temperature, confusion, odd behavior, or a convulsion after the first immunization, pertussis vaccine should be left out of subsequent vaccinations.

DPT and DPaT vaccines

Immunization against whooping cough is usually given in a combined form with a triple vaccine, known as DPT, that also protects against diphtheria and tetanus. Immunization in children is highly effective. Traditionally, the whooping cough vaccine has contained the *Bordetella* organism that has been killed by heat so that it cannot cause the disease. This is called whole cell vaccine, and it fairly often causes minor to moderate local reactions. A few unusually sensitive individuals have had seizures.

Because of concerns over these side effects, other whooping cough vaccines have been developed since the late 1970s and early 1980s. These contain purified extracts of the *Bordetella* organism and thus are called acellular vaccines. Several of these have been licensed for use in the United States. When combined with diphtheria and tetanus toxoids they are called DPaT vaccines. This is now the preferred form.

Acellular whooping cough vaccines are recommended for all children from two months onward. For most children of 15 months or more, however, the older DPT is an acceptable alternative.

> *See also:* **Antibiotics; Bacteria; Common cold; Fevers; Immunization; Oxygen; Pneumonia; Vaccinations**

X rays

Questions and Answers

If X rays are so dangerous, why are they still so widely used?

Modern X-ray equipment and strict safety precautions are used, and doses of X rays given in the majority of X-ray examinations are reduced to an absolute minimum. In theory, even the smallest X-ray dose carries a slight hazard, so it is a doctor's responsibility to ensure that X rays are taken only when the information obtained will be of benefit to a patient.

In the last week of pregnancy, my obstetrician said that she needed an X ray of my pelvis. Although I agreed, I worry that the X ray could have harmed my baby.

Your obstetrician was probably worried that your pelvis might have been too small for the baby to pass through safely, and was right to resolve her doubts by taking an X ray rather than risk waiting for problems to develop during labor. In this situation, an X ray was the definitive way of obtaining an answer, and worth any slight risk taken. During the first trimester the fetus is at greatest risk of damage from X rays; in late pregnancy X rays are considered relatively safe.

My brother has had many tests, and is about to have an X ray of the brain called a carotid angiogram. How is this done?

A contrast medium is injected into the carotid artery, filling the blood vessels of the brain and outlining them clearly when X rays are taken. The most comfortable and convenient way of injecting the contrast is through a long, very fine plastic catheter or tube, inserted into the femoral artery in the groin. The tube is manipulated under X-ray control until its tip lies in the artery to be studied.

A chance discovery gave medicine one of its most valuable diagnostic tools: a window into the inside of the body known simply as X rays. Their use enables early and accurate detection of internal injury and disease.

On November 8, 1895, Professor Wilhelm Conrad Röntgen, while conducting an experiment at the University of Würzburg, Germany, made a chance discovery that became a legend. For the purposes of the experiment his laboratory was in total darkness, and the electrical apparatus that he was studying had been enclosed in a lightproof black cardboard cover. Yet, as he passed an electric current through his apparatus, he became aware of a faint glow coming from a piece of chemically treated paper that was lying on a nearby workbench.

Professor Röntgen had discovered how to produce invisible, mysterious rays (he named them X rays), which had not only penetrated the opaque cardboard cover but had caused the fluorescent paper to glow. Later he discovered that the rays from his apparatus could also blacken a photographic plate and produce a permanent image using the fluorescent paper. He investigated other properties of the rays and found that they could penetrate many solid objects. He placed his hand in the path of the X rays and saw for the first time an image of his own bones suddenly appear on the fluorescent paper. Today, more than 100 years later, X rays are an indispensable aid to modern diagnostic medicine, and indeed most hospitals spend more money

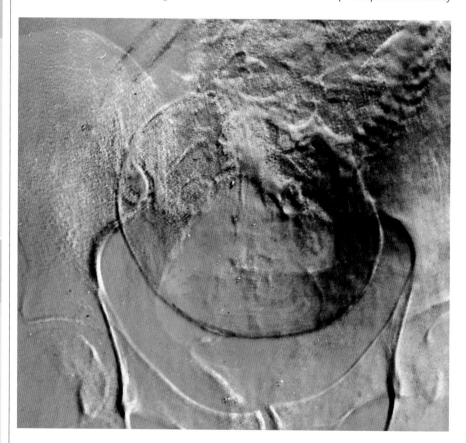

▲ *Computer color enhancement techniques add detail to X rays. Here an eight-month fetus can be seen in an ideal position, ready for birth. X rays during the last part of pregnancy are relatively safe.*

Questions and Answers

I twisted my knee months ago playing baseball. It has been troubling me ever since, and keeps locking. I'm due to have an arthrogram. What will it show?

Air and a contrast medium are injected into the knee joint under local anesthesia, giving a clear view of the joint. If you have torn a cartilage, the arthrogram will confirm this.

I hear differing opinions on the value of mammography. Is it valuable or a waste of time?

With the earlier and cruder equipment available, mammography did not much reduce the death rate from breast cancer. Now, the WHO agrees that, especially for older women, it saves many lives. With the development of high-tech full field digital mammography screening, and the use of MRI screening, we can anticipate a very high detection rate in even the earliest breast cancers.

My young daughter is to have a kidney X ray. Will it be painful, and is the dye injection risky?

In an IVU examination, an injection of a contrast medium containing iodine is given, usually into a vein in the arm. Young children understandably dislike injections, but the procedure itself will be entirely painless. Do tell the radiologist if your child has asthma, or any allergies that you know about, since an allergy to the contrast sometimes occurs.

How is it that X rays can be used to fight cancer?

X radiation can be dangerous because it damages all living cells. However, it particularly damages those cells that grow and divide profusely, as in cancer. Careful use of X rays has made it possible to destroy cancerous cells, or retard their development, while exposing healthy cells to as little radiation as possible.

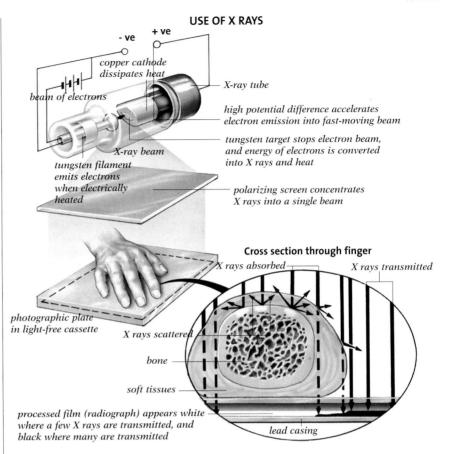

USE OF X RAYS

- ve + ve

copper cathode dissipates heat

beam of electrons

X-ray tube

high potential difference accelerates electron emission into fast-moving beam

tungsten target stops electron beam, and energy of electrons is converted into X rays and heat

X-ray beam

tungsten filament emits electrons when electrically heated

polarizing screen concentrates X rays into a single beam

photographic plate in light-free cassette

X rays scattered

Cross section through finger

X rays absorbed

X rays transmitted

bone

soft tissues

processed film (radiograph) appears white where a few X rays are transmitted, and black where many are transmitted

lead casing

▲ *X rays radiate outward from a tungsten target. They pass through the soft tissues of the body, but are absorbed by the bones. The shadow cast by the bones is caught by the photographic plate.*

on scanning departments than on any other department. The latest sophisticated technology provides a safe and reliable means of detecting disease at an early stage, and of monitoring treatment efficiently and effectively.

What are X rays?

X rays belong to the same family as light waves and radio waves, and, like radio waves, are invisible. They are produced artificially by bombarding a small tungsten target with electrons in a device called an X-ray tube. X rays travel in straight lines and radiate outward from a point on the target in all directions. In an X-ray machine, the X-ray tube is surrounded by a lead casing, except for a small aperture through which the X-ray beam emerges.

Each of the body's tissues absorbs X rays in a predictable way, and this is the property of X rays that enables them to be used in medicine to form images of the body. Bones are dense and contain calcium, which absorbs X rays well. Soft tissues, such as skin, fat, blood, and muscle, absorb X rays much less efficiently. When, for example, an arm is placed in the path of an X-ray beam, the X rays pass readily through the soft tissues but penetrate the bones less easily; the arm casts a shadow. X rays blacken photographic film, so the shadow cast by the bones appears white, while the shadow of the soft tissues is a dark shade of gray.

The X-ray examination

An X-ray image, or radiograph, is a demonstration of the anatomy of the part of the body under examination, and it is now possible to make a detailed inspection of almost any part of the body with X rays. X rays are of greatest use in the diagnosis and follow-up of disease and disorders that alter the structure of the body. Sometimes changes in structure are so dramatic that they

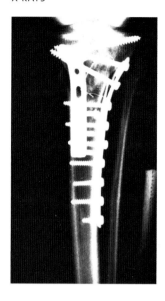
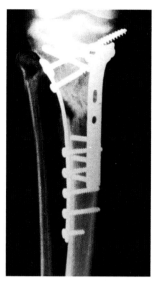

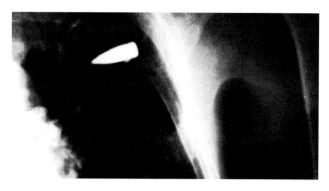

▲ *This dramatic X ray shows a bullet lodged in someone's upper chest: luckily the X ray shows no severe injury such as a punctured lung or damaged heart.*

◄ *After badly breaking both legs in a motorcycle accident, this victim had to have his bones pinned and bolted together.*

are immediately obvious even to the untrained observer, for example, in the case of broken bones. Frequently, however, the changes are more subtle, and may be apparent only to the trained eye of a radiologist (a doctor who specializes in the interpretation of X-ray images).

Before an X-ray examination, instructions about any special preparations that may be necessary are given to the patient when the appointment for the examination is made. In the case of examinations of the abdominal region, for example, it is often preferable for the patient to take laxatives and a special diet for two days beforehand, since emptying the intestines results in radiographs of much improved quality.

When the patient arrives at the X-ray department, the radiographer who will be taking the X rays explains the procedure. The patient undresses to expose the area concerned, and removes any objects, such as jewelry or dentures, that might produce an image on the radiograph. The position of the patient when the X ray is taken is chosen to provide the best demonstration of the part under examination, though this position may have to be modified if the patient is sick or in severe pain. Each X-ray film is carried in a flat cassette, and the patient lies, sits, or stands so that the area of interest is in contact with the cassette. It is essential to avoid movement while an X ray is taken; movement results in a blurred image. Every effort is made, therefore, to keep the patient comfortable, to use the shortest feasible exposure time (usually a mere fraction of a second), and, if necessary, to support or immobilize the region of interest with foam pads or a cloth bandage. To take an X ray, the radiographer leaves the room and presses an exposure button on the control panel to execute the X ray. Although the control panel is situated behind a protective screen, the radiographer is still able to see and talk to the patient at all times. If it is necessary for someone to remain in the room while X rays are taken, exposure to X rays is prevented by wearing a lead apron.

Special techniques

For most purposes, a standard X-ray examination is all that is required. Special techniques are available, however, that enable areas not adequately seen on standard radiographs to be studied in greater

detail. In general, these more sophisticated techniques necessitate the use of contrast media; substances that cause the tissue concerned to become opaque. The use of contrast media (which are eliminated from the body by the kidneys) can enhance views of the gallbladder and bile ducts, and the urinary and digestive tracts. When a contrast medium is injected directly into blood vessels (a procedure known as an angiograph), the arteries and veins are clearly outlined, and any abnormalities revealed. Likewise, using a contrast medium to highlight the fluid that surrounds the spinal cord is useful in detecting a nerve compressed by a disk or by a tumor.

By using a suspension of barium sulphate (an inert, chalky mixture that is opaque to X rays), it is possible to visualize the alimentary tract throughout its length. During a barium swallow examination, the patient is given a glass of flavored barium to drink. The patient's swallowing mechanism can be studied, abnormalities of the esophagus can be detected, and the stomach is clearly outlined. During the examination, the image is viewed continuously on a monitor, and the patient lies on a tilt table so that, with careful maneuvering, each part of the stomach and duodenum can be studied in turn.

Opacification of the urinary tract is achieved by intravenous injection of a solution with iodine; this is rapidly eliminated by the kidneys. Like barium, iodine is opaque to X rays, and if X-ray films are taken at various intervals after the injection, the kidneys, ureters, and bladder are clearly shown. This technique is intravenous urography (IVU or IVP) and is of great importance in the diagnosis of many types of kidney disease.

Digital radiography

Many X-ray departments have succeeded in abandoning the use of photographic films, which caused severe storage problems and involved great expense. Digital radiography involves the use of cassettes containing, in place of film, fine-grain, reusable, scintillating screens on which images are formed by the X rays. These screens can then be scanned by a computer scanner and the images saved as digital graphics files. Or the X-ray images can be converted directly to graphic files. A single small hard drive can store many thousands of high-quality images that in film form would have

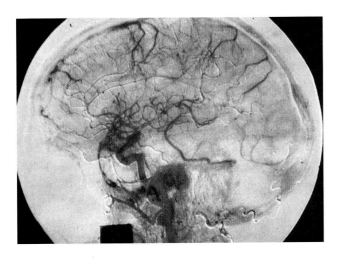

▲ *When contrast media are injected into the carotid artery, the blood vessels of the brain show up on X-ray film. The yellow band is the outline of the skull.*

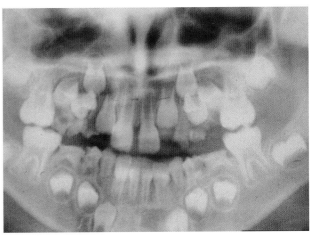

▲ *A technique called orthopantomography takes a panoramic view of the teeth: a child's second set of teeth can be seen coming through quite clearly.*

occupied a whole room. A major additional advantage is that individual images can be called up on a computer monitor in seconds. With such systems it is also easy to make backup copies that can be stored remotely in case of loss of the originals.

Dental X rays

X-ray techniques simplify the diagnosis of a wide range of important dental problems, and are now in everyday use. Tooth decay can be difficult to detect, especially in the spaces between the back teeth and in other inaccessible recesses. Decay, root disease, abscesses, and infections can all be visibly demonstrated with X rays, which will confirm a diagnosis at an early stage, reveal the extent of any disease, and help determine the most suitable form of treatment. A basic X-ray examination is now a routine part of a dental checkup. The equipment used is a low-powered X-ray unit, often linked to the dentist's chair. Small films (called bitewing films) are gripped in the mouth next to the teeth to be examined. More complex conditions, such as fractures of the jaw, tumors, cysts, and problems with abnormalities of growth and development of teeth, will require a much more detailed

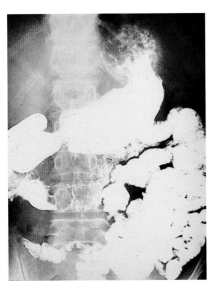

▼ *After barium liquid is swallowed, the digestive tract can be seen on an X ray. The stomach, the duodenum, and the rest of the small intestines are all shown.*

examination. A valuable technique is orthopantomography, in which an X-ray machine moves around the jaw of the patient while the X ray is taken, producing a panorama of the teeth and jaws. This technique shows both upper and lower jaws, any unerupted teeth, and the position and relationship of all the teeth on a single X-ray film.

When the two jaws do not fit together well, a side view of the face and jaws may be taken, showing the relationship of the teeth, jaws, and soft tissue. The pictures help the orthodontist to plan treatment, which may involve plates, braces, or corrective surgery.

CAT scanning

The most advanced application of X rays is computerized axial tomography, commonly known as CAT scanning or CT scanning. This is a highly sophisticated X-ray procedure developed independently by the American physicist Allan Cormack (1924–1998) and the British electrical engineer Godfrey Hounsfield (1919–2004); it won them jointly the 1979 Nobel Prize for physiology or medicine. The invention of the CAT scanner was one of the half-dozen most important medical advances of the 20th century.

X-ray tomography was in use long before the CAT scanner was invented. It was a method of using a swinging X-ray tube and film holder to record an image of a thin slice of the body. The results were crude, and many consecutive exposures, each involving a full dose of radiation, had to be made to provide useful information about the location and size of radiopaque objects and tissues. The major advance that made the modern CAT scanner possible was the realization that a computer could be used to store data from a large number of the separate X-ray slices and then correlate the data to synthesize a detailed image of a cross section of the inside of the body. The CAT scanner uses low-energy X-ray sources to send narrow beams of X radiation through the body to small detectors on the opposite side. These detectors are highly sensitive, and output an electrical signal that varies with the total density of the tissue through which the X rays pass. With each pulse of X rays, the resulting output from the detector is stored in a computer along with the orientation of the corresponding beam.

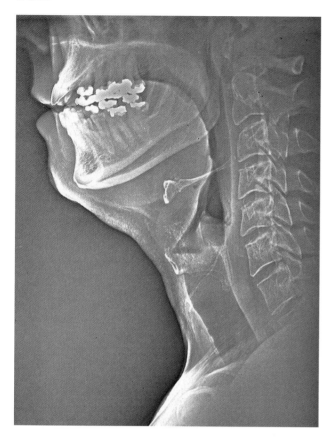

▲ *As X-ray technology advances, so the uses of X rays multiply. Special photographic techniques allow both the body outline and internal features to be captured. Here the voice box is being examined.*

The total radiation dose to the patient in the course of a CT scan is about the same as that of a conventional chest X ray. The computer is thus supplied with large numbers of pairs of data, the exact orientation of each of the numerous axes of X-ray projection, and, for each axis, the exact amount of attenuation caused by the bodily tissues. By solving large numbers of differential equations, the computer is able to determine the density of the tissue at every point at which the axes intersect, that is, at every point within the plane under examination.

CAT scanning provides a level of resolution and detail that was unobtainable by earlier forms of X ray, and was a major breakthrough in the noninvasive diagnosis of disease. It enables images to be made of structures, such as the brain, that are surrounded by bone. Conventional X rays are unable to show any detail in such structures. In addition, the CAT scanner has the advantage that it can show body planes in any desired orientation. The mass of data stored in the computer can be used to build up images in any required plane. Images can be viewed on a monitor screen, and records of these can be made on transparent photographic film. The basic idea behind CAT scanning has been seminal in allowing the development of a family of scanners using sources other than X rays. These include the MRI scanner, the ultrasound scanner, and the positron emission scanner.

Radiotherapy

Not only is the X-ray technique a valuable diagnostic tool; it is also an invaluable weapon against cancer. X rays can damage all living cells, but cells that are growing and dividing profusely, like cancer cells, are damaged more easily than normal cells, and are slow to recover. Radiotherapy is thus an important method of treatment in many types of cancer. Sometimes it is used on its own, as, for example, in the treatment of cervical cancer or leukemia, in order to destroy abnormal cells. It is also used in conjunction with other methods. For example, during the treatment of breast cancer, in which the malignant tumor is surgically removed, radiotherapy may be used to destroy any remaining tumor cells. Finally, it is used as a palliative measure to relieve symptoms of cancers too advanced to be cured. For example, in the case of cancer of the esophagus, radiotherapy may be used to facilitate swallowing, or, in the case of a brain tumor, to relieve the severity of a patient's headaches.

Both the dosage and the length of exposure take into account that radiation can also damage healthy cells. Side effects can be extremely unpleasant; they include fatigue, vomiting, and loss of hair in irradiated areas. Most side effects can be alleviated by treatment with drugs.

Some cancers are sensitive to radiotherapy, particularly tumors of the lymph glands and testes, and a complete cure is often possible. The cure rate for other types of cancer is also high, depending on how early treatment is started.

Hazards of X rays

The early pioneers of radiology had no idea how dangerous excessive exposure to X rays could be, and they therefore took no precautions at all when working with X rays. They discovered to their cost that large doses of radiation cause skin burns and dermatitis, cataract formation in the eyes, the appearance of various types of cancer, and damage to the reproductive organs resulting in genetic abnormalities in their children.

Now there is a much more complete understanding of the nature of the hazards of radiotherapy, which can be reduced to a minimum. Modern X-ray film, equipment, and techniques are designed to produce high-quality images at the lowest possible radiation dose to the patient. The danger of genetic damage can be minimized by shielding the patient's reproductive organs from an X-ray beam whenever possible with a sheet of lead.

Any nonurgent X-ray examinations of women who are of childbearing age are usually carried out only during the first 10 days of the menstrual cycle (this is called the ten-day rule), during which the possibility of pregnancy is unlikely.

Outlook

With technological advances in equipment, in terms of safety and effectiveness, of both X-ray scans and radiotherapeutic equipment, most of the time benefits to patients will far outweigh any risk of serious side effects. X rays will probably continue to be an invaluable tool in modern medicine.

See also: **Burns; Diet; Fractures; Genetics; Leukemia; Slipped disk**

Zest

Questions and Answers

An eager relish to get the most from life, a lively will to tackle its problems—zest is an aspect of people's well-being, largely determined by personality type and genetic inheritance, that fluctuates with their health and state of mind.

I don't sleep as well as I used to. This situation leaves me tired and irritable during the day, and I don't have the zest for life that I once had. What can I do?

Try to find out what is interfering with your sleep. Perhaps you are subconsciously depressed or anxious about something. Perhaps you are not getting enough leisure time, so that you take work worries to bed with you. If you can't resolve the problem yourself within two weeks, ask your doctor for help. However, don't start taking sleeping drugs, which may end up by making the situation worse.

I feel very sluggish these days. Would vitamin pills help?

No, probably not. You must first find out why you are less full of life than you used to be. It could be something physical, such as anemia. However, it might equally be something mental, like a nagging worry or unresolved problem. If necessary, get your doctor to help sort it out with you.

Since my husband died I have become miserable. I used to be such a lively person. Will I ever get back my zest for living?

Yes, you will eventually. Grief and bereavement are very draining, and you are unlikely to feel much zest for anything while grief remains with you. Although grief is a very natural thing, it can sometimes go on longer than is really necessary—it becomes a kind of habit. Perhaps you need to give yourself a better chance to get out of it by mixing more with other people, going to parties, and so on, even if you don't feel much like doing so at first. Buy yourself some new clothes; try doing something different or going somewhere completely new. It's surprising how quickly things can change once you make the first all-important move.

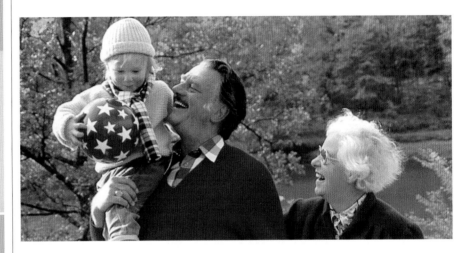

▲ *Zest for living, which allows people to draw vitality from nature and those around them, need never desert them. Grandchildren can be a source of inspiration for the elderly.*

Strictly speaking, "zest" is not a medical term, but it is a word used by both doctor and patient when discussing lethargy, depression, illness, or even behavior or attitude. The term "zest" means great interest, keen enjoyment, and an enthusiastic relish for life. Zest is not something all people have or even should have, but when it is missing from a normally lively person it may be cause for concern.

Physical well-being

A loss of zest may be symptomatic of impending sickness, anxiety, depression, or even poor eating habits or excessive living. If a person feels that his or her zest for life has disappeared, then it is time to sit back and take stock. Is a balanced diet being enjoyed, or has sluggishness come about through overindulgence and lack of exercise? What about alcohol? It is easy to get into a state of subintoxication in which the brain is seldom free from the numbing effects of alcohol. Even sleeping pills and tranquilizers can dampen a person's energy if taken on a regular basis, and the most lively of people may find their joie de vivre waning. A temporary course of drugs such as antibiotics may have a similar effect.

Regular sleep and exercise, plenty of play, and a vacation (at least once a year) involving a complete change of scene are important if a person is going to keep his or her energy levels high.

All in the mind

Of course, sickness and bereavement do drain a person's resources, and it often takes much time and adjustment before zest for life returns. However, zest is not just a matter of physical condition and enthusiasm; it is very much a state of mind. If a person's lifestyle is flat, excitement is missing, or work is boring and undemanding, then this may affect the mental and emotional state, producing an attitude of bored indifference. Only by objectively assessing all aspects of the life can one determine those aspects of it that need changing.

Once the first steps have been made, zest may return fairly quickly. However, there may be a medical cause behind the loss of zest, so this should be discussed with a doctor. Simply talking it through may be all that is needed.

> *See also:* Alcoholism; Antibiotics; Depression; Exercise

FIRST AID HANDBOOK

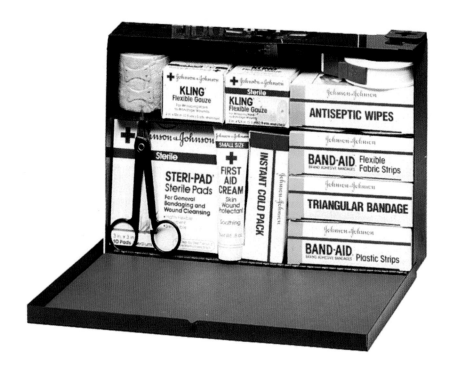

This section will give you all the basic information that you need
to deal with the more common emergencies. It gives a
quick and easy step-by-step guide to emergency first aid.

The aim of all first aid is to keep the patient alive, to protect him or her from
further harm, and to be as reassuring as possible.
In short, the first aid provider's task is to safeguard the victim until
a doctor or nurse arrives to take over.

First you should ensure that the patient is still breathing and try to restore
breathing if necessary. Then you should control any bleeding and treat
for unconsciousness. Next you need to protect the patient
by immobilizing any fractures, treating any burns, dressing
any wounds, and, finally, minimizing shock. Throughout this
process you need to comfort the victim.

Always make sure that you have an accessible record of your doctor's telephone
number, and never hesitate to call the emergency services—it is usually better,
except in extreme emergencies, to telephone an ambulance rather than
drive a patient to the hospital yourself.

Artificial respiration

- Hold patient's head back
- Pinch patient's nose and take a deep breath
- Place your mouth over patient's mouth and breathe into patient
- Check for pulse
- Repeat this procedure, regulating your puffs by the rise and fall of the patient's chest

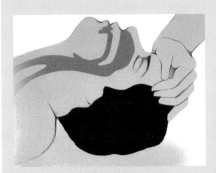

1. To ensure that patient's tongue does not block the throat, place a hand on the forehead and gently tip head back.

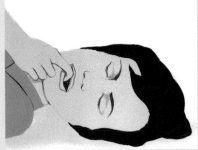

2. If there is an obstruction, turn the head to one side. Use your forefinger to clear out mouth. Tip head back again.

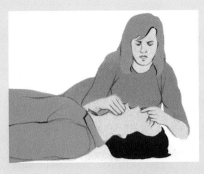

3. If the mouth is closed, grasp chin and pull open gently. Pinch the nose firmly shut and take a deep breath.

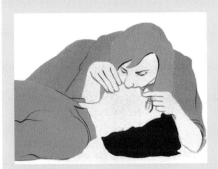

4. Place your mouth over patient's mouth, ensuring a firm seal. Give four breaths in fairly rapid succession.

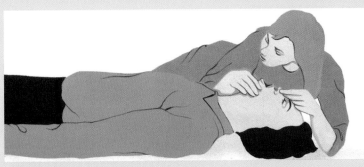

5. Remove mouth. You should feel and hear air leaving the patient's mouth, and the chest will sink. If there is a pulse but no breathing, give two breaths, enough to raise the chest. Continue breaths, about 12 per minute, until breathing resumes.

Take note

- In the case of a young child or baby, cover the mouth and nose. Don't blow too hard—give two slow breaths, just enough to raise the child's chest. If there is a pulse, continue giving breaths, one every three seconds for a baby, one every four seconds for a child.
- If the mouth is injured, hold the mouth shut by applying pressure underneath the chin. Give breaths into the nose and allow mouth to open for exhalation. Repeat.
- If treatment is interrupted (e.g., if the patient vomits), restart by giving four quick breaths, which will supply oxygen immediately.
- An alternative method of opening the patient's mouth is to place a hand under the neck and raise it slightly—the mouth should open on its own.
- To clear an obstruction in the patient's mouth, use a small, hard object if it is available, to keep your finger from being bitten.

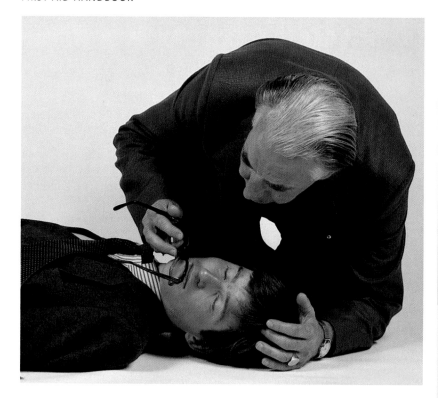

▲ *Before attempting artificial respiration, make sure that the victim has actually stopped breathing. Establish this by holding a pair of eyeglasses in front of his or her mouth: if the glass mists over, then the victim is still breathing.*
Note: If there is any possibility that the patient has suffered trauma or fracture, do not move the neck.

Dos and don'ts

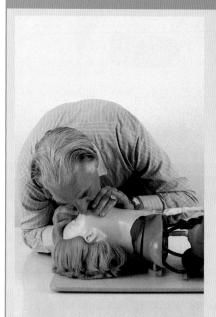

DO keep fingers and hands clear of the patient's lips and neck at all times—they could obstruct breathing.

DON'T blow too hard—just raise the patient's chest visibly; otherwise, you may damage the lung tissue.

DON'T try to drain water or fluid from the lungs of a person who may have drowned. The victim's first need is for oxygen, and air will bubble through liquid in the windpipe.

DON'T practice on a person who is breathing normally. If you enroll in a first aid class, there will be lifelike mannequins provided.

DON'T be worried if the person vomits; this is common. Stop your breathing for long enough to turn his or her head and clear the mouth, then resume by giving the patient four quick breaths.

Checklist

1. Send any onlookers for medical aid. Do not allow people to crowd around or interfere while first aid treatment is being given.

2. Loosen any tight clothing. If possible, the patient should be lightly and loosely covered to prevent heat loss, but the contour of the chest should remain clearly visible.

3. Sometimes it is enough to tilt the patient's head back. He or she may have stopped breathing because of a simple blockage, and holding the head back may free the airway. If this is the case, the patient will probably start to gasp for breath. Placed him or her in the recovery position and take precautions to minimize shock (see Shock).

4. Throughout the first aid treatment, keep checking that the patient's head is tilted back and be sure to keep his or her nose firmly pinched. It is easy to overlook these things if you are concentrating on giving artificial respiration.

5. Check periodically to see if the patient has started to breathe naturally. If breathing has not resumed, begin giving artificial respiration again, starting with four quick breaths and then resuming single puffs. If the patient's breathing has started, keep the head fully back and watch carefully in case the breathing stops again. Once the respiration is steady and natural, treat the patient for unconsciousness (see Unconsciousness).

6. Continue giving artificial respiration until the patient's breathing starts spontaneously or medical help arrives and is able to take over. People have been known to survive for up to eight hours after treatment has begun, so don't give up.

7. If the patient's heartbeat has stopped, heart compression will have to be used (see CPR). The only acceptable indication of a stopped heart is the complete lack of a pulse. Heart compression is a difficult technique to learn and apply, so try to attend a first aid course to supplement the information given here.

8. The risk of contracting HIV through mouth-to-mouth resuscitation is extremely remote, but there are special mouthpieces available that can be used as a safeguard.

Bites and stings

- Various bites and stings need different treatment
- Animal bites need to be washed thoroughly
- Snakebites need special care
- Bee stings have to be removed
- Jellyfish stings need to have tentacles removed

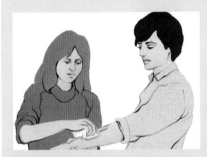

1. Animal bites should be treated like ordinary wounds (see Wounds), except that only the wound itself should be washed thoroughly. Consult a doctor to check for infection.

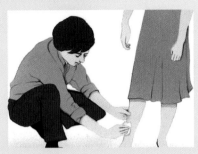

2. If the patient has been bitten by a venomous snake, wipe venom from the wound and bandage a pad tightly onto the wound. Keep patient absolutely still. Seek medical aid.

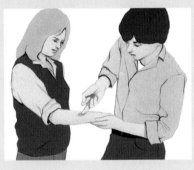

3. Bee and wasp stings are often left in the wound and continue to pump in venom after the insect has gone. Scrape the sting out with a credit card. Wash the wound and cover.

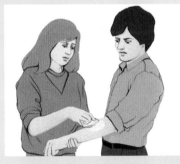

4. If jellyfish tentacles stick, wash with diluted ammonia or alcohol. Remove tentacles with a gloved hand. Soothe wound with calamine lotion. Seek medical aid.

Dos and don'ts

DO clean a bite or sting with warm water and, if possible, unperfumed soap. Then apply a mild antiseptic.

DO reassure the victim of a snakebite. People are often frightened by the idea of snake venom. Remind them that many people have been bitten by far more venomous snakes and have lived to tell the tale. If you have been bitten by a snake in a foreign country, try to remember what it looked like—a good description will save a great deal of medical time.

DO apply calamine lotion or cream to insect bites or stings, including those from gnats and fleas. Antihistamine cream is no longer recommended for home use.

DO get medical help quickly in the following instances:
1. Stings inside the mouth
2. The patient is allergic
3. Signs of shock—pallor, sweating, collapse, and breathing difficulties
4. Stinging by swarms of insects

DON'T apply vinegar to wasp stings or ammonia to bee stings, since these are no longer considered useful remedies.

DON'T use tweezers to remove a bee sting. This will only put pressure on the sting itself and cause it to release more venom. Use a fingernail or credit card.

DON'T treat snakebites by cutting the area, trying to suck out the venom, or applying a tourniquet. These "wild West" treatments can actually aggravate the wound.

Prickly plants

- Plants with prickles and thorns do not sting, but if they break the skin, infections such as tetanus can result. Thorns should be pulled out with fine tweezers. If they are deeply embedded, apply a small dressing and see a doctor or nurse.
- Stings from poison ivy should be washed with hot water and soap. Calamine lotion may help to relieve the discomfort. Cacti can leave fine needles embedded in the skin. Press adhesive bandage or tape onto the affected area, then lift off to remove prickles.

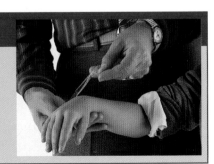

Take note

- In the case of a sting inside the mouth, medical aid should be sought immediately. The mouth may swell and breathing can be impaired as a result. While you are waiting for help, swelling can be minimized by using cold mouthwashes, sucking ice cubes, or even eating popsicles.

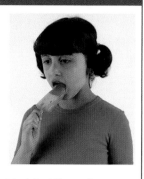

- The risk of infection is high with any animal bite, so always consult a doctor. This is particularly important if there is even the slightest risk of rabies. If the attacking animal was thought to be rabid, go to the hospital immediately. Report the animal to the local health department so that it can be caught and tested. People helping a victim should take care not to infect themselves.

- If jellyfish tentacles stick to a sting, cover with vinegar and flour, or with wet sand. Using the flat of a knife blade, scrape the sand off the area and wash with rubbing alcohol.

- If you cannot scrape a bee sting out using a fingernail or credit card, you can use a sterilized needle or pin. Hold the pointed end in the blue part of the flame from a lighter or match; this will sterilize the point.

- Ticks are parasites that feed on humans, dogs, and other warm-blooded vertebrates. Some ticks are harmless, but others can transmit disease to humans. A tick must be removed promptly. Cover it with mineral oil or alcohol to immobilize it, and then gently remove with a pair of tweezers, ensuring that the head is completely removed. Wash the area with soap and water, and cover with a bandage. Consult a doctor if fever, rash, or aches and pains occur.

▼ *A picnic in the backyard is one of the delights of childhood. However, it is important for parents to be aware that the undergrowth may contain creatures that bite or sting. Wearing shoes or sandals is a sensible measure.*

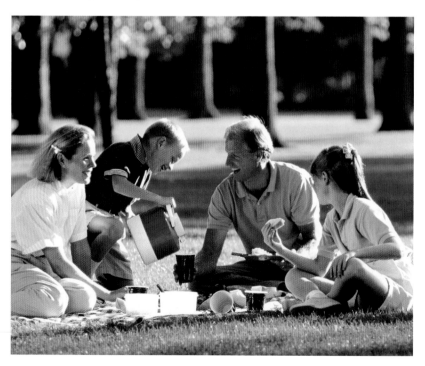

Checklist

1. Make sure that the patient does not scratch the affected area. The irritation and itchiness can be very annoying, but scratching or rubbing often only makes it more intolerable. It also helps to spread the venom, and it certainly increases the chances of developing an infection. A rash may take some time to appear; if a rash does occur, calamine lotion or 1 percent hydrocortisone can help to reduce irritation.

2. Any pain resulting from bites and stings usually resolves itself quickly within the following hour or two. If you do want to take some sort of painkiller, acetaminophen or ibuprofen may speed up the relief of pain. The pain caused by venomous snakebites tends to get progressively worse for some time after the incident, so it is important to give the patient anti-snakebite serum (antivenin) as soon as possible. This should be accompanied by other drugs, such as epinephrine or steroids, to prevent an adverse reaction to the serum. These should always be administered by a doctor.

3. The risk of infection is always high, particularly with bites. If the punctured area becomes red, swollen, harder, or more painful over the next couple of days, it is probably infected, and a doctor should be consulted. It is always sensible to call the emergency service or visit a doctor in the case of animal bites and snakebites, because infections or other complications are likely.

4. Shock can be caused by any form of bite or sting, no matter how minor. It is especially likely if the victim is elderly or very young, but any patient may suffer an allergic reaction to the venom, or just be very frightened. Always treat for shock (see Shock). Send for medical help as quickly as possible, but do not leave the patient alone. Keep the affected area immobilized.

5. Although plant and animal poisons have different constituents, they all contain a substance called histamine, which can produce symptoms that vary from rashes to serious breathing difficulties. In more severe cases, a doctor may administer an antihistamine by either pill or injection. Antihistamine is effective in alleviating the irritation and itching from bites or stings. It blocks the action of the chemical histamine, which the body releases in an allergic response to certain substances.

Bleeding

- Wear protective plastic gloves
- Apply pressure to the wound with your hand to stop the bleeding
- Unless it is known that there is a fracture, raise the injured part to diminish the force of the blood flow at the injury
- Maintain pressure even after a clot has formed
- Move the limb as little as possible, since there may be further injuries

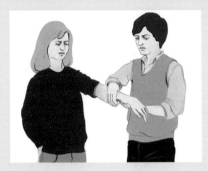

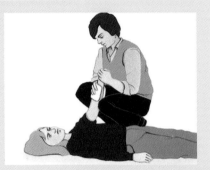

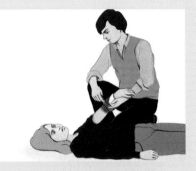

1. Stanch the bleeding by placing your gloved hand immediately over the wound and applying firm pressure; or, if this is easier and equally effective, pinch the edges of the wound firmly together.

2. Lay the patient down and raise his or her arm. Maintaining pressure all the time, use your free hand to make any available material (such as a handkerchief) into a pad. Hold firmly over the wound.

3. Still maintaining pressure, find other material (such as a belt, scarf, or tie) that will act as a bandage. Wrap this tightly around the pad, and secure it with a very firm knot.

What to do in an emergency

Coughing up blood
Place patient in recovery position (see Unconsciousness), but if breathing is difficult, prop up him or her on pillows. If you know from which side the blood is coming, let the patient lie toward that side. Clean away any blood from the mouth. Get medical aid quickly. Any blood coughed up must be reported to a doctor.

Vomiting blood
Place the patient in the recovery position. Clear away any vomit from the mouth. Get medical aid or an ambulance urgently. Keep the vomit for a doctor to examine.

Blood that collects for some time in the stomach before being vomited will be acted on by digestive juices, which will alter its color to brown or black. If red blood is vomited, the bleeding is probably severe and fast.

Slight but sustained bleeding in the stomach will give rise not to vomiting but to black, tarry-looking stools. This situation also requires medical attention.

Internal bleeding
Pain or discomfort can be deceptively slight. If the patient shows signs of shock (faintness, pallor, coldness, sweating, thirst, fast and weak pulse and breathing), place him or her in the recovery position or with the head low and legs raised. Loosen tight clothes and cover him or her with a blanket. Give no additional heat, and nothing by mouth. Send for urgent medical help or an ambulance.

Take note

- Keep checking on a bleeding patient for signs of shock. In an extreme case, he or she will be faint, pale, cold, sweating, and thirsty with a rapid, shallow pulse and breathing rate. At worst, breathing is labored and gasping.
- If any of the above signs appear in a patient without visible injury, suspect internal bleeding.
- Be suspicious of an external blow that has left no significant mark on the skin, but has had the force to imprint a pattern of bruising from overlying objects, such as a buckle or pocket contents. In such a case there may be internal damage with bleeding.
- Stomach bleeding is obvious if the patient vomits blood. The color of the blood depends on how long it has been in the stomach. It may be brown or black and resemble coffee grounds; this indicates that stomach acids have broken it down. Red blood indicates a severe type of internal hemorrhage.

Different types of bleeding

Bleeding from a palm
Keep the patient's arm raised. Make a thick pad from material available and get the patient to clench his or her fist around this. Make an improvised bandage, wrap it firmly around the pad, and knot it securely at the back of the hand.

Nosebleed
Make the patient sit up and bend forward, and pinch the lower half of his or her nose just above the nostrils between finger and thumb for at least 10 minutes without letting go. If necessary, the patient can spit out any blood from the mouth into a bowl. When bleeding has lessened, tip the head backward, maintaining pressure with finger and thumb. Do not let the patient blow his or her nose or sniff. A nosebleed after a blow on the head could be due to a skull injury, so, if appropriate, get immediate medical help.

Bleeding from a tooth socket
This might happen after a tooth extraction. Make the patient bite hard for at least 10 minutes on a thick pad placed over, but not into, the socket. If the patient cups his or her hand under the chin, with the elbow resting on a table, this will help to maintain pressure and be less tiring. Bleeding from the mouth usually looks worse than it is.

Bleeding from the tongue
Sit the patient up, bending forward. Grip the tongue firmly between finger and thumb with a clean handkerchief. Keep up the pressure for 10 minutes, letting the patient take the grip him- or herself.

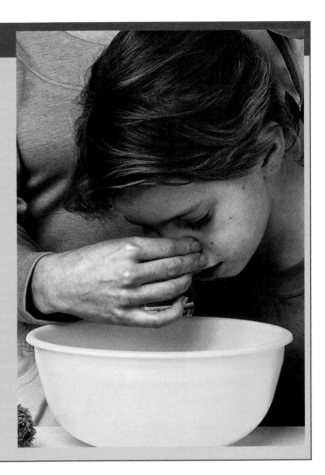

Dos and don'ts

DO tie the bandage firmly, much more so than you would to secure an ordinary dressing. Once the affected area has been bandaged, check the circulation and ensure that the bandage is not too tight. Check by pressing an area of skin until it looks pale. On release, the color should return at once, if it does not, the bandage is too tight and should be loosened. Circulation should be checked every 10 minutes or so. Watch for signs that the patient's fingers or toes are becoming pale and cold and unable to move. Even with severe bleeding, never apply a tourniquet.

DO get the patient to lie down, or at least sit down, as soon as possible, and then make sure he or she is not moved again.

DON'T waste time washing your hands or looking for orthodox sterile dressings. Speed is the priority; the risk of hemorrhage is far greater than the risk of infection.

DON'T ask the patient to use his or her hand to exert pressure—he or she may be too weak to do so.

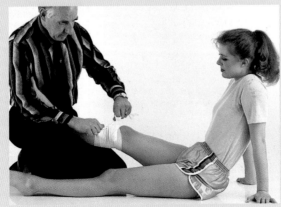

Checklist

1. The risk of shock is high when the patient has lost a lot of blood, so keep him or her warmly but loosely covered; stay with the patient and give reassurance. Keep checking for signs of shock: they are restlessness or irritability; altered consciousness; nausea; pale or ashen, cool, moist skin; rapid breathing; and rapid pulse. Shock can be life-threatening.

2. In severe cases of bleeding, get emergency medical care or call an ambulance immediately and give details of the accident.

3. Let the patient lie quietly and avoid any movement of the injured part; keep the limb elevated and immobilized. Lying down can help minimize pain.

4. Keep a close watch on the bandage. If there are signs of renewed bleeding, do not remove it, but apply more pressure; make another pad and bandage and apply these over the first bandage.

Burns

- If there are flames, smother with cloth or water, and get medical aid

In the event of ordinary household burns:
- To cool the burn, cover it with a thick cloth soaked in cold water or place it in a cold tub
- When the burn is cool, cover it with a clean, dry dressing, and guard against shock
- Lay patient down and call the ambulance or a doctor

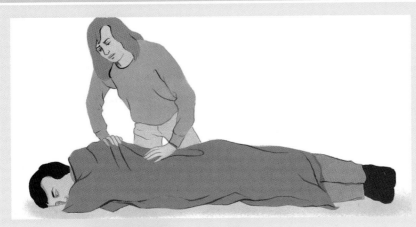

If the patient's clothes are on fire, lay him or her down and smother the flames by pressing down with any thick cloth (towel, curtain, rug, or jacket) that is nearby. Protect the patient's face by bringing the cloth down to fan the fire away from the head and toward the feet. Wrap the cloth firmly around the patient, but don't roll him or her around on the floor. This would expose other parts of the body to the flames. Once the fire is out, pull away charred or smoldering cloth. Leave anything sticking to the skin alone.

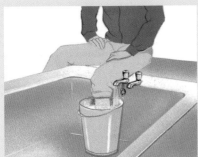

1. Plunge the burned limb into cold water and keep the cold tap running. Immerse it for at least 10 minutes. Or cover the area with a thick cloth soaked in water. Keep it damp.

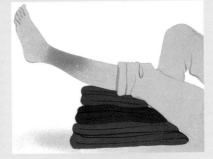

2. In severe cases, keep the patient lying down. If the face is burned, have the patient sit up. Elevate a burned limb to reduce swelling. A leg can be kept high by placing it on pillows.

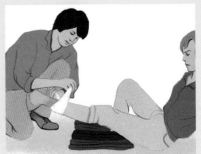

3. Cover the burned area with a clean, dry dressing (see Wounds), which is bandaged or strapped on lightly once the area has been well cooled. Do not apply lotions or ointments.

Dos and don'ts

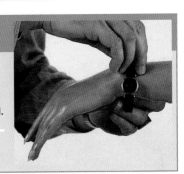

DO remove anything that might constrict if the burned part swells—for example, rings.

DO keep a burned limb elevated to reduce swelling.

DO get someone whose clothes are on fire to cover the face, drop to the floor, and roll around.

DON'T pull away anything that is stuck to the area that has been burned, and never apply any creams or ointments to the burn.

Take note

- Scalds are due to moist heat, such as steam or boiling water. Clothes saturated in steam, boiling water, or hot fat will continue to burn the skin unless they are taken off quickly. For a scalded throat, cool fast with mouthfuls of cold water or by sucking ice.
- Dry heat burns come from flames or from contact with hot objects. Friction can cause burns, as in sliding down a rope using firmly closed hands. Electricity can also cause deep burns.
- Corrosive chemicals such as strong acids can burn severely. For chemical burns, dilute and wash away the substance with lots of water until you are confident that it has all gone. Remove any contaminated clothing. For chemicals in the eye turn the patient, lying down, on the affected side. Gently pull open the eyelids. Pour streams of water into and over the eye to wash out the chemical. Cover with a clean, dry pad. Seek medical help. It is important to act as quickly as possible.
- The significant damage in burns is beneath the skin where the heat is retained. Apart from tissue destruction, the major effect is dilation of the blood vessels, which allows plasma to ooze from them, forming blisters. If the skin surface has been destroyed there will be no cover to hold in the fluid, and the plasma loss can be considerable. The risk of shock is high and must be guarded against. Fluid loss can be offset by frequently giving the patient small amounts of sweetened water.

Checklist

1. Get anyone who has been badly burned or scalded to the hospital as soon as possible. In young children and infants, even small burns should be regarded as very serious. Call an ambulance: it is speedier and allows the patient to remain lying down. If he or she continues to complain of severe pain during transit to the hospital, keep a cold wet cloth on the burned area. Reassure the patient at all times during the journey.

2. With any large burn there is a real risk of shock, and you should follow the advice given in the section on shock in this handbook. In such cases the depth of the burn is not as significant as the surface area affected: the greater the area of skin involved, the greater the volume of plasma oozing from the damaged vessels, and the higher the risk of shock.

3. The burn can be cooled either by immersing it in cold water (never use ice water or put ice directly on the skin), putting it under gently running cold water, or covering it with a cold, clean, wet dressing. If a blister forms, leave it alone. Avoid breathing or coughing on the burn, as this could contaminate it. After the burn has been cooled, pat the area dry and cover it with a dry, clean (preferably sterile) nonadhesive dressing Avoid using fluffy materials; plastic wrap can be used as a temporary dressing.

4. Burns offer an exception to the general first-aid rule of not giving anything by mouth to the injured person. Here you may give the patient about half a glassful of tepid water every 15 or 20 minutes. The water may be sweetened slightly, but remember that fluids can cause vomiting when the patient is suffering from shock. The liquid helps to replace body fluids that have been lost as a result of plasma loss caused by the burn.

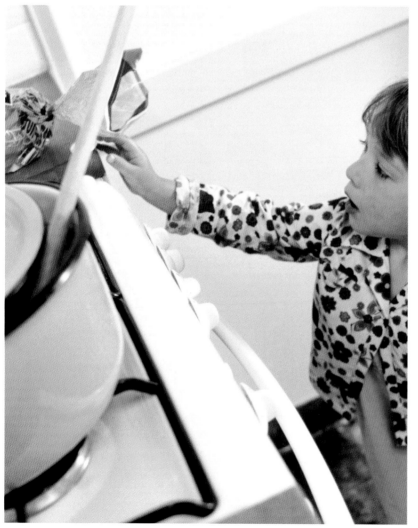

◀ *This child is in danger of suffering a serious but common injury: a bad scald. Make sure that kettles, teapots, saucepans, and the like are kept well out of the reach of inquisitive hands—away from the edge of a table or work surface. Don't place hot containers on placemats, tablecloths, or dish towels, where they can be pulled off easily, and never leave cookies or candies near teapots or kettles. A child will simply be blind to the dangers and, in his or her haste to reach the cookies, may knock the boiling liquid over and sustain an injury.*

Car accidents

- Search the area for any people thrown from the vehicles
- Establish an order of priority for treatment among the victims
- Treat patients for breathing, bleeding, and unconsciousness
- Delegate traffic control to an onlooker
- Send for emergency services, giving thorough details of the accident

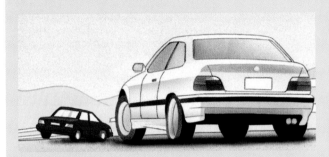

1. Stop your car a short distance away and park well into the side of the road. Turn on hazard lights and headlights to help you see exactly what has happened.

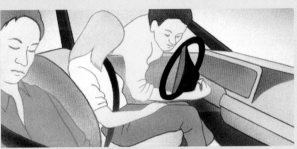

2. Extinguish any smoke coming from vehicles, but leave victims in position unless fire is a risk. Prevent further damage by immobilizing vehicles.

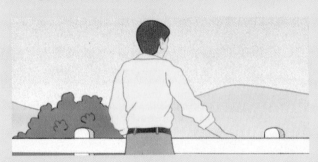

3. Look for victims who might have been thrown from the vehicles—for example, into ditches or over fences. If you have a cellular phone, call the emergency services.

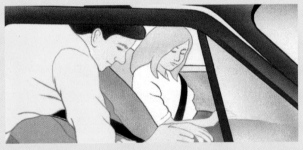

4. Treat victims in order of priority. Deal with breathing, bleeding, and unconsciousness in that order (see Bleeding; Unconsciousness). Move the victims as little as possible.

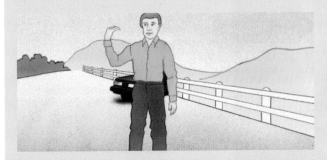

5. Use any onlookers as traffic controllers. Have them stand about 200 yards (65 meters) from the site of the accident and make sure they are clearly visible to oncoming drivers.

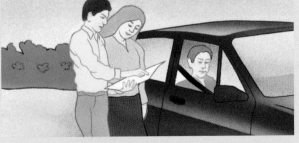

6. Send the first available person for emergency services, giving information about the location, number of vehicles involved, and details of any injured people.

Always be prepared

You should always carry a first aid kit in your car. Many of the accident victims who die before reaching the hospital could have been saved if simple first-aid measures had been taken promptly, so being prepared can be extremely vital. If you carry your own kit, you will be able to give thorough first aid to the victims of an accident that you come across; the kit will also be available should you be involved in an accident yourself.

The first aid kit should be kept in a clearly marked waterproof case, preferably in the glove compartment. The kit should include the following:

- packs of gauze and cotton
- 2- and 3-in. (5- and 7.5-cm) bandages
- medium and large sterile dressings
- a large flashlight (renew batteries every 2 to 3 months)
- a pair of protective rubber gloves
- a large pair of scissors
- pen and paper for messages

If possible, you should also carry a small fire extinguisher.

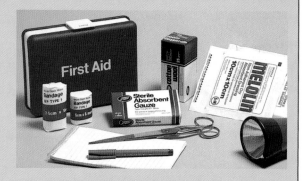

Checklist

1. While you are waiting for the emergency services to arrive, try to discourage other motorists and passersby from hanging around unless they can offer expert or practical help.

2. Keep the area between your car and the crash clear at all times so that the emergency services can stop safely near the accident.

3. Stay with the accident victims until the paramedics arrive. Watch the victims carefully to ensure that breathing does not stop, bleeding does not resume, and no one loses consciousness. Try to be calm and reassuring.

4. Use any spare time to gather information for the emergency services. Collect names and addresses from the least injured victims and take a note of the vehicle licence plates. If victims are unconscious, look for any medical information they may have on them in the way of bracelets, necklaces, or cards. Give the information to the police and paramedics when they arrive, along with any first aid measures that you have taken and any other useful observations.

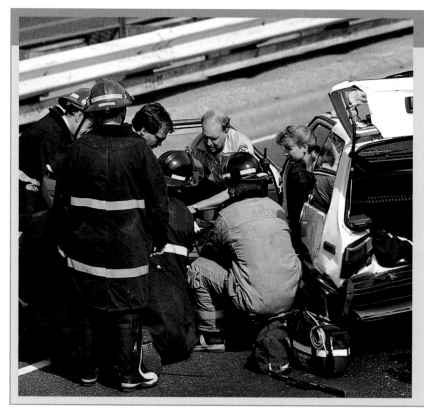

Dos and don'ts

DO ensure that there are no more accident victims in the area. Park your car a short distance away and well off the road. Make sure that the passing traffic is aware that an accident has occurred by asking onlookers to control the traffic.

DO check that all the vehicles are safe— switch off the ignition, apply the brakes, and, if possible, put the car in gear.

DO use any available material, such as car mats or coats, to keep the victims warm. If they are suffering from shock, however, you must avoid overheating them.

DON'T move accident victims from vehicles unless there is a danger of fire. It is a natural human tendency, but you may waste valuable time and even exacerbate existing injuries. The rescue services have special tools to cut people out of damaged vehicles, and this difficult task is best left for them to deal with.

DON'T ever smoke anywhere near the location of the car crash—leaking gasoline may catch fire.

Choking

- As long as the patient can cough vigorously, do not interfere
- If the patient cannot cough, alternate blows to the back with abdominal thrusts
- Should the patient collapse, give artificial respiration
- When airways are completely blocked, try to remove the obstruction
- Have a doctor examine the patient if blows or thrusts have been used

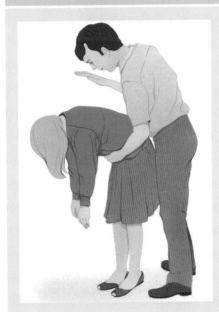

1. If the patient is not able to dislodge the object by coughing, bend him or her over and slap with the heel of your hand between the shoulder blades.

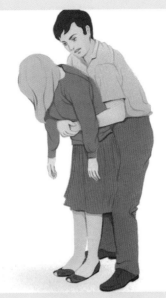

2. If four backslaps fail to loosen the object, give abdominal thrusts. Should the obstruction remain, try alternating back slaps with thrusts.

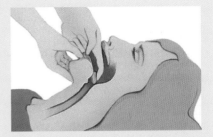

3. If the patient's airways are obstructed and you cannot get air into the lungs by artificial respiration, you must find and remove the object (see Artificial Respiration). Place a curved finger into the mouth, ensuring that the patient does not bite you, and probe the area gently. Do not ram the finger straight in, since this might push the object deeper into the throat. Start at the side of the cheek, moving the finger to the back of the mouth, then hook the finger forward to dislodge the object. Pull the object out quickly, so that the patient cannot suck it back into the throat.

Dos and don'ts

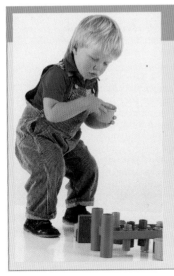

DO stay with the patient, even if he or she is able to speak and cough.

DO try to keep the patient as calm as possible. If the irritating object is in the throat, the trachea (windpipe), which is encircled by muscles, will react by going into spasm. Any anxiety on the part of the patient could increase the tension of the muscles, and the problem will worsen, since the object causing the obstruction is held more tightly.

DO give very hard blows high on the back if this is necessary. Most people do not appreciate how hard these should be to dislodge the object. If you have had to give back blows or abdominal thrusts, ensure that the patient is checked by a doctor. Both processes can cause internal damage.

DO make sure that small children are provided with safe toys. Avoid those with any small parts that can be easily removed and inhaled. Keep all small objects well out of a baby's or toddler's reach. At these ages, most children are particularly likely to put anything into their mouths.

DON'T resort to backslaps and abdominal thrusts before allowing the patient to try to dislodge the object by coughing vigorously. The object may be dislodged easily.

Take note

- If the patient can still speak to you, despite coughing, stand by. Encourage but do not interfere. Advise him or her to try separate heavy coughs with slow inhalation.
- Should this technique fail, bend the patient forward and give him or her a hard blow between the shoulder blades with the heel of your hand. If one blow fails, try up to four blows. This can be done when the patient is standing or sitting. If the patient is on the ground, turn him or her on one side.
- Bend a child over your lap or lay him or her along a thigh. Lay a baby along your arm, head down, and supporting the head and chest.
- If the object is still in place and the older child or adult is weakening, give abdominal thrusts. Encircle patient's waist from behind. Place one fist, thumb side first, halfway between the navel and lower end of the breastbone. Cup your hand over the fist and give a hard thrust (inward and a little upward). This may shoot the obstruction into or out of the mouth. If one thrust fails, try up to four.
- If the patient is on the ground, turn him or her onto his or her back and kneel astride his or her thighs. Place the heel of one hand halfway between the navel and the lower end of the breastbone. Place the heel of the other hand over the first, and continue as above.
- In the case of a baby, hold him or her faceup and head down. Support the head. Place your other hand along the end of his or her sternum and press with your fingers up to four times.
- If necessary, alternate five back blows with five abdominal thrusts.
- If the patient stops breathing, start artificial respiration.

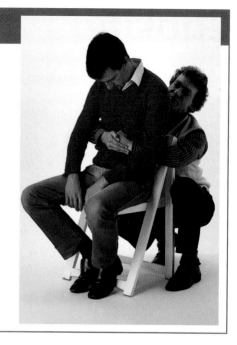

Checklist

1. When something "goes down the wrong way," it can obstruct the back of the throat or it could have moved a little farther down and be blocking the windpipe.

2. If the obstructing object comes free and moves into the patient's mouth, seize it and pull it out quickly so that the patient's next sudden breath will not suck it back in again.

3. If the patient feels faint or vomits, put him or her in the recovery position (see Unconsciousness).

4. If you have used the abdominal thrust, you must watch your patient carefully, even if he or she seems fit again.

5. Even if the patient seems fine, he or she should be seen by a doctor or sent to the hospital for observation as soon as possible, particularly if he or she is still coughing intermittently. In rare cases, the thrust damages an internal organ and medical treatment will then be necessary. This is a calculated risk you must take—the alternative might be suffocation and death.

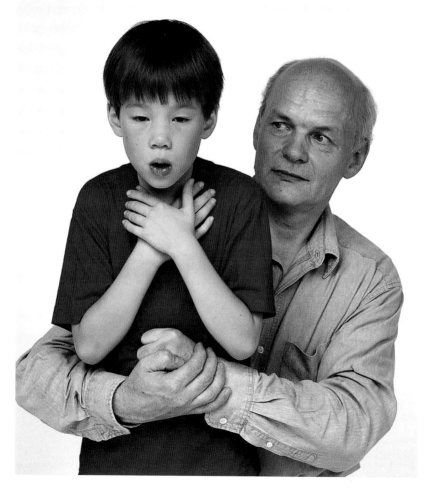

◄ *If a child is choking and four backslaps have failed to dislodge the object, encircle the child's waist from behind, cup your hand over your fist, and give a hard thrust.*

Convulsions

- Call an ambulance immediately
- Don't try to control thrashing limbs; surround patient with cushions
- When the jerking stops, keep the head tipped well back
- If the patient is uninjured and safe to move, place him or her in the recovery position

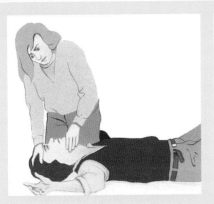

1. The patient lies rigid. To ensure a clear airway, the head should be tipped well back. Any tight clothes should already have been eased. Remember that the patient may have sustained an injury in falling.

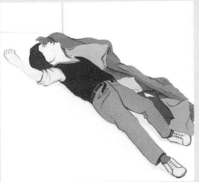

2. When convulsions start, do not attempt to control thrashing limbs. Instead, surround the patient with soft buffers to protect him or her from self-inflicted injuries and move dangerous objects out of reach.

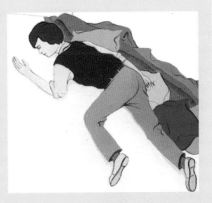

3. The patient stops jerking and relaxes, but remains unconscious. Keep the head tilted back, and look for injuries. If it is safe to do so, put the patient on one side in the recovery position.

Fever convulsions

- A child aged six months to five years with a high fever may have a brief convulsion.
- Tip the head back, and put him or her in the recovery position. Take off his or her clothes and cool him or her with a cold, wet sponge. Check his or her temperature with a thermometer in the armpit and try to reduce it by 1 or 2 degrees.
- Get medical attention as soon as possible. After recovery, keep the child lightly covered.

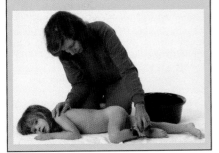

Dos and don'ts

DO check if the person has a medical tag stating that he or she is epileptic.

DO stay by the person's side until his or her recovery or until expert medical attention has arrived.

DO ease any tight clothing at the start of the convulsion. Tip the person's head well back to ensure that he or she does not choke during the attack.

DO mop away any froth that has come from the patient's mouth during the course of the convulsion.

DON'T try to control jerking or thrashing limbs. Just try to prevent self-inflicted injuries by moving furniture and other hard objects out of the way.

DON'T attempt to push anything between the teeth.

Take note

- An epileptic attack or a child's feverish convulsion may be alarming, but generally such seizures are short-lived.
- Most attacks of convulsion come without warning and the patient will usually fall unconscious. He or she may cry out and not be aware of doing so.
- The patient begins jerking limbs and face or thrashing about—this can last 30 seconds. There may be frothing at the mouth and breath holding, and the patient may bite his or her tongue, or may be incontinent.
- When the patient stops jerking, he or she will remain unconscious for some minutes. When the patient comes to, perhaps drowsily, he or she may wave any helping hands away. Many epileptics prefer to take care of themselves after an attack.
- Unless there are familiar people to look after the patient, you should get him or her to the hospital—by ambulance, if this is at all possible.

CPR (cardiopulmonary resuscitation)

- CPR, or heart compression, should be learned through formal instruction
- If the patient is not breathing, begin CPR, which alone may be sufficient to start circulation and promote sufficient air flow; this is more effective with two people
- Continue to alternate heart compression and respiration until the patient shows signs of recovery or until medical help arrives

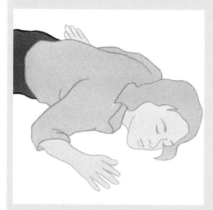

1. Start by sending someone for help. If the patient is breathing, place him or her in the recovery position (above). If there is no movement, no breathing, and no response to any stimulus, start heart compression at once. Do not waste time trying to find a pulse in the neck or doing artificial respiration.

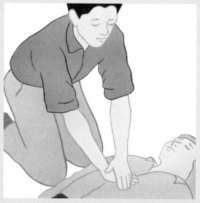

2. Kneel beside the patient, placing the heel of one hand on top of the other. Using the full weight of your body, apply pressure to the lower part of the breastbone, clear of the victim's ribs. If you are alone, the rate of compression should be 100 per minute, giving two breaths after every 30 compressions.

With two rescuers

If CPR is prolonged, two people will be needed to sustain the treatment. Effective heart compression needs a lot of energy, so get help. One rescuer should perform artificial resuscitation while the other carries out heart compression (see Artificial Respiration). The ratio should be 30 compressions and two breaths for adults but 15 compressions and two breaths for children and infants. The two rescuers should switch tasks every two minutes.

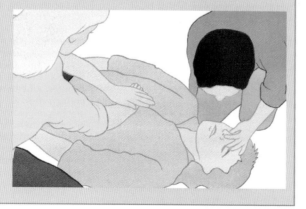

Take note

- Cardiopulmonary resuscitation is a life-support technique that is difficult to carry out effectively without proper training. Thus, although CPR can be performed following the instructions described here, the procedure is best learned by following a formal first-aid course.
- When attempting resuscitation, always follow the basic ABC of priorities: airway, breathing, and circulation.
- When performing CPR, position your shoulders directly over your hands and keep your arms straight and elbows locked, so that the whole of your body weight goes into each compression. Make sure that compressions are carried out smoothly and evenly.
- If you are performing heart compression on children, you will need much less force. With very small children, during resuscitation you may find it more effective to blow into both nose and mouth simultaneously.

Checklist

1. Make sure that the patient is lying down on a firm, level surface. CPR is much less effective if the patient is in a sitting position or if he or she is lying on a soft surface such as mattress.

2. To find the correct position for your hands to enable you to perform heart compressions, search for the notch at the lower end of the patient's breastbone, where it meets the ribs. Put your middle finger on the notch and your index finger next to your middle finger. Place the heel of one hand above your middle finger and your other hand directly on top of the first hand.

3. Use only the heel of your hand when making heart compressions, not the fingers. To keep your fingers out of the way, interlock them together or stick them up and away from the hand.

4. Recheck for signs of circulation and breathing only after you have done three cycles of 30 compressions and two rescue breaths. The check should last no more than 10 seconds.

Electric shock

- Turn the electricity off at the fuse box
- Do not touch the victim until you have done this
- Check that the victim is breathing
- Use artificial respiration if necessary
- Check for bleeding and bone fractures
- Treat any burns by cooling
- Send for medical help urgently

GENERAL POINTS

- The vast majority of electrical injuries occur in the home, so make sure that your electrical appliances and home wiring are in good working order.
- Do not touch a shock victim until he or she has been separated from the current, or the electricity supply has been turned off. Otherwise, you too may receive a shock.
- If you cannot turn the current off, use a dry implement made of nonconductive material, such as a broom or chair, to separate the victim from the live apparatus. Act quickly.
- When the victim is free, check that he or she is breathing. He or she may need artificial respiration at once (see Artificial Respiration).
- Try to ascertain the extent of the injury. A severe shock will cause burns and even cuts and fractures if the victim has fallen or been thrown. Use a dry dressing to protect cuts and burns (see Wounds). If burns are minor, cool them (see Burns).
- Immediately call for an ambulance. Stay with the victim. Watch for signs of collapse (pallor and sweating) until the ambulance arrives. Place the victim in the recovery position.

Dos and don'ts

DO turn off the main electricity supply before starting any work on the house wiring circuit, and always disconnect any appliance that you are about to repair.

DON'T ever handle any switches, plugs, or appliances with wet hands. If plugs or appliances become wet, unplug them and dry them off well before plugging them back in.

DON'T try to overload sockets with adapters. Try to have only one appliance per socket, and remember to disconnect plug when not in use.

DON'T ever try to rescue the victim of a high-voltage shock unless he or she has been thrown at least 50 feet (15 meters) away from the source. This type of hazard exists in some factories and roadside pylons.

If you discover the victim of an electric shock, do not touch him or her until he or she is separated from the current, as you may receive an equally forceful shock yourself. Turn off the electricity supply immediately. If this is not possible, separate the victim from the live apparatus by means of a dry implement made of nonconductive material—the wooden handle of a broom is ideal. Once the victim is free, check to see if he or she is breathing: the victim may need urgent artificial respiration.

Checklist

1. After sending for an ambulance, keep a close eye on the patient. Do not allow crowds to gather around him or her; do make sure he or she is warm and comfortable; and watch for signs of deterioration.

2. If the victim stops breathing at any time, then give artificial respiration either until he or she starts breathing again or until the ambulance arrives.

3. If the heart stops beating, give heart compression. This is best learned in a first aid class, but in a life-or-death situation follow the steps given in this first aid handbook (see CPR).

4. If the victim's breathing and heartbeat appear to recover, then lay the victim on his or her stomach, turn the head to one side, and draw up the arm and leg on that side— that is, place the victim in the recovery position (see Unconsciousness).

Falls

- Don't try to pick the patient up immediately, but check for injuries
- If a fracture is suspected, don't move the patient
- If the patient is uninjured, help him or her onto all fours, placing a stool in front of the patient. Get him or her to bend one knee and lean forward. Move to one side, and help the patient to push him- or herself up

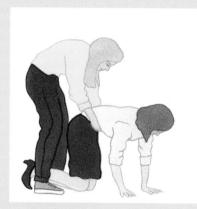

1. Clear the area of any extraneous objects. If the patient has use of arms and legs, turn him or her facedown. Stand over the patient's legs and help him or her onto all fours.

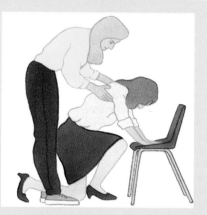

2. Place a stool or chair in front of the patient. Help the patient to put his or her hands on the seat. Still straddling the patient's legs, get him or her to bend one knee and lean forward.

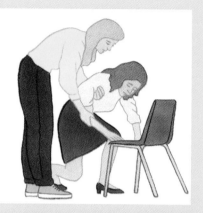

3. Move to one side of the patient. Put one hand in the armpit on that side and the other on the elbow. Gently help the patient to push him- or herself up, using the chair for additional support.

Take note

- Before trying to pick the patient up, it is essential to ascertain whether he or she is conscious—and if so, to ask him or her if there is any pain—and to establish whether he or she has sustained any injuries. Check for bleeding, wounds, or fractures (see Fractures).
- Consider whether it is safe to move the patient. This will not be advisable if there is any chance of a fracture—a fall from a height, a blow to the back, or pain in the back or neck may indicate a fractured spine. If you suspect this, don't move the victim. Make him or her comfortable and call for medical help.
- If you have decided that the patient can be moved but you need help, spread out a blanket and with someone's aid, roll him or her onto the center. Rolling each edge toward the patient, grasp the blanket firmly, one person at each end, and carry him or her to a couch or bed.

Dos and don'ts

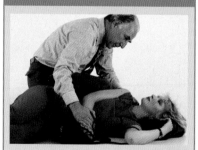

DO examine the patient carefully for injuries; give treatment when appropriate. When lifting him or her, have regard for your own back: lift correctly and as gently as possible.

DON'T attempt to move the patient if there is the slightest chance that he or she may have sustained a fracture. Leave the patient where he or she is until expert help arrives.

Checklist

1. If the patient's condition is uncertain, get a doctor, especially if the patient is unconscious, has difficulty moving a part of the body, or seems to have developed a psychological change—owing to a blow to the head, for example.

2. If the patient's legs are weak, get the patient to sit on the floor and place a low stool behind him or her. Have the patient place his or her hands on the seat and bend forward; the patient can then use his or her arms to push up and sit on the stool. Put a higher stool or chair behind the first one; repeat the maneuver to get him or her sitting on this one. The elderly and the weak, in particular, may need more help in getting up after a fall.

3. Ask yourself why the patient fell. If general weakness was the cause, discuss medication or the need for a walker with the doctor.

Fractures

- Keep the patient still and cover him or her with a blanket
- Attend to such injuries as an open wound or bleeding before dealing with the fracture
- If necessary, protect the broken bone
- Stay with the patient, and make him or her comfortable until professional help arrives

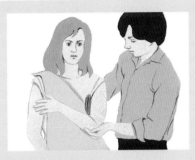

1. Simple arm sling: support elbow, keeping hand raised. Pass bandage between chest and arm.

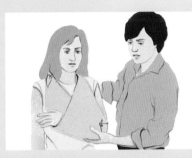

2. Bring bandage over forearm and around back of neck; tie together over hollow above clavicle. Pin at the elbow.

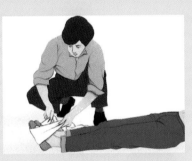

3. Figure-eight bandage: place patient's feet together. Lay middle of bandage across the soles of the feet.

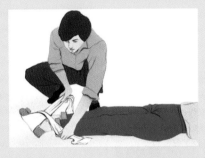

4. Bring ends of bandage to front of feet and cross over insteps. Wrap again by carrying ends to back of ankles.

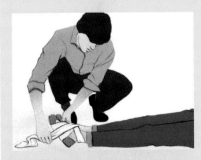

5. Cross ends and bring them back to front of ankle. Cross again. Take ends back under soles; tie ends in place.

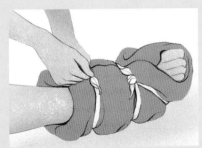

6. Foot-and-ankle bandage: use folded cloth or flat cushion around ankle and foot, then tie with narrow bandages.

445

Immobilizing fractures

Jaw:
Gently clear mouth of any blood or dentures. Put thick pad under and around jaw. (Patient's cupped hand can support it temporarily.) Secure by placing bandage over pad; bring ends up over ears and tie on top of patient's head.

Clavicle:
Keep point of elbow supported until sling can hold it; support arm on side of fracture with a sling (see page 445, figures 1 and 2). Place soft pad under armpit. Secure upper arm against chest: place wide bandage over arm and across back and chest, and tie under armpit on unaffected side.

Leg:
Keep patient lying down. Place padding between legs from groin to just above ankles. Put bandage around knees and tie on side. Make figure-eight bandage around feet and ankles (see page 445, figures 3, 4, and 5).

Arm:
If elbow can be bent without pain, place pad in armpit and support forearm with sling (see page 445, figures 1 and 2). Ensure that forearm slopes slightly upward. If elbow is straight and painful to bend, keep patient lying down. Place padding between arm and body. Secure arm to body with three wide bandages (as for clavicle, figures 1 and 2).

Foot and ankle:
Wrap folded cloth around foot. Secure with narrow bandages (see page 445, figure 6).

Checklist

1. In the case of a broken backbone, the fracture of a vertebra might create loose pieces of bone that could enter the spinal cord, causing permanent paralysis and loss of feeling. If there is any possibility of such a fracture, leave the patient as you found him or her and wait for professional assistance.

2. Deciding whether someone has broken a bone can be difficult—many of the classical features of a fracture can also indicate other injuries, such as a sprain. For example, an initial symptom that is common in a fracture is pain. Yet a severe contusion, without a break, can be extremely painful, and sometimes a major fracture hurts only a little. Restricted movement of the injured part and swelling of tissues in the area can be symptomatic of both sprains and fractures. Also, many fractures retain the broken bone ends in good anatomic position so that another classical feature, deformity, is not always present.

3. In diagnosing a fracture, the history of the injury should be taken into account. The likelihood of bone damage is high if there was a considerable force, such as a hard blow or a fall. Yet this can be deceptive, too, since diseased bones—or, in the elderly, brittle ones—can break relatively easily. However, anyone who administers first aid can do no harm by suspecting a fracture when circumstances suggest it, and thus acting accordingly.

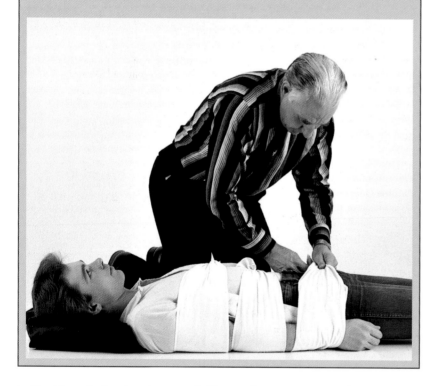

▶ *If a triangular bandage is not available, an adequate emergency sling can be rapidly improvised from clothing. The patient's arm can be placed inside the shirt, supported by the fastened buttons. A necktie can be used, or the hem of the patient's jacket can be taken up over the fractured arm and then pinned to a lapel.*

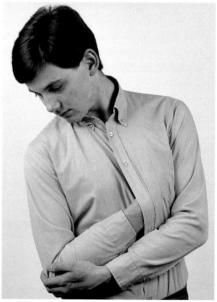

Heart attack

- Call or send for an ambulance immediately
- Place the patient in a resting position
- Keep the upper part of the body raised
- Loosen any tight clothing at neck and waist
- If breathing stops, give artificial respiration
- Keep patient warm by covering with a blanket

When a person suffers a heart attack, prompt action is of crucial importance. Make sure you perform the following in the correct order:

1. Call or send someone for an ambulance. Specify the nature of the problem.

2. Give the patient an aspirin.

3. Place the patient in a resting position at once—in bed, on a sofa, or in an armchair.

4. Loosen clothes at the neck and waist.

5. If the patient appears very breathless, let him or her sit up against a headboard banked with pillows. The headboard can be improvised with a light chair set upside down against the wall.

6. If there is nothing suitable against which the patient can rest, use your body as a prop.

7. Keep him or her loosely covered. Open the window so that the room is well ventilated.

8. Alleviate the patient's fears by keeping a calm and sympathetic attitude, and express confidence about recovery.

9. Reassure the patient that medical help has been sent for and that it will arrive shortly.

10. Remain with the patient to provide comfort, but avoid fussing and prevent others from crowding around.

11. If the patient loses consciousness and stops breathing, begin performing artificial respiration at once (see Artificial Respiration).

12. If the heart stops beating, the patient will also need heart compression (see CPR).

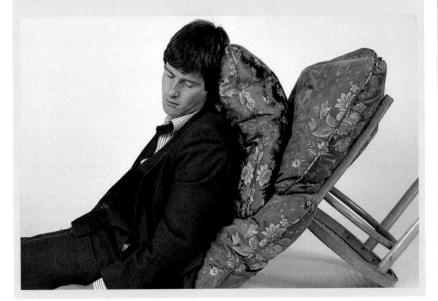

Take note

- The heart muscle depends on small arteries for the blood supply that keeps it going. If these vessels have become so narrow that they cannot provide the extra blood needed when a person exerts him- or herself or feels a strong emotion, the result is a pain in the chest. The condition is known as angina. The pain is viselike and sometimes spreads to the neck, shoulders, and arms.
- During a severe heart attack a clot blocking one of the arteries cuts off the blood from part of the heart muscle. Known as coronary thrombosis, the attack results in intense pain. The patient collapses, is pale, sweats, and has a fast, weak, and sometimes irregular pulse.
- In some cases, symptoms are mild and similar to those of indigestion. When in doubt, treat as a heart attack.
- Heart failure is different from the above conditions. Here, a weakened heart muscle causes the normal pumping action to become inadequate. Blood flowing into the heart from the lungs is not fully propelled forward and the lungs become congested. There is no pain, but the patient's breathing is very wet and bubbly and he or she may cough up watery, blood-tinged sputum.

Checklist

1. Following treatment and recovery, the patient may or may not be at risk of having further attacks, either soon after or in the years after the initial occurrence. It is difficult to make an accurate prediction.

2. What is certain is that the patient decreases his or her chances of a repetition of the attack and can live out the remainder of a normal life span if he or she closely follows the doctor's advice.

3. Particular care should be taken with diet, and, if the patient is a smoker, he or she should give up smoking.

4. The patient should always seek and follow a doctor's advice about starting on a healthy exercise program. This may help to prevent further attacks.

Hypothermia

- Exposure to cold can cause lasting damage to the body's tissues
- Complications associated with exposure include frostbite and hypothermia
- The extremities—nose, fingers, and toes—are most affected
- Any attempt at rapid rewarming can cause further tissue damage

Exposure

Symptoms of exposure include physical and mental slowing down, a decrease in reasoning power, mood changes, slurred speech, shivering, and cramps, followed by possible collapse. Once any symptoms are detected, stop the patient from moving and get him or her to take shelter. Remove any wet clothing and replace with blankets, a sleeping bag, or fresh clothing. Cover the patient's head and face, but leave the mouth, nose, and eyes free. If the patient is conscious, give him or her warm, sweet drinks, but never administer alcohol.

Frostbite

If subjected to intense cold, the tissues under the skin may freeze. Freezing is caused by the formation of tiny ice particles and disruption of the blood supply brought on by clumps of red blood cells that then block the vessels. When frostbite (numb, white tissue) is suspected, remove wet clothing and constricting objects (such as a ring) from the affected area. Apply a dry, protective cover after dabbing away any moisture. If possible, immerse the part in warm, not hot, water. Or, use a warm blanket. Do not rub area.

Hypothermia

A patient with hypothermia is extremely cold all over, with puffy skin that is white or blue—except for a child, who looks pink. The heartbeat will be slow and weak. When this occurs, keep the patient in bed in the recovery position. Cover the patient with blankets, but keep them loose. Do not use hot water bottles or an electric blanket, since excessive heat may damage the patient. Make sure that all open windows are shut and then warm the room with any available heater. If the patient is conscious, give him or her warm, sweet drinks.

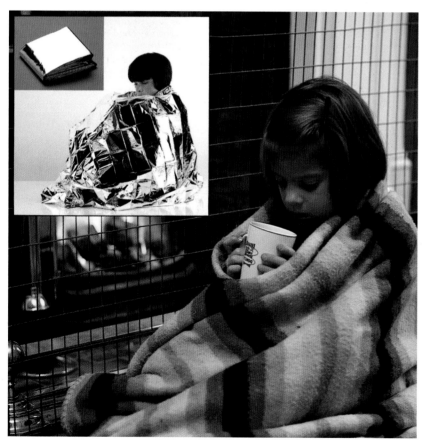

Dos and don'ts

DO cover the head in extreme cold to protect against excessive loss of body heat.

DO ensure that the young and elderly sleep in warm conditions, since they are particularly vulnerable to low temperatures.

DO use suitable protective clothing in extremely cold conditions. On long trips, take high-energy foods (such as chocolate and glucose) and flasks of hot, sweet drinks.

DON'T give a patient alcohol; it encourages the body to lose rather than retain heat.

◄ *Children who go on camping or hiking expeditions in which they risk exposure to cold or damp weather should be supplied with thermal blankets; they are excellent at retaining the body's heat, take up very little space, and are light to carry. Warming a cold child in front of a fire is effective in cases of chill and slight exposure—for example, after a soaking—but victims of severe exposure and frostbite should never be put near a roaring fire: rapid reheating may cause further tissue damage.*

Poisoning

- Call an ambulance and a Poison Control Center
- A conscious patient should be given fluids
- If patient is unconscious, put in the recovery position
- If he or she is not breathing, give artificial respiration

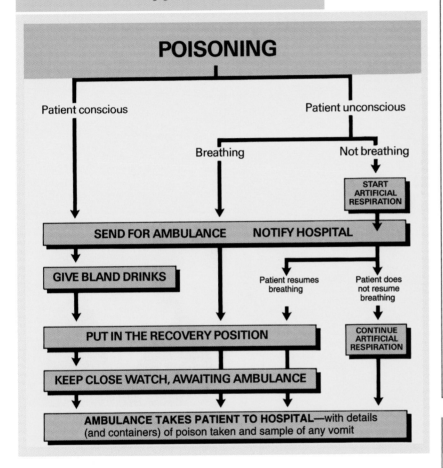

POISONING

Patient conscious — Patient unconscious

Breathing — Not breathing

→ START ARTIFICIAL RESPIRATION

SEND FOR AMBULANCE — **NOTIFY HOSPITAL**

GIVE BLAND DRINKS

Patient resumes breathing — Patient does not resume breathing

PUT IN THE RECOVERY POSITION — **CONTINUE ARTIFICIAL RESPIRATION**

KEEP CLOSE WATCH, AWAITING AMBULANCE

AMBULANCE TAKES PATIENT TO HOSPITAL—with details (and containers) of poison taken and sample of any vomit

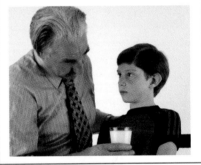
Pesticides

- Pesticides are variable in their action. The more dangerous ones, if used as sprays, can cause harm if swallowed, breathed in, or absorbed through the skin.
- The effects of pesticide poisoning can be cumulative, causing headaches, muscle ache, weakness, sweating, lassitude, vomiting, and difficulty in, or even cessation of, breathing.
- Get the patient out of the spray area and put him or her to rest. Wearing gloves, remove any contaminated clothing and thoroughly wash his or her skin. Check the pesticide container label for advice (always keep pesticides in the original containers—apart from being a safety measure, it usually gives instructions on what to do in an emergency).
- Summon medical help immediately and, if necessary, give artificial respiration (see Artificial Respiration).

Shock

- Shock is caused by many types of severe injury—it is due to failure of the circulation
- Always tend to major injuries first
- Minimize shock by laying the patient down at the site of the accident, keeping his or her head low and legs raised
- Loosen tight clothing and keep the patient lightly covered

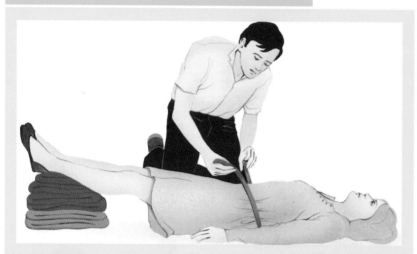

1. Stop bleeding (see Bleeding). If possible, treat patient on the spot. Lay him or her down with head low and legs raised about 12 in. (46 cm). Keep movement to a minimum.

2. Loosen tight clothing. Dress wounds with clean, dry material (see Wounds). If injuries allow, place the patient in the recovery position (see Unconsciousness).

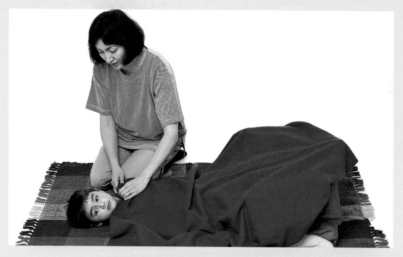

3. In cold conditions in which the person might shiver, cover loosely, but do not allow the skin to warm up. Do not cover routinely. As you give first aid, explain what you are doing so that the patient is reassured. Stay with the patient until medical aid arrives.

Take note

- Shock is usually caused by a severe loss of body fluid. This may be in the form of internal or external bleeding, or it may be due to the loss of blood plasma as a result of damage from a serious burn.
- Body fluid loss causes the heart to beat faster and weakly, and the blood pressure to fall. As a consequence, the entire body receives an inadequate supply of oxygen.
- First aid should be given to prevent shock, even if the victim looks and feels fine. Always treat for breathing, bleeding, burns, and fractures, in that order.
- A badly shocked victim will look bluish, pale, cold, and sweaty, and may appear to be mentally slow. Breathing will be shallow and the pulse fast and feeble.

Checklist

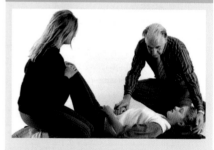

1. Keep a careful watch on the patient to make sure that he or she is breathing properly, does not start—or resume—bleeding, and does not vomit. Lightly cover with blankets so that the patient remains cool, but is not cold. Do not heat with hot water bottles or electric blankets—these will draw blood away from the vital organs where it is needed.

2. Do not give the victim any food, drink, or medication. Stimulants, such as alcohol and cigarettes, should be avoided completely.

3. Even if the patient seems to be unconscious, do not talk to bystanders about his or her condition. He or she may well hear you and understand what is being said. The patient needs to be reassured, not made more anxious.

Sprains and strains

- Let the patient rest the injured part in the most comfortable position, slightly raised if possible
- Cover the affected area with a cold compress, keeping it in position for approximately 30 minutes
- Protect the area with a pad of wool or cotton cloth
- Bandage from well below hurt area to well above

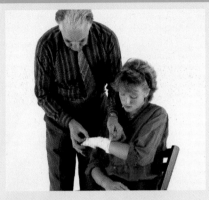

Checklist

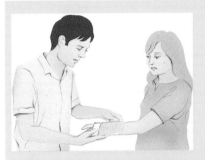

1. Spraining means damaging the ligaments around a joint. Apply a cold compress, then remove it and cover the area with a pad.

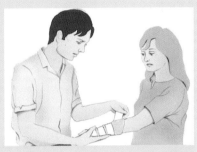

2. Starting well below the damaged joint, firmly wrap a bandage up and around the joint, leaving a few strips of padding visible.

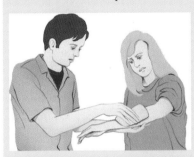

3. A strain involves a muscle in any part of the body. Apply a cold compress, then remove it and cover the area with a thick pad.

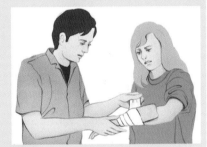

4. Wrap an elasticized bandage around the injured area. Do this firmly but not tightly, and cover the padding completely.

1. The strain or sprain needs rest and support in the form of a firm bandage. An elasticized bandage is best, but it is easy to make such a bandage so tight that it damages the underlying nerves and blood vessels. A thick cotton pad protects the area from this sort of constriction. If any part of the affected limb becomes cold, numb, or puffy, the bandage is probably too tight and should be loosened.

2. If pain is severe, but there is clearly no other injury, the patient may have aspirin, acetaminophen, or ibuprofen. However, if the pain seems too severe and you have the slightest doubt about a possible fracture, get medical aid urgently.

3. Sprains and strains can be more of a problem than people realize. Bandaging supports the limb and reduces pain, but movement is very limited. Several days may elapse before normal activity can be resumed. Check with your doctor before you do anything strenuous.

Take note

- In both strains and sprains the muscle or ligament has been overstretched by a powerful movement. Sometimes small blood vessels will also be torn and a bruise forms. The area will be painful, discolored, and swollen.
- Swelling can be minimized by cooling the area with a cold compress for up to 72 hours after the accident. After this, no amount of cooling will help to reduce the swelling.
- To make a cold compress: use thick cloth, such as a folded towel; soak it in cold water; wring it out so it is just moist; place on the sore area; keep in place for about half an hour; moisten if it begins to dry out too much.
- If you think there is the slightest chance that the patient has fractured a bone, treat as for fractures (see Fractures). Many doctors do exactly this until they have the results of an X ray.

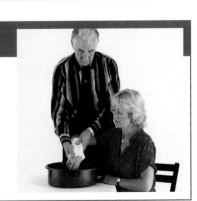

Unconsciousness

- If the patient is not breathing, begin artificial respiration immediately
- Clear the patient's mouth of any vomit, blood, or displaced dentures
- Control any bleeding; check for other wounds and for possible fractures
- If it is safe to move the patient, move him or her gently into the recovery position
- If possible, stay with the patient and send someone for medical help

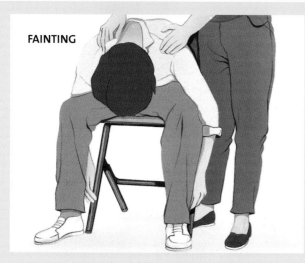

FAINTING

1. When a seated person feels faint and it is impossible to lay him or her down (for example, in a concert hall), tell him or her to bend all the way forward, with the head between the legs, and to try to relax completely. Do not leave the patient in case he or she loses consciousness.

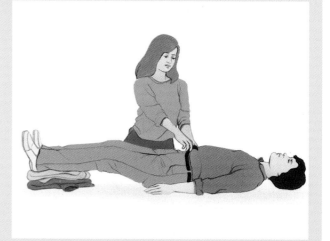

2. If possible, lay the patient down, with legs raised at least 12 in. (30 cm). Loosen tight clothing at neck. If the patient is conscious, tell him or her to take deep, slow breaths. As the patient recovers, give him or her cold water to drink. Ask him or her to stay still for 5 minutes before trying to sit up slowly.

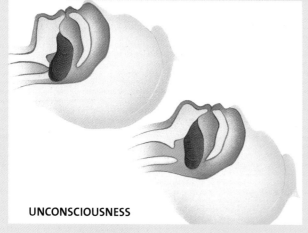

UNCONSCIOUSNESS

1. In an unconscious person, the tongue may sometimes flop backward and obstruct the opening of the windpipe. Bend the head back, without twisting the neck: the tongue will be carried up with the jaw and the airway will open. Give artificial respiration if necessary.

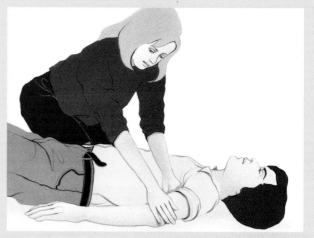

2. Stop bleeding (see Bleeding), dress wounds (see Wounds), and check for fractures (see Fractures) by feeling firmly but gently with hands flat, from one end of the body to the other for any swellings. If you suspect a fracture, avoid moving the patient; otherwise put him or her in recovery position.

Dos and don'ts

DO remember to check the patient's breathing before you do anything else. If he or she is lying on the back, the tongue may be obstructing the airways, and this must be treated as an emergency.

DO remove anything, such as a pillow, from under the patient's head if he or she is having any difficulty breathing.

DO follow the routine to safeguard breathing, stop bleeding, and protect against further harm before you move the patient into the recovery position.

DON'T twist or turn the neck when moving the head, in case there has been some injury to the upper part of the spinal column.

DON'T try to make an unconscious person drink. The fluid would run into the windpipe. Even if the patient responds vaguely to touch, his or her ability to swallow may be impaired.

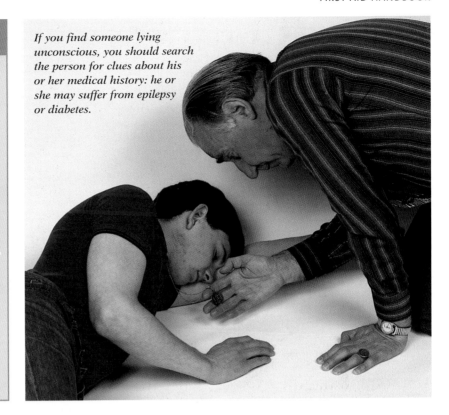

If you find someone lying unconscious, you should search the person for clues about his or her medical history: he or she may suffer from epilepsy or diabetes.

Take note

● Examine the patient to see if he or she is breathing. If not, then begin artificial respiration immediately (see Artificial Respiration).
● If the patient is breathing noisily and with some difficulty, use a curved finger to scoop the mouth clear of any obstruction in the airway, such as vomit or blood. Bend the head back and keep it in this position.
● Look for any severe bleeding. Control it at once (see Bleeding).
● Check for any other wounds. Cover them at once with a dressing (you may have to improvise one; see Wounds).
● Search for any possible fractures (see Fractures). If you suspect a fracture (which would be made worse by moving the patient), leave him or her as is. Note that a fractured spine is almost impossible to discern in an unconscious patient, but the circumstances (for example, a fall from a height or a blow to the back) may suggest it. If so, **do not move the patient under any circumstances.**
● If it is safe to move the patient, turn him or her gently into the recovery position (see below).
● Send for medical help.

RECOVERY POSITION

Checklist

1. The cause of the patient's unconsciousness may be unknown. This is for the doctor to diagnose and to treat. Your first responsibility is to call for medical aid and to administer first aid, if necessary.

2. Even if there is no sign of emergency at first, keep watching the patient carefully in case his or her breathing stops and needs artificial respiration, or the patient vomits. If he or she does vomit, clear his or her mouth using a curved finger.

3. If the patient is unknown to you and you will not harm him or her with your movements, search for any cards, bracelets, or other medical tags that may tell you if the patient suffers from a condition such as diabetes. Also search the person for any drugs that may indicate what could have led to a drug overdose. These items should be handed to the doctor or paramedics.

4. If you suspect that the patient has a fracture, and medical help will be delayed, or you have to transport the patient to the hospital, immobilize the part that has been fractured.

Wounds

- Elevate the injured part of the body; make sure the patient keeps still
- If bleeding is heavy, apply pressure on the wound with your hand until bleeding subsides
- Wash the wound, then put gauze over it, then a thick pad, and finally a firm bandage
- Protect the patient against shock and seek medical attention

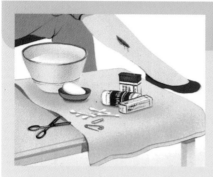

1. For dressing a wound you need several articles from a first aid box: cotton, gauze, bandages. You will also need soap and warm water.

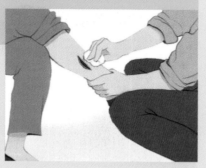

2. Elevate the wound. Wash it and skin around it. Use cotton moistened with water and soap; flush with clear water. Work outward from the wound.

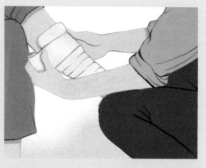

3. Put gauze over the wound, covering beyond the wound area. Place thick pad over the gauze. Bandage dressing firmly, preferably with a pressure bandage.

MAKING A RING PAD

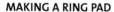

1. Use a long, thin, twisted fold of cloth such as a large handkerchief. Form one end into a circle.

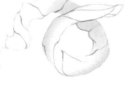

2. Hold the circle and slip the end through the loop. Keep looping the long, free end around the circle.

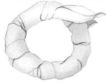

3. When all the cloth is used up, it forms a firm, thick ring that protects the wound when it is bandaged.

OBJECTS IN WOUNDS

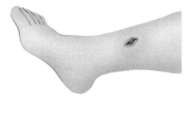

1. If an object is lying on the surface of a wound, brush it away with a clean piece of gauze. However, if an object has become embedded, you must leave it undisturbed. It will be removed properly when medical assistance becomes available.

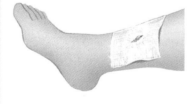

2. Carefully cover the wound with a piece of sterile gauze; it should be sufficiently large so that it extends well beyond the area of the wound itself. If the piece of gauze is too small, it may slip and a part of the wound may become exposed.

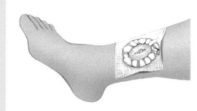

3. Make a ring pad (see box, left) from a large handkerchief or a small towel and place this around the object in the wound. This will prevent the object from being pressed on by the thick pad and bandage that you will place over it. Once the wound has been bandaged, expert medical advice should be sought.

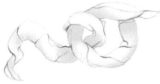

Take note

- Get the patient to sit or lie down and elevate the injured part of the body.
- Temporarily protect the wound with the cleanest cover that you can find. Wash your hands and collect the material needed: soap, water, cotton balls, gauze, bandages (or improvised substitutes). Place them on a clean surface nearby.
- Wash the wound and the skin around it. Use cotton moistened with water and soap; follow with clear water. Use a clean piece of cotton for each separate stroke, moving the cotton outward from the wound.
- Put nonstick gauze over the wound; make sure it is large enough to extend well beyond the wounded area and cover the cleaned skin.
- On top of the gauze, gently set a thick pad of cotton.
- Bandage firmly (but not too tightly). Each successive bandage turn should overlap the previous one by two-thirds of its width.
- Keep the wounded part at rest.
- Protect the patient against shock (see Shock).

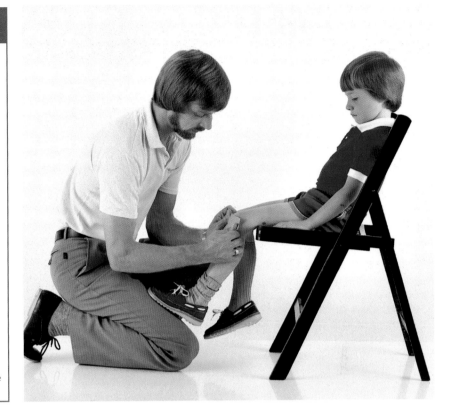

Dressings

- Convenient, ready-made, all-in-one dressings come with the gauze and the pad attached to the bandage.
- Adhesive dressings are either in continuous strips to be cut to size or in different sizes of single dressings. They are useful for dressing small, superficial wounds. After partly peeling off the protective cover, apply the gauze pad that is now exposed onto the wound, then pull away the cover.
- Tubular gauze is fitted over toes and fingers by means of a metal or plastic applicator.
- An improvised gauze dressing can be made from most smooth, clean materials such as a handkerchief, pillowcase, or towel (but not fluffy cotton). One or two folded handkerchiefs can serve as a pad. Cloths folded lengthwise (a handkerchief, scarf, sock, stocking, and so on) can serve as bandages. Make sure that the material is large enough to extend at least 1 in. (2.5 cm) beyond the edges of the wound.

Dressing an eye wound

- For an eye wound, bandage or tape a large, soft, clean pad over the whole eye, without putting any pressure on it. Never use fluffy material as a bandage.
- If it hurts the patient to move his or her eye, cover both eyes, because the two automatically move together.
- Seek medical help immediately— trying to remove foreign bodies may do more damage.

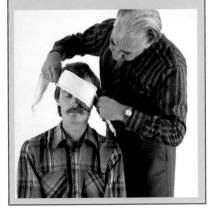

Checklist

1. The slight bleeding of most wounds is soon brought under control by the pressure of ordinary dressings and bandaging. However, if the patient's bleeding is severe, it will have to be controlled by applying pressure on the wound with your hand (see Bleeding).

2. In the case of wounds, the aim of first aid is to protect the wound from becoming infected and damaged. The person administering first aid should limit his or her help to cleaning around the wound (if circumstances permit) and to covering it.

3. In giving first aid, do not use antiseptic or antibiotic lotions and creams. These may interfere with the healing process.

4. With any wound there is the risk of tetanus, and the deeper the cut, the higher the risk. Tetanus vaccinations are given routinely in childhood, but immunity lasts only five to 10 years. Even if the patient has been immunized in the last 10 years, he or should consult a doctor to determine whether a tetanus booster is needed.

MEDICAL GLOSSARY

A

ABDOMEN The abdominal cavity that lies between the diaphragm and the pelvis, containing the stomach and intestines, as well as the kidneys, liver, and pancreas. The front wall is a muscular sheet, and the internal surface is lined by the peritoneum.

ABLATION The deliberate removal of tissue, such as a growth, for treatment purposes.

ABORTION "Spontaneous abortion" is the medical term for a miscarriage—the loss of an embryo, or fetus, before 28 weeks. The term "therapeutic abortion" refers to the surgical termination of pregnancy.

ABSCESS A cavity containing pus.

ACHONDROPLASIA Genetic disorder causing severe limitation of skeletal growth.

ACIDOSIS Abnormally high level of acidity in the blood, often as a result of kidney failure, diabetes, or poisoning.

ACNE Skin condition affecting face, neck, chest, and back, resulting in blackheads.

ACQUIRED IMMUNODEFICIENCY SYNDROME *See* AIDS.

ACROMEGALY Abnormal enlargement of face, hands, and feet as a result of a tumor of the pituitary gland.

ACUPUNCTURE Traditional Chinese medical technique in which fine needles are inserted into specific sites on the body along a series of energy lines, or meridians, in order to treat a disorder or relieve pain.

ACUTE Term used to characterize a medical condition that develops over a short time.

ADDISON'S DISEASE Failure of the adrenal glands, leading to low blood pressure, increased pigmentation of the skin, and possible collapse.

ADENOIDS Small masses of lymphatic tissue, found in the pharynx at the back of the nose, which are prone to swell up during childhood.

ADIPOSE Term meaning "fatty," used to describe tissue composed of fat cells.

ADRENAL GLANDS Two glands situated on top of the kidneys, of which the outer layer (the cortex) is responsible for the production of cortisone, and the inner core (the medulla) for the production of epinephrine.

AFTERBIRTH The placenta and other fetal tissues expelled from the uterus after childbirth.

AIDS (acquired immunodeficiency syndrome) A disease that causes fatal depression of the immune system owing to infection with HIV.

ALBINISM Condition characterized by a lack of pigment in hair, eyes, or skin.

ALBUMINURIA Presence of albumen (a form of protein) in the urine, usually the result of kidney disease, or of renal complications of another disease such as heart failure. Also called proteinuria.

ALCOHOLISM Addiction to alcohol, which can lead to deterioration in psychological and physical health, family life, and social position.

ALLERGEN A substance that causes an allergy.

ALLERGY Hypersensitive reaction, such as wheezing or rashes, to a foreign substance that stimulates the immune system.

ALOPECIA Hair loss. Alopecia areata is a disease with no known cure. It leads to patchy hair loss on the scalp.

ALTITUDE SICKNESS Headache, breathlessness, and weakness found in people who have not acclimatized to the reduced barometric pressure found at high altitudes.

ALVEOLUS The word "alveolus" means a small hollow, cavity, or socket. It can apply to a tooth socket, but in the lungs, alveoli are tiny air sacs through which gases diffuse in and out of the bloodstream.

AMEBIC DYSENTERY Inflammation of the intestines, caused by infestation with the amoeba *Entamoeba histolytica*, and characterized by blood-flecked diarrhea.

AMENORRHEA The absence of menstruation during pregnancy, or as a result of emotional disturbance or hormonal imbalance.

AMNIOCENTESIS An obstetric procedure in which a sample of the amniotic fluid surrounding a fetus is taken for testing.

AMNIOTIC FLUID The clear fluid surrounding a fetus in the uterus.

AMYOTROPHIC LATERAL SCLEROSIS (ALS) A progressive disease characterized by weakness in the muscles, and caused by degeneration of cells in the spinal cord. It is one form of motor neuron disease.

ANALGESIC Any drug that relieves pain.

ANAPHYLACTIC SHOCK Severe allergic reaction leading to collapse.

ANEMIA A lack of hemoglobin in the blood, often caused by a decrease in red cell production, by destruction of red cells, or by blood loss.

ANESTHESIA Pain relief given for the purpose of treatment or surgery. It can be administered as gas or injection that leads to unconsciousness (general anesthesia), or by injection in or around the affected part (local anesthesia).

ANEURYSM A dilation (widening) of a blood vessel as a result of a weakening in its wall.

ANGINA A cramplike pain often felt in the chest, arms, and legs that results from narrowing of the arteries. This narrowing starves the heart muscle of oxygen.

ANGIOGRAM An X-ray picture of blood vessels made after the injection of a contrast medium.

ANOREXIA NERVOSA An emotional disorder in which an abnormal drive to be thin leads to self-starvation, emaciation, and even death. The disorder is most often found in adolescents, predominantly in girls. Compare with bulimia.

ANTACID A medicine that neutralizes the effects of stomach acid.

ANTIBIOTIC Drug that acts against bacteria and other infecting organisms. Antibiotics are derived from naturally occurring substances made by other organisms. Examples include penicillin and tetracycline.

ANTIBODY A protein produced in the blood that attaches itself to invading organisms (or other foreign substances), making the foreign substances susceptible to destruction by immune system cells, especially phagocytes.

ANTICOAGULANT Any drug that delays or prevents coagulation (clotting) of the blood.

ANTICONVULSANT A drug that is used to prevent seizures.

ANTIGEN A substance that triggers the immune system into producing antibodies. *See* antibody.

ANTIHISTAMINE A drug that counteracts the effects of histamine in the body.

AORTA The main vessel in the arterial network.

AORTIC VALVE The heart valve between the left ventricle and the aorta.

APHASIA Loss of ability to speak or understand speech or the meaning of words.

APPENDECTOMY Surgical removal of an appendix.

ARTERIOGRAM An X-ray picture of arteries taken with the help of a radiopaque medium.

ARTERIOLE The smallest vessel of the arterial system.

ARTERY Blood vessels carrying oxygen-rich blood from the heart to the tissues.

ARTHRITIS Inflammation leading to pain and swelling of joints.

ARTIFICIAL INSEMINATION The insertion of sperm into the vagina or uterus by mechanical means rather than by sexual intercourse.

ASBESTOSIS Lung disease resulting from the effects of inhaled asbestos.

ASPHYXIA Lack of oxygen in the blood due to restricted respiration. Strangulation, inhalation of toxic fumes, and drowning are possible causes.

ASPIRIN A valuable mild painkiller and anti-inflammatory drug that works by blocking the production of prostaglandins. Aspirin reduces the risk or severity of thrombosis.

ASTHMA Respiratory disorder caused by narrowing of the bronchial tubes, leading to breathlessness and wheezing.

ASTIGMATISM Nonspherical curvature of the cornea causing visual blurring that is most severe in a particular meridian (orientation).

ATHEROMA Soft fatty substance laid down in the walls of the arteries, leading to narrowing, reduced blood flow, and sometimes heart attacks, strokes, or gangrene.

ATHEROSCLEROSIS The most common disease of arteries, featuring hardening of the walls and the deposition of atheroma in the lining. Atherosclerosis is the cause of heart attacks and strokes and is the major cause of death in the western world.

ATHLETE'S FOOT Common chronic fungal infection of the foot, usually found between the toes. Also called tinea pedis.

ATRIUM One of the two (left and right) low-pressure pumping chambers of the heart.

ATROPHY Wasting of an organ or tissue.

ATTENTION DEFICIT DISORDER *See* hyperactivity.

AUTISM A condition in which the sufferer is abnormally self-absorbed, and unable to relate to people or deal with everyday events.

AUTONOMIC NERVOUS SYSTEM The part of the nervous system that controls automatic functions, such as heartbeat and sweating.

AZT The trademark drug used to inhibit HIV.

B

BACTERIA Small, single-celled organisms that cause infection. Bacteria vary in shape, being spheric (cocci), rod-shaped (bacilli), spiral (spirochetes), or comma-shaped (vibrios).

BASAL METABOLIC RATE A measure of the basic level of the body's metabolic processes. The rate is raised by thyroid overactivity and lowered by thyroid underactivity.

BCG (bacille Calmette-Guérin) A form of tuberculosis (TB) bacterium that is able to stimulate immunity without causing disease, and is used as a vaccination against TB.

BEDSORES Painful ulcers that develop on the skin of bedridden patients, such as stroke victims. Also called decubitus ulcers or pressure sores.

BEHAVIOR THERAPY Psychological technique that aims to alter abnormal behavior patterns.

BENIGN Term used to describe tumors that do not spread to other parts of the body. Compare with malignant.

BENZODIAZEPINES A class of drugs used as sedatives and mild tranquilizers and for the short-term treatment of insomnia. They have largely replaced barbiturates for these purposes.

BETA-BLOCKERS A family of drugs that block the effects of epinephrine, principally used to treat heart disorders and high blood pressure.

BILE Greenish-brown fluid produced by the liver that carries away the liver's waste products and helps to break down fats in the small intestine, which it enters via the bile duct.

BILHARZIA *See* schistosomiasis.

BIOPSY A sample of tissue taken from the body for microscopic examination.

BIORHYTHMS Physiological functions that vary over time in a rhythmic way, of which the menstrual cycle is a good example.

BIPOLAR DISORDER A mental disorder that fluctuates between deep depression and excessive elation. Also called manic depression.

BLADDER The hollow, muscular organ in the pelvis that acts as a reservoir for urine.

BLOOD CLOTTING The vital mechanism whereby components of the blood solidify after any damage, thereby stopping bleeding.

BLOOD GROUPS A system of classifying blood according to the identifying chemical markers on the red blood cells. Classification is vital in order to ensure compatibility for blood transfusion, thereby avoiding adverse reaction.

BLOOD PRESSURE The pressure of blood in the larger arteries. The peak pressure with each heartbeat is called the systolic pressure, and the running pressure between beats is called the diastolic pressure. It is written as, for instance 120/80. These figures are of pressure in terms of the height in millimeters of a column of mercury. Blood pressure is a function of the force of the heart muscle contraction as affected by the resistance offered by the arteries.

BLUE BABY A baby born with a heart defect that results in a lack of oxygen in the blood and a characteristic bluish complexion.

BM STRIP A simple test for blood sugar levels used by many diabetics.

BOIL An abscess in the skin, usually arising from a hair follicle infected with the bacterium *Staphyloccocus aureus*.

BOTULISM A rare but highly dangerous form of food poisoning caused by the toxin produced by the bacterium *Clostridium botulinum*, which thrives in improperly canned or improperly preserved foods.

BRADYCARDIA An abnormally slow heartbeat, which in an adult is anything below 60 beats per minute.

BREAST PUMP An electric or hand pump used to express milk from a nursing mother.

BREATHLESSNESS Shortness of breath leading to rapid conscious breathing.

BREECH BIRTH Birth where the baby is born feet, knees, or buttocks first.

BRONCHIAL TUBES The airways that connect the trachea to the lungs.

BRONCHIECTASIS Persistent infection in the lungs due to destruction of lung tissue.

BRONCHITIS Inflammation of the bronchial tubes, characterized by coughing and difficulty in breathing.

BRONCHOGRAM X ray using contrast medium to outline the bronchial tubes.

BRONCHOSCOPE Instrument for looking into the lungs via the trachea and bronchial tubes.

BUBONIC PLAGUE The most common form of plague, characterized by painful buboes (large inflammatory swellings) and fever.

BUERGER'S DISEASE A disease causing blockages in arteries of the legs and arms that may lead to gangrene and loss of limbs. It occurs mainly in young men who smoke.

BULIMIA Disorder characterized by gross overeating, and often followed by self-induced vomiting. Associated with anorexia nervosa.

BUNION Inflammation and painful swelling over the joint at the base of the big toe.

BURN Any area of tissue that is destroyed or damaged by heat, electricity, chemicals, gases, or radiation.

BURSA (pl. bursae) Fibrous, fluid-filled sac acting as a cushion between some tendons, or the skin and bones beneath them.

BYSSINOSIS A respiratory disease primarily affecting workers in the cotton industry. Caused by inhalation of cotton-fiber dust.

C

CALCIFICATION The accumulation of calcium in tissue; a normal process in bone.

CALORIE A unit used by dieticians to express the amount of energy taken into the body from digested food. A calorie is defined as the amount of heat that will raise 1,000 ml (1 liter) of water by 1 degree Celsius. In physics, a calorie is the amount of heat that will raise 1 ml of water by 1 degree Celsius.

CANCER Any sort of malignant tumor that spreads by setting up new foci of tumor (metastases) in different parts of the body instead of being confined to where it grew.

CAPILLARIES The tiny blood vessels that connect the arterioles to the venules, and the sites at which the contents of the blood pass through to the tissues.

CARBOHYDRATE One of the three basic food types. Carbohydrates are the sugars and starches (chemical combinations of sugars) found in cereals and potatoes.

CARBUNCLE A large boil with numerous pockets of pus.

CARCINOGEN Any cancer-causing substance.

CARCINOID SYNDROME A rare condition characterized by facial flushes and diarrhea, caused by an intestinal or lung tumor called a carcinoid.

CARCINOMA The most common form of tumor, occurring in the lining membrane of such organs as the lungs, breasts, and stomach. Compare with sarcoma.

CARDIAC ARREST A cessation of the heart's pumping action. The most common cause is heart attack, but other causes are anaphylactic shock, hypothermia, and electric shock.

CARDIOVASCULAR Of or pertaining to the heart and blood vessels.

CARRIER A person who has an infectious disease without having any of its symptoms, and who is able to transmit the disease to other people.

CARTILAGE Gristly connective tissue that forms an important part of the skeletal system, such as the joints.

CAT SCAN (computerized tomography; or computerized assisted tomography) An X-ray technique that creates detailed pictures of the body's internal structures by producing detailed images of tissue composition in cross section.

CATARACT An area of opaque tissue that develops in the internal lens of the eye and impairs sight.

CATARRH An increase in mucus, usually due to inflammation of the mucous membrane.

CATATONIA Extreme muscular immobility suffered by some patients with schizophrenia.

CATHETER Any tube passed into the body for diagnostic or treatment purposes.

CELIAC DISEASE A condition leading to malabsorption of food from the intestines, caused by sensitivity of the intestinal lining to gluten. Also called sprue.

CEREBELLUM The part of the brain that coordinates movement and maintains balance.

CEREBRAL HEMORRHAGE Bleeding into the brain, causing stroke.

CEREBRAL PALSY Disturbance in the function of the brain and nervous system as a result of injury often caused through lack of oxygen during birth.

CEREBROSPINAL FLUID Fluid that bathes and cushions the brain and spinal cord.

CEREBRUM The largest, uppermost, and most complex part of the brain, dealing with the sensory, motor, and intellectual functions, including speech and memory.

CERVICAL SMEAR A specimen taken from the secretions and superficial cells of the cervix for laboratory investigation.

CERVIX Any neck, but usually the neck of the uterus, which is the central channel which opens during labor to allow childbirth.

CESAREAN SECTION Surgery to remove a baby from the uterus through an incision in the abdominal wall.

CHEMOTHERAPY The use of chemical compounds to destroy cancer cells.

CHICKEN POX An extremely infectious disease common during childhood, of which the symptoms include a rash of fluid-filled spots.

CHILBLAINS Hot, red, itchy patches of skin on toes or fingers caused by exposure to cold.

CHIROPODY Care of the feet, with particular emphasis on the care of nails and the removal of hard skin, corns, warts, and calluses.

CHIROPRACTIC A therapy based on the belief that an individual's health is directly related to the condition of his or her spinal column. Treatment does not include drugs or surgery, but centers on the manipulation of the patient's spine. A practitioner is termed a chiropractor.

CHOLANGITIS Inflammation of the bile ducts.

CHOLECYSTECTOMY Surgery to remove the gallbladder.

CHOLECYSTITIS Inflammation of the gallbladder.

CHOLECYSTOGRAM An X-ray picture of the gallbladder.

CHOLERA An acute bacterial infection of the small intestine, characterized by diarrhea and vomiting, and caused by ingestion of foods and drinks that have been contaminated with the feces of those infected with the bacterium.

CHOLESTEROL A fatty substance that is essential to the structure of cell walls. However, when present in the blood in excessive quantities (usually owing to a diet too rich in animal fats), it is laid down in the walls of arteries, causing atheroma. Cholesterol can also crystallize as gallstones in the bladder.

CHROMOSOMES Threadlike structures within the cell nucleus that carry genetic information. Humans have 23 pairs of chromosomes, plus one pair of sex chromosomes.

CHRONIC Term used to describe an illness that persists over a long period of time.

CIRCUMCISION Removal of the foreskin from the penis, for religious or health reasons, or both.

CIRRHOSIS Liver disease resulting from a continuing process of liver cell destruction.

CLEFT PALATE Congenital abnormality of the palate in which the two sides of the palate fail to fuse, leaving a gap between them.

CLINICAL PATHOLOGY The laboratory-based study of disease.

CLITORIS A small erectile organ on the exterior of the vulva, analogous to the penis.

CLUBFOOT Deformity of the foot present from birth in which the sole is turned inward. Medical name is talipes.

COAGULATION The process in which blood solidifies to form a clot.

COLD SORE A painful sore on the lips that usually arises when the immune system is under stress, for example, during a cold. Caused by the herpes simplex virus.

COLIC An attack of pain in the abdomen that comes in waves.

COLITIS Painful inflammation of the large intestine (colon) leading to diarrhea and occasional bleeding.

COLON The tube stretching from the end of the small intestine through to the rectum. Also called large intestine.

COLOR BLINDNESS Inability to distinguish between some colors, most commonly between red and green.

COLOSTOMY The temporary or permanent surgical rerouting of the colon through the abdominal wall in order to create an artificial anus—used to relieve a blockage in the intestine, such as a cancerous growth.

COMA A state of profound unconsciousness, commonly brought on by head injuries, blood clots, poisoning, or strokes.

COMPOUND FRACTURE A fracture that breaks through the skin.

CONCEPTION The fertilization of the ovum by the sperm, leading to embryo formation.

CONCUSSION A brief loss of consciousness owing to a head injury; often followed by temporarily disturbed vision and loss of memory.

CONDOM A sheath slipped over the erect penis to prevent conception and transmission of STDs such as HIV.

CONGENITAL Term used to describe disease or abnormality which is present from birth, but which is not necessarily hereditary.

CONGESTIVE CARDIAC FAILURE Inefficient heart action that leads to a buildup of pressure in the veins and lungs, resulting in breathlessness and edema.

CONJUNCTIVA The mucous membrane lining the inner surface of the eyelids and the white part of the eyeball.

CONJUNCTIVITIS Inflammation of the conjunctiva due to infection or allergy, causing red eyes and a thick discharge.

CONNECTIVE TISSUE The basic cement and packaging of the body that holds the organs in place and fills spaces. Fibers of the protein collagen provide strength; the protein elastin provides elasticity.

CONSTIPATION Difficulty in passing feces, usually because they are too hard and dry.

CONTAGIOUS Term used to describe a disease that can be contracted from other people by physical contact.

CONTRACEPTION Any method of preventing pregnancy.

CONTRAST MEDIUM A radiopaque substance injected into the body in order to enhance detail on X rays.

CONVULSION A seizure. Sudden involuntary spasms, with or without loss of consciousness, due to abnormal cerebral stimulation.

CORNEA The transparent outer lens of the eye.

CORONARY THROMBOSIS The blockage of a coronary (heart) artery with a clot, leading to a heart attack.

CORPUS LUTEUM The yellowish mass of tissue that forms at the point of rupture after the ovary releases an egg. It produces the sex hormone progesterone.

CORTISONE A hormone produced by the adrenal glands.

CPR (cardiopulmonary resuscitation) A resuscitation technique used both to support the circulation after the heart has stopped beating, and to stimulate the heart back into action. Also called heart massage.

CREUTZFELDT-JAKOB DISEASE (CJD) An uncommon but inevitably fatal spongy degeneration of the brain caused by a protein molecule called a prion that can be acquired by eating beef from animals suffering from bovine spongiform encephalopathy (BSE).

CRIB DEATH The sudden, unexplained death of an apparently healthy baby. Also called sudden infant death syndrome.

CROUP Acute viral infection of the respiratory tract in children, causing fever and a characteristic harsh cough.

CRYOSURGERY Surgery carried out by destroying tissue with cold temperatures, or otherwise using low-temperature objects as surgical instruments.

CURETTAGE Scraping out of any hollow space, such as an abscess cavity.

CYST Any abnormal fluid-filled cavity.

CYSTIC FIBROSIS Hereditary disease, appearing in infancy and characterized by excessive mucus, breathing difficulties, and abnormal secretion and function of many of the other secretory glands of the body.

CYSTITIS A painful inflammatory infection of the bladder.

CYSTOGRAM An X-ray picture of the bladder.

CYSTOSCOPY Looking into the bladder using a special narrow optical viewing tube passed through the urethra.

CYTOLOGY The study of cells, particularly the microscopic examination of cells in such substances as sputum, cervical smears, and urine, to see if cancer cells are present.

CYTOTOXIC Term used to describe drugs that destroy cancerous cells.

D

D & C (dilatation and curettage) Surgery to scrape away the lining of the uterus.

DANDRUFF Scaling of the scalp. Acute dandruff is called seborrheic dermatitis.

DECONGESTANT A drug used to reduce congestion of the air passages.

DEEP VEIN THROMBOSIS A clot in the deep veins of the legs, causing swelling and discoloration of the skin. It may cause a life-threatening pulmonary embolism.

DEFIBRILLATOR A machine that delivers an electric shock to the chest in an attempt to reestablish proper rhythm of the heartbeat.

DEHYDRATION Excessive loss of fluid from the body, normally accompanied by an imbalance in the levels of sodium, potassium, and chloride.

DELIRIUM A state of altered consciousness in which a patient is unaware of his or her surroundings, or finds them strange or frightening—usually brought about by fever, shock, or drug abuse.

DELIRIUM TREMENS (DTs) Acute reaction caused by cessation of excessive intake of alcohol over a long period of time.

DEMENTIA A state of disordered brain function due to generalized loss of brain cells, often in old age. Memory is lost early, and in the final stages of dementia patients may be completely disoriented, unable to care for themselves, and incontinent.

DENTAL CARIES Tooth decay caused by bacterial action, and prevented by effective dental hygiene.

DERMATITIS Inflammation of the skin.

DERMATOLOGY The branch of medicine concerned with diseases of the skin.

DIABETES One of two conditions that cause excessive urination, but "diabetes" usually refers to diabetes mellitus.

DIABETES INSIPIDUS A metabolic disorder caused by deficient production of the antidiuretic hormone (called ADH), or by the failure of the kidney to respond to ADH.

DIABETES MELLITUS Complex metabolic disorder primarily caused by deficient production of insulin in the pancreas.

DIAGNOSIS The identification of disease based on observation of the patient's signs and symptoms. Compare with prognosis.

DIALYSIS Artificial method of taking over the function of the kidneys in order to keep the blood free from waste products, or to purify it of poisons and drugs.

DIAPHRAGM The sheet of muscle that forms a barrier between the contents of the chest and those of the abdomen.

DIARRHEA Increased frequency of defecation with liquid or unformed stools.

DIASTOLE The period during which the heart is relaxing between heartbeats. Compare with systole.

DIASTOLIC PRESSURE See blood pressure.

DIPHTHERIA An acute infectious disease characterized by the formation of a membrane in the throat that can obstruct breathing.

DIPLOPIA Double vision.

DIURETIC A drug prompting increased urine production.

DIVERTICULUM (pl. diverticula) Any pouchlike outward protrusion from a tubular or saccular organ such as the bladder, stomach, or intestine.

DNA (deoxyribonucleic acid) The genetic material that is passed from generation to generation in the chromosomes.

DOWN SYNDROME The most common chromosome abnormality, in which there are three number 21 chromosomes instead of just two. The condition is characterized by mental retardation and multiple defects. Formerly called mongolism.

DUCTUS ARTERIOSUS The vascular channel in the fetus that bypasses the lungs by joining the left pulmonary artery to the aorta. It generally closes after birth when the oxygen supply is provided by the lungs.

DUODENAL ULCER A breakdown in the lining of the duodenum due to the effects of stomach acid.

DUODENUM The first segment of the small intestine as it leaves the stomach.

DWARFISM Abnormal shortness of stature.

DYSENTERY Severe diarrhea due to an infection, often with blood present in the matter evacuated.

DYSLEXIA A pathological impairment of the ability to read.

DYSMENORRHEA Severe menstrual pains.

DYSPAREUNIA Pain during sexual intercourse.

DYSPEPSIA Indigestion; usually resulting from the effects of stomach acid.

DYSPNEA Breathlessness; often a symptom of heart and lung disease.

DYSURIA Pain during the passing of urine; often a symptom of an infection of the urethra.

E

ECG (Electrocardiogram) A graph showing the sequence of electrical changes occurring in the heart during a succession of heartbeats. Characteristic changes in the graph are helpful in diagnosing heart disorders.

ECHOCARDIOGRAM An ultrasound technique used to build up a moving picture of the heart.

ECLAMPSIA A rare complication of pregnancy characterized by high blood pressure and seizures.

ECT (electroconvulsive therapy) An electric shock to the brain given under anesthesia in order to produce a convulsion. Used to relieve symptoms of clinical depression.

ECTOPIC PREGNANCY A pregnancy developing outside the uterus, usually in one of the fallopian tubes.

ECZEMA Any superficial dermatitis, characterized by a red, scaly, itchy, and sometimes weeping skin rash.

EDEMA Any swelling of tissues due to an increase in fluid content.

EEG (electroencephalogram) A multi-channel recording of the electrical activity of the brain.

ELECTROLYTES Soluble mineral compounds that conduct electric currents, of which the body has a large number. These include sodium, potassium, calcium, magnesium, and chloride, and they must be kept within narrow limits for the normal function of cells, especially nerve cells.

ELECTROLYTES AND UREA The name of a common blood test whereby the levels of important minerals (electrolytes) in the body are measured, also the level of urea.

ELEPHANTIASIS Massive swelling of the legs or areas of the trunk or head due to blockage of the lymph vessels by a tiny worm called *Wuchereria bancrofti*.

EMBOLISM The result of a blood vessel's becoming blocked by an embolus.

EMBOLUS A foreign object, usually part of a thrombus, a tumor, or other tissue, or a mass of air, that drifts in the bloodstream until it becomes lodged in a blood vessel. *See also* embolism.

EMBRYO The early stages of a baby's development in the uterus, from the second week or so after conception until the seventh or eighth week of pregnancy. Compare with fetus.

EMPHYSEMA A chronic lung disease, resulting from overenlargement of the lung's air spaces, that causes the destruction of the lung tissue.

ENCEPHALITIS (pl. encephalides) Inflammation of the brain.

ENDEMIC Term used to describe a disease that is native to a particular area or population. Compare with epidemic, epizootic, and pandemic.

ENDOCARDITIS Infection on the inner surface of the heart, usually occurring only when there is already some minor abnormality of structure.

ENDOCRINE SYSTEM The system of endocrine glands (pituitary, thyroid, parathyroid, and adrenal) that produces the body's hormones.

ENDOSCOPY Examination of any part of the interior of the body by a narrow rigid, or flexible optical viewing device which is introduced via a natural anatomical opening or through a short incision.

ENDOTRACHEAL TUBE A tube that is passed into the windpipe to enable artificial ventilation by means of a respirator.

ENEMA Fluid passed into the rectum by syringe in order to help treat constipation.

ENTERITIS Infection of the intestines, leading to diarrhea and abdominal colic.

ENURESIS Passing urine without control, usually during sleep—a condition that occurs commonly in childhood.

ENZYMES Protein catalysts necessary for the innumerable biochemical reactions that occur in living cells and elsewhere in the body. Almost all the genes are codes for the production of enzymes.

EPIDEMIC A widespread outbreak of an infectious disease. Compare with endemic, epizootic, and pandemic.

EPILEPSY A disease of the nervous system that causes recurrent convulsions due to an overwhelming electrical discharge in the brain.

EPINEPHRINE A hormone produced by the adrenal glands that has many effects that together produce a bodily state appropriate for coping with sudden physical emergency. The hormone is produced synthetically as a treatment for cardiac arrest, anaphylactic shock, and acute asthma. It is also known as adrenaline.

EPISIOTOMY A cut made to widen the external opening of the vagina in order to ease childbirth.

EPIZOOTIC An outbreak of infectious disease that spreads through an entire species of animal in the same geographic area.

ESOPHAGUS The muscular canal that leads from the back of the throat down to the stomach.

ESTROGEN One of the two important female hormones. Variations in estrogen levels occur during the menstrual cycle and are responsible for many of the changes that occur in the uterus.

EUSTACHIAN TUBE The tube that connects the middle ear (the part of the ear inside the eardrum) to the back of the throat.

EXFOLIATION The process whereby cells are lost from the surface of any lining or surface layer, such as the lining of the gut or the skin.

EXPECTORANT A drug (e.g., acetylcysteine) designed to promote expectoration.

EXPECTORATION The ejection of mucus, sputum, and other fluids from the lungs by coughing or spitting.

F

FALLOPIAN TUBES The two tubes arising out of the uterus and ending near the ovaries through which eggs produced in the ovaries normally pass on their way to the womb. Also called oviducts.

FAMILY PLANNING Strategic contraception.

FAT One of the three basic food types. It is the most concentrated provider of energy, and is stored in the body as adipose tissue.

FECES The residue after the nutrient value of food has been absorbed by the small intestine—ejected from the body through the anus.

FERTILIZATION The process whereby a sperm enters an egg and fuses with it to start the process of cell division that may end in the production of an embryo.

FETUS Human conceptus growing in the uterus—usually so called from the seventh or eighth week of pregnancy. Compare with embryo.

FEVER A high body temperature, above the normal 98.6°F (37°C). Most infectious illnesses cause fever, which is a sign that the body's temperature-regulating mechanism has been reset by the infection.

FIBROIDS Benign fibromuscular tumors which grow in the uterus, and which may cause heavy menstruation and disturbances in urination.

FIBROSING ALVEOLITIS A disease whereby the alveoli of the lungs become closed by scar tissue so that they no longer allow oxygen to pass into the blood.

FIBROSIS A proliferation of fibrous connective tissue, as part of the formation of scar tissue after injury or infection, or other tissue disease.

FISSURE A split in the skin or other surface.

FISTULA An abnormal channel leading from one body cavity to another, or from an internal organ to the skin.

FLATULENCE The presence of excessive gas in the stomach or intestines.

FOLLICLE A small sac or tubular gland.

FONTANELLES The gaps between the developing bones of a baby's skull— covered and protected by soft membranous tissue and skin.

FORAMEN An opening, usually referring to the opening in a bone through which blood vessels or nerves pass.

FORCEPS Instrument used during surgery that picks up tissue in a pincerlike fashion. Obstetric forceps are used to assist in difficult births.

FORENSIC MEDICINE The branch of pathology that deals with unnatural or criminal injury or deaths.

FORMALIN Solution of formaldehyde in water used for preserving tissue after removal for examination.

FRACTURE Term used to describe an injury to a bone in which the continuity of the tissue is broken.

FROSTBITE Traumatic tissue injury due to cold.

FROZEN SECTION Tissue taken during surgery on which a very rapid microscopic examination is carried out in order to determine the course of the operation.

FUNGAL INFECTION An inflammatory infection caused by a fungus.

G

GALLBLADDER A saclike organ attached to the liver that collects bile and then discharges it into the intestine in response to a fatty meal.

GANGLION A small fibrous swelling on the wrist or the back of the hand. Also the knots of nervous tissue that act as relay stations in the nervous system.

GANGRENE Death of tissue following a breakdown in the blood supply.

GASTRECTOMY The surgical removal of the stomach.

GASTRIC ULCER A break in the inner lining of the stomach, usually resulting from the effects of stomach acid.

GASTRITIS Inflammation of the mucosa of the stomach, causing indigestion and vomiting.

GASTROENTEROLOGY The branch of medicine concerning the stomach, intestines, liver, and pancreas.

GASTROSCOPY Inspection of the inside of the stomach and duodenum using a flexible endoscope passed through the mouth.

GENES The biological units that determine inherited characteristics such as eye color. Each characteristic is controlled by one or more genes passed on from one's parents.

GENETICS The study of genes and inherited characteristics and diseases.

GERIATRICS Branch of medical and social science dealing with the health of the elderly.

GERMAN MEASLES See rubella.

GINGIVITIS Inflammation of the gums.

GLAND Any organ that produces a secretion.

GLANDULAR FEVER See infectious mononucleosis.

GLAUCOMA An eye disease caused by excessive pressure of fluid in the eye, which may lead to loss of sight.

GLUCOSE A simple sugar that is the main source of energy for the body's cells.

GLUTEN A protein constituent of wheat and wheat products, and the constituent responsible for producing celiac disease.

GLYCOGEN A form of glucose stored in the liver and muscles and released as needed for energy.

GOITER A visible swelling of the thyroid gland.

GONORRHEA A sexually transmitted

disease that produces a greenish-yellow urethral or vaginal discharge.

GOUT Swollen painful joints. Gout especially affects the joint at the base of the big toe, and is caused by excessive accumulation of uric acid.

GRAFT Transfer of a piece of tissue to another site, or replacement of diseased tissue with tissue from another individual. Artificial tissue may also be used.

GRAND MAL SEIZURE Epileptic convulsion characterized by jerking movements and loss of consciousness. Compare with petit mal seizure.

GRANULOMA Term used by pathologists to describe some forms of localized inflammation or infection.

GREENSTICK FRACTURE A partial fracture of a child's bone, which, because the bone is so pliable, splits rather than breaks.

GROUP THERAPY Treatment of psychological problems by discussion within a group of people and under the direction of a trained therapist.

GROWTHS Popularly used to refer to tumors both benign and malignant.

GYNECOLOGIST A specialist in the diseases of the female reproductive system.

H

HALITOSIS Bad- or foul-smelling breath.

HALLUCINATION An imaginary sensation perceived through any of the five senses—the result of drug use, alcohol withdrawal, severe illness, or schizophrenia.

HALLUCINOGENIC Term describing a drug that produces hallucinations.

HAMMERTOE A common deformity usually affecting the second toe (the one next to the big toe) in which the toe is permanently flexed in a clawlike position.

HAMSTRING MUSCLE The group of three muscles at the back of the thigh.

HAY FEVER Runny nose and coldlike symptoms owing to pollen allergy.

HEART ATTACK A sudden, acutely painful, distressing, and often fatal event in which part of the heart muscle is deprived of its blood supply and dies, because of blockage of a branch of one of the coronary arteries. In those who survive, the dead tissue is replaced by scar tissue but the heart is usually weakened in its pumping power.

HEARTBURN A burning sensation behind the sternum, caused by stomach acid in the esophagus.

HEART FAILURE A condition in which the heart can no longer pump enough blood to meet the metabolic requirements of the body.

HEART MASSAGE *See* CPR.

HEART MURMUR Any of several sounds heard in addition to the regular heartbeat.

HEAT EXHAUSTION Condition caused by loss of body fluids due to prolonged exposure to high temperature, causing cramps, nausea, and finally loss of consciousness. Compare with heatstroke.

HEATSTROKE The medical term for sunstroke. A severe and sometimes fatal condition resulting from the collapse of the body's ability to regulate its temperature, due to prolonged exposure to hot sunshine or high temperatures. Also called heat hyperprexia.

HEMATOMA A trapped mass of blood in the tissues of an organ or in the skin.

HEMATURIA Blood in the urine.

HEMIPLEGIA Paralysis of one half of the body.

HEMODIALYSIS The use of a kidney machine to remove waste products from the blood after a patient's kidneys have ceased functioning.

HEMOGLOBIN The oxygen-carrying substance in red blood cells.

HEMOPHILIA An inherited disorder of blood clotting due to absence of one of the factors needed for clotting (factor VIII). Generally only males are affected, though females may be carriers.

HEMORRHAGE Medical term for bleeding.

HEMORRHOIDS Varicosity in the blood vessels of the anus that can give rise to bleeding and discomfort. Also called piles.

HEPATITIS Inflammation of the liver, usually caused by one of the hepatitis viruses.

HERNIA A weakness in the muscular wall of the abdomen that allows tissue (often the small intestine) to push through.

HERPES A group of viruses responsible for cold sores, chicken pox, shingles, and genital sores.

HIATUS HERNIA Condition in which the stomach pushes up through the diaphragm through the hole occupied by the gullet.

HIV (human immunodeficiency virus) The retrovirus that causes AIDS.

HODGKIN'S DISEASE Cancerlike disease of the lymph nodes.

HOMEOPATHY Treatment of disease involving minute doses of a substance that produces symptoms similar to those of the disease itself.

HORMONE One of the complex chemicals produced in the body that regulate the body's metabolism and functions.

HORMONE REPLACEMENT THERAPY (HRT) Synthetic or natural hormones that were used to counteract hormonal deficiency during menopause. HRT carries a slightly higher risk of heart disease, strokes, and breast cancer.

HYDATID DISEASE A disease caused by larval forms of tapeworms, and characterized by cysts in the liver and other organs.

HYDROCEPHALUS Increase in volume of the cerebrospinal fluid within the brain's ventricles. In children it may lead to enlargement of the head, and it is often associated with spina bifida.

HYMEN The thin membrane which partly covers the entrance to the vagina, and which may be torn or stretched during first sexual intercourse or by the use of tampons.

HYPERACTIVITY A term used to describe excessive activity in children, associated with brain damage, epilepsy, and psychiatric trouble, but only very rarely with food allergy. Also known as attention deficit hyperactivity disorder.

HYPERSENSITIVITY Tendency to experience allergic reactions, especially to drugs.

HYPERTENSION Raised blood pressure, which puts extra strain on the heart and arteries, thereby increasing the risk of heart attacks, strokes, and kidney damage.

HYPERTHYROIDISM Overactivity of the thyroid gland that can lead to weight loss, tremor, protrusion of the eyes, hyperactivity, moist skin, and jumpiness.

HYPERTROPHY Abnormal enlargement of an organ or tissue in order to meet extra demands made on it by the body.

HYPERVENTILATION Abnormally rapid breathing, leading to dizziness, tingling in the hands, or even loss of consciousness.

HYPOCHONDRIA Neurotic preoccupation with one's own health and with disease.

HYPODERMIC Term meaning literally "under the skin," as in hypodermic injections.

HYPOGLYCEMIA An abnormally low level of sugar in the blood, causing such symptoms as confusion, coma, trembling, and sweating, and even death.

HYPOTENSION Low blood pressure.

HYPOTHALAMUS The area at the base of the brain that controls many of the body's automatic and hormone-related activities.

HYPOTHERMIA Abnormally low body

temperature—below 95°F (35°C)—usually caused by prolonged exposure to cold, and leading to a faint heart rate, pallor, and eventual collapse.

HYPOTHYROIDISM Underactivity of the thyroid gland, leading to weight gain and thick, dry skin.

HYPOXIA A low level of oxygen in the tissues as a result of lung or heart disease.

HYSTERECTOMY Removal of the uterus.

I

IATROGENIC Term used to describe a condition caused by medical treatment.

ICHTHYOSIS A skin condition in which the skin is abnormally thick and scaly.

IDIOPATHIC Denoting a disease or symptom of which the cause is unknown.

ILEOSTOMY Surgery performed to bring the end of the ileum onto the surface of the abdomen, creating a stoma through which intestinal contents can be discharged.

ILEUM Medical term for the small intestine. Absorbs nutrients.

ILEUS Obstruction of the ileum.

IMMUNE SYSTEM The complex system by which the body defends itself against infection.

IMMUNIZATION Preparing the body to fight and prevent an infection through the injection of material from the infecting organism, or by using an attenuated (non-disease-causing) strain of the organism itself.

IMMUNOGLOBULIN *See* antibody.

IMMUNOSUPPRESSIVE DRUGS Drugs that suppress the immune system.

IMPACTED TEETH Teeth that are jammed in position beneath the gum and thereby fail to grow from the jaw into the mouth properly.

IMPETIGO An acute staphylococcal skin infection characterized by pustules and yellowish crusts.

IMPOTENCE Failure to achieve or sustain an erection of the penis.

IN VITRO FERTILIZATION (IVF) A method of enabling women who are unable to conceive to bear children by fertilizing egg cells with sperm outside the body ("in vitro" literally means "in glass," i.e., in an artificial environment), and then inserting some of the fertilized eggs in the uterus. Popularly called test-tube babies.

INCONTINENCE Failure to control the bladder or bowel movements, or both.

INCUBATION PERIOD The period between exposure to a contagious or similar infection and the first appearance of any symptoms of the disease.

INDIGESTION A nonmedical term used to describe pain, discomfort, and other symptoms arising from the stomach or intestines after the intake of food.

INDUCTION (OF LABOR) Procedure in which labor is started artificially.

INFARCTION Tissue damage due to a blockage in blood supply.

INFECTIOUS MONONUCLEOSIS Viral infection causing swollen lymph nodes and a sore throat. Also called glandular fever.

INFERTILITY Inability of a couple to conceive and reproduce after a reasonable period of time (about a year to 18 months).

INFLAMMATION A reaction of the body's tissues to injury or illness, characterized by redness, heat, swelling, and pain—a mechanism of defense and repair.

INGROWN TOENAIL Inflammation of the soft tissues at the edge of the nail with swelling, so that the tissue extends over the edges of the nail, causing an appearance of ingrowing. Nail edges never grow sideways.

INHALERS Aerosol or powder-dispersing containers that release doses of drugs for inhalation—used in the treatment of asthma and other respiratory disorders.

INOCULATION Administration of a vaccine in order to produce immunization.

INSULIN A hormone secreted in the pancreas that regulates blood sugar levels.

INTENSIVE CARE UNIT (ICU) A hospital unit that provides specialized treatment for severe medical and surgical disorders.

INTERFERON A protein produced by the body cells when triggered by a virus infection—used as a drug to treat certain diseases.

INTERTRIGO Irritated skin in body folds, such as under the breasts.

INTESTINES The long continuous tube connecting stomach to anus. The first part (small intestine or ileum) absorbs nutrients; the second (large intestine or colon) processes the waste.

INTRAUTERINE DEVICE (IUD) A small device inserted into the uterus in order to prevent pregnancy.

INTRAVENOUS (IV) Within or into a vein.

IRRADIATION Exposure to any form of radiant energy, such as light, heat, and X rays, for therapeutic or diagnostic purposes.

IRRIGATION The process of washing out a wound or body cavity—for example, the colon—with fluid.

IRRITABLE BOWEL SYNDROME A common condition that is characterized by episodes of abdominal pain and disturbance of the intestines (constipation or diarrhea). Also called irritable or spastic colon.

ISCHEMIA Condition in which tissue receives an inadequate blood supply.

ISOTOPE SCANNING A diagnostic technique based on the detection of radiation emitted by radioactive isotopes introduced into the body. Also called radionuclide scanning.

J

JAUNDICE Yellowness of the skin most commonly due to liver conditions, such as hepatitis, in which bile does not pass through the liver properly, resulting in its accumulation in the blood.

JUGULAR LINE A fine tube placed in the jugular vein for the purpose of measuring pressure in the heart (jugular venous pressure, or JVP) and giving drugs.

JUGULAR VEINS The veins that drain blood from the head.

K

KELOID An excessive thickening of skin around a scar.

KERATIN The protein that makes up the outer layers of the skin, nails, and hair.

KERATITIS Inflammation of the cornea.

KETONES Acid waste products from the burning of fats by the body's cells.

KIDNEY FAILURE Malfunction of the kidneys, causing waste products such as urea to accumulate in the blood.

KIDNEY MACHINE A machine that artificially cleans the blood of waste products using a process called dialysis.

KNOCK-KNEE A deformity in which the legs bend inward at the knees so that they knock each other on walking. Medical name is genu valgum.

KWASHIORKOR A disease in children caused by a protein-deficient diet, resulting in retarded growth, edema, lassitude, and diarrhea. It is common in most parts of Africa.

KYPHOSIS Outward curvature of the dorsal part of the spine.

L

LABOR The process of childbirth, which starts with the first contractions of the uterus proceeding to full opening of the neck of the uterus (first stage), then the birth of the baby (second stage), and ends with the passage of the placenta from the uterus.

LACTATION Milk production by the breasts.

LAMINECTOMY Surgical removal of the arch of a vertebra to gain access to the spinal cord. It is usually performed to treat injury, or remove a tumor or slipped disk.

LANOLIN A naturally occurring substance that softens and lubricates skin.

LAPAROSCOPY The use of a special endoscope that is passed through the abdominal wall in order to view the abdominal organs.

LAPAROTOMY Surgical incision to open the abdominal cavity. In practice, the term means an exploratory operation for diagnostic purposes.

LARYNGITIS Inflammation of the mucous membrane lining the larynx, caused by an infection or irritation, and accompanied by hoarseness or complete loss of voice.

LARYNX The organ of the voice, sited in the air passage between the pharynx and the trachea.

LASSA FEVER A frequently fatal viral disease occurring in sub-Saharan Africa.

LAVAGE The process of washing out hollow organs such as the stomach.

LAXATIVE Medicine that stimulates the intestines to open, relieving constipation.

LAZY EYE Dimmed vision in an eye that otherwise appears structurally normal. Also called amblyopia.

LEAD POISONING The effect of toxic levels of lead present in the body either by ingestion or by inhalation, producing convulsions, weight loss, poor coordination, and mental impairment.

LEGIONNAIRES' DISEASE A bacterial pneumonia caused by infection with the bacterium *Legionella pneumophila*.

LEPROSY A chronic but not especially contagious disease of the skin and nerves produced by the bacterium *Mycobacterium leprae*.

LEPTOSPIROSIS Acute infectious disease caused by the organism *Leptospira interrogans*, and transmitted to humans via the urine of rats and dogs. Symptoms include jaundice and fever. The most serious form is called Weil's disease.

LESION An area of tissue in which the structure and function are altered or impaired owing to injury or disease.

LEUKEMIA A blood disease in which cancerous change in the bone marrow produces abnormal numbers and forms of immature white blood cells.

LEUKOCYTOSIS An excess of white cells in the blood, often due to infection.

LEUKOPENIA A lack of white blood cells, often the result of blood disease or as a side effect of anticancer or other drugs, and causing a reduced resistance to infection.

LEUKOPLAKIA A condition featuring white patches of thickened mucous membrane, especially in the mouth. Can proceed to cancer.

LEUKORRHEA Whitish vaginal discharge.

LEUKOTOMY Surgical removal of some of the connections to the brain's frontal lobes in order to relieve psychiatric symptoms. Also called lobotomy.

LICHEN PLANUS A nonmalignant, chronic skin disease characterized by thick, hardened red patches.

LIGAMENT One of the many strong fibrous bands, usually forming parallel bundles, which hold the bones together at a joint, and which also support the organs.

LIGHT THERAPY Exposure of the skin to infrared and ultraviolet rays for therapeutic purposes, as in the treatment of SAD.

LINCTUS A medicine for the relief of coughs.

LINIMENT An oily preparation rubbed into the skin to relieve pain in the underlying muscle.

LIPOMA A benign fatty tumor.

LIVER The largest gland of the body, situated in the upper right-hand corner of the abdomen just beneath the diaphragm. It is a highly complex gland, with more than 500 functions. These include the production of bile, the conversion and storage of many substances vital for the body's well-being (such as glycogen and urea), and the detoxification of ingested substances, such as alcohol and various drugs.

LIVER FAILURE Inability of the liver to fulfill its function, causing fatigue, anorexia, jaundice, coma, and death.

LIVER FUNCTION TEST A common blood test in which the level of various substances helps to indicate how well the liver is working.

LOBOTOMY *See* leukotomy.

LOCHIA The discharge that flows from the vagina after childbirth.

LORDOSIS An abnormal degree of forward curvature of the lower part of the spine, which results in excessive curvatures elsewhere in the spine.

LOWER-BACK PAIN Ache or pain in the lower back caused by muscular strain or disk trouble.

LUMBAGO *See* lower-back pain.

LUMBAR DISK A condition in which the central part of the disks that lie between the vertebrae bursts or becomes displaced and presses against the nerves of the spinal cord. Also called slipped disk.

LUMBAR PUNCTURE The introduction of a hollow needle into the spinal canal in order to remove cerebrospinal fluid for examination. Also called spinal tap.

LUNG FUNCTION TESTS Diagnostic tests performed to determine the volume of air that can be inhaled into and exhaled from the lungs.

LUPUS ERYTHEMATOSUS A chronic inflammatory disease of the connective tissue, affecting the skin and various internal organs. It is an autoimmune disease. *See* systemic lupus erythematosus.

LYMPH Pale watery fluid which carries, among other things, leukocytes around the body's tissues, and which is filtered by the lymph nodes.

LYMPH NODE A small structure that filters infection; part of the lymphatic system.

LYMPHATIC SYSTEM A network of vessels transferring lymph from the tissue fluids to the bloodstream. Lymph nodes occur at intervals along the lymphatic vessels.

LYMPHOCYTE A type of white blood cell produced in the bone marrow and present mainly in the lymph and blood. Lymphocytes are involved in immunity.

M

MALABSORPTION Failure of the small intestine to absorb nutrients properly.

MALARIA Serious infectious illness common in the tropics, caused by four species of the organism *Plasmodium*, which is passed to humans via an infected anopheles mosquito. Typical symptoms are fever and an enlarged spleen.

MALIGNANT Term used to describe tumors that spread into surrounding tissues and elsewhere in the body. The term is also used to describe other dangerous diseases or states.

MALNUTRITION A nutritional deficiency due to the lack of the basic elements of a balanced diet. Usually brought on by a severe shortage of food, it can also sometimes be caused by inadequate absorption of food or an intake of inappropriate food. The term "malnutrition" also increasingly refers to the kind of excessive eating that causes obesity.

MALOCCLUSION Improper alignment of the upper and lower teeth on biting.

MAMMOGRAPHY X-ray pictures of the breast, used to help detect tumors.

MANIA A state of excessive and sometimes dangerous excitement, in which patients lack insight into their behavior.

MANIC DEPRESSION *See* bipolar disorder.

MANTOUX TEST A skin test used to determine exposure to infection with tuberculosis.

MARFAN'S SYNDROME An inherited condition causing elongation of the bones, and often accompanied by cardiovascular abnormalities.

MARROW The soft matter found in the middle of bones that plays a vital function in the formation of blood. Also called bone marrow.

MASTECTOMY Surgical removal of a breast, usually in cases of breast cancer.

MASTITIS Inflammation of breast tissue, which may occur soon after the birth of a child (acute mastitis) or which may describe chronic fibrous changes in the breast (chronic mastitis).

MASTOIDITIS Inflammation of the air-containing sinuses in the bone behind the ear.

MEASLES An acute, highly contagious viral disease which occurs principally in childhood, and which is characterized by red eyes, fever, and a rash. Also called morbilli and rubeola.

MECKEL'S DIVERTICULUM A pouch found in the wall of the small intestine in 1 or 2 percent of the population, and usually asymptomatic.

MECONIUM The first feces of a baby, usually dark green or black in color, and consisting of epithelial cells, mucus, and bile.

MEGACOLON Abnormal enlargement of the large intestine, usually as a result of constipation.

MELANIN The black or dark brown pigment that is present in the skin, hair, and eyes.

MEMBRANE Any thin layer of tissue.

MÉNIÈRE'S DISEASE A chronic disease of the inner ear, found in older people and characterized by recurrent deafness, buzzing in the ears, and vertigo.

MENINGES (sing. meninx) The three membranes that surround the brain and spinal cord.

MENINGITIS (pl. meningitides) Any infection of the meninges.

MENOPAUSE The cessation of menses.

MENORRHAGIA Excess menses.

MENSES The flow of blood that occurs during menstruation. Also called period.

MENSTRUATION The period of bleeding as the uterus sheds its lining each month during a woman's reproductive years.

MENTAL RETARDATION A low or very low level of mental ability, which is usually congenital.

METABOLISM The chemical processes that enable the body to work.

METASTASIS (pl. metastases) The process by which tumor cells spread from the site of the original tumor to remote parts of the body. Also the name given to such a secondary tumor.

MICROSURGERY The minute surgical dissection and manipulation of human tissue.

MICTURATING CYSTOGRAM An X-ray picture of the bladder taken while the patient is passing urine.

MIDWIFERY Qualified supervision of pregnancy and childbirth. Compare with obstetrics.

MIGRAINE Recurrent severe headaches, associated with nausea and visual disturbance.

MINERALS Metallic elements, such as sodium, that are vital to many of the body's functions.

MISCARRIAGE Loss of an embryo or fetus from the uterus before 28 weeks of pregnancy, but usually occurring during the first 16 weeks. Medical term is spontaneous abortion.

MITRAL STENOSIS An obstructive lesion in the valve between the left atrium and ventricle, usually due to rheumatic fever.

MOLE A pigmented spot on the skin.

MONGOLISM *See* Down syndrome.

MORBILLI *See* measles.

MORNING SICKNESS Nausea and vomiting widely experienced in early pregnancy (from the sixth to the 12th week), but not necessarily only in the mornings.

MORPHINE A narcotic painkiller derived from a type of poppy.

MOTION SICKNESS Condition arising from erratic movement that upsets the organs of balance, leading to nausea, vomiting, and vertigo.

MOTOR Pertaining to action or movement.

MOTOR NEURON DISEASE One of various

progressive diseases that cause degeneration of the spinal cord.

MUCOSA (pl. mucosae) Various types of moist membrane that line the tubular structures, cavities, and organs of the body. Also called mucous membrane.

MUCOUS MEMBRANE *See* mucosa.

MUCUS Viscous substance secreted by the mucous membranes as a lubricant and barrier against damage and infection.

MULTIPLE SCLEROSIS (MS) Chronic disease of the nervous system. Characterized by loss of the myelin sheath surrounding the nerves, it produces many symptoms, including weakness and loss of coordination. Its course is episodic, with frequent remissions.

MUMPS An acute viral disease primarily affecting the parotid glands in the cheeks.

MUSCLE Powerful tissue that is responsible for all movement.

MUSCULAR DYSTROPHY (MD) A group of inherited diseases causing progressive atrophy of groups of muscles.

MYASTHENIA GRAVIS Rare autoimmune disease featuring weakness of isolated muscle groups, especially in the face and neck.

MYCOSIS Infection by fungi.

MYELOMA Malignant disease of the bone marrow.

MYOCARDITIS Severe inflammation of the heart muscle.

MYOPATHY Any disease of muscle.

N

NARCOTIC A drug that dulls the senses; used to induce sleep or as a painkiller.

NATUROPATHY A system of health care that relies on natural substances, exercise in water, and a natural environment in order to maintain health and effect cures.

NAUSEA The sensation of wanting to vomit.

NECROSIS Death of tissue.

NEOPLASM Term used to refer to tumors, both benign and malignant.

NEPHRECTOMY Surgical removal of a kidney.

NEPHRITIS (adj. nephritic) Any inflammation of the kidneys.

NERVES Bundles of nerve cells enclosed in conducting tissue that carry messages between the brain and the other organs.

NERVOUS BREAKDOWN An informal term to describe a sudden emotional disorder that disrupts normal functioning.

NEURAL Of or pertaining to the nerves.

NEURALGIA Pain felt along a nerve.

NEUROFIBROMA A fibrous tumor of the nervous tissue.

NEUROFIBROMATOSIS Congenital condition characterized by multiple neurofibromas, and accompanied by areas of abnormal pigmentation of the skin.

NEUROLOGY Branch of medicine concerned with the treatment of diseases of the nervous system.

NEUROSIS An emotional disorder such as mild depression, anxiety, or any of the phobias.

NEUROSURGEON A surgeon who operates on the brain, the spinal cord, and other parts of the nervous system.

NOCTURIA Passing urine during the night.

NONSPECIFIC URETHRITIS (NSU) Inflammation of the lining of the urethra caused by germs or agencies other than those commonly known to cause urethritis. The condition formerly described as nonspecific urethritis is now known to be a chlamydial infection.

NUCLEAR MEDICINE The use of radioactive substances to assist in the investigation and treatment of disease.

NUCLEUS The central part of any cell (except red blood cells), which contains the genetic material.

NYSTAGMUS Neurological disorder in which the eyes jerk rapidly and uncontrollably, usually from side to side.

O

OBESITY An excessive amount of body fat.

OBSESSION An unhealthy preoccupation.

OBSTETRICIAN A doctor specializing in the care of women during pregnancy and childbirth.

OBSTETRICS The branch of medicine concerned with pregnancy and childbirth.

OCCLUSION Blockage of a tube in the body.

OCCUPATIONAL THERAPY (OT) The rehabilitation of patients after illness, accidents, or psychiatric breakdown.

ONCOLOGY The branch of medicine concerned with the diagnosis and treatment of cancer.

OOPHORECTOMY Surgical removal of the ovaries, sometimes performed in conjunction with a hysterectomy.

OPHTHALMOLOGY The branch of medicine concerned with the diagnosis and treatment of eye disease.

OPHTHALMOSCOPE Instrument used to inspect the inner eye and retina.

OPTIC NERVE Either of the pair of nerves that carry visual stimuli from the retina to the brain.

OPTOMETRY The practice of testing sight and prescribing corrective lenses.

ORCHITIS Inflammation of the testis.

ORTHODONTICS The branch of dentistry concerned with straightening irregular teeth and making sure that the teeth of the upper and lower jaws align correctly.

ORTHOPEDICS Branch of surgery concerned with the diseases and injuries of bones and the muscles, tendons, and ligaments attached to them.

OSTEOARTHRITIS A long-term inflammatory disease that leads to the destruction of one or more joints.

OSTEOLOGY The branch of anatomy concerned with the bones.

OSTEOMALACIA Softening of the bones, usually caused by a deficiency of calcium and vitamin D.

OSTEOMYELITIS Local or generalized infection of the bone or bone marrow, causing muscle spasms, pain, and fever.

OSTEOPATHY A therapeutic system that, although reliant on orthodox methods of medical treatment (such as drugs, surgery, and irradiation), is based on a much closer interaction between skeletal structure and body function than is found in conventional medicine.

OSTEOPOROSIS A condition in which the bones become thin and brittle.

OTITIS Inflammation or infection of the ear; otitis media is inflammation of the middle ear and is common in children.

OTOSCOPE Instrument used to examine the outer and middle ear.

OTOSCOPY The use of an otoscope to look into the ear and inspect the patient's eardrum.

OVARY The female organ in which eggs are made and stored. Sited inside the abdomen at the ends of the fallopian tubes.

OVULATION Release of one or more ova from an ovary. Unless the egg is fertilized, this usually occurs about 14 days prior to the onset of the next menstrual period.

P

PACEMAKER An electrical device used to regulate a very slow heartbeat (heart block).

PAGET'S DISEASE A disease characterized by bone deformation, usually found in the elderly.

PALLIATIVE Treatment that relieves symptoms rather than providing a cure.

PALPATE To feel for abnormalities with the hands during a physical examination.

PALPITATION Pounding or racing of the heart rate under conditions of stress, or as a result of coronary disease.

PANCREAS The organ at the back of the abdomen, which is responsible for producing the digestive juices. It also produces the hormone insulin.

PANCREATITIS Inflammation of the pancreas, which may produce severe abdominal pain and eventual collapse.

PANDEMIC Any disease that spreads over a very wide area, and sometimes worldwide. Compare epidemic.

PAP SMEAR A simple method of detecting cervical cancer that involves the staining of a sample of exfoliated cells taken from the cervix. Also called Papanicolaou smear.

PAPILLEDEMA A condition in which raised pressure in the fluid around the brain leads to visible swelling of the optic nerve within the eye.

PARALYSIS Inability to move a part or all of the body, caused by disease or injury of the nervous system.

PARAPLEGIA A condition in which the legs are paralyzed owing to disease or injury in the spinal cord.

PARASITE An organism that lives on another living organism. Viruses, bacteria, and fungi are all parasites, as are larger organisms such as worms, lice, and fleas.

PARATHYROID One of four glands found behind the thyroid that control the level of calcium in the body.

PARATYPHOID FEVER A disease caused by food contaminated with a salmonella bacterium. Symptoms resemble those of typhoid fever.

PARKINSON'S DISEASE A disease of the nervous system, characterized by tremor and slowness of movement.

PARONYCHIA See whitlow.

PAROTITIS Inflammation or infection of the parotid glands in the cheek, most commonly due to mumps.

PATENT DUCTUS ARTERIOSUS (PDA) Failure of the ductus arteriosus to close after birth, which places an additional workload on the left side of the heart.

PATHOGEN Any organism that causes disease.

PATHOLOGY The study of the causes, characteristics, and effects of disease.

PEDIATRICS The branch of medicine

concerned with the treatment of children and childhood diseases.

PENICILLIN An effective antibiotic derived from the fungus *Penicillium*.

PEPTIC ULCER An ulcer in the stomach or duodenum resulting from the effects of stomach acid. *Helicobacter pylori* infection is often associated with peptic ulcers; the bacterium interferes with the mucus layer in the stomach so that acidic juices can erode the lining.

PERCUSSION A diagnostic method involving tapping part of the body to determine the condition of internal organs.

PERICARDITIS Inflammation of the fibrous sac holding the heart.

PERICARDIUM The fibrous sac that surrounds the heart.

PERISTALSIS The rhythmic waves of muscular contraction that move food along the digestive tract.

PERITONEUM The membrane lining the abdominal cavity and covering the organs.

PERITONITIS Inflammation of the peritoneum.

PERNICIOUS ANEMIA Anemia resulting from a failure to absorb vitamin B12 from the intestine.

PESSARY A medicated vaginal suppository. Also a plastic ring inserted to treat prolapse of the uterus when surgery is inappropriate.

PETIT MAL SEIZURE Epileptic seizure that takes the form of a sudden, momentary loss of consciousness (or absences). Also called absence seizure.

pH (potential hydrogen) The scale of measurement for acidity.

PHALANGES The small bones that make up the fingers and toes.

PHARMACOLOGY The branch of medicine concerning the effects and properties of drugs.

PHARYNGITIS Inflammation of the pharynx.

PHARYNX The upper part of the throat at the back of the mouth and the nose.

PHEOCHROMOCYTOMA A rare tumor of the adrenal gland.

PHLEBITIS Inflammation of the veins, often associated with thrombosis.

PHLEGM Mucus produced by the nose and sinuses, or by the airways in the chest.

PHYSICAL THERAPY The physical rehabilitation of people recovering after an illness, accident, or surgery.

PHYSICIAN A person who is licenced to practice medicine, but who uses drugs and other treatments rather than surgery.

POSTMORTEM EXAMINATION An examination of a body after death, whereby direct inspection of the organs and microscopic examination of tissue specimens help to explain the cause of death.

POSTPARTUM HEMORRHAGE Bleeding after the birth of a baby.

PREECLAMPSIA Development of high blood pressure during pregnancy. The symptoms of the full condition are high blood pressure, edema, and protein in the urine.

PREMEDICATION Drugs given to patients in order to relax them before surgery.

PREMENSTRUAL SYNDROME (PMS) Irritability occurring before the onset of the monthly period; PMS is due to hormonal changes.

PRESSURE SORES *See* bedsores.

PROCTALGIA A pain in and around the anus.

PROCTITIS Inflammation of the rectal lining.

PROCTOSCOPE An instrument for inspecting the anal canal and rectum.

PROGNOSIS Assessment of the likely outcome of a disease. Compare diagnosis.

PROLAPSE The falling or sliding of an organ from its normal position.

PROPHYLACTIC A form of treatment designed to prevent disease.

PROSTAGLANDINS Chemical compounds that perform a range of hormonelike functions.

PROSTATE GLAND The gland at the base of the bladder in males which is involved in semen production, and which may enlarge later in life and obstruct urine flow.

PROSTHESIS Any artificial replacement for a part of the body.

PROSTRATION Profound collapse, often accompanied by low blood pressure.

PROTEIN The substance made from strings of amino acid molecules that forms the basic building blocks of the body.

PROTEINURIA *See* albuminuria.

PRURITUS Medical term for itching.

PSORIASIS A skin rash with red, scaly patches, found most commonly on the knees and elbows.

PSYCHIATRY The branch of medicine concerned with disorders of the mind.

PSYCHOANALYSIS A form of therapy in which the analyst helps the patient to explore his or her own unconscious mind in order to relieve psychiatric difficulties.

PSYCHOLOGY The study of the mechanisms by which the mind works.

PSYCHOSIS A severe psychiatric illness.

PSYCHOTHERAPY Treatment of emotional problems or psychiatric illness by discussion with a therapist, either on an individual basis or as part of a group.

PUBERTY The sequence of events that changes a child to an adult.

PULMONARY Of or pertaining to the lungs.

PURPURA Tiny spots of bleeding into the skin.

PUS Yellowish-white substance consisting of the debris of bacteria and white blood cells.

PYLORIC STENOSIS Obstruction at the outlet of the stomach, occurring in adults as the result of an ulcer, or as a congenital problem in babies.

PYREXIA Medical term for a fever.

Q

Q FEVER A feverish illness of cattle, goats, and sheep caused by the organism *Coxiella burnetii*.

QUARANTINE Keeping animals or people isolated from the community at large because of the risk of spreading an infectious disease.

R

RABIES A potentially fatal viral disease affecting the nervous system—passed to humans by bites from infected (rabid) animals, and characterized by hydrophobia (fear of water).

RADIATION SICKNESS Sickness arising from exposure to ionizing radiation, characterized by symptoms ranging from nausea and vomiting to fetal damage and cancer, depending on the length of exposure.

RADIOLOGY The use of X rays in order to produce pictures of internal structures and thus diagnose disease.

RADIOTHERAPY The use of X rays to treat disease.

REFERRED PAIN Pain felt at a site remote from the source of the pain.

REFRACTORY A word commonly used by doctors to describe the failure of a condition to respond to treatment.

RELAPSE The return of an illness after apparent recovery.

REMISSION A period free from the symptoms of a chronic illness.

RESUSCITATION The technique used to bring critically ill patients back from the brink of death; in particular the use of artificial respiration and chest compression after cardiac arrest.

RETINA The delicate, multilayered membrane of the eye that receives visual stimuli from the outside world.

RETINAL DETACHMENT The separation of the retina from the back of the eye.

RETROVIRUS A family of viruses, including HIV, which contain RNA, and which are able to produce DNA, using their RNA as a template, and incorporate this into the genome of infected cells.

RH (RHESUS) FACTOR An inherited substance present on the red blood cells that characterizes membership of the Rh blood group system. The importance of the Rh group is that a fetus with a different group from its mother may have its red blood cells destroyed by her antibodies.

RHEUMATIC FEVER A feverish illness following an infection by a streptococcus, which may lead to heart damage.

RHEUMATISM A nonmedical term referring to aches and pains of the joints and related tissues.

RHEUMATOID ARTHRITIS Inflammation of the joints, which may also effect internal organs.

RHINITIS Inflammation of the lining of the nose, usually due to a cold or hay fever.

RICKETS Deficiency disease that affects children during skeletal growth, causing soft and deformed bones and caused by an inability to process calcium due to a deficiency in vitamin D.

RNA (ribonucleic acid) Together with DNA, one of the two substances that carry the inherited genetic instructions in cells. In humans, DNA supplies the genetic codes, and RNA helps to decode them.

RODENT ULCER An ulcer found on the face that is, in fact, a mild form of skin cancer capable of eating away tissue unless removed.

ROSEOLA A common minor viral infection in children and babies that causes a rash.

RUBELLA A virus infection which usually produces only rash and fever, but which can severely damage the fetus in early pregnancy. Also called German measles.

S

SAD (seasonal affective disorder) A mood disorder associated with the decrease in hours of sunlight during the autumn and winter.

SAFER SEX Sexual intercourse in which the risk of transmitting viruses such as HIV is reduced by using protective measures such as condoms. There is no such thing as safe sex.

SALINE A simple salt solution, commonly administered intravenously.

SALIVA Fluid present in the mouth and secreted by the salivary glands as an aid to digestion.

SALIVARY GLANDS One of the three pairs of glands that secrete fluids (including saliva) into the mouth to aid digestion.

SALMONELLA A genus of bacteria that causes typhoid, paratyphoid, and certain kinds of food poisoning.

SALPINGECTOMY Surgical removal of the fallopian tubes.

SALPINGITIS An inflammation of the fallopian tubes, which is usually a symptom of pelvic inflammatory disease.

SALVE Healing or soothing medicated ointment.

SARCOMA A malignant tumor arising in muscle, bone, or other connective tissue.

SCABIES Skin infection caused by mites.

SCARLET FEVER An acute, but now rare, infectious childhood illness characterized by sore throat, fever, swollen lymph nodes, and a pronounced red rash. Also called scarlatina.

SCHISTOSOMIASIS A common tropical parasitic infestation, afflicting over 200 million people worldwide. Also called bilharzia.

SCHIZOPHRENIA A psychotic illness featuring delusions, hallucinations, and a variety of thought disorders that usually start in the late teens or early adult life.

SCIATICA Pain running down the leg, arising from irritation of the sciatic nerve, usually due to disk trouble.

SCLEROSIS Hardening of any body tissue.

SCOLIOSIS A lateral curvature of the spine.

SEASONAL AFFECTIVE DISORDER See SAD.

SEBACEOUS GLANDS Glands that lubricate and protect the skin.

SEBORRHEA Abnormally high production of sebum leading to dandruff and acne.

SEBUM The oily substance produced by the sebaceous glands.

SEDATIVE A drug that decreases functional activity and has a generally calming effect.

SEMEN The fluid which is discharged by the male when he ejaculates, and which contains spermatozoa and secretions from other glands such as the prostate.

SENILE DEMENTIA The loss of mental capacity in the elderly due to the death of brain cells.

SENILITY Old age. Often used incorrectly to refer to the presence of various mental and physical disorders common in old age.

SEPSIS Infection with bacteria.

SEPTICEMIA Invasion of the blood by infectious microorganisms, causing fever and chills. Also called blood poisoning.

SEROTONIN Naturally occurring substance found in the brain, blood, and intestines that elevates mood and has many other actions.

SEX HORMONES Hormones that control sexual functions and their development, such as the menstrual cycle and the production of eggs or sperm. There are three main types: androgen hormones (male sex hormones, of which testosterone is the most important); estrogen (female sex hormones); and progesterone (important in the female reproductive cycle).

SÉZARY SYNDROME An intensely irritating form of dermatitis with severe skin shedding, caused by skin infiltration with T cells.

SEXUAL INTERCOURSE The reproductive act, in which the male penis penetrates the female vagina, culminating in the ejaculation of semen. Medical name is coitus.

SHINGLES A skin rash that follows the underlying distribution of nerves. Due to infection with the varicella zoster virus, which also causes chicken pox.

SHOCK A critical drop in blood pressure that, if untreated, may lead to coma and death.

SIAMESE TWINS Identical twins in which the embryo has not split in half, resulting in the twins' being joined. Also called conjoined twins.

SICKLE CELL A crescent-shaped red blood cell containing the abnormal hemoglobin that causes sickle-cell anemia.

SICKLE-CELL ANEMIA An incurable inherited disease in which abnormal hemoglobin causes the red blood cells to become distorted, resulting in joint pain, thrombosis, fever, and chronic anemia.

SIDE EFFECT An undesirable effect accompanying the desired effect of a drug.

SIDS See crib death.

SILICOSIS Lung disease due to exposure to the silicon dioxide present in stone dust.

SINUS An air-filled cavity within the facial bones, connected to the nostrils.

SINUSITIS Infection of the sinuses.

SKIN GRAFT Skin transplanted from one part of the body to another in order to repair damage or to correct a deformity.

SLEEPING SICKNESS A disease of tropical Africa caused by the presence in the blood of minute protozoans called trypanosomes, which are transmitted by the tsetse fly. It runs a slow course, and is fatal if left untreated. Also called African trypanosomiasis.

SLIPPED DISK Backward protrusion of pulpy material from the center of an intervertebral disk with painful pressure on emerging spinal nerves.

SMALLPOX An acute and often fatal disease which produced a rash and a fever, but which is now eradicated.

SMEGMA The secretions of glands under the foreskin of the penis.

SPASTIC COLON See irritable bowel syndrome.

SPASTICITY A neurological term used to describe resistance of a limb to passive movement. Usually accompanied by weakness, it is caused by damage to nerves in the brain or spinal cord.

SPECULUM An instrument that can be inserted into a body opening (such as the vagina) for the purposes of examination.

SPEECH THERAPY Treatment and counseling to correct speech difficulties.

SPERM See spermatozoon.

SPERMACIDES Contraceptive preparations that kill sperm.

SPERMATOZOON (pl. spermatozoa) Male germ cell that is produced in the testes and carried in the semen. Also called sperm.

SPHINCTER Any muscular ring around any body orifice, which closes it off, as in the anus.

SPHYGMOMANOMETER Instrument used to measure blood pressure.

SPINA BIFIDA Congenital defect in which part of the backbone fails to close, exposing the spinal cord. Often associated with hydrocephalus, it may cause paralysis of the legs.

SPINAL CORD The cord of nervous tissue which runs down from the brain inside the central bony canal of the backbone, and from which all the nerves to the body below the brain branch off.

SPINE The column of bone and cartilage that extends from the base of the skull to the pelvis, contains the spinal cord, and supports the trunk and head.

SPLEEN An organ in the upper left-hand corner of the abdomen, responsible for filtering worn-out blood cells.

SPLINT A device for holding a joint in a suitable position to prevent deformity, or to support a limb after a fracture.

SPONDYLITIS Painful inflammation of the spine, often leading to disabling fusion of adjacent vertebrae.

SPRAIN A common injury to joints in which the ligaments that hold them together become overstretched or torn.

SPRUE A malabsorption disease of the small intestine.

SPUTUM The secretions of the bronchial tubes.

SQUINT Condition in which one eye is not properly aligned. Also called strabismus.

STEATORRHEA Excessive fat in the feces.

STENOSIS A narrowed or blocked tube or passage in the body. The term is often used to describe blockages in the arteries or across the valves of the heart.

STERILIZATION Surgery to prevent eggs from reaching the woman's uterus, or sperm from being emitted in a man. Also means the killing of all infective microorganisms on surgical equipment.

STERNUM The breastbone.

STEROIDS Complex chemical molecules, such as the sex hormones; sometimes used to describe cortisone and those drugs that have a cortisonelike effect.

STETHOSCOPE Instrument used for listening to the sounds of the heart, the lungs, and other internal organs.

STIMULANT A drug that stimulates the brain.

STOMA An artificial opening in a body organ or channel (e.g., the intestine).

STOMACH PUMP Equipment used for washing out the stomach, for example, after a drug overdose or poisoning.

STOMATITIS Inflammation of the lining of the mouth.

STRABISMUS See squint.

STRANGULATED HERNIA A hernia in which the contents of the small intestine have become stuck, constricting the blood supply and posing the risk of gangrene.

STREPTOCOCCUS A type of bacterium.

STREPTOMYCIN An antibiotic, used mainly against tuberculosis.

STRICTURE A local narrowing in any tubular structure.

STROKE Sudden loss of an area of brain function, causing a defect in movement, sensation, vision, speech, comprehension, or personality. Strokes commonly affect one side of the body only.

STY An infection around the root of an eyelash.

SUBLINGUAL Term meaning "under the tongue"—a route by which drugs may be given.

SUDDEN INFANT DEATH SYNDROME (SIDS) See crib death.

SULFONAMIDES A group of drugs that are effective against bacteria.

SUNSTROKE See heatstroke.

SUPPOSITORIES Drugs that are inserted into the rectum or vagina.

SUPPURATION Formation of pus as a result of infection.

SURGEON A doctor specially trained in treating diseases by operation.

SUTURE The medical name for a wound stitch.

SYMPTOMS The characteristics of an illness.

SYNCOPE Sudden loss of consciousness. Also called fainting.

SYNDROME A number of specific features that together characterize a disorder.

SYNOVIAL MEMBRANES The membranes that line and lubricate the joints.

SYNOVITIS Inflammation of the synovial membranes.

SYPHILIS A sexually transmitted and inheritable disease caused by the organism *Treponema pallidum*.

SYSTEMIC LUPUS ERYTHEMATOSUS (SLE) A disease involving many of the body's organs, including the skin, joints, and kidneys.

SYSTOLE The time during which the heart is contracting. Each heartbeat is a systole. Compare with diastole.

SYSTOLIC PRESSURE See blood pressure.

T

T CELL A type of white blood cell that is involved in immunity.

TACHYCARDIA An abnormally fast heart rate.

TEARS The watery, salty secretion of the lacrimal glands that keeps the cornea and conjuctiva of the eye moist.

TELANGIECTASIA Conspicuously widened small blood vessels often seen in the skin; also known as broken veins.

TEMPORAL ARTERITIS Inflammation of the forehead arteries causing acute pain, tenderness, redness, and the risk of incipient blindness unless urgently treated with steroid drugs.

TENDON Fibrous cord that binds muscles onto bones and transmits the force of their contraction.

TENDONITIS Inflammation of a tendon, usually caused by injury.

TENNIS ELBOW Inflammation of the tendons on the outer side of the elbow as a result of overuse of the arm.

TENOSYNOVITIS Inflammation of the sheath surrounding a tendon.

TERATOGENESIS Malformation of a fetus due to genetic or environmental causes.

TEST-TUBE BABY *See* in vitro fertilization.

TESTES (sing. testis) The male sexual organs responsible for the production of both sperm and male sex hormone.

TESTOSTERONE The male sex hormone produced by the testes.

TETANUS A disease of the nervous system caused by a toxin produced by the bacterium *Clostridium tetani*, which contaminates wounds.

TETANY A condition in which the muscles of the hands and feet go into uncontrollable spasm.

THALASSEMIA An inherited abnormality of the hemoglobin that produces severe anemia in affected children.

THALIDOMIDE A type of tranquilizer and sleeping drug that produced deformity in babies when taken by pregnant women; now used strictly as a treatment for leprosy.

THORAX Medical term for the chest.

THROAT Nonmedical term for the pharynx.

THROMBOCYTE Blood platelet, necessary for blood clotting.

THROMBOSIS The formation of a blood clot within an artery or a vein. While such clotting is a normal reaction in a damaged blood vessel, it occurs in an intact vessel only if it is diseased. Thrombosis in arteries leading to the heart muscle can cause a heart attack, and a thrombus in one of the arteries supplying the brain is a common cause of stroke.

THROMBUS (pl. thrombi) A blood clot.

THRUSH *See* yeast.

THYMUS A flat organ in the neck that processes immune system T cells early in life but later shrinks.

THYROID The gland in the neck that produces the hormone thyroxine, which is important in controlling the body's metabolism.

TIC Involuntary twitching or spasm.

TINEA Fungal skin infection of which athlete's foot is a common example.

TINNITUS Ringing or buzzing in the ears.

TISSUE Collection of similar cells and connecting substance to make material from which organs and other structures are formed.

TISSUE TYPING A series of tests to evaluate compatibility of tissues, necessary when transplanting organs.

TONSILLECTOMY Surgical removal of the tonsils.

TONSILS Two patches of lymphoid tissue that lie at the back of the throat on either side.

TOPICAL APPLICATION The application of a drug directly onto a surface, for example, the eyes, gums, tongue, vagina, or anal canal; or an internal surface during surgery.

TOURNIQUET A device that stops the blood flow to a limb by constricting it.

TOXEMIA Blood poisoning caused by bacterial toxins circulating in the bloodstream. *See* preeclampsia.

TOXICOLOGY The study of toxins.

TOXINS Poisons produced by germs.

TRACHEOSTOMY The opening in the windpipe produced by a tracheotomy.

TRACHEOTOMY Surgical procedure whereby an opening is made in the windpipe to ease breathing in diseases of the larynx, or to enable people to remain on respirators for prolonged periods.

TRACTION Use of a system of weights to pull broken bones into place.

TRANQUILIZER A nonmedical term used to describe drugs that act on the nervous system to produce a calming effect.

TRANSFUSION Intravenous administration of fluids, especially blood or plasma.

TRANSPLANT The transfer of any piece of living tissue from one location in the body to another, or from one body to another.

TRAUMA (literally "damage") Any physical injury or severe emotional shock.

TREMOR A regular, involuntary rhythmic shaking of some part of the body.

TRICHINOSIS Infestation with the larvae of *Trichinella spiralis*, usually acquired by eating infected pork products.

TRICHOMONIASIS VAGINALIS A vaginal infection caused by *Trichomonas vaginalis*, characterized by a greenish, odorous discharge.

TRISOMY The presence of an additional chromosome in an individual's cells, so that there are three rather than two of a particular number. The most common disorder associated with a trisomy is Down

syndrome, which is also known as trisomy 21 syndrome.

TROPICAL DISEASES Diseases endemic in undeveloped areas where standards of hygiene, sanitation, and public health administration are low. These areas are found mainly in the tropics, but environmental temperatures are not the fundamental factor.

TUBERCULOSIS (TB) A bacterial infection which most often produces disease in the lungs, but which may affect other organs.

TUMOR A benign or malignant growth.

TWINS Two offspring resulting from one pregnancy. Identical (or monovular) twins develop from a single ovum that divides early in its development. Binovular twins develop separately from two ova.

TYPHOID FEVER A bacterial fever that is caused by ingestion of food, water, and milk contaminated with *Salmonella typhi*, with symptoms resembling those of typhus (typhoid means "typhus-like"): fever, diarrhea, and a rash.

TYPHUS A disease spread by tics, lice, or fleas, producing fever, rash, and, in severe cases, death.

U

ULCER A break in a smooth lining membrane or surface—for example, in the skin or stomach—that fails to heal and may become inflamed.

ULCERATIVE COLITIS A disease causing chronic diarrhea as a result of inflammation and ulceration of the lining of the colon.

ULTRASOUND Sound waves of very high frequency used to produce images of the body's internal structures.

UMBILICAL CORD The cord that carries blood, nutrients, and oxygen from a mother to her unborn child.

UMBILICUS The point on the abdomen where the umbilical cord once joined the fetal abdomen. Also called navel.

UREA A white, soluble waste product of protein formed in the liver and excreted in the urine.

UREMIA A high level of urea in the blood.

URETER One of the two tubes carrying urine from the kidney to the bladder.

URETHRA The tube that carries urine from the bladder out of the body.

URETHRITIS Infection of the urethra.

URIC ACID A breakdown product of DNA found in urine.

URINE The product of the kidneys, containing many of the waste products accumulated in the body.

UROLOGY The branch of medicine concerned with the diseases and treatment of the urinary system of both men and women, and the male genital organs.

UTERUS The organ found in all female mammals that contains and nourishes unborn offspring. Also called womb.

UVEITIS Inflammation affecting the middle part of the eye (the iris and related structures).

V

VACCINATION The administration of a vaccine to prevent one of the infectious diseases.

VAGINA The female genital passage that leads to the uterus.

VAGINISMUS Spasm of the muscles that surround the vagina, causing rejection of sexual intercourse.

VAGOTOMY Surgical cutting of the vagus nerve, usually in order to reduce acid secretion. Formerly used in the treatment of ulcers.

VAGUS NERVE One of a pair of cranial nerves that exert control on the throat, esophagus, larynx, bronchi, lungs, heart, stomach, and intestines.

VALVE A mechanism that allows fluid (such as blood) to flow only one way down a tube.

VARICOSE VEIN A distended and twisted vein.

VAS DEFERENS The tube that carries sperm from the testes to the ejaculatory duct.

VASECTOMY The surgical severing of the vasa deferentia in order to produce sterility.

VASOCONSTRICTION Narrowing of the blood vessels, due to either external factors such as cold, fear, and stress, or to the action of internal secretions such as epinephrine and serotonin.

VEIN A vessel carrying blood from the body tissues to the heart.

VENTRICLE One of the two lower chambers of the heart that receive blood from the atria; also one of the four fluid-filled cavities in the brain.

VENTRICULAR FIBRILLATION Rapid, chaotic beating of the heart, which, if uncorrected, causes death.

VERRUCA (pl. verrucae) A wart.

VERTIGO Dizziness and spinning sensation.

VIREMIA The presence of a virus in the blood.

VIRILISM A condition in which a female starts to acquire male sexual characteristics as a result of a hormonal imbalance.

VIRULENCE The relative capacity of a microorganism to cause disease, assessed according to such factors as incidence of infection among a population, and the rate of mortality.

VIRUS A small infective agent that consists of a protein shell containing a core of DNA or RNA. Viruses require animal cells to reproduce within living cells. They do not respond to antibiotic treatment.

VISCERA Collective term used to describe the internal organs.

VITAL CAPACITY The largest volume of air that can be expelled after a maximal inspiration.

VITAMINS A group of substances that cannot be synthesized by the body but are essential, in tiny amounts, for its healthy growth and development. Vitamins are usually present in a balanced diet, but can also be taken in pill form.

VITILIGO A skin disorder characterized by loss of pigment and patches of pale skin.

VOLVULUS A condition in which part of the digestive tract twists around on itself, cutting off its own blood supply.

VULVA The female external genitalia, including the area of the labia, the clitoris, and the urethral opening.

VULVITIS Inflammation of the vulva.

W

WART Common, infectious, but harmless growths on the skin caused by viruses. Often found on the hand, where they form small swellings. Plantar wart is a wart on the sole of the foot.

WASSERMANN REACTION Formerly the most commonly used blood test to detect evidence of previous infection with syphilis.

WASTING Loss of muscle substance due to illness or prolonged lack of use, especially in cases where the nerve supply to the muscle has failed.

WEANING The gradual substitution of solid foods for milk in an infant's diet.

WEIL'S DISEASE *See* leptospirosis.

WHIPLASH INJURY An injury to the neck that is often sustained in car accidents, where sudden deceleration causes the neck to jerk backward and forward violently.

WHITLOW Infection of the nail bed, resulting in a collection of pus in the nail fold. Also called paronychia.

WHOOPING COUGH An infectious disease of the airways that is common in children who have not been vaccinated against it. There is a characteristic whooping sound after the cough. Also called pertussis.

WOMB *See* uterus.

XYZ

X CHROMOSOME A sex chromosome. Females carry a pair of X chromosomes, whereas males carry one X chromosome and one Y chromosome.

X RAY A method of passing electromagnetic radiation through the various tissues of the body and projecting the resulting image onto photographic film. Those tissues that are more radiopaque (allow fewer X rays to pass through them), such as bone, show up as shadows on the film. Used for diagnostic purposes.

Y CHROMOSOME *See* X chromosome.

YEAST Types of fungi, some of which can cause infections of the skin or mucous membranes. The most common disease-causing yeast is *Candida albicans*.

YELLOW FEVER A serious viral disease that is spread from person to person by mosquitoes, causing fever and jaundice.

FURTHER RESEARCH

BIBLIOGRAPHY

American Red Cross. *First Aid: Responding to Emergencies*, revised 4th edition. Yardley, PA: StayWell, 2007.

Duyff, Roberta Larson. *American Dietetic Association Complete Food and Nutrition Guide*, 3rd edition. New York: Wiley, 2006.

Griffith, H. Winter. *Complete Guide to Symptoms, Illness, and Surgery*, revised 5th edition. New York: Perigee, 2006.

Kolata, Gina. *Ultimate Fitness: The Quest for Truth about Exercise and Health*. New York: Farrar, Straus, and Giroux, 2003.

Lipsky, Martin S., ed. *American Medical Association Concise Medical Encyclopedia*. New York: Random House, 2006.

Litin, Scott, ed. *Mayo Clinic Family Health Book*, 4th edition. Des Moines, IA: Time Inc., 2009.

Marieb, Elaine N., and Katja Hoehn. *Human Anatomy and Physiology*, 8th edition. San Francisco: Benjamin Cummings, 2010.

Steinberg, Laurence. *You and Your Adolescent: The Essential Guide for Ages 10-25*. New York: Simon & Schuster, 2011.

Subbarao, Italo, Jim Lyznicki, and James J. James, eds. *American Medical Association Handbook of First Aid and Emergency Care*, revised and updated edition. New York: Random House, 2009.

Warrell, David A., et al. *Oxford Textbook of Medicine*, 5th edition. New York: Oxford University Press, 2010.

INTERNET RESOURCES

Accident Prevention Corporation
www.safetyman.com

Addiction Search
www.addictionsearch.com

Administration on Aging
www.aoa.gov

Aerobics and Fitness Association of America
www.afaa.com

AIDS
www.aids.org

Alcohol and Drug Problems Association
www.adpana.com

Alternative Medicine Foundation
www.amfoundation.org

Alzheimer's Association
www.alz.org

American Academy of Allergy, Asthma, and Immunology
www.aaaai.org

American Academy of Child and Adolescent Psychiatry
www.aacap.org

American Academy of Family Physicians
http://familydoctor.org

American Academy of Pediatrics
www.aap.org

American Alternative Medicine Association
www.joinaama.com

American Cancer Society
www.cancer.org

American College of Sports Medicine
www.acsm.org

American Council on Science and Health
www.acsh.org

American Diabetes Association
www.diabetes.org

American Dietetic Association
www.eatright.org

American Geriatrics Society
www.americangeriatrics.org

American Health Care Association
www.ahcancal.org

American Heart Association
www.heart.org

American Liver Foundation
www.liverfoundation.org

American Lung Association
www.lungusa.org

American Medical Association
www.ama-assn.org

American Pain Society
www.ampainsoc.org

American Psychiatric Association
www.psych.org

American Psychological Association
www.apa.org

American Red Cross
www.redcross.org

American Social Health Association
www.ashastd.org

American Society for Reproductive Medicine
www.asrm.org

American Society of Alternative Therapists
www.asat.org

Association for Behavioral and Cognitive Therapies
www.abct.org

Birth Defect Research for Children
www.birthdefects.org

Body Positive
www.bodypositive.com

Brain Injury Association of America
www.biausa.org

CancerCare
www.cancercare.org

CancerNet
www.cancernet.com

Centers for Disease Control and Prevention
www.cdc.gov

Child Development Institute
www.childdevelopmentinstitute.org

Council for Responsible Nutrition
www.crnusa.org

Diabetes Exercise and Sports Association
www.diabetes-exercise.org

Dietary Guidelines for Americans
www.cnpp.usda.gov/dietaryguidelines.htm

Eating Disorder Referral and Information Center
www.edreferral.com

Gay and Lesbian Medical Association
www.glma.org

Harvard School of Public Health
www.hsph.harvard.edu

HealthCentral
www.healthcentral.com

Juvenile Diabetes Research Foundation International
www.jdrf.org

KidsHealth
http://kidshealth.org

Learning Disabilities Association of America
www.ldanatl.org

Leukemia and Lymphoma Society
www.leukemia.org

MayoClinic
www.mayoclinic.com

MedHelp
www.medhelp.org

MedlinePlus
www.nlm.nih.gov/medlineplus

MyPlate
www.choosemyplate.gov

National Alliance on Mental Illness
www.nami.org

National Association of Anorexia Nervosa and Associated Disorders
www.anad.org

National Campaign to Prevent Teen and Unplanned Pregnancy
www.thenationalcampaign.org

National Cancer Institute
www.cancer.gov

National Council on the Aging
www.ncoa.org

National Institutes of Health
www.nih.gov

National Library of Medicine
www.nlm.nih.gov

National Mental Health Consumers' Self-Help Clearinghouse
www.mhselfhelp.org

National Women's Health Information Center
www.womenshealth.gov

Nutrition Source
www.hsph.harvard.edu/ nutritionsource

Planned Parenthood
www.plannedparenthood.org

Sexuality Information and Education Council of the United States
www.siecus.org

Sports Medicine on the Web
www.sportsmedicine.com

Stop Bullying Now
www.stopbullyingnow.hrsa.gov

TeenGrowth
www.teengrowth.com

Women's Health Resource
www.imaginis.com

HOTLINES

AIDS Hotline
800-342-AIDS (800-342-2437)

Al-Anon/Alateen
888-4AL-ANON (888-425-2666)

American Pregnancy Hotline
888-672-2296

American Trauma Society
800-556-7890

Center for the Prevention of School Violence
800-299-6504

Childhelp (Child Abuse)
800-4-A-CHILD (800-422-4453)

Gay & Lesbian National Hotline
888-THE-GLNH (888-843-4564)

Hate Crime Hotline
800-616-HATE (800-616-4283)

Mental Health InfoSource
800-447-4474

National Domestic Violence Hotline
800-799-SAFE (800-799-7233)

National Drug Abuse Hotline
800-662-HELP (800-662-4357)

National Eating Disorders Association
800-931-2237

National Health Information Center
800-336-4797

National Runaway Hotline
800-231-6946

National Sexually Transmitted Diseases Hotline
800-227-8922

National Suicide Prevention Lifeline
800-273-TALK (800-273-8255)

National Youth Crisis Hotline
800-448-4663

Self-Injury Hotline
800-DONT-CUT (800-366-8288)

Smokers' Helpline
800-NO-BUTTS (800-662-8887)

TalkZone (Peer Counselors)
800-475-TALK (800-475-2855)

INDEX

PICTURE CREDITS